Advanced Biomarkers for Neurological Diseases

Advanced Biomarkers for Neurological Diseases

Editor: Noah Benge

AMERICAN
MEDICAL PUBLISHERS
www.americanmedicalpublishers.com

AMERICAN
MEDICAL PUBLISHERS
www.americanmedicalpublishers.com

Cataloging-in-Publication Data

Advanced biomarkers for neurological diseases / edited by Noah Benge.
p. cm.
Includes bibliographical references and index.
ISBN 979-8-88740-311-3
1. Nervous system--Diseases. 2. Biochemical markers. 3. Neurology. I. Benge, Noah.
RC346 .A38 2023
616.8--dc23

American Medical Publishers,
41 Flatbush Avenue,
1st Floor, New York,
NY 11217, USA

ISBN 979-8-88740-311-3 (Hardback)

Contents

Preface IX

Chapter 1 **Role of Neuroimaging as a Biomarker for Neurodegenerative Diseases** 1
Soichiro Shimizu, Daisuke Hirose, Hirokuni Hatanaka, Naoto Takenoshita, Yoshitsugu Kaneko, Yusuke Ogawa, Hirofumi Sakurai and Haruo Hanyu

Chapter 2 **Biomarkers of Spinal and Bulbar Muscle Atrophy (SBMA)** 7
Giorgia Querin, Peter Bede, Veronique Marchand-Pauvert and Pierre-Francois Pradat

Chapter 3 **Past and Future of Neurotrophic Growth Factors Therapies in ALS: From Single Neurotrophic Growth Factor to Stem Cells and Human Platelet Lysates** 16
Flore Gouel, Anne-Sophie Rolland, Jean-Christophe Devedjian, Thierry Burnouf and David Devos

Chapter 4 **Biomarker Supervised G-CSF (Filgrastim) Response in ALS Patients** 27
Siw Johannesen, Bettina Budeus, Sebastian Peters, Sabine Iberl, Anne-Louise Meyer, Tina Kammermaier, Eva Wirkert, Tim-Henrik Bruun, Verena C. Samara, Wilhelm Schulte-Mattler, Wolfgang Herr, Armin Schneider, Jochen Grassinger and Ulrich Bogdahn

Chapter 5 **An Overview of MicroRNAs as Biomarkers of ALS** 42
Greig Joilin, P. Nigel Leigh, Sarah F. Newbury and Majid Hafezparast

Chapter 6 **Metabolomics Biomarkers: A Strategy Toward Therapeutics Improvement in ALS** 51
Débora Lanznaster, Denis Reis de Assis, Philippe Corcia, Pierre-François Pradat and Hélène Blasco

Chapter 7 **Biological Significance of microRNA Biomarkers in ALS – Innocent Bystanders or Disease Culprits?** 58
Sophie Foggin, Raquel Mesquita-Ribeiro, Federico Dajas-Bailador and Rob Layfield

Chapter 8 **Diagnostic Challenge and Neuromuscular Junction Contribution to ALS Pathogenesis** 66
Maria-Letizia Campanari, Annis-Rayan Bourefis and Edor Kabashi

Chapter 9 **Circadian Rhythm Dysfunction Accelerates Disease Progression in a Mouse Model with Amyotrophic Lateral Sclerosis** 74
Zhilin Huang, Qiang Liu, Yu Peng, Jiaying Dai, Youna Xie, Weineng Chen, Simei Long, Zhong Pei, Huanxing Su and Xiaoli Yao

Chapter 10 **Diaphragmatic Neurophysiology and Respiratory Markers in ALS** 84
Mamede de Carvalho, Michael Swash and Susana Pinto

Chapter 11 **Positron Emission Tomography Molecular Imaging Biomarkers for Amyotrophic Lateral Sclerosis** 92
Sheena Chew and Nazem Atassi

Chapter 12 **Unbiased MRI Analyses Identify Micropathologic Differences Between Upper Motor Neuron-Predominant ALS Phenotypes** 104
Venkateswaran Rajagopalan and Erik P. Pioro

Chapter 13 **Tracking a Fast-Moving Disease: Longitudinal Markers, Monitoring, and Clinical Trial Endpoints in ALS** 112
Rangariroyashe Hannah Chipika, Eoin Finegan, Stacey Li Hi Shing, Orla Hardiman and Peter Bede

Chapter 14 **Ethical Principles in Patient-Centered Medical Care to Support Quality of Life in Amyotrophic Lateral Sclerosis** 130
Dorothée Lulé, Andrea Kübler and Albert C. Ludolph

Chapter 15 **Imaging Cerebral Activity in Amyotrophic Lateral Sclerosis** 138
Malcolm Proudfoot, Peter Bede and Martin R. Turner

Chapter 16 **A Systematic Review of Suggested Molecular Strata, Biomarkers and their Tissue Sources in ALS** 151
Udaya Geetha Vijayakumar, Vanessa Milla, Mei Yu Cynthia Stafford, Anthony J. Bjourson, William Duddy and Stephanie Marie-Rose Duguez

Chapter 17 **Suboptimal Baseline Serum Vitamin B12 is Associated with Cognitive Decline in People with Alzheimer's Disease Undergoing Cholinesterase Inhibitor Treatment** 168
Hsiao Shan Cho, Li Kai Huang, Yao Tung Lee, Lung Chan and Chien Tai Hong

Chapter 18 **The Impact of Cognitive and Behavioral Symptoms on ALS Patients and their Caregivers** 173
Jashelle Caga, Sharpley Hsieh, Patricia Lillo, Kaitlin Dudley and Eneida Mioshi

Chapter 19 **Amyotrophic Lateral Sclerosis and Primary Biliary Cirrhosis Overlap Syndrome** 180
Haibo Zhang, Yaling Liu, Zhenfei Li, Na Liang, Xiaomeng Zhou, Xiangyu Nie, Ting Zhang and Weijing Qi

Chapter 20 **The Clinical and Radiological Spectrum of Hippocampal Pathology in Amyotrophic Lateral Sclerosis** 186
Foteini Christidi, Efstratios Karavasilis, Georgios Velonakis, Panagiotis Ferentinos, Michail Rentzos, Nikolaos Kelekis, Ioannis Evdokimidis and Peter Bede

Chapter 21 **Metabolic Disturbances in the Striatum and Substantia Nigra in the Onset and Progression of MPTP-Induced Parkinsonism Model** 197
Yi Lu, Xiaoxia Zhang, Liangcai Zhao, Changwei Yang, Linlin Pan, Chen Li, Kun Liu, Guanghui Bai, Hongchang Gao and Zhihan Yan

Chapter 22 **Structural Connectivity Alterations in Amyotrophic Lateral Sclerosis: A Graph Theory Based Imaging Study** 207
Etienne Fortanier, Aude-Marie Grapperon, Arnaud Le Troter, Annie Verschueren, Ben Ridley, Maxime Guye, Shahram Attarian, Jean-Philippe Ranjeva and Wafaa Zaaraoui

Chapter 23 **Developing a Neuroimaging Biomarker for Amyotrophic Lateral Sclerosis: Multi-Center Data Sharing and the Road to a "Global Cohort"** 219
Robert Steinbach, Nayana Gaur, Beatrice Stubendorff, Otto W. Witte and Julian Grosskreutz

Permissions

List of Contributors

Index

Preface

The diseases of the central or peripheral nervous system are called neurological disorders. These disorders include epilepsy, Alzheimer's disease, and other dementias. Cerebrovascular diseases such as stroke, migraine, multiple sclerosis, Parkinson's disease, etc. are also considered as neurological diseases. A biomarker or biological marker is a cell, tissue, or body fluid cell that can be measured and evaluated to indicate a pharmacological response to a normal biological process, pathogenic process, or therapeutic intervention. Biomarkers characterize the progression of the disease from the earliest natural signs of the disease. Biomarkers assess the disease susceptibility and severity enabling prediction of outcomes, deciding interventions, and assessing the therapeutic responses. Based on clinical applications, biomarkers can be categorized as molecular biomarkers, cellular biomarkers, or imaging biomarkers. This book aims to shed light on some of the unexplored aspects of biomarkers. It presents researches and studies performed by experts across the globe on the topic in detail. It attempts to assist those with a goal of furthering their studies in the field of biomarkers and biomarker development.

After months of intensive research and writing, this book is the end result of all who devoted their time and efforts in the initiation and progress of this book. It will surely be a source of reference in enhancing the required knowledge of the new developments in the area. During the course of developing this book, certain measures such as accuracy, authenticity and research focused analytical studies were given preference in order to produce a comprehensive book in the area of study.

This book would not have been possible without the efforts of the authors and the publisher. I extend my sincere thanks to them. Secondly, I express my gratitude to my family and well-wishers. And most importantly, I thank my students for constantly expressing their willingness and curiosity in enhancing their knowledge in the field, which encourages me to take up further research projects for the advancement of the area.

Editor

1

Role of Neuroimaging as a Biomarker for Neurodegenerative Diseases

Soichiro Shimizu, Daisuke Hirose, Hirokuni Hatanaka, Naoto Takenoshita, Yoshitsugu Kaneko, Yusuke Ogawa, Hirofumi Sakurai and Haruo Hanyu*

Department of Geriatric Medicine, Tokyo Medical University, Tokyo, Japan

Correspondence:
Soichiro Shimizu
soichiroshimizu@gmail.com

It has recently been recognized that neurodegenerative diseases are caused by common cellular and molecular mechanisms including protein aggregation and inclusion body formation. Each type of neurodegenerative disease is characterized by the specific protein that aggregates. In these days, the pathway involved in protein aggregation has been elucidated. These are leading to approaches toward disease-modifying therapies. Neurodegenerative diseases are fundamentally diagnosed pathologically. Therefore, autopsy is essential for a definitive diagnosis of a neurodegenerative disease. However, recently, the development of various molecular brain imaging techniques have enabled pathological changes in the brain to be inferred even without autopsy. Some molecular imaging techniques are described as biomarker in diagnostic criteria of neurodegenerative disease. Magnetic resonance imaging (MRI), single photon emission computed tomography (SPECT), positron emission tomography (PET), and amyloid imaging are described in the diagnostic guidelines for Alzheimer's disease in the National Institute on Aging-Alzheimer's Association. MRI, dopamine transporter (DAT) imaging, and ^{123}I-metaiodobenzyl-guanidine (MIBG) myocardial scintigraphy listed in the guidelines for consensus clinical diagnostic criteria for dementia with Lewy bodies are described as potential biomarkers. The Movement Disorder Society Progressive Supranuclear Palsy Study Group defined MRI, SPECT/PET, DAT imaging, and tau imaging as biomarkers. Other diagnostic criteria for neurodegenerative disease described neuroimaging findings as only characteristic finding, not as biomarker. In this review, we describe the role of neuroimaging as a potential biomarker for neurodegenerative diseases.

Keywords: amyloid, biomarker, DAT, dementia, MIBG, neuroimaging, tau

INTRODUCTION

Each neurodegenerative disease type is characterized by the specific protein that aggregates. Recently, extensive research has been performed on disease-modifying therapies for neurodegenerative diseases (i.e., Alzheimer's disease, tauopathies, etc.), which are expected to be developed in the near future. Simple and practical biomarkers specific for each neurodegenerative disease are urgently required for their accurate diagnosis and facilitate the development of disease-modifying interventions. A recent study demonstrated the potential clinical utility of plasma biomarkers in predicting brain amyloid-β burden (1). However, in daily clinical setting, plasma biomarkers are not available yet and analyzing the cerebrospinal fluid (CSF) of all patients may be difficult (2–4).

In many diagnostic criteria for neurodegenerative disease, characteristic findings in neuroimaging are mentioned. Moreover, only few recent diagnostic criteria for neurodegenerative diseases have mentioned neuroimaging techniques as biomarkers that can estimate pathological changes occurring in the brains of neurodegenerative disease patients (2, 3, 5, 6).

The current mini-review addresses the roles of neuroimaging techniques described as biomarkers on diagnostic criteria for individual neurodegenerative diseases as research topics. Even though there were numerical findings of neuroimaging technique of neurodegenerative disease, we omitted those of not described in diagnostic criteria. For example, about prion disease, hyperintensity in cortex and basal ganglia on FLAIR and DWI are widely known as characteristic magnetic resonance imaging (MRI) finding of prion disease in daily clinical setting. However, this characteristic MRI finding is not described in diagnostic criteria for prion disease which is widely used (7).

In this review, we defined the characteristic neuroimaging findings described in diagnostic criteria from Level A and B based on evidence level as follows:

Level A: able to use the research criteria; described as biomarkers in diagnostic criteria.
Level B: supportive biomarker of clinical diagnosis; described as supportive biomarkers for research criteria in diagnostic criteria.
Level C: supportive of clinical diagnosis; not described as biomarkers but characteristic finding in diagnostic criteria.

Table 1 shows a summary of neuroimaging techniques used as biomarkers, as described in various diagnostic criteria.

Magnetic Resonance Imaging

Magnetic resonance imaging is one of the most widely used neuroimaging techniques for the diagnosis of neurodegenerative diseases. However, among the diagnostic criteria for neurodegenerative diseases, only two diagnostic guidelines, namely, for Alzheimer disease (AD) (2, 3) and for dementia with Lewy bodies (DLB) (5) state characteristic MRI findings as biomarkers.

The National Institute on Aging-Alzheimer's Association (NIA-AA) diagnostic guidelines for AD state disproportionate atrophy on structural MRI in the medial, basal, and lateral temporal lobes, as well as the medial parietal cortex, as a biomarker of neuronal degeneration or injury (2, 3) (Level A).

The latest diagnostic guidelines of DLB (5) state the absence of or minimal atrophy of the medial temporal lobe on MRI as a supportive biomarker that is consistent with DLB, which assists in the diagnostic evaluation, but does not have clear diagnostic specificity (Level B). Hippocampus is strongly correlated at autopsy with tangles rather than plaque or Lewy body-associated pathology (8). Many studies reported the coexistence of DLB and AD pathology in patients. Most patients with DLB also demonstrate AD pathology (5, 9). Therefore, it should be emphasized that if patients have medial temporal lobe atrophy, DLB should not be denied.

The movement disorder society (MDS) clinical diagnostic criteria for progressive supranuclear palsy (PSP) that has recently been established state a characteristic MRI finding, namely, predominant midbrain atrophy relative to the pons, as a supportive feature, but not a biomarker of PSP (10) (Level C). On the other hand, the MDS-endorsed PSP Study Group classified various neuroimaging techniques into five classes of biomarkers for Richardson's syndrome (PSP-RS) and the other variant syndromes of PSP (vPSP), which were defined by evidence levels. However, to our knowledge, the top two level evidence biomarkers (i.e., 5: definitive and 4: supportive of pathological diagnosis) have not been described in the literature. On the other hand, characteristic MRI findings on PSP are described in detail as classified biomarkers (level 1: research tool, level 2: supportive of clinical diagnosis, and level 3: supportive of early clinical diagnosis) for individual PSP clinical subtypes (Levels A–C). Although details have been omitted from this review, basal ganglia and thalamic atrophy, and rates of whole-brain and midbrain atrophy are mentioned as representative examples of biomarkers for PSP-RS, and midbrain

TABLE 1 | Summary of neuroimaging techniques used as biomarkers.

Imaging technique	Disease	Evidence level	Actual description in diagnostic criteria
MRI	AD	A	Atrophy in temporal lobe sand medial parietal cortex
	DLB	B	Absence of or minimal medial temporal lobe atrophy
	PSP[a]	A–C	Characteristic image findings described for each subtype
SPECT/PET	AD	A	Hypometabolism in temporoparietal cortex
	DLB	B	Hypoperfusion/metabolism in occipital lobe and posterior cingulate island sign on FDG-PET
	PSP[a]	A–C	Frontal lobe hypoperfusion, frontal lobe and midbrain hypometabolism, and frontal hypometabolism
DAT imaging	DLB	A	Reduced dopamine transporter uptake in basal ganglia
	PSP[a]	A–C	Reduced striatal DAT/D2 receptor and reduced brain stem DAT
MIBG	DLB	A	Abnormal (low uptake) on MIBG myocardial scintigraphy
Amyloid PET	AD	A	Positive PET amyloid imaging
Tau PET	PSP[a]	B	THK5351 uptake in midbrain and globus pallidus
			[^{18}F]AV-1451 uptake in midbrain, thalamus, basal ganglia, and dentate nucleus of the cerebellum

[a]Not described in diagnostic criteria, but defined as a biomarker by the MDS-endorsed PSP Study Group.
Evidence levels are different depend on clinical subtypes.
MRI, magnetic resonance imaging; SPECT, single photon emission computed tomography; PET, positron emission tomography; DAT imaging, dopamine transporter imaging; MIBG, ^{123}Iodine-metaiodobenzylguanidine myocardial scintigraphy; AD, Alzheimer's disease; DLB, dementia with Lewy bodies; PSP, progressive supranuclear palsy; MDS, movement disorder society; FDG, ^{18}fluorodeoxyglucose.
Level A: able to use the research criteria; described as biomarkers in diagnostic criteria.
Level B: supportive biomarker of clinical diagnosis; described as supportive biomarkers for research criteria in diagnostic criteria.
Level C: supportive of clinical diagnosis; not described as biomarkers but characteristic finding in diagnostic criteria.

atrophy is mentioned as a biomarker of vPSP. Furthermore, it is noteworthy that not only structural MRI findings but also findings displayed on functional MRI and diffusion tensor imaging are described. Details of the MRI findings are described elsewhere (6).

Other diagnostic criteria for neurodegenerative diseases also describe characteristic findings on MRI, but there are no descriptions of biomarkers. Frontotemporal lobar degeneration (FTLD) has three clinical subtypes (11), which demonstrate various pathological changes (e.g., FTLD-tau, FTLD-TDP, FTLD-UPS, and FTLD-FUS FTLD-ni) (12). The diagnostic criteria for FTLD that is most commonly used (11) mentions MRI findings of individual clinical subtypes as characteristics, rather than as biomarkers (Level C). As FTLD is caused by various pathological changes, it is difficult to consider neuroimaging data, including those from MRI, as biomarkers. Recent diagnostic criteria for the behavioral variant of frontotemporal dementia (bvFTD) (13) mentioned frontal or anterior temporal atrophy displayed on MRI or computed tomography as characteristic findings suggesting a diagnosis of bvFTD.

A second consensus statement on the diagnosis of multiple system atrophy (MSA) mentioned atrophy displayed on MRI of the putamen, middle cerebellar peduncle, pons, or cerebellum as an additional feature suggestive of MSA-P or MSA-C, but not as a biomarker (14) (Level C).

However, many past studies showed, coexistence of several pathological changes is not rare in elderly patients (5, 9, 15). Therefore, existence of individual pathological change is suggested due to the above MRI characteristic findings, however, it should be noted that coexistence of other pathological changes cannot be denied.

Single Photon Emission Computed Tomography (SPECT) and Positron Emission Tomography (PET)

Recently, among the nuclear medicine imaging techniques, SPECT and PET have been used for the diagnosis of neurodegenerative diseases in the daily clinical setting and are the most commonly used new neuroimaging techniques.

The NIA-AA diagnostic guidelines for AD describe decreased ^{18}fluorodeoxyglucose (FDG) uptake on PET in the temporoparietal cortex as a biomarker of neuronal degeneration or injury (2, 3) (Level A).

The most recent diagnostic criteria for DLB (5) mentioned hypoperfusion/hypometabolism by SPECT/PET in the occipital lobe and the posterior cingulate island sign on FDG-PET imaging as supportive biomarkers (Level B). An autopsy-confirmed study suggested that FDG-PET occipital hypometabolism was able to differentiate DLB from AD with high accuracy (16). Larger studies on patients earlier in the course of the disease suggested a sensitivity (70%) and specificity (74%) slightly lower than required for an indicative biomarker, although better than that reported for SPECT (65 and 64%, respectively) (17, 18). On the other hand, our past study showed that there was no significant perfusion differences in medial occipital lobe between AD and DLB (19). In any case, compared with dopamine transporter (DAT) imaging ^{123}Iodine-metaiodobenzylguanidine (MIBG) cardiac scintigraphy described below, occipital hypoperfusion has low sensitivity and specificity. Therefore, it is understandable that it stayed in only one of the supportive biomarker with most resent diagnostic criteria. Relative preservation of the metabolic activities of the posterior cingulate cortex and midcingulate cortex on FDG-PET (the cingulate island sign) has been described in DLB (20), associated with less concurrent neurofibrillary pathology, but with no difference in amyloid-beta (Aβ) load relative to AD (21).

In the recent MDS clinical diagnostic criteria for PSP, predominant midbrain hypometabolism relative to the pons displayed on FDG-PET is described as a supportive feature, rather than a biomarker (10) (Level C). On the other hand, the MDS PSP Study Group defined SPECT frontal hypoperfusion as a level 1 biomarker (research tool), FDG-PET frontal and midbrain hypometabolism as a level 2 biomarker (supportive of clinical diagnosis), and FDG-PET frontal hypometabolism as a class 3 biomarker (supportive of early clinical diagnosis) for PSP-RS (6) (Levels A–C).

Recent diagnostic criteria for bvFTD (13) stated frontal or anterior temporal hypoperfusion or hypometabolism displayed on PET or SPECT as characteristic neuroimaging data suggestive of bvFTD (Level C). This criteria states that functional imaging changes may provide additional sensitivity, suggesting that behavioral and functional abnormalities may precede structural imaging changes in bvFTD.

The second consensus statement on MSA stated hypometabolism on FDG-PET in the putamen, brainstem, and cerebellum as additional features of possible MSA-P and hypometabolism on FDG-PET in the putamen as an additional feature of possible MSA-C, rather than as biomarkers (14) (Level C).

Dopamine Transporter Imaging

DAT imaging use a ligand that binds to the presynaptic dopamine transporter, can be used to analyze the integrity of the nigrostriatal projection pathway. ^{123}I-2β-carbomethoxy-3β-(4-iodophenyl)-*N*-(3-fluoropropyl) nortropane (^{123}I-FP-CIT) is the ligand for DAT-SPECT that is most widely used. ^{123}I-FP-CIT has been used in a large number of trials to identify the *in vivo* loss of dopamine transporters in the striatum of patients with presynaptic parkinsonism (22, 23). Therefore, Parkinson syndrome including Parkinson's disease (PD) that has the dysfunction of the nigrostriatal projection pathway showed reduced DAT uptake. In other words, DAT imaging is not suitable for differentiation of presynaptic Parkinson syndrome. Therefore, the recent clinical diagnostic criteria for PD by the MDS did not mention DAT imaging as biomarker or characteristic imaging finding of PD (24). DAT imaging requires attention to use in the following cases, patients with an infarction in the basal ganglia, patients who are unable to stop the use of medications that affect DAT uptake (e.g., cocaine, amphetamines, bupropion, selective serotonin reuptake inhibitors, etc.) (25).

However, DAT imaging is useful for differentiating DLB from other dementias. The latest diagnostic guidelines of DLB state reduced dopamine transporter (DAT) uptake in the basal ganglia displayed on SPECT or PET as indicative biomarkers (5) (Level A). However, there are no biomarkers available for the clinical diagnosis of Lewy body-associated pathology. DAT imaging was described as a useful indirect method for determining Lewy body-associated pathology. Reduced DAT uptake in the basal ganglia has been confirmed by SPECT or PET imaging. The utility of DAT imaging in distinguishing DLB from AD is well established, with a sensitivity of 78% and a specificity of 90% (26).

In the recent MDS clinical diagnostic criteria for PSP, postsynaptic striatal dopaminergic degeneration, as demonstrated for example by ^{123}I-iodobenzamide (IBZM)-SPECT or ^{18}F-desmethoxyfallypride (DMFP)-PET, is described as a supportive feature rather than as a biomarker (10) (Level C). However, the MDS PSP Study Group defined reduced striatal DAT/D2 receptor levels and reduced brainstem DAT levels as level 2 biomarkers for PSP-RS (Level B), and reduced striatal DAT as a level 1 biomarker for some types of vPSP (6) (Level A).

The second consensus statement on the diagnosis of MSA states presynaptic nigrostriatal dopaminergic denervation displayed on SPECT or PET as an additional feature suggestive of MSA-P, but not as a biomarker (14) (Level C).

^{123}Iodine-Metaiodobenzylguanidine Myocardial Scintigraphy

MIBG is a physiologic analog of noradrenaline used to determine the location, integrity, and function of postganglionic noradrenergic neurons. Lewy body disease including DLB and PD presents an impairment of adrenergic function and consequently an abnormal MIBG myocardial syntigraphy (27). MIBG myocardial scintigraphy requires attention to patients with heart disease, diabetes, or thyroid disease, or patients taking any drugs known to affect the accumulation of MIBG (28).

The latest diagnostic guidelines of DLB state abnormal (low uptake) MIBG myocardial scintigraphy as an indicative biomarker (5) (Level A). MIBG myocardial scintigraphy quantifies postganglionic sympathetic cardiac innervation, which is reduced in Lewy body disease (27, 29). The sensitivity and specificity values of MIBG myocardial scintigraphy for discriminating probable DLB from probable AD rise from 69 and 87%, respectively, in severely demented patients to 77 and 94%, respectively, in mildly demented patients (30).

The recent clinical diagnostic criteria for PD by the MDS described the presence of either olfactory loss or cardiac sympathetic denervation on MIBG myocardial scintigraphy as supportive criteria, but not as a biomarker (24) (Level B).

In MSA, which is an α-synucleinopathy similar to PD, the diagnostic criteria (14) also does not state MIBG myocardial scintigraphy as supportive diagnostic criteria (Level C). The reason is that there is no consensus on the usefulness of MIBG myocardial scintigraphy for diagnosing MSA. Many reports using MIBG myocardial scintigraphy have shown preserved sympathetic postganglionic neurons in MSA, in contrast to in PD (31). On the other hand, some studies have shown denervation in patients with MSA displayed on MIBG myocardial scintigraphy (32).

Aβ Imaging

Interest in the use of Aβ imaging for the diagnosis of AD has been increasing. Aβ imaging is a tool expected to be new possibilities for the early detection, intervention, and prevention of AD. NIA-AA diagnostic guidelines for AD showed that biomarkers of brain Aβ protein deposition are low CSF Aβ42 and positive PET amyloid imaging (2, 3) (Level A). In addition, the diagnostic criteria do not specify the particular amyloid imaging tracer to be used. Studies with ^{11}C-Pittsburgh compound-B (^{11}C-PiB), the first and most widely studied PET Aβ ligand, indicated that Aβ imaging may enable the earlier diagnosis of AD (33, 34). However, owing to the 20-min half-life of ^{11}C, ^{11}C-PiB can only be used in large PET centers with their own on-site cyclotron and radiopharmacy facilities. ^{18}F is a more suitable radioisotope for widespread clinical use as its longer half-life of 110 min enables distribution from a production site to multiple PET centers. Recently, ^{18}F-labeled tracers have been developed, which are starting to be used clinically. The actual ^{18}F-labeled tracers being used are as follows: flutemetamol (GE Healthcare), florbetapir (Amyvid, Eli Lilly), florbetaben (Neuraceq, Piramal Imaging), and ^{18}F-AZD4694 (recently renamed NAV4694) (Astra-Zeneca, Navidea) are derived from stilbene. The above ^{18}F-labeled tracers except NAV4694 have been approved by the Food and Drug Administration. Correlations have been shown between levels of biomarker CSF Aβ42 and PET signals using ^{11}C-PiB as a tracer for Aβdeposits in the brain (35) and comparable studies have been performed for ^{18}F-labeled amyloid tracers (36, 37). A systematic review found no marked differences in the diagnostic accuracy among flutemetamol, florbetapir, and florbetaben (38). These three tracers perform better when used to differentiate between patients with AD and healthy controls. Furthermore, a study showed that NAV4694 displays high cortical binding and low nonspecific white matter binding in AD patients (39).

On the other hand, NIA-AA diagnostic guidelines for AD described, "guidelines do not advocate the use of AD biomarker tests for routine diagnostic purposes at the present time" (2, 3). At the present time, amyloid imaging should be used for research criteria of AD, taking into consideration that it is not possible at all facilities. Further studies using amyloid imaging are required to identify the tracer with the highest sensitivity and specificity, and to identify the positioning of Aβ imaging in clinical use. However, we believe that amyloid imaging, particularly ^{18}F-labeled tracers, contribute to the early diagnosis of AD.

Tau Imaging

The advances of molecular imaging in recent years have led to the development of promising tau-specific PET tracers. In recent years, hot topics were shifted from general neuroimaging to molecular imaging of the neurodegeneration related to tau protein (40).

Unfortunately, tau imaging has not been stated as a biomarker in any diagnostic criteria for neurodegenerative diseases. However, the MDS PSP study group defined two tau-specific tracers (i.e., ^{18}F-THK5351 and ^{18}F-AV1451) as a biomarker of PSP-RS (6) (Level B). Because very few articles have been published on this subject, it has been suggested to have low reliability.

However, tau imaging is expected to become an important biomarker of tau pathology in the future. There are six different isoforms of tau, formed by alternative mRNA splicing of the microtubule-associated protein tau (*MAPT*) gene. More importantly, the inclusion or exclusion of exon 10 results in either 4 repeats (4R) or 3 repeats (3R) of the microtubule-binding domain being transcribed in the tau protein, respectively (41). The 3R/4R ratio is 1:1 under physiological conditions and in patients with AD, tangle predominant senile dementia, and chronic traumatic encephalopathy. 3R isoforms are dominant in FTD and 4R isoforms are dominant in corticobasal degeneration, PSP, and argyrophilic grain disease (42).

The radiotracers used to image tau neurofibrillary tangle deposition in living AD patient brains are ^{18}F-FDDNP (43), ^{18}F-AV1451 (44), ^{11}C-PBB3 (45), and ^{18}F-THK5351 (46). These tracers are now available for clinical assessment of patients with various tauopathies, including AD, as well as in healthy subjects.

However, PET tracers used for tau imaging still have some problems that remain to be resolved. These tracers often show "off-target" binding. Recently, it has become clear that these tracers detected the distribution of not only tau but also other proteins (47). For example, ^{18}F-THK5351 has been confirmed to also bind to monoamine oxidase B (48). Moreover, ^{18}F-AV1451 is well known to bind to calcifications, iron, melanin, and blood vessels (49). Therefore, further studies of a large number of patients, with consideration of the results of pathological analyses are required. Even considering the above issues, we believe that with further research, tau imaging will become a useful biomarker in the near future.

CONCLUSION

In this review, we introduced the various neuroimaging techniques described in the current diagnostic criteria for neurodegenerative diseases and the possibility of new neuroimaging techniques as biomarkers. We believe that further advances in these neuroimaging techniques will lead to useful biomarkers that can accurately predict the pathological changes occurring in various neurodegenerative diseases.

AUTHOR CONTRIBUTIONS

SS, DH, Hi.H, NT, YK, and YO wrote the manuscript. HS and Ha.H critically reviewed the manuscript.

ACKNOWLEDGMENTS

We are grateful to the medical editors of the Department of International Medical Communications of Tokyo Medical University for reviewing the manuscript.

REFERENCES

1. Nakamura A, Kaneko N, Villemagne VL, Kato T, Doecke J, Doré V, et al. High performance plasma amyloid-β biomarkers for Alzheimer's disease. *Nature* (2018) 554(7691):249–54. doi:10.1038/nature25456
2. Jack CR, Albert MS, Knopman DS, McKhann GM, Sperling RA, Carrillo MC, et al. Introduction to the recommendations from the National Institute on Aging-Alzheimer's Association workgroups on diagnostic guidelines for Alzheimer's disease. *Alzheimers Dement* (2011) 7(3):257–62. doi:10.1016/j.jalz.2011.03.004
3. McKhann GM, Knopman DS, Chertkow H, Hyman BT, Jack CR, Kawas CH, et al. The diagnosis of dementia due to Alzheimer's disease: recommendations from the National Institute on Aging-Alzheimer's Association workgroups on diagnostic guidelines for Alzheimer's disease. *Alzheimers Dement* (2011) 7(3):263–9. doi:10.1016/j.jalz.2011.03.005
4. Shaw LM, Vanderstichele H, Knapik-Czajka M, Clark CM, Aisen PS, Petersen RC, et al. Cerebrospinal fluid biomarker signature in Alzheimer's disease neuroimaging initiative subjects. *Ann Neurol* (2009) 65:403–13. doi:10.1002/ana.21610
5. McKeith IG, Boeve BF, Dickson DW, Halliday G, Taylor JP, Weintraub D, et al. Diagnosis and management of dementia with Lewy bodies: fourth consensus report of the DLB consortium. *Neurology* (2017) 89(1):88–100. doi:10.1212/WNL.0000000000004058
6. Whitwell JL, Höglinger GU, Antonini A, Bordelon Y, Boxer AL, Colosimo C, et al. Radiological biomarkers for diagnosis in PSP: where are we and where do we need to be? *Mov Disord* (2017) 32(7):955–71. doi:10.1002/mds.27038
7. WHO. *WHO Manual for Strengthening Diagnosis and Surveillance of Creutzfeldt-Jakob Disease*. Geneva, switzerland (1998).
8. Burton EJ, Barber R, Mukaetova-Ladinska EB, Robson J, Perry RH, Jaros E, et al. Medial temporal lobe atrophy on MRI differentiates Alzheimer's disease from dementia with Lewy bodies and vascular cognitive impairment: a prospective study with pathological verification of diagnosis. *Brain* (2009) 132(Pt 1):195–203. doi:10.1093/brain/awn298
9. Ballard C, Ziabreva I, Perry R, Larsen JP, O'Brien J, McKeith I, et al. Differences in neuropathologic characteristics across the Lewy body dementia spectrum. *Neurology* (2006) 67(11):1931–4. doi:10.1212/01.wnl.0000249130.63615.cc
10. Höglinger GU, Respondek G, Stamelou M, Kurz C, Josephs KA, Lang AE, et al. Clinical diagnosis of progressive supranuclear palsy: the movement disorder society criteria. *Mov Disord* (2017) 32(6):853–64. doi:10.1002/mds.26987
11. Neary D, Snowden JS, Gustafson L, Passant U, Stuss D, Black S, et al. Frontotemporal lobar degeneration: a consensus on clinical diagnostic criteria. *Neurology* (1998) 51(6):1546–54. doi:10.1212/WNL.51.6.1546
12. Mackenzie IR, Neumann M, Bigio EH, Cairns NJ, Alafuzoff I, Kril J, et al. Nomenclature and nosology for neuropathologic subtypes of frontotemporal lobar degeneration: an update. *Acta Neuropathol* (2010) 119(1):1–4. doi:10.1007/s00401-009-0612-2
13. Rascovsky K, Hodges JR, Knopman D, Mendez MF, Kramer JH, Neuhaus J, et al. Sensitivity of revised diagnostic criteria for the behavioural variant of frontotemporal dementia. *Brain* (2011) 134(Pt 9):2456–77. doi:10.1093/brain/awr179
14. Gilman S, Wenning GK, Low PA, Brooks DJ, Mathias CJ, Trojanowski JQ, et al. Second consensus statement on the diagnosis of multiple system atrophy. *Neurology* (2008) 71(9):670–6. doi:10.1212/01.wnl.0000324625.00404.15
15. Toledo JB, Cairns NJ, Da X, Chen K, Carter D, Fleisher A, et al. Clinical and multimodal biomarker correlates of ADNI neuropathological findings. *Acta Neuropathol Commun* (2013) 2013(1):65. doi:10.1186/2051-5960-1-65
16. Minoshima S, Foster NL, Sima AA, Frey KA, Albin RL, Kuhl DE. Alzheimer's disease versus dementia with Lewy bodies: cerebral metabolic distinction with autopsy confirmation. *Ann Neurol* (2001) 50(3):358–65. doi:10.1002/ana.1133
17. Lobotesis K, Fenwick JD, Phipps A, Ryman A, Swann A, Ballard C, et al. Occipital hypoperfusion on SPECT in dementia with Lewy bodies but not AD. *Neurology* (2001) 56(5):643–9. doi:10.1212/WNL.56.5.643
18. O'Brien JT, Firbank MJ, Davison C, Barnett N, Bamford C, Donaldson C, et al. 18F-FDG PET and perfusion SPECT in the diagnosis of Alzheimer and Lewy body dementias. *J Nucl Med* (2014) 55(12):1959–65. doi:10.2967/jnumed.114.143347
19. Shimizu S, Kanetaka H, Hirao K, Fukasawa R, Namioka N, Hatanaka H, et al. Neuroimaging for diagnosing dementia with Lewy bodies: what is the best neuroimaging technique in discriminating dementia with Lewy bodies from Alzheimer's disease? *Geriatr Gerontol Int* (2017) 17(5):819–24. doi:10.1111/ggi.12794
20. Lim SM, Katsifis A, Villemagne VL, Best R, Jones G, Saling M, et al. The 18F-FDG PET cingulate island sign and comparison to 123I-beta-CIT SPECT for

diagnosis of dementia with Lewy bodies. *J Nucl Med* (2009) 50(10):1638–45. doi:10.2967/jnumed.109.065870

21. Graff-Radford J, Murray ME, Lowe VJ, Boeve BF, Ferman TJ, Przybelski SA, et al. Dementia with Lewy bodies: basis of cingulate Island sign. *Neurology* (2014) 83(9):801–9. doi:10.1212/WNL.0000000000000734
22. Benamer TS, Patterson J, Grosset DG, Booij J, de Bruin K, van Royen E, et al. Accurate differentiation of parkinsonism and essential tremor using visual assessment of [123I]-FP-CIT SPECT imaging: the [123I]-FP-CIT study group. *Mov Disord* (2000) 15(3):503–10. doi:10.1002/1531-8257(200005)15:3<503::AID-MDS1013>3.0.CO;2-V
23. Booij J, Speelman JD, Horstink MW, Wolters EC. The clinical benefit of imaging striatal dopamine transporters with [^{123}I]FP-CIT SPET in differentiating patients with presynaptic parkinsonism from those with other forms of parkinsonism. *Eur J Nucl Med* (2001) 28:266–72. doi:10.1007/s002590000460
24. Postuma RB, Berg D, Stern M, Poewe W, Olanow CW, Oertel W, et al. MDS clinical diagnostic criteria for Parkinson's disease. *Mov Disord* (2015) 30(12):1591–601. doi:10.1002/mds.26424
25. Djang DS, Janssen MJ, Bohnen N, Booij J, Henderson TA, Herholz K, et al. SNM practice guideline for dopamine transporter imaging with 123I-ioflupane SPECT 1.0. *J Nucl Med* (2012) 53:154–63. doi:10.2967/jnumed.111.100784
26. McKeith I, O'Brien J, Walker Z, Tatsch K, Booij J, Darcourt J, et al. Sensitivity and specificity of dopamine transporter imaging with 123I-FP-CIT SPECT in dementia with Lewy bodies: a phase III, multicentre study. *Lancet Neurol* (2007) 6(4):305–13. doi:10.1016/S1474-4422(07)70057-1
27. Treglia G, Cason E. Diagnostic performance of myocardial innervation imaging using MIBG scintigraphy in differential diagnosis between dementia with Lewy bodies and other dementias: a systematic review and a meta-analysis. *J Neuroimaging* (2012) 22(2):111–7. doi:10.1111/j.1552-6569.2010.00532.x
28. Solanski KK, Bomanji J, Moyes J, Mather SJ, Trainer PJ, Britton KE. A pharmacological guide to medicines which interfere with the biodistribution of radiolabelled meta-iodobenzylguanidine (MIBG). *Nucl Med Commun* (1992) 13:513–21. doi:10.1097/00006231-199207000-00006
29. Nakajima K, Okuda K, Yoshimura M, Matsuo S, Wakabayashi H, Imanishi Y, et al. Multicenter cross-calibration of I-123 metaiodobenzylguanidine heart-to-mediastinum ratios to overcome camera-collimator variations. *J Nucl Cardiol* (2014) 21(5):970–8. doi:10.1007/s12350-014-9916-2
30. Yoshita M, Arai H, Arai T, Asada T, Fujishiro H, Hanyu H, et al. Diagnostic accuracy of 123I-meta-iodobenzylguanidine myocardial scintigraphy in dementia with Lewy bodies: a multicenter study. *PLoS One* (2015) 10(3):e0120540. doi:10.1371/journal.pone.0120540
31. Courbon F, Brefel-Courbon C, Thalamas C, Alibelli MJ, Berry I, Montastruc JL, et al. Cardiac MIBG scintigraphy is a sensitive tool for detecting cardiac sympathetic denervation in Parkinson's disease. *Mov Disord* (2003) 18(8):890–7. doi:10.1002/mds.10461
32. Nagayama H, Hamamoto M, Ueda M, Nagashima J, Katayama Y. Reliability of MIBG myocardial scintigraphy in the diagnosis of Parkinson's disease. *J Neurol Neurosurg Psychiatry* (2005) 76(2):249–51. doi:10.1136/jnnp.2004.037028
33. Rowe CC, Ng S, Ackermann U, Gong SJ, Pike K, Savage G, et al. Imaging beta-amyloid burden in aging and dementia. *Neurology* (2007) 68(20):1718–25. doi:10.1212/01.wnl.0000261919.22630.ea
34. Klunk WE, Engler H, Nordberg A, Wang Y, Blomqvist G, Holt DP, et al. Imaging brain amyloid in Alzheimer's disease with Pittsburgh compound-B. *Ann Neurol* (2004) 55(3):306–19. doi:10.1002/ana.20009
35. Weigand SD, Vemuri P, Wiste HJ, Senjem ML, Pankratz VS, Aisen PS, et al. Transforming cerebrospinal fluid Aβ42 measures into calculated Pittsburgh compound B units of brain Aβ amyloid. *Alzheimers Dement* (2011) 7(2):133–41. doi:10.1016/j.jalz.2010.08.230
36. Schipke CG, Koglin N, Bullich S, Joachim LK, Haas B, Seibyl J, et al. Correlation of florbetaben PET imaging and the amyloid peptide Aß42 in cerebrospinal fluid. *Psychiatry Res* (2017) 265:98–101. doi:10.1016/j.pscychresns.2016.10.011
37. Toledo JB, Bjerke M, Da X, Landau SM, Foster NL, Jagust W, et al. Nonlinear association between cerebrospinal fluid and florbetapir F-18 β-amyloid measures across the spectrum of Alzheimer disease. *JAMA Neurol* (2015) 72(5):571–81. doi:10.1001/jamaneurol.2014.4829
38. Morris E, Chalkidou A, Hammers A, Peacock J, Summers J, Keevil S. Diagnostic accuracy of (18)F amyloid PET tracers for the diagnosis of Alzheimer's disease: a systematic review and meta-analysis. *Eur J Nucl Med Mol Imaging* (2016) 43(2):374–85. doi:10.1007/s00259-015-3228-x
39. Rowe CC, Pejoska S, Mulligan RS, Jones G, Chan JG, Svensson S, et al. Head-to-head comparison of 11C-PiB and 18F-AZD4694 (NAV4694) for β-amyloid imaging in aging and dementia. *J Nucl Med* (2013) 54(6):880–6. doi:10.2967/jnumed.112.114785
40. Yeung AW, Goto TK, Leung WK. The changing landscape of neuroscience research, 2006-2015: a bibliometric study. *Front Neurosci* (2017) 11:120. doi:10.3389/fnins.2017.00120
41. Niblock M, Gallo JM. Tau alternative splicing in familial and sporadic tauopathies. *Biochem Soc Trans* (2012) 40(4):677–80. doi:10.1042/BST20120091
42. Liu F, Gong CX. Tau exon 10 alternative splicing and tauopathies. *Mol Neurodegener* (2008) 3:8. doi:10.1186/1750-1326-3-8
43. Shoghi-Jadid K, Small GW, Agdeppa ED, Kepe V, Ercoli LM, Siddarth P, et al. Localization of neurofibrillary tangles and beta-amyloid plaques in the brains of living patients with Alzheimer disease. *Am J Geriatr Psychiatry* (2002) 10(1):24–35. doi:10.1097/00019442-200201000-00004
44. Chien DT, Bahri S, Szardenings AK, Walsh JC, Mu F, Su MY, et al. Early clinical PET imaging results with the novel PHF-tau radioligand [F-18]-T807. *J Alzheimers Dis* (2013) 34(2):457–68. doi:10.3233/JAD-122059
45. Maruyama M, Shimada H, Suhara T, Shinotoh H, Ji B, Maeda J, et al. Imaging of tau pathology in a tauopathy mouse model and in Alzheimer patients compared to normal controls. *Neuron* (2013) 79(6):1094–108. doi:10.1016/j.neuron.2013.07.037
46. Harada R, Okamura N, Furumoto S, Furukawa K, Ishiki A, Tomita N, et al. 18F-THK5351: a novel PET radiotracer for imaging neurofibrillary pathology in Alzheimer disease. *J Nucl Med* (2016) 57(2):208–14. doi:10.2967/jnumed.115.164848
47. Kikuchi A, Okamura N, Hasegawa T, Harada R, Watanuki S, Funaki Y, et al. In vivo visualization of tau deposits in corticobasal syndrome by 18F-THK5351 PET. *Neurology* (2016) 87(22):2309–16. doi:10.1212/WNL.0000000000003375
48. Ng KP, Pascoal TA, Mathotaarachchi S, Therriault J, Kang MS, Shin M, et al. Monoamine oxidase B inhibitor, selegiline, reduces 18F-THK5351 uptake in the human brain. *Alzheimers Res Ther* (2017) 9(1):25. doi:10.1186/s13195-017-0253-y
49. Choi JY, Cho H, Ahn SJ, Lee JH, Ryu YH, Lee MS, et al. "Off-target" 18F-AV-1451 binding in the basal ganglia correlates with age-related iron accumulation. *J Nucl Med* (2018) 59(1):117–20. doi:10.2967/jnumed.117.195248

2

Biomarkers of Spinal and Bulbar Muscle Atrophy (SBMA)

Giorgia Querin[1,2], Peter Bede[1,2,3], Veronique Marchand-Pauvert[1] and Pierre-Francois Pradat[1,2,4]*

[1] Laboratoire d'Imagerie Biomédicale, CNRS, INSERM, Sorbonne Université, Paris, France, [2] APHP, Département de Neurologie, Centre Référent SLA, Hôpital Pitié-Salpêtrière, Paris, France, [3] Computational Neuroimaging Group, Academic Unit of Neurology, Trinity College Dublin, Dublin, Ireland, [4] Northern Ireland Centre for Stratified Medicine, Biomedical Sciences Research Institute Ulster University, C-TRIC, Altnagelvin Hospital, Londonderry, United Kingdom

Correspondence:
Giorgia Querin
giorgia.querin@gmail.com

Spinal and bulbar muscular atrophy (SBMA), also known as Kennedy's disease, is a rare, X-linked, late onset neuromuscular disorder. The disease is caused by a CAG trinucleotide repeat expansion in the first exon of the androgen receptor gene. It is characterized by slowly progressive lower motor neurons degeneration, primary myopathy and widespread multisystem involvement. Respiratory involvement is rare, and the condition is associated with a normal life expectancy. Despite a plethora of therapeutic studies in mouse models, no effective disease-modifying therapy has been licensed for clinical use to date. The development of sensitive monitoring markers for the particularly slowly progressing pathology of SBMA is urgently required to aid future clinical trials. A small number of outcome measures have been proposed recently, including promising biochemical markers, which show correlation with clinical disability and disease-stage and progression. Nevertheless, a paucity of SBMA-specific biomarker studies persists, delaying the development of monitoring markers for pharmaceutical trials. Collaborative efforts through international consortia and multicenter registries are likely to contribute to the characterization of the natural history of the condition, the establishment of disease-specific biomarker panels and ultimately contribute to the development of disease-modifying drugs.

Keywords: SBMA, biomarkers, clinical trials, multisystem involvement, outcome measures

INTRODUCTION

Spinal and bulbar muscular atrophy (SBMA), also known as Kennedy's disease, is a rare, X-linked, adult onset, neuromuscular disorder (1) characterized by slowly progressive lower motor neuron (LMN) degeneration, skeletal muscle pathology and by a spectrum of multi-organ involvement (2–4). The disease is caused by a CAG repeat expansion in the first exon of the androgen receptor (AR) gene encoding for a poly-glutamine (polyQ) tract. A repeat number higher than 38 is considered pathogenic (5). PolyQ-AR toxicity is hormone-dependent and CAG repeat size inversely correlates with age of symptom onset but not with disease progression rates (6, 7). Heterozygous female carriers of the mutation only present subtle signs of neuromuscular involvement such as muscle cramps and hand tremor (8, 9). The disease is rare, with an estimated prevalence of 3.5/100,000 male inhabitants in southern Europe (10, 11) but the presence of a founder effect is retained to cause considerable differences in the distribution of the disease in various geographical regions (12, 13). Subjects with minimal symptoms and the relatively limited awareness of the condition make it likely that the real prevalence of SBMA is underestimated.

Despite several promising therapeutic studies (14), no disease-modifying treatment currently exists for SBMA. Similarly to SMA, the lack of sensitive monitoring markers for the slow progression rates of SBMA is one of main the barriers to successful clinical trials (15, 16). The objective of this work is the systematic review of candidate biomarkers in SBMA and the appraisal of their potential in clinical management and pharmaceutical trials.

THE NEUROLOGICAL PRESENTATION

Limb weakness is present in 97% of SBMA cases. It usually appears at the of age of 35–40 and starts typically proximally in the lower limbs (2, 3, 6, 17). However, tremors, muscle cramps, myalgia, gynecomastia, and exercise intolerance are often reported long before the onset of frank limb weakness (17, 18). Clinical signs of LMN involvement, such as fasciculations, muscle cramps, and atrophy are invariably present. Proximal muscles are predominantly affected, leading to difficulties in climbing stairs and getting up from a sitting position. Motor impairment is usually slowly progressive (19) and survival is only slightly reduced (6, 17). In addition to limb muscle wasting, fasciculations, and decreased deep tendon reflexes, clinical features often include a high-frequency postural hand tremor and postural leg tremor (20).

Bulbar impairment occurs in about 10–30% of patients at the onset of the disease (17), but it is present in the majority of the patients at later stages. It slowly progresses over time and may lead to aspiration pneumonia, which is a frequent cause of death in SBMA (6). Dysphagia is due to impaired oro-pharyngeal phase of deglutition (21), and is associated with tongue's muscles weakness, fasciculations, and atrophy (21). Dysarthria is characterized by hypernasality secondary to incomplete soft palate elevation and is associated with dysphonia. Speech impairment can evolve into markedly reduced intelligibility. Facial weakness and asymmetry, perioral fasciculations, myokymia, and jaw drop are also common clinical features (21–23). Recurrent laryngospasms have been noted in up to 47% of SBMA patients (24).

The presence of a distal sensory neuropathy is a hallmark feature of the disease (25) which has been described in post-mortem studies (26), sural nerve biopsies (27), and neurophysiology (28). The sensory neuropathy may be asymptomatic or manifests in distal numbness and paraesthesia in the lower limbs and reduced sensation for vibration. Neurophysiological examination readily detects reduced or absent sensory action potentials (SAPs) (28, 29). Degeneration of small myelinated and unmyelinated fibers may explain the high incidence of neuropathic pain (30) in SBMA.

MULTISYSTEM INVOLVEMENT

Complex multi-organ involvement is a hallmark feature of SBMA. The core non-neurological features of SBMA include gynecomastia, testicular atrophy, reduced fertility and erectile dysfunction. Dysfunction of the AR protein leads to partial androgen insensitivity (31), manifesting in erectile dysfunction (3), gynecomastia and reduced fertility (31, 32). Testosterone and dehydro-epiandrosterone sulfate (DHEAS) are elevated in up to 38% of patients (32). The Androgen Sensitivity Index (ASI) (LH × testosterone), which reflects androgen resistance, is found to be increased in almost half of the patients (3, 32). DHEAS is thought to correlate with CAG repeat number as well as disease duration (32). Metabolic syndrome with increased BMI, elevated serum cholesterol, triglycerides, and fasting glucose is also a key feature of the disease (3, 31–33) and insulin resistance is associated with disease severity (34). Liver involvement with steatosis and sometimes inflammation has been described (33), but the risk of progression to liver fibrosis is unclear. Recurrent urinary symptoms and incomplete bladder emptying may affect more than the third of male SBMA patients even in the absence of benign prostatic hyperplasia, which is likely to be explained by pelvic floor and bulbuocanvernosus muscle dysfunction (3). While there is no evidence of a primary cardiomyopathy in SBMA (35), Brugada-like ECG abnormalities have been reported in almost half of the patients in a large Japanese cohort (36). Obstructive sleep apnea (OSA), poor sleep quality and periodic limb movements in sleep have also been reported (37).

BIOMARKERS IN SBMA

A biomarker is a parameter that can be measured accurately and reproducibly and used as an indicator of normal biological processes, pathogenic processes, or pharmacologic responses to a therapeutic intervention (WHO definition, 1998). An ideal biomarker should have a predictive value and capture subtle changes over relatively short periods of time. Additional requirements to biomarkers include cost-effectiveness, non-invasiveness, and reproducibility (38, 39). It is generally agreed that no single biomarker is suitable for diagnostic, prognostic and monitoring roles and a panel of several markers may be better suited as multirole indicators (40). SBMA is a rare and slowly progressing condition, therefore the development of sensitive outcome measures would enable smaller sample-size and shorter duration of pharmaceutical trials (41, 42).

BIOMARKERS OF NEUROLOGICAL INVOLVEMENT IN SBMA

In recent years, an unprecedented interest has developed in the standardized assessment of neuromuscular performance in SBMA, evaluation of novel therapeutic strategies (14) and in the launch of national SBMA registries (42, 43). Many of the commonly used instruments, such as the MRC score, respiratory function parameters, the modified Norris scale, ALSFRS-r, Quantitative Myasthenia Gravis Score etc. are non-specific to

SBMA, yet remain widely utilized. As these tools have been developed for other conditions, new batteries of tests have been recently proposed to specifically appraise disability in SBMA (**Table 1**).

6-Minute-Walk-Test (6MWT)

The 6-minute-walk-test (6MWT) was proposed as an accurate marker of disease progression (44). It measures the distance a person can walk within 6 min and is regarded as a composite proxy of cardiopulmonary and neuromuscular abilities (61). Due to its relative simplicity and cost-effectiveness it has been widely adopted as an outcome measure in several neuromuscular conditions, such SMA and myopathies (62, 63). The 6MWT is traditionally considered the most reliable marker of motor impairment in SBMA, it reliably captures a 10% decline over 1 year (44) and has been used as a primary outcome measure in clinical trials (45, 57). A shorter version of the test, the "2-MWT," also exists and is thought to be reliable (63).

Adult Myopathy Assessment Tool (AMAT)

The Adult myopathy assessment tool (AMAT) is a performance-based instrument composed of functional and endurance subscales (46). AMAT provides a comprehensive evaluation of motor function, and muscle fatigue, which is a key facet of disability in SBMA (64). One of the strengths of AMAT is that it can also be applied to non-ambulatory patients. It is widely used in both SBMA registers (43) and in clinical trials (47, 52).

SBMA Functional Rating Scale (SBMAFRS)

The SBMA functional rating scale (SBMAFRS) SBMAFRS is a recently validated scale (48, 49), which has been developed from the ALSFRS-r (65) and specifically adapted for the disability profile of SBMA. It is a questionnaire-based scale that measures physical function in activities of daily living (ADL) and consists of five main domains measuring bulbar, upper-limb, lower-limb, truncal, and respiratory function. The SBMAFRS has proven to be more sensitive than the ALSFRS-r in evaluating SBMA patients with moderate motor deficits (48).

1234-Scale

The 1234-scale is another questionnaire-based scale based on the ALSFRS-r, which focuses on SBMA-associated motor disability (50). It includes items such as the ability to do push-ups, ability to run and to stand up from a squatting position. The 1234-scale has shown good internal validity and high reliability (50), but its sensitivity as a monitoring marker has not been confirmed.

Quantitative Muscle Strength Assessment (QMA)

Manual muscle testing (MMT) is commonly used to describe muscle weakness in neuromuscular conditions even though it is highly evaluator-dependent (66). A number of more objective techniques are available to evaluate muscle strength quantitatively in the four limbs (67). Grip strength measured by a handheld dynamometer is one of the simplest and most reproducible QMA parameters. Significant changes in grip strength have been observed in a 3-year longitudinal study of SBMA (19), but progressive changes have not been captured over a 1-year follow-up (44). QMA of maximal voluntary isometric muscle strength has been repeatedly proposed as an outcome measure for clinical trials (46, 47, 52, 54), but its efficacy as a biomarker is limited by considerable inter-centers variability.

Videofluoroscopy (VF)

Videofluoroscopy (VF) is routinely used to evaluate dysphagia in a range of neurological conditions. In SBMA, VF can reliably detect the impairment of the oral phase of deglutition confirming large amount of oral barium residue (56). VF has been previously used in clinical trials (51, 55, 68), but the lack of standardization makes it less suitable for robust multicenter studies.

Fiber Endoscopic Evaluation of Swallowing

Fiber endoscopic evaluation of swallowing has also been assessed as a candidate biomarker of bulbar impairment, but the diagnostic and prognostic value of the technique is yet to be validated (21).

Tongue Pressure

Tongue pressure measurements using an electronic device has been proposed as a biomarker of dysphagia in SBMA, and has been shown to be a low-cost and reliable way of detecting tongue weakness early in the course of the disease (54). An important limitation is that it is susceptible to a ceiling effect in subjects with severe bulbar impairment. Nevertheless, it has been used successfully in a trial of head-lift exercises as a possible rehabilitation strategy in SBMA-associated dysphagia (55).

Electrophysiology

Standard electrophysiology measures are routinely used in the diagnostic work-up of SBMA, but they exhibit limited sensitivity to longitudinal changes (28). This is somewhat unexpected given the correlation between CAG repeat numbers and electrophysiological parameters (29). Quantitative Motor Unit Number Estimation (MUNE) techniques have emerged as a promising way of quantifying motor neuron loss in a number of motor neuron diseases (69, 70). Significant MUNE reductions have been shown in SBMA patients both in cross-sectional and longitudinal study designs, making it one of the most promising candidate outcome measures (58, 59). MUNIX is a more recent, non-invasive method of quantifying motor neuron loss, that has already been utilized in ALS (71), peripheral neuropathies (72), and more recently in adult SMA patients (16). The motor unit size index (MUSIX) (CMAP amplitude/MUNIX) is increasingly accepted as a measure of compensatory collateral sprouting. This technique has not been tested in SBMA yet, but is likely be a promising tool in the evaluation of longitudinal motor neurons loss.

Quantitative Muscle MRI

While quantitative muscle MRI would be an obvious candidate marker of disease progression in SBMA, there is a surprising scarcity of such studies. Existing studies have shown that muscle imaging can effectively detect muscle pathology in distal leg muscles which is less obvious on clinical assessment (60).

TABLE 1 | Research studies considering motor and bulbar skills-related outcome measures.

Primary outcome measure	Reference number	Authors	Other outcome measures in the study	Type of study	Number of patients	Duration of follow-up
MOTOR SKILLS-RELATED OUTCOME MEASURES						
6MWT	(44)	Takeuci et al.	Modified Norris score, ALSFRS-R, grip strength	Observational, longitudinal study	35 at baseline, 24 at follow-up	12 months
	(45)	Querin et al.	MMT, ALSFRS-R, FVC	Pilot, unblinded pharmacological trial (Clenbuterol)	20	12 months
AMAT	(46)	Harris-Love et al.	QMA, 2MWT, ADL assessment, SF-36v2	Observational, cross-sectional study	55	/
	(47)	Shrader et al.	QMA, STS test, Timed up and Go test, Balance tests, SF-36v2, Beck depression scale, serum CK, IGF-1 and testosterone	Randomized, evaluator-blinded pharmacological trial (Physical exercise)	50	12 weeks
SBMAFRS	(48)	Hashizume et al.	ALSFRS-R, Modified Norris Score	Observational, longitudinal study	80	12 months
	(49)	Querin et al.	MMT, 6MWT, ALSFRS-R	Observational, longitudinal study	60	8 weeks
1234 scale	(50)	Lu et al.	ALSFRS-R	Observational, longitudinal study	81	32 months
ALSFRS-R	(51)	Banno et al.	VF, MMT, FVC, serum CK, AST, ALT, Beck depression scale, 1C2-positive cells in scrotal skin biopsies	Randomized, double-blinded pharmacological trial (Leuprorelin)	50	48+96 weeks
QMA	(52)	Fernández-Rhodes et al.	AMAT, MMT, 2MWT, SF-36v2, IIEF, MUNE, CMAP VF, FVC, serum CK and testosterone	Randomized, double-blinded pharmacological trial (Dutasteride)	50	24 months
Hand grip strength	(53)	Hijikata et al.	Modified QMG score, ALSFRS-R, SBMAFRS, 15-foot timed-walk test, rise-from-bed test, swallowing questionnaires, FVC, Multidimensional Fatigue Inventory, urinary 8-OHdG	Randomized, double-blinded pharmacological trial (Creatine Monohydrate)	45	8 weeks
BULBAR FUNCTION-RELATED OUTCOME MEASURES						
Tongue pressure	(54)	Mano et al.	Modified Norris score, ALSFRS-R, QMA, grip strength, MMT, modified QMG score, VF, swallowing questionnaires, timed walk test	Observational, cross-sectional study (validity of tongue pressure as marker of dysphagia)	47	/
	(55)	Mano et al.	VF, modified QMG score, ALSFRS-R, serum CK and testosterone	Non-randomized, interventional study (head lift exercises)	6	12 weeks
VF	(56)	Hashizume et al.	ALSFRS-R, SBMAFRS, swallowing questionnaires, Limbs Norris score, Bulbar Norris score	Observational, longitudinal study	111	30 days
	(57)	Katsuno et al.	ALSFRS-R, 6MWT, modified QMG score, 1C2-positive cells in scrotal skin biopsies, serum CK and testosterone, ALSAQ-5 score	Randomized, double-blinded pharmacological trial (Leuprorelin)	204	12 months
FEES	(21)	Warnecke et al.	MMT, modified Rankin scale	Observational, cross-sectional study	10	/
INSTRUMENTAL OUTCOME MEASURES						
MUNE	(58)	Suzuki et al.	Limbs Norris score, Bulbar Norris score, ALSFRS-R, grip strength	Observational, longitudinal study	52	12 months
	(59)	Lehky et al.	CMAP, SMUP	Observational, cross-sectional study	54	/
CMAP and SNAPs	(29)	Suzuki et al.	Limbs Norris score, Bulbar Norris score, ALSFRS-R, spinal cord tissue specimens	Observational, cross-sectional study	106	/
Muscle MRI	(60)	Hamano et al.	/	Observational, cross-sectional study	3	/

ALSFRS-R, Amyotrophic Lateral Sclerosis functional rating scale-revised; MMT, manual muscle testing; FVC, forced vital capacity; QMA, quantitative muscle assessment, 2 or 6MWT, 2 or 6 minutes-walk-test; ADL, activity of daily living; DXA, Dual-energy X-ray absorptiometry, urinary 8-OHdG, 8-hydroxydeoxyguanosine; VF, videofluoroscopy; AMAT, adult myopathy assessment tool; IIEF, International Index of erectile function; MUNE, motor unit number estimate; CMAP, compound motor action potential; CK, creatine-kinase; QMC score, quantitative myasthenia gravis score; SMUP, single motor unit potential.

Spinal Cord Imaging

Spinal cord imaging has seen unprecedented advances in recent years and has been applied successfully to other motor neuron diseases such as ALS (73–75), and SMA (15) to characterize gray (76) and white matter pathology (77). There is an ongoing study to test its efficacy in SBMA patients (NCT02885870).

Quantitative Brain Imaging

Quantitative brain imaging studies demonstrated white matter alterations in the corticospinal tracts (CST), limbic system (78, 79), brainstem and cerebellum (80). Voxel-based morphometry (VBM) of SBMA cohorts revealed gray matter atrophy in the frontal lobes and in the brainstem (78–81). Frontal hypometabolism has been detected by positron-emission-tomography (PET) (82). These studies confirm the multisystem nature of SBMA-associated pathology, and that neurodegeneration is not limited to LMNs but involve the CSTs and widespread cerebral regions. Despite imaging evidence of extra-motor involvement, neuropsychological studies have only detected subtle frontal dysfunction in small study populations (83, 84) which were not confirmed in larger cohorts (85, 86).

BIOMARKERS OF MULTISYSTEM INVOLVEMENT IN SBMA

Increased Serum CK Levels

Increased serum CK levels have been reported by almost every SBMA study and support the hypothesis of a primary myopathy in SBMA (87, 88). Elevated serum CK levels can be detected prior to symptom onset (89) and may be most marked around disease manifestation (18, 19). Nevertheless, no correlation was found between serum CK levels and age of onset, CAG repeat numbers, disease duration or rate of progression (6, 19). As a result, CK levels are thought to be useful as part of the diagnostic workup, but of limited use in monitoring disease progression.

Transaminases Levels

Transaminases levels have also consistently been shown to be raised in SBMA including the pre-symptomatic phase of the disease (89), but they do not correlate with the progression of the neurological symptoms. The clinical significance of raised transaminases in SBMA is a topic of debate and its prognostic value remains to be established (33).

Serum Creatinine Level

Serum creatinine level has also been proposed as a potential biomarker (90) despite its lack of specificity to SBMA. It tends to be reduced in the pre-symptomatic and symptomatic phases of the disease (91) and correlate well with parameters of motor impairment (6, 19, 91).

Proxies of Metabolic Syndrome and Insulin Resistance

Proxies of metabolic syndrome and insulin resistance are considered closely associated with primary molecular disease mechanisms. The homeostasis model assessment of insulin resistance (HOMA-IR) index correlated significantly with motor function parameters in one study (34), but this relationship has

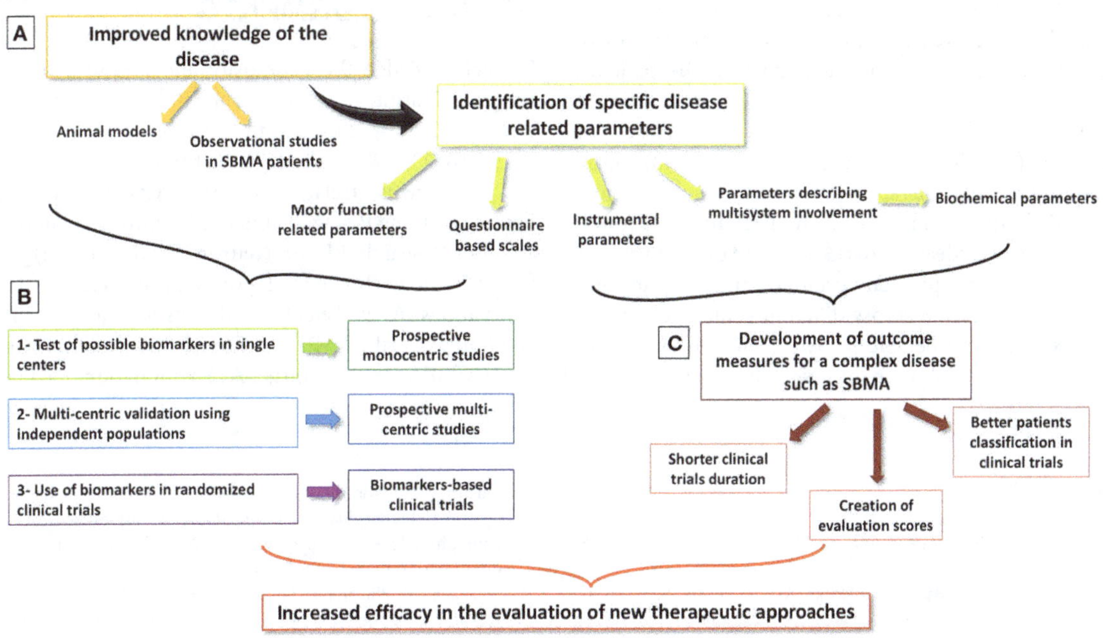

FIGURE 1 | Milestones of biomarker development in SBMA. **(A)** Better knowledge of SBMA through animal models and observational studies allows the identification of possible biomarkers of disease status and of its progression. **(B)** Different steps are needed to develop and validate a biomarker in order to make it a reliable outcome measure in clinical trials. **(C)** Considered the complexity of SBMA and its multi-system presentation, the development of global biomarkers, including both motor function and biochemical parameters, is warranted with the aim of improving the efficacy of upcoming clinical trials.

not been confirmed by others (32). **Hormones levels** and **ASI** (Androgen Sensitivity Index) have also been repeatedly proposed as markers of SBMA. Free testosterone levels correlate with muscle strength in one study (2) but it does not correlate with CAG repeat numbers or disease progression according to others (57). DHEAS levels have been linked to disease duration (91).

Skin Biopsies

Skin biopsies have been performed in some clinical trials to evaluate changes in the frequency of anti-polyQ antibody-positive cells after treatment (57). This index may be sensitive to changes during pharmacological treatment but the methodology is inherently invasive and poorly harmonized across different centers.

Adipose Tissue Quantification

A recent study proposed adipose tissue quantification using whole-body MRI and reported significant subcutaneous fat accumulation in SBMA patients. This correlated both with CAG repeat lengths, disease duration and progression rates (32). These data suggest that adipose tissue MRI may be an additional marker of multisystem involvement in SBMA.

DISCUSSION AND FUTURE PERSPECTIVES

Interest in SBMA biomarkers has grown steadily in recent years, fuelled both by accruing knowledge about pathogenesis and novel therapeutic strategies (14, 42). SBMA is now widely recognized as a multisystem syndrome (3). A multitude of studies focus on multi-organ involvement, and the systemic phenotype is now considered just as relevant as the neurological manifestations. It is increasingly recognized that non-neurological features of the disease have an equally important impact on the patients' quality of life (3, 31–34, 87, 88, 91, 92). Until now, clinical trials on SBMA focused almost exclusively on the treatment of motor symptoms (14, 45, 47, 51–53, 55, 57, 68, 92, 93), but a shift to targeted molecular therapies (94) and focus on systemic processes are likely to be witnessed in the near future. From a clinical trial perspective, ideal biomarkers should undergo robust validation, sensitivity and specificity profiling, and sampling and measurement harmonization across different centers. Crucially, candidate markers should be able to detect the subtle changes expected after the administration of a specific treatment (95). Given the particularly slow progression rates observed in SBMA, the definition of an effective outcome measures is challenging. The integration of neurological, metabolic, and endocrine indicators seems essential into composite biomarker panels in addition to functional scales. Serum creatinine levels appear to correlate strongly with motor impairment and HOMA-IR index with disease duration (34). The convincing validation of these parameters and their use as effective outcome measures in clinical trials will require robust multicenter study designs (96) (**Figure 1**).

Furthermore, the comparison of the specificity profile of candidate biomarkers seems essential to define their roles in clinical applications. The establishment of national and international SBMA registers is a clear priority which will be an invaluable resource for future SBMA research (42). As in other neurodegenerative conditions (95, 96), the integration of clinical, molecular, imaging and neurophysiological markers may be required for assessing the efficacy of disease-modifying interventions (95, 96). To conclude, we underline the relevance of considering both motor (muscle force evaluation, questionnaire based scales, and performed tasks) and biochemical parameters as possible outcome measures for a multi-system and complex pathology as SBMA. Beyond their monitoring roles, validated biomarkers will also aid patient stratification upon entry into pharmacological trials (97).

AUTHOR CONTRIBUTIONS

The paper was drafted by GQ and PB and has been reviewed for intellectual content by VM-P and P-FP.

ACKNOWLEDGMENTS

We acknowledge the generosity and kindness of our patients for participating in research on SBMA worldwide. Peter Bede is supported by the Health Research Board (HRB—Ireland; HRB EIA-2017-019), the Irish Institute of Clinical Neuroscience IICN—Novartis Ireland Research Grant, the Iris O'Brien Foundation, the Perrigo Clinician-Scientist Research Fellowship, and the Research Motor Neuron (RMN-Ireland) Foundation. Pierre-Francois Pradat is supported by the French Association for Myopathies (AFM-Telephon), the Institute for Research in Brain and Spinal Cord (IRME) the French Association for Research in ALS (ARSLA) and the Target ALS Foundation.

REFERENCES

1. Fischbeck KH. Kennedy disease. *J Inherit Metab Dis.* (1997) 20:152–8. doi: 10.1023/A:1005344403603
2. Rhodes LE, Freeman BK, Auh S, Kokkinis AD, La Pean A, Chen C, et al. Clinical features of spinal and bulbar muscular atrophy. *Brain* (2009) 132:3242–51. doi: 10.1093/brain/awp258
3. Querin G, Bertolin C, da Re E, Volpe M, Zara G, Pegoraro E, et al. Non-neural phenotype of spinal and bulbar muscular atrophy: results from a large cohort of Italian patients. *J Neurol Neurosurg Psychiatry* (2016) 87:810–6. doi: 10.1136/jnnp-2015-311305
4. Querin G, Sorarù G, Pradat PF. Kennedy disease (X-linked recessive bulbospinal neuronopathy): a comprehensive review from pathophysiology to therapy. *Rev Neurol (Paris)* (2017) 173:326–37. doi: 10.1016/j.neurol.2017.03.019
5. La Spada AR, Wilson EM, Lubahn DB, Harding AE, Fischbeck KH. Androgen receptor gene mutations in X-linked spinal and bulbar muscular atrophy. *Nature* (1991) 352:77–9. doi: 10.1038/352077a0
6. Atsuta N, Watanabe H, Ito M, Banno H, Suzuki K, Katsuno M, et al. Natural history of spinal and bulbar muscular atrophy (SBMA): a study of 223 Japanese patients. *Brain* (2006) 129:1446–55. doi: 10.1093/brain/awl096

7. Chahin N, Klein C, Mandrekar J, Sorenson E. Natural history of spinal-bulbar muscular atrophy. *Neurology* (2008) 70:1967–71. doi: 10.1212/01.wnl.0000312510.49768.eb
8. Sorarù G, D'Ascenzo C, Polo A, Palmieri A, Baggio L, Vergani L, et al. Spinal and bulbar muscular atrophy: skeletal muscle pathology in male patients and heterozygous females. *J Neurol Sci.* (2008) 264:100–5. doi: 10.1016/j.jns.2007.08.012
9. Ishihara H, Kanda F, Nishio H, Sumino K, Chihara K. Clinical features and skewed X-chromosome inactivation in female carriers of X-linked recessive spinal and bulbar muscular atrophy. *J Neurol.* (2001) 248:856–60. doi: 10.1007/s004150170069
10. Guidetti D, Sabadini R, Ferlini A, Torrente I. Epidemiological survey of X-linked bulbar and spinal muscular atrophy, or Kennedy disease, in the province of Reggio Emilia, Italy. *Eur J Epidemiol.* (2001) 17:587–91. doi: 10.1023/A:1014580219761
11. Lund A, Udd B, Juvonen V, Andersen PM, Cederquist K, Davis M, et al. Multiple founder effects in spinal and bulbar muscular atrophy (SBMA, Kennedy disease) around the world. *Eur J Hum Genet.* (2001) 9:431–6. doi: 10.1038/sj.ejhg.5200656
12. Lund A, Udd B, Juvonen V, Andersen PM, Cederquist K, Ronnevi LO, et al. Founder effect in spinal and bulbar muscular atrophy (SBMA) in Scandinavia. *Eur J Hum Genet.* (2000) 8:631–6. doi: 10.1038/sj.ejhg.5200517
13. Tanaka F, Doyu M, Ito Y, Matsumoto M, Mitsuma T, Abe K, et al. Founder effect in spinal and bulbar muscular atrophy (SBMA). *Hum Mol Genet.* (1996) 5:1253–7. doi: 10.1093/hmg/5.9.1253
14. Weydt P, Sagnelli A, Rosenbohm A, Fratta P, Pradat PF, Ludolph AC, et al. Clinical trials in spinal and bulbar muscular atrophy-past, present, and future. *J Mol Neurosci.* (2016) 58:394–400. doi: 10.1007/s12031-015-0682-7
15. El Mendili M-M, Lenglet T, Stojkovic T, Behin A, Guimarães-Costa R, Salachas F, et al. Cervical spinal cord atrophy profile in adult SMN1-linked SMA. *PLoS ONE* (2016) 11:e0152439. doi: 10.1371/journal.pone.0152439
16. Querin G, Lenglet T, Debs R, Stojkovic T, Behin A, Salachas F, et al. The motor neuron number index (MUNIX) profile of patients with adult spinal muscular atrophy (SMA). *Clin Neurophysiol.* (2018) 129:2333–40. doi: 10.1016/j.clinph.2018.08.025
17. Fratta P, Nirmalananthan N, Masset L, Skorupinska I, Collins T, Cortese A, et al. Correlation of clinical and molecular features in spinal bulbar muscular atrophy. *Neurology* (2014) 82:2077–84. doi: 10.1212/WNL.0000000000000507
18. Finsterer J, Soraru G. Onset manifestations of spinal and bulbar muscular atrophy (Kennedy's Disease). *J Mol Neurosci.* (2016) 58:321–9. doi: 10.1007/s12031-015-0663-x
19. Hashizume A, Katsuno M, Banno H, Suzuki K, Suga N, Mano T, et al. Longitudinal changes of outcome measures in spinal and bulbar muscular atrophy. *Brain* (2012) 135:2838–48. doi: 10.1093/brain/aws170
20. Nishiyama A, Sugeno N, Tateyama M, Nishiyama S, Kato M, Aoki M. Postural leg tremor in X-linked spinal and bulbar muscular atrophy. *J Clin Neurosci.* (2014) 21:799–802. doi: 10.1016/j.jocn.2013.07.026
21. Warnecke T, Oelenberg S, Teismann I, Suntrup S, Hamacher C, Young P, et al. Dysphagia in X-linked bulbospinal muscular atrophy (Kennedy disease). *Neuromuscul Disord.* (2009) 19:704–8. doi: 10.1016/j.nmd.2009.06.371
22. Sumner CJ, Fischbeck KH. Jaw drop in Kennedy's disease. *Neurology* (2002) 59:1471–2. doi: 10.1212/01.WNL.0000033325.01878.13
23. Finsterer J. Perspectives of Kennedy's disease. *J Neurol Sci.* (2010) 298:1–10. doi: 10.1016/j.jns.2010.08.025
24. Sperfeld A-D, Hanemann CO, Ludolph AC, Kassubek J. Laryngospasm: an underdiagnosed symptom of X-linked spinobulbar muscular atrophy. *Neurology* (2005) 64:753–4. doi: 10.1212/01.WNL.0000151978.74467.E7
25. Antonini G, Gragnani F, Romaniello A, Pennisi EM, Morino S, Ceschin V, et al. Sensory involvement in spinal-bulbar muscular atrophy (Kennedy's disease). *Muscle Nerve* (2000) 23:252–8. doi: 10.1002/(SICI)1097-4598(200002)23:2<252::AID-MUS17>3.0.CO;2-P
26. Nagashima T, Seko K, Hirose K, Mannen T, Yoshimura S, Arima R, et al. Familial bulbo-spinal muscular atrophy associated with testicular atrophy and sensory neuropathy (Kennedy-Alter-Sung syndrome): autopsy case report of two brothers. *J Neurol Sci.* (1988) 87:141–52. doi: 10.1016/0022-510X(88)90240-7
27. Sobue G, Hashizume Y, Mukai E, Hirayama M, Mitsuma T, Takahashi A. X-linked recessive bulbospinal neuronopathy: a clinicopathological study. *Brain* (1989) 112:209–32. doi: 10.1093/brain/112.1.209
28. Ferrante MA, Wilbourn AJ. The characteristic electrodiagnostic features of Kennedy's disease. *Muscle Nerve* (1997) 20:323–9.
29. Suzuki K, Katsuno M, Banno H, Takeuchi Y, Atsuta N, Ito M, et al. CAG repeat size correlates to electrophysiological motor and sensory phenotypes in SBMA. *Brain* (2008) 131:229–39. doi: 10.1093/brain/awm289
30. Manganelli F, Iodice V, Provitera V, Pisciotta C, Nolano M, Perretti A, et al. Small-fiber involvement in spinobulbar muscular atrophy (Kennedy's disease). *Muscle Nerve* (2007) 36:816–20. doi: 10.1002/mus.20872
31. Dejager S, Bry-Gauillard H, Bruckert E, Eymard B, Salachas F, LeGuern E, et al. A comprehensive endocrine description of Kennedy's disease revealing androgen insensitivity linked to CAG repeat length. *J Clin Endocrinol Metab.* (2002) 87:3893–901. doi: 10.1210/jcem.87.8.8780
32. Rosenbohm A, Hirsch S, Volk AE, Grehl T, Grosskreutz J, Hanisch F, et al. The metabolic and endocrine characteristics in spinal and bulbar muscular atrophy. *J Neurol.* (2018) 265:1026–36. doi: 10.1007/s00415-018-8790-2
33. Guber RD, Takyar V, Kokkinis A, Fox DA, Alao H, Kats I, et al. Nonalcoholic fatty liver disease in spinal and bulbar muscular atrophy. *Neurology* (2017) 89:2481–90. doi: 10.1212/WNL.0000000000004748
34. Nakatsuji H, Araki A, Hashizume A, Hijikata Y, Yamada S, Inagaki T, et al. Correlation of insulin resistance and motor function in spinal and bulbar muscular atrophy. *J Neurol.* (2017) 264:839–47. doi: 10.1007/s00415-017-8405-3
35. Querin G, Melacini P, D'Ascenzo C, Morandi L, Mazzini L, Silani V, et al. No evidence of cardiomyopathy in spinal and bulbar muscular atrophy. *Acta Neurol Scand.* (2013) 128:e30–2. doi: 10.1111/ane.12140
36. Araki A, Katsuno M, Suzuki K, Banno H, Suga N, Hashizume A, et al. Brugada syndrome in spinal and bulbar muscular atrophy. *Neurology* (2014) 82:1813–21. doi: 10.1212/WNL.0000000000000434
37. Romigi A, Liguori C, Placidi F, Albanese M, Izzi F, Uasone E, et al. Sleep disorders in spinal and bulbar muscular atrophy (Kennedy's disease): a controlled polysomnographic and self-reported questionnaires study. *J Neurol.* (2014) 261:889–93. doi: 10.1007/s00415-014-7293-z
38. Strimbu K, Tavel JA. What are biomarkers? *Curr Opin HIV AIDS* (2010) 5:463–6. doi: 10.1097/COH.0b013e32833ed177
39. Fleming TR, Powers JH. Biomarkers and surrogate endpoints in clinical trials. *Stat Med.* (2012) 31:2973–84. doi: 10.1002/sim.5403
40. Bede P, Querin G, Pradat PF. The changing landscape of motor neuron disease imaging: the transition from descriptive studies to precision clinical tools. *Curr Opin Neurol.* (2018) 31:431–8. doi: 10.1097/WCO.0000000000000569
41. Scotton C, Passarelli C, Neri M, Ferlini A. Biomarkers in rare neuromuscular diseases. *Exp Cell Res.* (2014) 325:44–9. doi: 10.1016/j.yexcr.2013.12.020
42. Pennuto M, Greensmith L, Pradat P-F, Sorarù G. 210th ENMC International Workshop: Research and clinical management of patients with spinal and bulbar muscular atrophy, 27-29 March, 2015, Naarden, The Netherlands. *Neuromuscul Disord.* (2015) 25:802–12. doi: 10.1016/j.nmd.2015.06.462
43. Pareyson D, Fratta P, Pradat P, Sorarù G, Finsterer J, Vissing J, et al. Towards a European registry and biorepository for patients with spinal and bulbar muscular atrophy. *J Mol Sci.* (2016) 58:394–400. doi: 10.1007/s12031-015-0704-5
44. Takeuchi Y, Katsuno M, Banno H, Suzuki K, Kawashima M, Atsuta N, et al. Walking capacity evaluated by the 6-minute walk test in spinal and bulbar muscular atrophy. *Muscle Nerve* (2008) 38:964–71. doi: 10.1002/mus.21077
45. Querin G, D'Ascenzo C, Peterle E, Ermani M, Bello L, Melacini P, et al. Pilot trial of clenbuterol in spinal and bulbar muscular atrophy. *Neurology* (2013) 80:2095–8. doi: 10.1212/WNL.0b013e318295d766
46. Harris-Love MO, Fernandez-Rhodes L, Joe G, Shrader JA, Kokkinis A, La Pean Kirschner A, et al. Assessing function and endurance in adults with spinal and bulbar muscular atrophy: validity of the adult myopathy assessment tool. *Rehabil Res Pract.* (2014) 2014:873872. doi: 10.1155/2014/873872
47. Shrader JA, Kats I, Kokkinis A, Zampieri C, Levy E, Joe GO, et al. A randomized controlled trial of exercise in spinal and bulbar muscular atrophy. *Ann Clin Transl Neurol.* (2015) 2:739–47. doi: 10.1002/acn3.208

48. Hashizume A, Katsuno M, Suzuki K, Banno H, Suga N, Mano T, et al. A functional scale for spinal and bulbar muscular atrophy: cross-sectional and longitudinal study. *Neuromuscul Disord.* (2015) 25:554–62. doi: 10.1016/j.nmd.2015.03.008
49. Querin G, DaRe E, Martinelli I, Bello L, Bertolin C, Pareyson D, et al. Validation of the Italian version of the SBMA functional rating scale as outcome measure. *Neurol Sci.* (2016) 37:1815–21. doi: 10.1007/s10072-016-2666-y
50. Lu M, Guo H, Fan D. Kennedy's disease 1234 scale: preliminary design and test. *J Clin Neurosci.* (2017) 40:185–9. doi: 10.1016/j.jocn.2017.02.007
51. Banno H, Katsuno M, Suzuki K, Takeuchi Y, Kawashima M, Suga N, et al. Phase 2 trial of leuprorelin in patients with spinal and bulbar muscular atrophy. *Ann Neurol.* (2009) 65:140–50. doi: 10.1002/ana.21540
52. Fernández-Rhodes LE, Kokkinis AD, White MJ, Watts CA, Auh S, Jeffries NO, et al. Efficacy and safety of dutasteride in patients with spinal and bulbar muscular atrophy: a randomised placebo-controlled trial. *Lancet Neurol.* (2011) 10:140–7. doi: 10.1016/S1474-4422(10)70321-5
53. Hijikata Y, Katsuno M, Suzuki K, Hashizume A, Araki A, Yamada S, et al. Treatment with creatine monohydrate in spinal and bulbar muscular atrophy: protocol for a randomized, double-blind, placebo-controlled trial. *JMIR Res Protoc.* (2018) 7:e69. doi: 10.2196/resprot.8655
54. Mano T, Katsuno M, Banno H, Suzuki K, Suga N, Hashizume A, et al. Tongue pressure as a novel biomarker of spinal and bulbar muscular atrophy. *Neurology* (2014) 82:255–62. doi: 10.1212/WNL.0000000000000041
55. Mano T, Katsuno M, Banno H, Suzuki K, Suga N, Hashizume A, et al. Head lift exercise improves swallowing dysfunction in spinal and bulbar muscular atrophy. *Eur Neurol.* (2015) 74:251–8. doi: 10.1159/000431088
56. Hashizume A, Banno H, Katsuno M, Hijikata Y, Yamada S, Inagaki T, et al. Quantitative assessment of swallowing dysfunction in patients with spinal and bulbar muscular atrophy. *Intern Med.* (2017) 56:3159–65. doi: 10.2169/internalmedicine.8799-16
57. Katsuno M, Banno H, Suzuki K, Takeuchi Y, Kawashima M, Yabe I, et al. Efficacy and safety of leuprorelin in patients with spinal and bulbar muscular atrophy (JASMITT study): a multicentre, randomised, double-blind, placebo-controlled trial. *Lancet Neurol.* (2010) 9:875–84. doi: 10.1016/S1474-4422(10)70182-4
58. Suzuki K, Katsuno M, Banno H, Takeuchi Y, Kawashima M, Suga N, et al. The profile of motor unit number estimation (MUNE) in spinal and bulbar muscular atrophy. *J Neurol Neurosurg Psychiatry* (2010) 81:567–71. doi: 10.1136/jnnp.2009.190462
59. Lehky TJ, Chen CJ, di Prospero NA, Rhodes LE, Fischbeck K, Floeter MK. Standard and modified statistical MUNE evaluations in spinal-bulbar muscular atrophy. *Muscle Nerve* (2009) 40:809–14. doi: 10.1002/mus.21399
60. Hamano T, Mutoh T, Hirayama M, Kawamura Y, Nagata M, Fujiyama J, et al. Muscle MRI findings of X-linked spinal and bulbar muscular atrophy. *J Neurol Sci.* (2004) 222:93–7. doi: 10.1016/j.jns.2004.04.028
61. ATS Committee on Proficiency Standards for Clinical Pulmonary Function Laboratories. ATS statement: guidelines for the six-minute walk test. *Am J Respir Crit Care Med.* (2002) 166:111–7. doi: 10.1164/ajrccm.166.1.at1102
62. Dunaway Young S, Montes J, Kramer SS, Marra J, Salazar R, Cruz R, et al. Six-minute walk test is reliable and valid in spinal muscular atrophy. *Muscle Nerve* (2016) 54:836–42. doi: 10.1002/mus.25120
63. Andersen LK, Knak KL, Witting N, Vissing J. Two- and 6-minute walk tests assess walking capability equally in neuromuscular diseases. *Neurology* (2016) 86:442–5. doi: 10.1212/WNL.0000000000002332
64. Meriggioli MN, Rowin J. Fatigue and abnormal neuromuscular transmission in Kennedy's disease. *Muscle Nerve* (2003) 27:249–51. doi: 10.1002/mus.10295
65. Cedarbaum JM, Stambler N, Malta E, Fuller C, Hilt D, Thurmond B, et al. The ALSFRS-R: a revised ALS functional rating scale that incorporates assessments of respiratory function. BDNF ALS Study Group (Phase III). *J Neurol Sci.* (1999) 169:13–21.
66. Bohannon RW. Manual muscle testing: does it meet the standards of an adequate screening test? *Clin Rehabil.* (2005) 19:662–7. doi: 10.1191/0269215505cr873oa
67. Hogrel JY, Ollivier G, Desnuelle C. Manual and quantitative muscle testing in neuromuscular disorders. How to assess the consistency of strength measurements in clinical trials? *Rev Neurol.* (2006) 162:427–36.
68. Banno H, Katsuno M, Suzuki K, Sobue G. Dutasteride for spinal and bulbar muscular atrophy. *Lancet Neurol.* (2011) 10:113–5. doi: 10.1016/S1474-4422(10)70324-0
69. Gooch C, Shefner J. MUNE. *Amyotroph Lateral Scler Other Mot Neuron Disord.* (2004) 5:104–7. doi: 10.1080/17434470410019889
70. Swoboda KJ, Prior TW, Scott CB, McNaught TP, Wride MC, Reyna SP, et al. Natural history of denervation in SMA: relation to age, SMN2 copy number, and function. *Ann Neurol.* (2005) 57:704–12. doi: 10.1002/ana.20473
71. Neuwirth C, Barkhaus PE, Burkhardt C, Castro J, Czell D, De Carvalho M, et al. Tracking motor neuron loss in a set of six muscles in amyotrophic lateral sclerosis using the Motor Unit Number Index (MUNIX): a 15-month longitudinal multicentre trial. *J Neurol Neurosurg Psychiatry* (2015) 86:1172–9. doi: 10.1136/jnnp-2015-310509
72. Delmont E, Benvenutto A, Grimaldi S, Duprat L, Philibert M, Pouget J, et al. Motor unit number index (MUNIX): is it relevant in chronic inflammatory demyelinating polyradiculoneuropathy (CIDP)? *Clin Neurophysiol.* (2016) 127:1891–4. doi: 10.1016/j.clinph.2015.12.002
73. El Mendili MM, Cohen-Adad J, Pelegrini-Issac M, Rossignol S, Morizot-Koutlidis R, Marchand-Pauvert V, et al. Multi-parametric spinal cord MRI as potential progression marker in amyotrophic lateral sclerosis. *PLoS ONE* (2014) 9:e95516. doi: 10.1371/journal.pone.0095516
74. Querin G, El Mendili MM, Lenglet T, Delphine S, Marchand-Pauvert V, Benali H, et al. Spinal cord multi-parametric magnetic resonance imaging for survival prediction in amyotrophic lateral sclerosis. *Eur J Neurol.* (2017) 24:1040–6. doi: 10.1111/ene.13329
75. Querin G, El Mendili MM, Bede P, Delphine S, Lenglet T, Marchand-Pauvert V, et al. Multimodal spinal cord MRI offers accurate diagnostic classification in ALS. *J Neurol Neurosurg Psychiatry* (2018) 20:jnnp-2017-317214. doi: 10.1136/jnnp-2017-317214
76. Paquin ME, El Mendili MM, Gros C, Dupont SM, Cohen-Adad J, Pradat PF. Spinal cord gray matter atrophy in amyotrophic lateral sclerosis. *AJNR Am J Neuroradiol.* (2018) 39:184–192. doi: 10.3174/ajnr.A5427
77. Agosta F, Rocca MA, Valsasina P, Sala S, Caputo D, Perini M, et al. A longitudinal diffusion tensor MRI study of the cervical cord and brain in amyotrophic lateral sclerosis patients. *J Neurol Neurosurg Psychiatry* (2009) 80:53–5. doi: 10.1136/jnnp.2008.154252
78. Kassubek J, Juengling FD, Sperfeld AD. Widespread white matter changes in Kennedy disease: a voxel based morphometry study. *J Neurol Neurosurg Psychiatry* (2007) 78:1209–12. doi: 10.1136/jnnp.2006.112532
79. Unrath A, Müller HP, Riecker A, Ludolph AC, Sperfeld AD, Kassubek J. Whole brain-based analysis of regional white matter tract alterations in rare motor neuron diseases by diffusion tensor imaging. *Hum Brain Mapp.* (2010) 31:1727–40. doi: 10.1002/hbm.20971
80. Pieper CC, Konrad C, Sommer J, Teismann I, Schiffbauer H. Structural changes of central white matter tracts in Kennedy's disease - a diffusion tensor imaging and voxel-based morphometry study. *Acta Neurol Scand.* (2013) 127:323–8. doi: 10.1111/ane.12018
81. Sperfeld AD, Bretschneider V, Flaith L, Unrath A, Hanemann CO, Ludolph AC, et al. MR-pathologic comparison of the upper spinal cord in different motor neuron diseases. *Eurol Neurol.* (2005) 53:74–7. doi: 10.1159/000084650
82. Lai T-H, Liu R-S, Yang B-H, Wang P-S, Lin K-P, Lee Y-C, et al. Cerebral involvement in spinal and bulbar muscular atrophy (Kennedy's disease): a pilot study of PET. *J Neurol Sci.* (2013) 335:139–44. doi: 10.1016/j.jns.2013.09.016
83. Kasper E, Wegrzyn M, Marx I, Korp C, Kress W, Benecke R, et al. Minor cognitive disturbances in X-linked spinal and bulbar muscular atrophy, Kennedy's disease. *Amyotroph Lateral Scler Frontotemporal Degener.* (2014) 15:15–20. doi: 10.3109/21678421.2013.837927
84. Soukup GR, Sperfeld AD, Uttner I, Karitzky J, Ludolph AC, Kassubek J, et al. Frontotemporal cognitive function in X-linked spinal and bulbar muscular atrophy (SBMA): a controlled neuropsychological study of 20 patients. *J Neurol.* (2009) 256:1869–75. doi: 10.1007/s00415-009-5212-5
85. Di Rosa E, Sorarù G, Kleinbub JR, Calvo V, Vallesi A, Querin G, et al. Theory of mind, empathy and neuropsychological functioning in X-linked Spinal and Bulbar Muscular Atrophy: a controlled study of 20 patients. *J Neurol.* (2015) 262:394–401. doi: 10.1007/s00415-014-7567-5

86. Marcato S, Querin G, Pick E, Kleinbub JR, Martinalli I, Bertolin C, et al. Not impaired neuropsychological performance and enhanced memory recall in patients with SBMA: a large sample comparative study. *Sci Rep.* (2018) 8:13627. doi: 10.1038/s41598-018-32062-5
87. Manzano R, Sorarú G, Grunseich C, Fratta P, Zuccaro E, Pennuto M, et al. Beyond motor neurons: expanding the clinical spectrum in Kennedy's disease. *J Neurol Neurosurg Psychiatry* (2018) 89:808–12. doi: 10.1136/jnnp-2017-316961
88. Rinaldi C, Bott LC, Fischbeck KH. Muscle matters in kennedy's disease. *Neuron* (2014) 82:251–3. doi: 10.1016/j.neuron.2014.04.005
89. Sorenson EJ, Klein CJ. Elevated creatine kinase and transaminases in asymptomatic SBMA. *Amyotroph Lateral Scler.* (2007) 8:62–4. doi: 10.1080/17482960600765040
90. Hijikata Y, Katsuno M, Suzuki K, Hashizume A, Araki A, Yamada S, et al. Impaired muscle uptake of creatine in spinal and bulbar muscular atrophy. *Ann Clin Transl Neurol.* (2016) 3:537–46. doi: 10.1002/acn3.324
91. Hijikata Y, Hashizume A, Yamada S, Inagaki T, Ito D, Hirakawa A, et al. Biomarker-based analysis of preclinical progression in spinal and bulbar muscular atrophy. *Neurology* (2018) 90:e1501–9. doi: 10.1212/WNL.0000000000005360
92. Hashizume A, Katsuno M, Suzuki K, Hirakawa A, Hijikata Y, Yamada S, et al. Long-term treatment with leuprorelin for spinal and bulbar muscular atrophy: natural history-controlled study. *J Neurol Neurosurg Psychiatry* (2017) 88:1026–32. doi: 10.1136/jnnp-2017-316015
93. Guber RD, Kokkinis AD, Schindler AB, Bendixen RM, Heatwole CR, Fischbeck KH, et al. Patient-identifed impact of symptoms in spinal and bulbar muscular atrophy. *Muscle Nerve* (2018) 57:40–4. doi: 10.1002/mus.25957
94. Rinaldi C, Malik B, Greensmith L. Targeted molecular therapies for SBMA. *J Mol Sci.* (2016) 58:335–42. doi: 10.1007/s12031-015-0676-5
95. Turner MR, Kiernan MC, Leigh PN, Talbot K. Biomarkers in amyotrophic lateral sclerosis. *Lancet Neurol.* (2009) 8:94–109. doi: 10.1016/S1474-4422(08)70293-X
96. Chiò A, Montalcini RL, Traynor BJ. Motor neuron disease in 2014: biomarkers for ALS—in search of the Promised Land. *Nat Rev Neurol.* (2015) 11:72–4. doi: 10.1038/nrneurol.2014.250
97. Pennuto M, Rinaldi C. From gene to therapy in spinal and bulbar muscular atrophy: are we there yet? *Mol Cell Encodcrinol.* (2018) 465:113–21. doi: 10.1016/j.mce.2017.07.005

3

Past and Future of Neurotrophic Growth Factors Therapies in ALS: From Single Neurotrophic Growth Factor to Stem Cells and Human Platelet Lysates

Flore Gouel[1†], Anne-Sophie Rolland[1†], Jean-Christophe Devedjian[1], Thierry Burnouf[2,3,4] and David Devos[1,5]*

[1] Department of Medical Pharmacology, Lille University, INSERM UMRS_1171, University Hospital Center, LICEND COEN Center, Lille, France, [2] Graduate Institute of Biomedical Materials and Tissue Engineering, College of Biomedical Engineering, Taipei Medical University, Taipei, Taiwan, [3] International PhD Program in Biomedical Engineering, College of Biomedical Engineering, Taipei Medical University, Taipei, Taiwan, [4] International PhD Program in Cell Therapy and Regeneration Medicine, College of Medicine, Taipei Medical University, Taipei, Taiwan, [5] Department of Neurology, Lille University, INSERM UMRS_1171, University Hospital Center, LICEND COEN Center, Lille, France

***Correspondence:**
David Devos
david.devos@chru-lille.fr

† These authors have contributed equally to this work

Amyotrophic lateral sclerosis (ALS) is a fatal neurodegenerative disease that typically results in death within 3–5 years after diagnosis. To date, there is no curative treatment and therefore an urgent unmet need of neuroprotective and/or neurorestorative treatments. Due to their spectrum of capacities in the central nervous system—e.g., development, plasticity, maintenance, neurogenesis—neurotrophic growth factors (NTF) have been exploited for therapeutic strategies in ALS for decades. In this review we present the initial strategy of using single NTF by different routes of administration to the use of stem cells transplantation to express a multiple NTFs-rich secretome to finally focus on a new biotherapy based on the human platelet lysates, the natural healing system containing a mix of pleitropic NTF and having immunomodulatory function. This review highlights that this latter treatment may be crucial to power the neuroprotection and/or neurorestoration therapy requested in this devastating disease.

Keywords: Amyotrophic lateral sclerosis, growth factors, therapeutic, stem cell, human platelet lysate

INTRODUCTION

Amyotrophic lateral sclerosis (ALS) is a fatal neurodegenerative disease affecting the upper and lower motor neurons in the cerebral cortex, brainstem and spinal cord that lead to a progressive, irreversible muscle paralysis, and swallowing and respiratory dysfunctions. Death eventually occurs 3–5 years after diagnosis (1). The majority of ALS cases (90%) are sporadic with unknown cause (2). To date, there is no curative treatment in ALS. Therefore, the development of new and effective treatment is highly urgent. Among the different approaches, the delivery of neurotrophic factors (NTFs) is explored since the 90's because NTFs are necessary to regulate several physiological processes such as neuronal differentiation and survival, axonal outgrowth and synapses maintenance (3–5), proliferation and differentiation of stem cells in the nervous system (6–9). Therefore, these trophic factors represent a promising therapeutic strategy to treat neurodegenerative diseases (10) such as ALS.

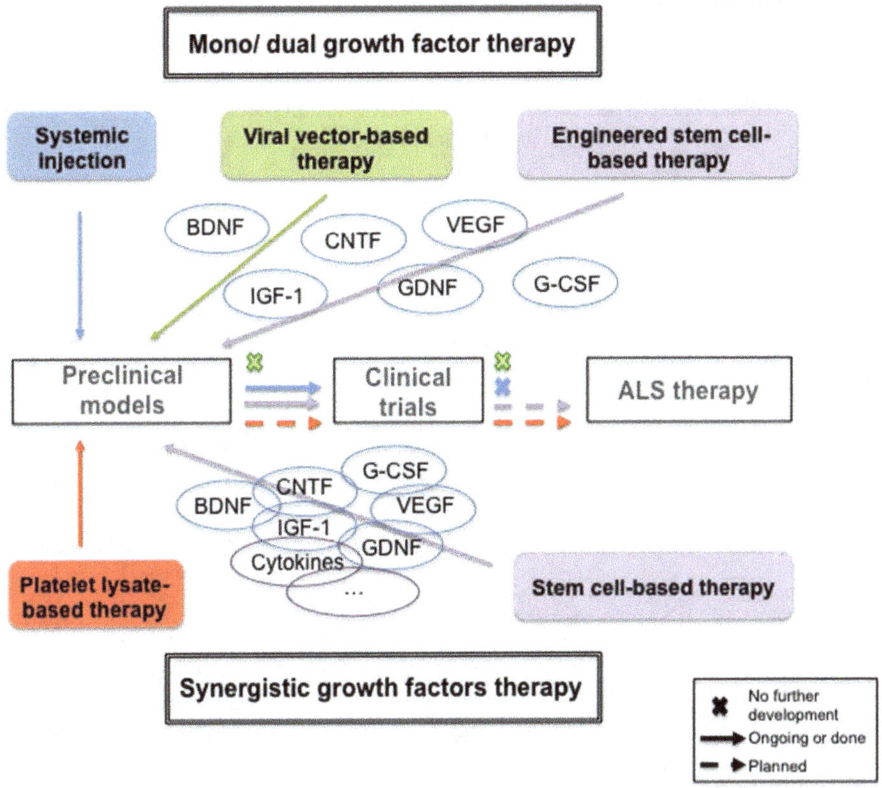

Graphical Abstract | From single to synergistic neurotrophic growth factors therapies.

PRECLINICAL EVIDENCE OF NEUROTROPHICS GROWTH FACTORS ABILITIES TO TREAT AMYOTROPHIC LATERAL SCLEROSIS (TABLE 1)

Recombinant NTFs Delivery by Injection

Some trophic factors have been demonstrated to promote cell survival and be protective in both *in vitro* and *in vivo* models of neuronal degeneration: Ciliary Neurotrophic Factor (CNTF), Brain-derived Neurotrophic Factor (BDNF), Glial-Derived Neurotrophic Factor (GDNF), Insulin-like Growth Factor 1 (IGF-1), Vascular Endothelial Growth Factor (VEGF), and Granulocyte-Colony Stimulating Factor (G-CSF). *In vivo* experiments performed in ALS models using single recombinant growth factors are described in this section.

CNTF, one of the first NTF studied in ALS models, injected intraperitonally in *pmn/pmn* mice, mouse model for human spinal motor neuron disease (11) or subcutaneously in wobbler mice (12) improved motor function and survival, and decreased neuronal degeneration and muscle atrophy (13). In addition, Mitsumoto et al. demonstrated a synergic effect of CNTF and BDNF, respectively, to arrest disease progression for 1 month (14).

The fusion protein BDNF with the c fragment of the tetanus toxin (BDNF-TTC) exhibited enhanced neuroprotective effect in SOD1^{G93A} ALS mice model, but no synergic effect was observed compared to TTC alone (55). Recently, motor function improvement and less neuronal loss were observed in SOD1^{G93A} mice treated with the flavonoid 7,8-dihydroxyflavone, a small-molecule mimicking the effect of BDNF (56). Two receptors binding the BDNF, p75^{NTR} and TrkB.T1, were highlighted in SOD1^{G93A}: a decreased of p75^{NTR} expression correlated with a delay of mortality and motor impairment (57); a deletion of the TrkB.T1 increased survival and delayed motor deficit (58).

Treatment with encapsuled GDNF-secreting cells in *pmn/pmn* mice did not impact motor neuron degeneration and lifespan (15). The authors suggest a combined treatment for GDNF with others NTFs. Recently, astrocytic GDNF triggered by the tumor necrosis factor α (TNFα) was highlighted in the SOD1^{G93A} mice, and found to limit motor neuron degeneration and disease progression (59).

Intraperitoneal (16) or intracerebroventricular (17) injection of VEGF at doses of 1 g/kg/d and 0.2 μg/kg/d in SOD1^{G93A} mice and rats, respectively, increased lifespan and improved motor performance. Similar data were observed in a sporadic model of ALS rats induced by excitotoxic administration of AMPA (60, 61).

Finally, protective properties of G-CSF were observed in SOD1^{G93A} mice when delivered continuously at dose of 30 μg/kg/d (18). Indeed, disease progression was reduced and

TABLE 1 | Different routes of NTFs delivery and therapies in pre-clinical models.

NTF	Delivery route	Model	Outcomes	References
RECOMBINANT NEUROTROPHIC GROWTH FACTORS				
CNTF	I.P	*pmn/pmn* mice (20–21 d)	MP+, S+	(11)
	S.C	Wobbler mice	MP+, MC+	(12–14)
BDNF	S.C	Wobbler mice	MP+	(14)
GDNF	S.C	*pmn/pmn* mice (15–18 d)	No effect	(15)
VEGF	I.P	SOD1^{G93A} mice (74 d)	MP+, DDO+, S+11 d	(16)
	I.C.V	SOD1$^{G93A/LSd}$ rats (60 d)	MP+, DDO+, S+10 d	(17)
	I.S.P	Excitotoxic model in rats	MP+, DDO+, S+10.5 d, +5 d	(18, 19)
Viral vector based gene therapy				
AAV-NTF				
IGF-1	I.M	SOD1^{G93A} mice (90 d)	MP+, S+22 d	(20)
	I.S.P	SOD1^{G93A} mice (60 d)	MP+, DDO+, S+12.3 d ♂	(21)
	In D.C.N	SOD1^{G93A} mice (88–90 d)	MP+, S+14 d	(22)
	I.M	SOD1^{G93A} mice (60 and 90 d)	MP+, DDO+, S+29 d and +15 d ♂, +24 d and +14 d ♀	(23)
	I.V	SOD1^{G93A} mice (90 d)	MP+, S+10 d	(24)
	I.C.V	SOD1^{G93A} mice (80–90 d)	DDO+, S+12 d	(25)
VEGF	I.C.V	SOD1^{G93A} mice (80–90 d)	DDO+, S+9 d ♂, +20 d ♀	(25)
	I.T	SOD1^{G93A} mice (90 d)	DDO+, S+12 d	(26)
GDNF	I.M	SOD1^{G93A} mice (90 d)	MP+, DDO+, S+16.6 d	(27)
	I.V	SOD1^{G93A} rats (25 d)	MP +/–, S–	(28)
G-CSF	I.S.P	SOD1^{G93A} mice (70 d)	MP+, DDO+, S+	(29)
Stem cell based therapy				
AAV-NTF				
hSC-NSC	I.S.P	SOD1^{G93A} rats (56–62 d)	MP+, DDO+, S+11 d	(30, 31)
gm hNSC line (VEGF)	I.T	SOD1^{G93A} mice (70 d)	DDO+, S+12 d	(32)
hSC-NPC	I.S.P	SOD1^{G93A} mice (40 d)	MP+, S+5 d	(33)
gm hNPC (GDNF)	I.S.P	SOD1^{G93A} rats (~80 d) rats (~80 d)	MP–, S–	(34, 35)
	Cortex	SOD1^{G93A} rats (~80 d) macaques	DDO+, S+14 d	(36)
hBM-MSC	I.S.P	SOD1$^{(G93A)dl}$ mice (28 w)	MP+	(37)
		SOD1^{G93A} mice	MP+	(38)
mBM-MSC	I.V	SOD1^{G93A} mice (90 d)	MP+, S+17.3 d	(39)
gm hBM-MSC (GDNF, VEGF, GNDF/IGF-1, BDNF)	I.M	SOD1^{G93A} rats (80 d)	MP+, S+28 d and +18 d for GDNF, + 13 d for VEGF, +28 d for GDNF/VEGF	(40, 41)
mBM	I.S.P and I.M	mdf/ocd mice (6 weeks)	MP+	(42, 43)
mASC	I.V	SOD1^{G93A} mice (76–77 d)	MP+, S–	(44)
hASC	I.V and I.C.V	SOD1^{G93A} mice (70 d)	MP+, DDO+, S+	(45)
hUCBC	I.V	SOD1^{G93A} mice (56 d, 66 d)	DDO+, S+21 d, +38.5 d, +23.8 d	(46–48)
		SOD1^{G93A} mice (60 and 90 d)	MP+, S+10 d	(49)
	I.T	SOD1^{G93A} mice	No effect	(50)
	I.S.P	SOD1^{G93A} mice (40 and 90 d)	MP+, S+6 d for 40 d mice	(51)
	I.C.V	SOD1^{G93A} (70 d) Wobbler mice (28 d)	MP+, S+18 d MP+	(52)
gm hUCBC (VEGF, GDNF, and/or NCAM)	I.V	SOD1$^{(G93A)dl}$ mice	MP+, S+	(53, 54)

I.P, intraperitoneal; I.M, intramuscular; I.V, intravenous; I.C.V, intracerebrovascular; I.S.P, intraspinal; I.T, intrathecal; S.C, subcutaneous; DCN, deep cerebellar nuclei; gm, genetically modified for expression of NTFs in brackets; hSC-NSC: human spinal cord-neural stem cell; m/hBM-MSC, murine/human bone marrow-mesenchymal stem cell; m/hASC, murine/human adipose derived MSC; hUCBC, human umbilical cord blood cells. Main results are summarized as follow: MP, motor performance; DDO, delay of disease onset; S, survival. The age of the model at the treatment is noted in brackets (d, days old; w, weeks). +, improvement; –, deterioration. ♂, male; ♀, female.

survival increased by rescuing motoneurons. Similar results were obtained with subcutaneous injection of pegfilgrastim, a more stable analog of G-CSF (19).

As protein infusion has known drawbacks (invasive method of delivery, protein stability over time, short half-life) others strategies, such as viral vector-based gene therapy and stem cell-based therapy have been developed to express NTFs of interest and avoid chronic injection.

NTFs Delivery by Viral Vector-Based Gene Therapy

Many studies focused on IGF-1. The intramuscular injection of adeno-associated viral (AAV)-IGF-1 in SOD1^{G93A} mice before or at the time of disease symptoms delayed disease onset and increased lifespan (20). Intraparenchymal spinal cord delivery was also tested, showing higher expression of IGF-1 but partial rescue (21), whereas a stereotaxic injection into the deep cerebellar nuclei significantly extended mice lifespan (22). Recently the injection of self-complementary adeno-associated viral vector 9 (scAAV9), a more efficient transducing agent for IGF-1, extended survival, and motor performance of SOD1^{G93A} mice when injected either intramuscularly (23) or intravenously (24). Also, the intracerebroventricular injection of AAV4-VEGF was studied and gave similar results than AAV4-IGF-1 by slowing disease progression. No combined effect of these 2 constructions was observed in SOD1^{G93A} mice (25). Similarly the intrathecal injection of scAAV9-VEGF showed positive impact on lifespan and motor performance in mice (26). The AAV-GDNF, injected intramuscularly in SOD1^{G93A} allowed expression of the protein at the sites of injection, a retrograde transport in anterior horn neurons, and was associated with a delay in the onset and the progression of the disease (27). However, the systemic injection of AAV9-GDNF in SOD1^{G93A} rats showed limited functional improvement and no survival extension (28). Finally the efficacy of intraspinal delivery was showed for AAV-G-CSF in SOD1^{G93A} mice with minimal systemic effects (29).

NTFs Delivery by Stem Cell-Based Therapy

Different types of stem cells exist—based on their source, clonogenic capacity, differentiation potential and availability—and exert a paracrine effect, suitable for therapy in neurodegenerative disease such the ALS (62–65). We mainly focus here on stem cells with potential clinical application, engineered or used as such, e.g., a mix of NTFs.

Neuroprotection With Neural Stem Cells (NSC) and Neural Progenitor Cells (NPC)

Human NSC graft into lumbar protuberance of SOD1^{G93A} rats was shown to delay the onset and the progression of the disease, with their integration into the spinal cord (30, 31). Similarly, the intraspinal administration of human NPC delayed the progression of the disease in SOD1^{G93A} mice (33).

NSC were also engineered to secrete specific one. Intrathecal transplantation of human NSC overexpressing VEGF in SOD1^{G93A} mice delayed the onset of the disease and increased survival with an integration and differentiation of NSC-VEGF into the spinal cord (32). Human neural progenitor cells NPC (hNPC) were also genetically modified to secrete GDNF. The transplantation of such engineered cells in SOD1 rats were integrated into the spinal cord, limited motoneuron degeneration but failed to improve motor function (34, 35). However, the transplantation of hPNC-GDNF into the cortex extended the survival of SOD1^{G93A} rats and was safe for primates (36).

Mesenchymal Stromal Cells (MSC)

Bone marrow (BM) MSC (BM-MSC), when injected intraspinally (37, 38) or intravenously (39) in SOD1^{G93A} mice, allowed decreased motoneurons degeneration, improved survival and motor function, prevented pro-inflammatory factors. Indeed, MSC display immunomodulatory properties by secreting anti-inflammatory cytokines such as TGF-β or IL-10 (66) Since neuroinflammatory markers were detected in neural tissues of ALS patients (67) promising results can be expected with MSC based therapy. Moreover, intramuscular transplantation of human BM-MSC genetically modified to secrete GDNF in SOD1^{G93A} rats, showed a decrease in motoneuron loss and an overall increased lifespan (40). In addition they demonstrated a synergic effect of the combined intramuscular delivery of hMSC-GDNF and hMSC-VEGF with an increased survival, protection of neuromuscular junction and motoneuron degeneration, greater than either growth factor delivered individually (41). Even though human BM-MSC injections have positive effects on the disease progression, it should be noted that the whole BM intraspinally transplanted showed a greater improvement of motor functions than BM-MSC in *mdf/ocd* mice (42) and increased motoneurons survival when intramuscularly transplanted (43).

Others reported positive results with adipose derived MSC when administrated by systemic (44), or intracerebroventricular administration (45).

Human Umbilical Cord Blood (hUCB)

The first study performed on SOD1^{G93A} mice irradiated and transplanted intravenously with hUBC mononuclear cells (MNC), showed a delay in the onset of symptoms and increased the survival (46, 47). Transplanted cells integrated regions of motoneuron degeneration and expressed neural markers (48). Recently, the efficiency of chronic intravenous injections of UCB MNC in symptomatic SOD1^{G93A} mice was demonstrated, with increased lifespan and reduced inflammatory effectors (49). Similarly, the intraspinal as the intracerebroventricular injection of hUCB in pre-symptomatic SOD1^{G93A} or wobbler mice increased survival and motor performance (51, 52). However, intrathecal administration of hUCB did not affect the lifespan of motor function of ALS mice (50).

Some authors engineered hUCB MNC to secrete some NTFs or to enhance homing at the site of degeneration (68, 69). Recently, transplanted hUCB transduced with AAV encoding VEGF, GDNF and/or neural cell adhesion molecule (NCAM), led to a high rate of SOD1^{G93A} mice survival and improved motor function. Moreover, transplanted cells were detected 1 month after grafting into the lumbar spinal cord (53, 54).

CLINICAL TRIALS WITH GROWTH FACTORS: EVIDENCE AND HYPOTHESIS FOR THE FAILURE

Regarding the promising effects obtained in ALS animal models, clinical trials were conducted to examine the neuroprotective effects of these growth factors therapies in ALS patients (**Table 2**).

Trials Involving NTFs Protein Systemic Injections

CNTF

In 90's the ALS CNTF Treatment study group published results obtained in phase I (70) and phase II/III (72) clinical trials where enrolled patients received subcutaneous administration of recombinant human CNTF (rHCNTF) at different doses, 15 or 30 μg/kg, three times a week for 9 months. The phase II/III randomized, placebo-controlled evaluated the safety, tolerability, and efficacy. No statistically difference between rHCNTF-treated patients and placebo-treated patients were observed and side effects were sufficiently severe to limit dosing in many patients. A second trial, same year, did not show any positive effect either (71).

One year later, Penn et al. published results of a phase I clinical trial with intrathecal pump delivery (73). The disease progression was not modified either but no systemic side effects were observed. Thus, intrathecal administration may be the preferred route of administration. To our knowledge, no further clinical study are under investigation.

BDNF

Due to a promising phase I/II clinical trial showing the safety and efficacy of subcutaneous administration of BDNF in 1995, a phase III was designed (74). Results failed to demonstrate an effect on survival but *post-hoc* analyses showed that those ALS patients with early respiratory impairment showed benefit (75). One year later a phase I trial showed the feasibility of intrathecal method of delivery (76) but two other trials conducted in 2003 and 2005 felt to detect any efficacy (77, 78).

IGF-1

In the late 90's, two clinical trials used IGF-1 at a dose of 0.1 mg/kg/d by subcutaneous delivery and found contradictory and opposite results (79, 80). In 2008, a phase III showed no benefit of this route of delivery in 2 years of trials (82). In a pilot study conducted in 2005, intrathecal administration had beneficial effect using high doses of IGF-1 (3 μg/kg every 2 weeks) but it was not placebo-controlled (81).

G-CSF

Ten years ago, two pilot clinical trials with subcutaneous G-CSF administration at a dose of 5 μg/kg/d reported a trend for slowing down the disease progression (84) and a delay in motor decline (83). A Phase II clinical trial is under investigation but results are not yet available.

VEGF

Three clinical trials assessed the safety, tolerability, and the possible motor function improvement as well as survival time of the intracerebroventricular administration of 4 μg/d VEGF. To our knowledge, no results are published.

6- Failure Hypothesis

Most of the clinical trials based on direct protein administration gave disappointing outcomes in view of the promising preclinical results. Different hypotheses can be raised to explain those failures (70–84):

- The route of administration: subcutaneous injection seems less efficient than the intrathecal one
- The minimal ability of these growth factors to cross the blood brain barrier
- The dose: highest safe dose in humans can be lower than those determined in animals, as the clinical trial with CNTF demonstrated
- The treatment start time: in animals, treatment start before the onset of the disease whereas in humans the diagnosis is performed at later stage
- The need of synergic association of numerous neurotrophic factors

Trials Involving Adeno-Associated Viral Gene Therapy

To our knowledge, there is no reported clinical trial using adeno-associated viral gene therapy despite promising results obtained with $SOD1^{G93A}$ mice. AAV2 and AAV9 are vectors having the greatest potential, one specific for neuron tissue, one passing the blood brain barrier and exhibiting neuronal tropisms, respectively. One of the drawbacks of genes therapies for ALS can be the safety. Indeed to stop delivery will not be possible if serious adverse events occur during the treatment.

Trials Involving Stem Cell Therapy

Twenty-two trials involving stem cells-based therapy are registered on ClinicalTrials.gov. Most of them use MSC from different origins and few have results available. This section is an overview of all the known clinical trials.

Neural Stem Cells

In 2012, two trials sponsored by Neuralstem used NSC by intraspinal injection. The phase I did not show any adverse events (85, 86), but the phase II has an unknown status on the ClinicalTrials.gov website.

Recently, published results of a phase I trial, proposing transplantation of human NSCs into the lumbar spinal cord, demonstrated the safety and reproducibility of this cell therapy. Moreover, because the brain tissue used was from natural miscarriages, ethical concerns may be eliminated (87). An ongoing clinical trial concern neuronal progenitor cells engineered to produce GDNF. This is a phase I/IIA trial, active but not recruiting. No results are available for now.

TABLE 2 | Clinical trials with growth factors.

NCT number	NTF	Delivery method	Phase and status of the trial	Cohort size	Outcomes	References	Year
PROTEIN INFUSION							
Not provided	CNTF	SC	Phase I, terminated	57	No adverse neurologic effects, safe, and tolerated	(70)	1995
Not provided		SC	Phase I, terminated	570	No beneficial effect, adverse events dose related, increased number of death at the highest dose, no beneficial effect on ALS progression	(71)	1996
Not provided		SC	Phase II/III	730	Disease progression not modified, minor adverse side effects	(72)	1996
Not provided		IT	Phase I	4	Pain syndromes dose-related, no systemic side effect, no improvement, or worsen of motor function	(73)	1997
Not provided	BDNF	SC	Phase I/II, terminated	283	Tolerated, Trend of improved survival, less deterioration of predicted FVC	(74)	1995
Not provided	BDNF	SC	Phase III	1 135	Disease progression not modified, Patients with early respiratory impairment and with altered bowel function showed benefit	(75)	1999
Not provided	BDNF	IT	Phase I/II, terminated	25	Well tolerated, feasible	(76)	2000
Not provided	BDNF	IT	Phase III, terminated	17	No adverse events, no effect	(77)	2003
Not provided	BDNF	IT	Phase II/III, terminated	13	No effect	(78)	2005
Not provided	IGF-1	SC	Not specify	266	Slowed the progression of functional impairment, slow the decline in health-related quality of life	(79)	1997
Not provided		SC	Not specify	183	Safe and well-tolerated, no effect	(80)	1998
Not provided		IT	Not specify	9	No serious adverse effect, modest beneficial effect	(81)	2005
NCT00035815		SC	Phase III, completed	330	No benefit	(82)	2008
Not provided	G-CSF	SC	Phase I, terminated	13	Safe, less decline of ALSFRS score	(83)	2009
Not provided		SC	Phase I, terminated	39	Safe, no significative effect on ALSFRS score	(84)	2010
NCT00397423		Not specify	Phase II, completed	40	Not available		
NCT01999803	VEGF	ICV	Phase I, terminated	15	Not available		
NCT02269436		ICV	Phase I, terminated	11	Not available		
NCT01384162		ICV	Phase I/II, terminated	15	Not available		
STEM CELLS							
NCT number	**Type of stem cells**	**Delivery method**	**Phase and status of the trial**	**Cohort size**	**Results**	**References**	**Year**
NCT01348451	NSC	ISP	Phase I	12	No major adverse events	(85, 86)	2012
NCT01730716	NSC	ISP	Phase II, unknown status	18	Not available		
NCT02943850	NPC	ISP	Phase I/IIa, active, not recruiting	18	Not available		
NCT01640067	NSC	ISP	Phase I, completed	6	Safe approach, no increase of disease progression	(87)	2015
NCT00781872	MSC	IT, IV	Phase I/II, terminated	19	Safe and feasible, ALS-FRS score stable the first 6 months	(88)	2010
NCT03085706	PBMC	ISP	Phase NA, completed	14	Not available		
NCT01933321	HSC	IT	Phase II/III, completed	14	Not available		
NCT01609283	MSC	IT	Phase I, active, not recruiting	27	Not available		
NCT01142856	MSC	IT	Phase I, completed	1	Not available		

(Continued)

TABLE 2 | Continued

NCT number	NTF	Delivery method	Phase and status of the trial	Cohort size	Outcomes	References	Year
NCT00855400	MSC	ISP	Phase I/II completed	11	No severe adverse event, no acceleration in the rate of decline, possible neurotrophic activity	(89)	2012
NCT02286011	MC	IM	Phase I, active, not recruiting	20	Not available		
NCT00855400	MC	ISP	Phase I, completed	11	Safe approach, no worsening of the disease	(90)	2016
NCT03268603	MSC	IT	Phase II, recruiting	60	Not available		
NCT01254539	MSC	ISP, IT	Phase I/II, completed	63	Infusion of MSC produces spinal changes unrelated with clinical events and disease worsening	(91)	2013
NCT01363401	MSC	IT	Phase I/II, completed	64	Possible benefit lasting at least 6 months with safety	(92)	2018
NCT02917681	MSC	IT	Phase I/II, recruiting	28	Not available		
NCT02987413	MSC	IT	Phase I, completed	3	Not available		
NCT02290886	MSC	IV	Phase I/II, active, not recruiting	52	Not available		
NCT01051882	MSC	IM or IT	Phase I/II, completed	12	Safe and tolerated, no serious adverse event, possible benefits on ALS-FRS score, and percentage of FVC	(93)	2016
NCT01777646	MSC	IM + IT	Phase IIa, completed	14			
NCT03280056	MSC	IT	Phase III, Recruiting	200	Not available		
NCT02017912	MSC	IM, IT	Phase II, completed	48	Not available		
NCT01759797	MSC	IV	Phase I/II, completed	6	No adverse events, ALS-FRS score reduced, FVC percentage reduced	(94)	2019
NCT01771640	MSC	IT	Phase I, completed	8			

FVC, force vital capacity; HSC, hematopoietic stem cells; I, intramuscular; ISP, intraspinal; IT, intrathecal; IV, intravenous; MC, mononuclear cell; MSC, mesenchymal stem cells; NPC, neuronal progenitor cells; NSC, neural stem cells; NTF, neurotrophic factor, PBMC, peripheral blood mononuclear cell; SC, subcutaneous.

Blood Cells

Two clinical trials, one using autologous peripheral blood mononuclear cell for intraspinal transplantation and one in phase II/III using hematopoietic stem cells for intrathecal injection were conducted and completed but no results were reported to our knowledge. One trial using autologous bone marrow mononuclear cells (90) for intraspinal injection showed the safety of the procedure.

Mesenchymal Stromal Cells

Among 14 clinical trials using MSCs from diverse origin such as bone marrow, adipose tissue or engineered to secrete particular NTFs, through diverse types of delivery (intrathecal, intraspinal, intramuscular, intravenous, or intraventricular), 5 have no published results, 4 are ongoing, and 5 are completed with published results. All of them are listed in the **Table 2** and the last 5 are detailed below and involved the use of the bone marrow derived MSCs.

In 2012, a phase I/II, using autologous bone marrow MSCs administered by intraspinal delivery, was conducted. No severe adverse event were observed, no acceleration of the disease progression noticed and an increase of the motoneurons in the treated segments compared with the untreated segments for patients who died for unrelated reasons to the procedure. Thus, this trial demonstrates the safety of intraspinal infusion of MSCs and suggests their neurotrophic activity (89). In 2013, a phase I/II confirmed the safety of BM-MSC infusion (91).

In 2016, two clinical trials in small groups of patients, phase I/II, used bone marrow MSCs engineered to secrete NTFs. Intramuscular transplantation for early ALS patients and intrathecal transplantation for progressive ALS patients were evaluated. They concluded that both route of administration are safe and provide indications of possible clinical benefits that need to be confirmed on a bigger cohort (93).

In 2018, a phase I/II trial was initiated to evaluate the safety and efficacy of these cells through intrathecal delivery. A possible benefit seems to last at least 6 months with apparent safety (92). A phase II is required to evaluate long-term efficacy and safety.

Finally, recent phase I/II trials showed safety and feasibility of intravenous and intrathecal transplantation of autologous bone marrow MSCs (94). Indeed, no adverse events were reported and the ALS-FRS score and the force vital capacity percentage were significantly reduced. Additional trials with bigger cohort are needed.

To conclude, stem cells-based therapy as a future therapy to treat ALS patients is premature due to the lack of results. As for the protein infusion, some questions need to be considered:

- The delivery method
- The timing of intervention
- The number of cells to transplant to obtain a therapeutic efficacy
- The capacity of transplanted cells to migrate to the area of interest and to mature in the hostile environment
- The evaluation of the long-term efficacy

Nevertheless, trophic factors remain essential for neuronal maintenance and survival and remain a promising candidate to treat ALS patients. Another source of those factors can be the natural healing system, namely the platelet lysate, and a continuous infusion into the brain by intracerebroventricular (ICV) injection can be a route of administration, avoiding the potential problem with the blood brain barrier crossing.

HOW TO IMPROVE GROWTH FACTORS THERAPEUTICS IN ALS: A NEW THERAPEUTIC APPROACH BASED ON THE HUMAN PLATELET LYSATE

The lack of clinical efficacy of single NTF infusion, despite a good diffusion, required increasing the dose to a point where they finally induced poor tolerance (i.e., µg). A single NTF was therefore unable to induce the complex set of signaling pathways required to promote efficient neuroprotection. Platelets constitute abundant, natural sources of physiological balanced mixtures of many growth factors [e.g., Platelet Derived Growth Factor (PDGF), VEGF, IGF-1, EGF, or TGFβ) (95) and are used to enhance wound healing and tissue repair (96). In addition, they express adhesion molecules, secret chemokines (97) giving thus neuroinflammatory property to the platelate lysate that could be of an additional interest in ALS therapy. Interestingly, it was demonstrated that ICV injection of human platelet lysates significantly reduced infarct volumes in rats with permanent middle cerebral artery occlusion, improved motor function and promoted endogenous neural stem cells proliferation (98). Similar results were obtained with platelet rich plasma in ischemic rats (99). Moreover, intranasal (IN) administration of platelet lysates was demonstrated to be neuroprotective in Alzheimer and Parkinson's disease animal models (100, 101). To pursue with the neuroprotective potential of platelets lysate in neurodegenerative diseases, we developed a heated low protein human purified platelet lysate (HPPL) preparation, compatible with ICV and IN intermittent administration, to deplete fibrinogen, avoid thrombogenic, and proteolytic activities. We demonstrated its neuroprotective effect in *in vitro* and *in vivo* model of Parkinson's disease and its anti-inflammatory properties (102). To extend the concept to ALS, HPPL was tested on a motoneuron-like model and strongly protected from apoptosis and oxidative stress (103). Higher neuroprotection was obtained with HPPL compare to single growth factor or combination of 4 (PDGF, BDNF, BFGF, VEGF) and involved specific signaling pathway such as Akt and MEK (103). These results give a real hope for neuroprotective therapy and need to be confirmed in *in vivo* ALS model with ICV or IN administration of HPPL.

AUTHOR CONTRIBUTIONS

FG and A-SR wrote the manuscript. J-CD, TB, and DD critically revised the manuscript. All authors read and approved the submitted version.

FUNDING

The authors wish to acknowledge support from the ARSLA charity (*Association pour la Recherche sur la Sclérose Latérale Amyotrophique et autres maladies du motoneurone*), I-SITE-ULNE Foundation, Credit Agricole Foundation, and SATT NORD.

REFERENCES

1. Wijesekera LC, Leigh PN. Amyotrophic lateral sclerosis. *Orphanet J Rare Dis.* (2009) 4:3. doi: 10.1186/1750-1172-4-3
2. Taylor JP, Brown RH, Cleveland DW. Decoding ALS: from genes to mechanism. *Nature.* (2016) 539:197–206. doi: 10.1038/nature20413
3. Korsching S. The neurotrophic factor concept: a reexamination. *J Neurosci.* (1993) 13:2739–48. doi: 10.1523/JNEUROSCI.13-07-02739.1993
4. Boonman Z, Isacson O. Apoptosis in neuronal development and transplantation: role of caspases and trophic factors. *Exp Neurol.* (1999) 156:1–15. doi: 10.1006/exnr.1999.7056
5. Hou ST, Jiang SX, Smith RA. Permissive and repulsive cues and signalling pathways of axonal outgrowth and regeneration. *Int Rev Cell Mol Biol.* (2008) 267:125–81. doi: 10.1016/S1937-6448(08)00603-5
6. Lamballe F, Smeyne RJ, Barbacid M. Developmental expression of trkC, the neurotrophin-3 receptor, in the mammalian nervous system. *J Neurosci.* (1994) 14:14–28. doi: 10.1523/JNEUROSCI.14-01-00014.1994
7. Tuttle R, O'Leary DD. Neurotrophins rapidly modulate growth cone response to the axon guidance molecule, collapsin-1. *Mol Cell Neurosci.* (1998) 11:1–8. doi: 10.1006/mcne.1998.0671
8. Lo DC. Instructive roles of neurotrophins in synaptic plasticity. *Prog Brain Res.* (1998) 117:65–70. doi: 10.1016/S0079-6123(08)64008-X
9. Cattaneo E, McKay R. Proliferation and differentiation of neuronal stem cells regulated by nerve growth factor. *Nature.* (1990) 347:762–5. doi: 10.1038/347762a0
10. Kotzbauer PT, Holtzman DM. Expectations and challenges in the therapeutic use of neurotrophic factors. *Ann Neurol.* (2006) 59:444–7. doi: 10.1002/ana.20794
11. Sendtner M, Schmalbruch H, Stöckli KA, Carroll P, Kreutzberg GW, Thoenen H. Ciliary neurotrophic factor prevents degeneration of motor neurons in mouse mutant progressive motor neuronopathy. *Nature.* (1992) 358:502–4. doi: 10.1038/358502a0
12. Mitsumoto H, Ikeda K, Holmlund T, Greene T, Cedarbaum JM, Wong V, et al. The effects of ciliary neurotrophic factor on motor dysfunction in wobbler mouse motor neuron disease. *Ann Neurol.* (1994) 36:142–8. doi: 10.1002/ana.410360205
13. Ikeda K, Wong V, Holmlund TH, Greene T, Cedarbaum JM, Lindsay RM, et al. Histometric effects of ciliary neurotrophic factor in wobbler mouse motor neuron disease. *Ann Neurol.* (1995) 37:47–54. doi: 10.1002/ana.410370110
14. Mitsumoto H, Ikeda K, Klinkosz B, Cedarbaum JM, Wong V, Lindsay RM. Arrest of motor neuron disease in wobbler mice cotreated with CNTF and BDNF. *Science.* (1994) 265:1107–1110. doi: 10.1126/science.8066451

15. Sagot Y, Tan SA, Hammang JP, Aebischer P, Kato AC. GDNF slows loss of motoneurons but not axonal degeneration or premature death of pmn/pmn mice. *J Neurosci.* (1996) 16:2335–41. doi: 10.1523/JNEUROSCI.16-07-02335.1996
16. Zheng C, Nennesmo I, Fadeel B, Henter J-I. Vascular endothelial growth factor prolongs survival in a transgenic mouse model of ALS. *Ann Neurol.* (2004) 56:564–7. doi: 10.1002/ana.20223
17. Storkebaum E, Lambrechts D, Dewerchin M, Moreno-Murciano M-P, Appelmans S, Oh H, et al. Treatment of motoneuron degeneration by intracerebroventricular delivery of VEGF in a rat model of ALS. *Nat Neurosci.* (2005) 8:85–92. doi: 10.1038/nn1360
18. Pitzer C, Krüger C, Plaas C, Kirsch F, Dittgen T, Müller R, et al. Granulocyte-colony stimulating factor improves outcome in a mouse model of amyotrophic lateral sclerosis. *Brain.* (2008) 131:3335–47. doi: 10.1093/brain/awn243
19. Rando A, Gasco S, de la Torre M, García-Redondo A, Zaragoza P, Toivonen JM, et al. Granulocyte colony-stimulating factor ameliorates skeletal muscle dysfunction in amyotrophic lateral sclerosis mice and improves proliferation of SOD1-G93A myoblasts *in vitro*. *Neurodegener Dis.* (2017) 17:1–13. doi: 10.1159/000446113
20. Kaspar BK, Lladó J, Sherkat N, Rothstein JD, Gage FH. Retrograde viral delivery of IGF-1 prolongs survival in a mouse ALS model. *Science.* (2003) 301:839–42. doi: 10.1126/science.1086137
21. Lepore AC, Haenggeli C, Gasmi M, Bishop KM, Bartus RT, Maragakis NJ, et al. Intraparenchymal spinal cord delivery of adeno-associated virus IGF-1 is protective in the SOD1G93A model of ALS. *Brain Res.* (2007) 1185:256–65. doi: 10.1016/j.brainres.2007.09.034
22. Dodge JC, Haidet AM, Yang W, Passini MA, Hester M, Clarke J, et al. Delivery of AAV-IGF-1 to the CNS extends survival in ALS mice through modification of aberrant glial cell activity. *Mol Ther.* (2008) 16:1056–64. doi: 10.1038/mt.2008.60
23. Lin H, Hu H, Duan W, Liu Y, Tan G, Li Z, et al. Intramuscular delivery of scAAV9-hIGF1 prolongs survival in the hSOD1G93A ALS mouse model via upregulation of D-amino acid oxidase. *Mol Neurobiol.* (2018) 55:682–95. doi: 10.1007/s12035-016-0335-z
24. Wang W, Wen D, Duan W, Yin J, Cui C, Wang Y, et al. Systemic administration of scAAV9-IGF1 extends survival in SOD1G93A ALS mice via inhibiting p38 MAPK and the JNK-mediated apoptosis pathway. *Brain Res Bull.* (2018) 139:203–10. doi: 10.1016/j.brainresbull.2018.02.015
25. Dodge JC, Treleaven CM, Fidler JA, Hester M, Haidet A, Handy C, et al. AAV4-mediated expression of IGF-1 and VEGF within cellular components of the ventricular system improves survival outcome in familial ALS mice. *Mol Ther.* (2010) 18:2075–84. doi: 10.1038/mt.2010.206
26. Wang Y, Duan W, Wang W, Di Wen, Liu Y, Liu Y, et al. scAAV9-VEGF prolongs the survival of transgenic ALS mice by promoting activation of M2 microglia and the PI3K/Akt pathway. *Brain Res.* (2016) 1648:1–10. doi: 10.1016/j.brainres.2016.06.043
27. Wang LJ, Lu YY, Muramatsu S, Ikeguchi K, Fujimoto K, Okada T, et al. Neuroprotective effects of glial cell line-derived neurotrophic factor mediated by an adeno-associated virus vector in a transgenic animal model of amyotrophic lateral sclerosis. *J Neurosci.* (2002) 22:6920–8. doi: 10.1523/JNEUROSCI.22-16-06920.2002
28. Thomsen GM, Alkaslasi M, Vit JP, Lawless G, Godoy M, Gowing G, et al. Systemic injection of AAV9-GDNF provides modest functional improvements in the SOD1G93A ALS rat but has adverse side effects. *Gene Ther.* (2017) 24:245–52. doi: 10.1038/gt.2017.9
29. Henriques A, Pitzer C, Dittgen T, Klugmann M, Dupuis L, Schneider A. CNS-targeted viral delivery of G-CSF in an animal model for ALS: improved efficacy and preservation of the neuromuscular unit. *Mol Ther.* (2011) 19:284–92. doi: 10.1038/mt.2010.271
30. Xu L, Yan J, Chen D, Welsh AM, Hazel T, Johe K, et al. Human neural stem cell grafts ameliorate motor neuron disease in SOD-1 transgenic rats. *Transplantation.* (2006) 82:865–75. doi: 10.1097/01.tp.0000235532.00920.7a
31. Xu L, Ryugo DK, Pongstaporn T, Johe K, Koliatsos VE. Human neural stem cell grafts in the spinal cord of SOD1 transgenic rats: differentiation and structural integration into the segmental motor circuitry. *J Comp Neurol.* (2009) 514:297–309. doi: 10.1002/cne.22022
32. Hwang DH, Lee HJ, Park IH, Seok JI, Kim BG, Joo IS, et al. Intrathecal transplantation of human neural stem cells overexpressing VEGF provide behavioral improvement, disease onset delay and survival extension in transgenic ALS mice. *Gene Ther.* (2009) 16:1234–44. doi: 10.1038/gt.2009.80
33. Knippenberg S, Rath KJ, Böselt S, Thau-Habermann N, Schwarz SC, Dengler R, et al. Intraspinal administration of human spinal cord-derived neural progenitor cells in the G93A-SOD1 mouse model of ALS delays symptom progression, prolongs survival and increases expression of endogenous neurotrophic factors. *J Tissue Eng Regen Med.* (2017) 11:751–64. doi: 10.1002/term.1972
34. Klein SM, Behrstock S, McHugh J, Hoffmann K, Wallace K, Suzuki M, et al. GDNF delivery using human neural progenitor cells in a rat model of ALS. *Hum Gene Ther.* (2005) 16:509–21. doi: 10.1089/hum.2005.16.509
35. Suzuki M, McHugh J, Tork C, Shelley B, Klein SM, Aebischer P, et al. GDNF secreting human neural progenitor cells protect dying motor neurons, but not their projection to muscle, in a rat model of familial ALS. *PLoS ONE.* (2007) 2:e689. doi: 10.1371/journal.pone.0000689
36. Thomsen GM, Avalos P, Ma AA, Alkaslasi M, Cho N, Wyss L, et al. Transplantation of neural progenitor cells expressing glial cell line-derived neurotrophic factor into the motor cortex as a strategy to treat amyotrophic lateral sclerosis. *Stem Cells.* (2018) 36:1122–31. doi: 10.1002/stem.2825
37. Vercelli A, Mereuta OM, Garbossa D, Muraca G, Mareschi K, Rustichelli D, et al. Human mesenchymal stem cell transplantation extends survival, improves motor performance and decreases neuroinflammation in mouse model of amyotrophic lateral sclerosis. *Neurobiol Dis.* (2008) 31:395–405. doi: 10.1016/j.nbd.2008.05.016
38. Boido M, Piras A, Valsecchi V, Spigolon G, Mareschi K, Ferrero I, et al. Human mesenchymal stromal cell transplantation modulates neuroinflammatory milieu in a mouse model of amyotrophic lateral sclerosis. *Cytotherapy.* (2014) 16:1059–72. doi: 10.1016/j.jcyt.2014.02.003
39. Uccelli A, Milanese M, Principato MC, Morando S, Bonifacino T, Vergani L, et al. Intravenous mesenchymal stem cells improve survival and motor function in experimental amyotrophic lateral sclerosis. *Mol Med.* (2012) 18:794–804. doi: 10.2119/molmed.2011.00498
40. Suzuki M, McHugh J, Tork C, Shelley B, Hayes A, Bellantuono I, et al. Direct muscle delivery of GDNF with human mesenchymal stem cells improves motor neuron survival and function in a rat model of familial ALS. *Mol Ther.* (2008) 16:2002–10. doi: 10.1038/mt.2008.197
41. Krakora D, Mulcrone P, Meyer M, Lewis C, Bernau K, Gowing G, et al. Synergistic effects of GDNF and VEGF on lifespan and disease progression in a familial ALS rat model. *Mol Ther.* (2013) 21:1602–10. doi: 10.1038/mt.2013.108
42. Pastor D, Viso-Leon MC, Jones J, Jaramillo-Merchan J, Toledo-Aral JJ, Moraleda JM, et al. Comparative effects between Bone Marrow and mesenchymal stem cell transplantation in GDNF expression and motor function recovery in a motorneuron degenerative mouse model. *Stem Cell Rev.* (2012) 8:445–58. doi: 10.1007/s12015-011-9295-x
43. Pastor D, Viso-Leon MC, Botella-Lopez A, Jaramillo-Merchan J, Moraleda JM, Jones J, et al. Bone marrow transplantation in hindlimb muscles of motorneuron degenerative mice reduces neuronal death and improves motor function. *Stem Cells Dev.* (2013) 22:1633–44. doi: 10.1089/scd.2012.0487
44. Marconi S, Bonaconsa M, Scambi I, Squintani GM, Rui W, Turano E, et al. Systemic treatment with adipose-derived mesenchymal stem cells ameliorates clinical and pathological features in the amyotrophic lateral sclerosis murine model. *Neuroscience.* (2013) 248:333–43. doi: 10.1016/j.neuroscience.2013.05.034
45. Kim KS, Lee HJ, An J, Kim YB, Ra JC, Lim I, et al. Transplantation of human adipose tissue-derived stem cells delays clinical onset and prolongs life span in ALS mouse model. *Cell Transplant.* (2014) 23:1585–97. doi: 10.3727/096368913X673450
46. Ende N, Weinstein F, Chen R, Ende M. Human umbilical cord blood effect on sod mice (amyotrophic lateral sclerosis). *Life Sci.* (2000) 67:53–9. doi: 10.1016/S0024-3205(00)00602-0
47. Chen R, Ende N. The potential for the use of mononuclear cells from human umbilical cord blood in the treatment of amyotrophic lateral sclerosis in SOD1 mice. *J Med.* (2000) 31:21–30.

48. Garbuzova-Davis S, Willing AE, Zigova T, Saporta S, Justen EB, Lane JC, et al. Intravenous administration of human umbilical cord blood cells in a mouse model of amyotrophic lateral sclerosis: distribution, migration, and differentiation. *J Hematother Stem Cell Res.* (2003) 12:255–70. doi: 10.1089/152581603322022990
49. Garbuzova-Davis S, Rodrigues MCO, Mirtyl S, Turner S, Mitha S, Sodhi J, et al. Multiple intravenous administrations of human umbilical cord blood cells benefit in a mouse model of ALS. *PLoS ONE.* (2012) 7:e31254. doi: 10.1371/journal.pone.0031254
50. Habisch HJ, Janowski M, Binder D, Kuzma-Kozakiewicz M, Widmann A, Habich A, et al. Intrathecal application of neuroectodermally converted stem cells into a mouse model of ALS: limited intraparenchymal migration and survival narrows therapeutic effects. *J Neural Transm.* (2007) 114:1395–406. doi: 10.1007/s00702-007-0748-y
51. Knippenberg S, Thau N, Schwabe K, Dengler R, Schambach A, Hass R, et al. Intraspinal injection of human umbilical cord blood-derived cells is neuroprotective in a transgenic mouse model of amyotrophic lateral sclerosis. *Neurodegener Dis.* (2012) 9:107–20. doi: 10.1159/000331327
52. Bigini P, Veglianese P, Andriolo G, Cova L, Grignaschi G, Caron I, et al. Intracerebroventricular administration of human umbilical cord blood cells delays disease progression in two murine models of motor neuron degeneration. *Rejuvenation Res.* (2011) 14:623–39. doi: 10.1089/rej.2011.1197
53. Islamov RR, Rizvanov AA, Mukhamedyarov MA, Salafutdinov II, Garanina EE, Fedotova VY, et al. Symptomatic improvement, increased life-span and sustained cell homing in amyotrophic lateral sclerosis after transplantation of human umbilical cord blood cells genetically modified with adeno-viral vectors expressing a neuro-protective factor and a neural cell adhesion molecule. *Curr Gene Ther.* (2015) 15:266–76. doi: 10.2174/1566523215666150126122317
54. Islamov RR, Rizvanov AA, Fedotova VY, Izmailov AA, Safiullov ZZ, Garanina EE, et al. Tandem delivery of multiple therapeutic genes using umbilical cord blood cells improves symptomatic outcomes in ALS. *Mol Neurobiol.* (2017) 54:4756–63. doi: 10.1007/s12035-016-0017-x
55. Calvo AC, Moreno-Igoa M, Mancuso R, Manzano R, Oliván S, Muñoz MJ, et al. Lack of a synergistic effect of a non-viral ALS gene therapy based on BDNF and a TTC fusion molecule. *Orphanet J Rare Dis.* (2011) 6:10. doi: 10.1186/1750-1172-6-10
56. Korkmaz OT, Aytan N, Carreras I, Choi J-K, Kowall NW, Jenkins BG, et al. 7,8-Dihydroxyflavone improves motor performance and enhances lower motor neuronal survival in a mouse model of amyotrophic lateral sclerosis. *Neurosci Lett.* (2014) 566:286–91. doi: 10.1016/j.neulet.2014.02.058
57. Turner BJ, Cheah IK, Macfarlane KJ, Lopes EC, Petratos S, Langford SJ, et al. Antisense peptide nucleic acid-mediated knockdown of the p75 neurotrophin receptor delays motor neuron disease in mutant SOD1 transgenic mice. *J Neurochem.* (2003) 87:752–63. doi: 10.1046/j.1471-4159.2003.02053.x
58. Yanpallewar SU, Barrick CA, Buckley H, Becker J, Tessarollo L. Deletion of the BDNF truncated receptor TrkB.T1 delays disease onset in a mouse model of amyotrophic lateral sclerosis. *PLoS ONE.* (2012) 7:e39946. doi: 10.1371/journal.pone.0039946
59. Brambilla L, Guidotti G, Martorana F, Iyer AM, Aronica E, Valori CF, et al. Disruption of the astrocytic TNFR1-GDNF axis accelerates motor neuron degeneration and disease progression in amyotrophic lateral sclerosis. *Hum Mol Genet.* (2016) 25:3080–95. doi: 10.1093/hmg/ddw161
60. Tovar-Y-Romo LB, Zepeda A, Tapia R. Vascular endothelial growth factor prevents paralysis and motoneuron death in a rat model of excitotoxic spinal cord neurodegeneration. *J Neuropathol Exp Neurol.* (2007) 66:913–22. doi: 10.1097/nen.0b013e3181567c16
61. Tovar-y-Romo LB, Tapia R. Delayed administration of VEGF rescues spinal motor neurons from death with a short effective time frame in excitotoxic experimental models *in vivo*. *ASN Neuro.* (2012) 4: e0008. doi: 10.1042/AN20110057
62. Czarzasta J, Habich A, Siwek T, Czaplinski A, Maksymowicz W, Wojtkiewicz J. Stem cells for ALS: an overview of possible therapeutic approaches. *Int J Dev Neurosci.* (2017) 57:46–55. doi: 10.1016/j.ijdevneu.2017.01.003
63. Mathieu P, Battista D, Depino A, Roca V, Graciarena M, Pitossi F. The more you have, the less you get: the functional role of inflammation on neuronal differentiation of endogenous and transplanted neural stem cells in the adult brain. *J Neurochem.* (2010) 112:1368–85. doi: 10.1111/j.1471-4159.2009.06548.x
64. Reekmans K, Praet J, Daans J, Reumers V, Pauwels P, Van der Linden A, et al. Current challenges for the advancement of neural stem cell biology and transplantation research. *Stem Cell Rev.* (2012) 8:262–78. doi: 10.1007/s12015-011-9266-2
65. Lewis CM, Suzuki M. Therapeutic applications of mesenchymal stem cells for amyotrophic lateral sclerosis. *Stem Cell Res Ther.* (2014) 5:32. doi: 10.1186/scrt421
66. Gugliandono A, Bramanti P, Mazzon E. Mesenchymal stem cells: a potential approach for Amyotrophic Lateral Sclerosis? *Stem Cells Int.* (2019) 2019:3675627. doi: 10.1155/2019/3675627
67. Beers DR, Appel SH. Immune dysregulation in amyotrophic lateral sclerosis: mechanisms and emerging therapies. *Lancet Neurol.* (2019) 18:211–20. doi: 10.1016/S1474-4422(18)30394-6
68. Rizvanov AA, Kiyasov AP, Gaziziov IM, Yilmaz TS, Kaligin MS, Andreeva DI, et al. Human umbilical cord blood cells transfected with VEGF and L(1)CAM do not differentiate into neurons but transform into vascular endothelial cells and secrete neuro-trophic factors to support neuro-genesis-a novel approach in stem cell therapy. *Neurochem Int.* (2008) 53:389–94. doi: 10.1016/j.neuint.2008.09.011
69. Rizvanov AA, Guseva DS, Salafutdinov II, Kudryashova NV, Bashirov FV, Kiyasov AP, et al. Genetically modified human umbilical cord blood cells expressing vascular endothelial growth factor and fibroblast growth factor 2 differentiate into glial cells after transplantation into amyotrophic lateral sclerosis transgenic mice. *Exp Biol Med.* (2011) 236:91–8. doi: 10.1258/ebm.2010.010172
70. A phase I study of recombinant human ciliary neurotrophic factor (rHCNTF) in patients with amyotrophic lateral sclerosis. The ALS CNTF Treatment Study (ACTS) Phase I-II Study Group. *Clin Neuropharmacol.* (1995) 18:515–32. doi: 10.1097/00002826-199512000-00004
71. Miller RG, Petajan JH, Bryan WW, Armon C, Barohn RJ, Goodpasture JC, et al. A placebo-controlled trial of recombinant human ciliary neurotrophic (rhCNTF) factor in amyotrophic lateral sclerosis. rhCNTF ALS Study Group. *Ann Neurol.* (1996) 39:256–60. doi: 10.1002/ana.410390215
72. A double-blind placebo-controlled clinical trial of subcutaneous recombinant human ciliary neurotrophic factor (rHCNTF) in amyotrophic lateral sclerosis. ALS CNTF Treatment Study Group. *Neurology.* (1996) 46:1244–9. doi: 10.1212/WNL.46.5.1244
73. Penn RD, Kroin JS, York MM, Cedarbaum JM. Intrathecal ciliary neurotrophic factor delivery for treatment of amyotrophic lateral sclerosis (phase I trial). *Neurosurgery.* (1997) 40:94–9; discussion: 99–100. doi: 10.1227/00006123-199701000-00021
74. Works in progress abstracts. *Ann Neurol.* (1995) 38:971–3. doi: 10.1002/ana.410380629
75. A controlled trial of recombinant methionyl human BDNF in ALS: The BDNF Study Group (Phase III). *Neurology.* (1999) 52:1427–33. doi: 10.1212/WNL.52.7.1427
76. Ochs G, Penn RD, York M, Giess R, Beck M, Tonn J, et al. A phase I/II trial of recombinant methionyl human brain derived neurotrophic factor administered by intrathecal infusion to patients with amyotrophic lateral sclerosis. *Amyotroph Lateral Scler Other Motor Neuron Disord.* (2000) 1:201–6. doi: 10.1080/14660820050515197
77. Kalra S, Genge A, Arnold DL. A prospective, randomized, placebo-controlled evaluation of corticoneuronal response to intrathecal BDNF therapy in ALS using magnetic resonance spectroscopy: feasibility and results. *Amyotroph Lateral Scler Other Motor Neuron Disord.* (2003) 4:22–6. doi: 10.1080/14660820310006689
78. Beck M, Flachenecker P, Magnus T, Giess R, Reiners K, Toyka KV, et al. Autonomic dysfunction in ALS: a preliminary study on the effects of intrathecal BDNF. *Amyotroph Lateral Scler Other Motor Neuron Disord.* (2005) 6:100–3. doi: 10.1080/14660820510028412
79. Lai EC, Felice KJ, Festoff BW, Gawel MJ, Gelinas DF, Kratz R, et al. Effect of recombinant human insulin-like growth factor-I on progression of ALS. A placebo-controlled study. The North America ALS/IGF-I Study Group. *Neurology.* (1997) 49:1621–30. doi: 10.1212/WNL.49.6.1621

80. Borasio GD, Robberecht W, Leigh PN, Emile J, Guiloff RJ, Jerusalem F, et al. A placebo-controlled trial of insulin-like growth factor-I in amyotrophic lateral sclerosis. European ALS/IGF-I Study Group. *Neurology.* (1998) 51:583–6. doi: 10.1212/WNL.51.2.583
81. Nagano I, Shiote M, Murakami T, Kamada H, Hamakawa Y, Matsubara E, et al. Beneficial effects of intrathecal IGF-1 administration in patients with amyotrophic lateral sclerosis. *Neurol Res.* (2005) 27:768–2. doi: 10.1179/016164105X39860
82. Sorenson EJ, Windbank AJ, Mandrekar JN, Bamlet WR, Appel SH, Armon C, et al. Subcutaneous IGF-1 is not beneficial in 2-year ALS trial. *Neurology.* (2008) 71:1770–5. doi: 10.1212/01.wnl.0000335970.78664.36
83. Zhang Y, Wang L, Fu Y, Song H, Zhao H, Deng M, et al. Preliminary investigation of effect of granulocyte colony stimulating factor on amyotrophic lateral sclerosis. *Amyotroph Lateral Scler.* (2009) 10:430–1. doi: 10.3109/17482960802588059
84. Nefussy B, Artamonov I, Deutsch V, Naparstek E, Nagler A, Drory VE. Recombinant human granulocyte-colony stimulating factor administration for treating amyotrophic lateral sclerosis: A pilot study. *Amyotroph Lateral Scler.* (2010) 11:187–93. doi: 10.3109/17482960902933809
85. Riley J, Federici T, Polak M, Kelly C, Glass J, Raore B, et al. Intraspinal stem cell transplantation in amyotrophic lateral sclerosis: a phase I safety trial, technical note, and lumbar safety outcomes. *Neurosurgery.* (2012) 71:405–16; discussion: 416. doi: 10.1227/NEU.0b013e31825ca05f
86. Glass JD, Boulis NM, Johe K, Rutkove SB, Federici T, Polak M, et al. Lumbar intraspinal injection of neural stem cells in patients with amyotrophic lateral sclerosis: results of a phase I trial in 12 patients. *Stem Cells.* (2012) 30:1144–51. doi: 10.1002/stem.1079
87. Mazzini L, Gelati M, Profico DC, Sgaravizzi G, Projetti Pensi M, Muzi G, et al. Human neural stem cell transplantation in ALS: initial results from a phase I trial. *J Transl Med.* (2015) 13:17. doi: 10.1186/s12967-014-0371-2
88. Karussis D, Karageorgiou C, Vaknin-Dembinsky A, Gowda-Kurkalli B, Gomori JM, Kassis I, et al. Safety and immunological effects of mesenchymal stem cell transplantation in patients with multiple sclerosis and amyotrophic lateral sclerosis. *Arch Neurol.* (2010) 10:1187–94. doi: 10.1001/archneurol.2010.248
89. Blanquer M, Moraleda JM, Iniesta F, Gómez-Espuch J, Meca-Lallana J, Villaverde R, et al. Neurotrophic bone marrow cellular nests prevent spinal motoneuron degeneration in amyotrophic lateral sclerosis patients: a pilot safety study. *Stem Cells.* (2012) 30:1277–85. doi: 10.1002/stem.1080
90. Ruiz-López FJ, Guardiola J, undIzura Verline, Gómez-Espuch J, uIniesta Fnderline, Blanquer Munderline, et al. Breathing pattern in a phase I clinical trial of intraspinal injection of autologous bone marrow mononuclear cells in patients with amyotrophic lateral sclerosis. *Respir Physiol Neurobiol.* (2016) 221:54–8. doi: 10.1016/j.resp.2015.11.007
91. García Santos JM, Blanquer Munderline, Torres del Río S, uIniesta Fnderline, uEspuch JGnderline, Pérez-Espejo MÁ, et al. Acute and chronic MRI changes in the spine and spinal cord after surgical stem cell grafting in patients with definite amyotrophic lateral sclerosis: post-infusion injuries are unrelated with clinical impairment. *Magn Reson Imaging.* (2013) 8:1298–308. doi: 10.1016/j.mri.2013.05.006
92. Oh KW, Noh MY, Kwon MS, Kim HY, Oh SI, Park J, et al. Repeated intrathecal mesenchymal stem cells for amyotrophic lateral sclerosis. *Ann Neurol.* (2018) 84:361–73. doi: 10.1002/ana.25302
93. Petrou P, Gothelf Y, Argov Z, Gotkine M, Levy YS, Kassis I, et al. Safety and clinical effects of mesenchymal stem cells secreting neurotrophic factor transplantation in patients with amyotrophic lateral sclerosis: results of phase 1/2 and 2a clinical trials. *JAMA Neurol.* (2016) 73:337–44. doi: 10.1001/jamaneurol.2015.4321
94. Nabavi SM, Arab L, Jarooghi N, Bolurieh T, Abbasi F, Mardpour S, et al. Safety, feasibility of intravenous and intrathecal injection of autologous Bone marrow derived mesenchymal stromal cells in patients with amyotrophic lateral sclerosis: an open label phase I clinical trial. *Cell J.* (2019) 20:592–8. doi: 10.22074/cellj.2019.5370
95. Nurden AT, Nurden P, Sanchez M, Andia I, Anitua E. Platelets and wound healing. *Front Biosci.* (2008) 13:3532–48. doi: 10.2741/2947
96. Burnouf T, Goubran HA, Chen TM, Ou KL, El-Ekiaby M, Radosevic M. Blood-derived biomaterials and platelet growth factors in regenerative medicine. *Blood Rev.* (2013) 27:77–89. doi: 10.1016/j.blre.2013.02.001
97. Nurden AT. The biology of the platelet with special reference to inflammation, wound healing and immunity. *Front Biosci.* (2018) 23:726–51. doi: 10.2741/4613
98. Hayon Y, Dashevsky O, Shai E, Varon D, Leker RR. Platelet lysates stimulate angiogenesis, neurogenesis and neuroprotection after stroke. *Thromb Haemost.* (2013) 110:323–30. doi: 10.1160/TH12-11-0875
99. Zhang Y, Ying G, Ren C, Jizhang Y, Brogan D, Liu Z, et al. Administration of human platelet-rich plasma reduces infarction volume and improves motor function in adult rats with focal ischemic stroke. *Brain Res.* (2015) 1594:267–73. doi: 10.1016/j.brainres.2014.10.035
100. Anitua E, Pascual C, Antequera D, Bolos M, Padilla S, Orive G, et al. Plasma rich in growth factors (PRGF-Endoret) reduces neuropathologic hallmarks and improves cognitive functions in an Alzheimer's disease mouse model. *Neurobiol Aging.* (2014) 35:1582–95. doi: 10.1016/j.neurobiolaging.2014.01.009
101. Anitua E, Pascual C, Perez-Gonzalez R, Orive G, Carro E. Intranasal PRGF-Endoret enhances neuronal survival and attenuates NF-kappaB-dependent inflammation process in a mouse model of Parkinson's disease. *J Control Release.* (2015) 203:170–80. doi: 10.1016/j.jconrel.2015.02.030
102. Chou ML, Wu JW, Gouel F, Jonneaux A, Timmerman K, Renn TY, et al. Tailor-made purified human platelet lysate concentrated in neurotrophins for treatment of Parkinson's disease. *Biomaterials.* (2017) 142:77–89. doi: 10.1016/j.biomaterials.2017.07.018
103. Gouel F, Do Van B, Chou ML, Jonneaux A, Moreau C, Bordet R, et al. The protective effect of human platelet lysate in models of neurodegenerative disease: involvement of the Akt and MEK pathways. *J Tissue Eng Regen Med.* (2017) 11:3236–40. doi: 10.1002/term.2222

4

Biomarker Supervised G-CSF (Filgrastim) Response in ALS Patients

*Siw Johannesen[1], Bettina Budeus[2], Sebastian Peters[1], Sabine Iberl[3], Anne-Louise Meyer[1], Tina Kammermaier[1], Eva Wirkert[1], Tim-Henrik Bruun[1], Verena C. Samara[4], Wilhelm Schulte-Mattler[1], Wolfgang Herr[3], Armin Schneider[2], Jochen Grassinger[3] and Ulrich Bogdahn[1]**

[1] Department of Neurology, University Hospital Regensburg, Regensburg, Germany, [2] Lifedatascience Consulting, Schriesheim, Germany, [3] Department of Hematology, Internal Medicine III, University Hospital Regensburg, Regensburg, Germany, [4] Stanford Neuroscience Health Center, Palo Alto, CA, United States

***Correspondence:**
Ulrich Bogdahn
uli.bogdahn@ukr.de

Objective: To evaluate safety, tolerability and feasibility of long-term treatment with Granulocyte-colony stimulating factor (G-CSF), a well-known hematopoietic stem cell factor, guided by assessment of mobilized bone marrow derived stem cells and cytokines in the serum of patients with amyotrophic lateral sclerosis (ALS) treated on a named patient basis.

Methods: 36 ALS patients were treated with subcutaneous injections of G-CSF on a named patient basis and in an outpatient setting. Drug was dosed by individual application schemes (mean 464 Mio IU/month, range 90-2160 Mio IU/month) over a median of 13.7 months (range from 2.7 to 73.8 months). Safety, tolerability, survival and change in ALSFRS-R were observed. Hematopoietic stem cells were monitored by flow cytometry analysis of circulating $CD34^{+}$ and $CD34^{+}CD38^{-}$ cells, and peripheral cytokines were assessed by electrochemoluminescence throughout the intervention period. Analysis of immunological and hematological markers was conducted.

Results: Long term and individually adapted treatment with G-CSF was well tolerated and safe. G-CSF led to a significant mobilization of hematopoietic stem cells into the peripheral blood. Higher mobilization capacity was associated with prolonged survival. Initial levels of serum cytokines, such as MDC, TNF-beta, IL-7, IL-16, and Tie-2 were significantly associated with survival. Continued application of G-CSF led to persistent alterations in serum cytokines and ongoing measurements revealed the multifaceted effects of G-CSF.

Conclusions: G-CSF treatment is feasible and safe for ALS patients. It may exert its beneficial effects through neuroprotective and -regenerative activities, mobilization of hematopoietic stem cells and regulation of pro- and anti-inflammatory cytokines as well as angiogenic factors. These cytokines may serve as prognostic markers when measured at the time of diagnosis. Hematopoietic stem cell numbers and cytokine levels are altered by ongoing G-CSF application and may potentially serve as treatment biomarkers for early monitoring of G-CSF treatment efficacy in ALS in future clinical trials.

Keywords: amyotrophic lateral sclerosis, granulocyte-colony stimulating factor, cytokines, hematopoietic stem and progenitor cells, HSPC, treatment

INTRODUCTION

Amyotrophic lateral sclerosis (ALS) is a life threatening neurodegenerative disorder characterized by premature loss of upper and lower motoneurons in the adult brain and spinal cord (1). The life time risk of ALS is below one in 400 individuals (2), the incidence is 2–3 per 100,000 in Europe (3). The unmet medical need in ALS patients is underlined by a median survival of 29.8 months from symptom onset, and of 15.8 months from diagnosis (4). Only modest treatment effects have been observed by riluzole (5) and edaravone (6).

In view of the great heterogeneity of disease etiology, neuronal damage likely results from many different pathologic changes, including neuroinflammation (3). Neurodegenerative processes with altered homeostasis, protein accumulation and cell death generates neuroinflammation, and central nervous system (CNS)-resident immune cells such as astrocytes and microglia trigger neuroinflammation and neurodegeneration (7). Inflammation may arise reactive to ALS-related CNS alterations, but also play an initial role and trigger both onset of disease and further accelerate progression of ALS (3). A complex, cytokine-mediated crosstalk between CNS and systemic immune cells regulates immune responses to either pro- or anti-inflammatory states, which evolve over time (7).

Granulocyte-colony stimulating factor (G-CSF) is a 20-kDa glycoprotein and a well characterized growth factor that plays a key role in production, mobilization, and differentiation of hematopoietic stem cells (8, 9). It is a widely used compound for treatment of neutropenia and for mobilization of $CD34^+$ hematopoietic stem cells prior to bone marrow transplantation. G-CSF enhances immunocompetence and has systemic anti-inflammatory effects (10). G-CSF is safe and well tolerated; most common side effects are moderate bone pain and musculoskeletal pain in 20–30% of patients, rarely splenomegaly and allergic reactions (11). Aside from hematopoietic functions, G-CSF acts as a neuronal growth factor in the CNS and possesses neuroprotective and -regenerative properties (12, 13). G-CSF passes the intact blood brain barrier, and its receptor is widely expressed within the CNS (12). G-CSF is thought to be neuroprotective through anti-apoptotic effects (12, 14), it induces neural differentiation, supports neurogenesis, contributes to re-endothelialization and arteriogenesis (12, 15). Systemic G-CSF induced hematopoietic stem cells may contribute on a direct cellular level in neurodegeneration by migration to the CNS (16, 17), where they may offer trophic support and modulate the local CNS immune system (17, 18). Observing G-CSF induced systemic hematopoietic stem cells may also shed light upon direct G-CSF effects on neural cells and stem cells as a surrogate system. Furthermore, G-CSF modulates monocyte function and attenuates the neuroinflammatory cascade (13). An interesting bone marrow-brain connection has been shown as G-CSF induced bone marrow derived cells migrate to CNS and express microglial phenotype in a mouse model of cranial irradiation. This was associated with a better functional outcome and suggested to facilitate neuroprotection by direct effects on resident CNS cells as well as modulation of cellular microenvironment in neurovascular niches (15). Angiogenic factors may promote neurogenesis through direct effects on neuronal cells (19) and indirectly by angiogenic support of the highly vascularized neurogenic zones. G-CSF improved motor function and survival in mouse models of ALS (20–22). Small trials with G-CSF treatment in ALS patients demonstrated excellent tolerability and safety (23–25), with modulation of immune parameters (26), and possible minor benefits detected by neuroimaging (27). In summary, G-CSF exerts multiple physiological effects within the CNS and may be a potent modulator of different functions relevant to ALS pathophysiology (13). Importantly, from *in vitro*, mouse model and human exploratory evidence the mode of action most relevant for potential treatment effects cannot with certainty be concluded.

Due to the paucity of available treatment options we provided individual, off-label G-CSF treatment to ALS patients. G-CSF, considering its multimodal systemic and CNS effects, may be a promising treatment option in view of the etiopathological and clinical heterogeneity of ALS. Biomarkers are measurable indicators of disease and/or intervention and may be useful in monitoring long-term degenerative or reparative processes within the CNS. In view of the above-discussed complexity of ALS, it seems unlikely that a single biomarker can sufficiently reflect treatment effects on disease progression. We therefore used a panel of pro- and anti-inflammatory blood parameters, angiogenic factors, as well as hematopoietic stem cell markers. Monitoring pro-differentiation and -mobilization effects on hematopoietic stem cells may serve as a proxy for G-CSF activity on neural stem cells in individual patients and/or reflect direct and indirect beneficial effects of mobilized hematopoietic stem cells. Observing a panel of peripheral cytokines may reveal system wide immune and inflammatory status relevant for peripheral-CNS crosstalk.

G-CSF is known to be a safe stem-cell mobilizing agent. We investigated whether the number of mobilized hematopoietic stem cells is different in G-CSF treated ALS patients of longer versus shorter survival. Secondly, we were interested in whether baseline cytokine levels are associated with survival of G-CSF treated ALS patients. Lastly, we sought to explore hematopoietic stem cells and cytokine level alterations during G-CSF treatment.

METHODS

Patients, Procedures and Ethics

Treatment with G-CSF was offered to 36 patients seen at the University of Regensburg with definite or probable ALS according to the revised El Escorial criteria (28). As this was not a prospective clinical trial, the use of formal exclusion criteria was not considered appropriate. However, neither patients with a current or past history of neurologic disease other than ALS, nor patients participating in any interventional study were offered this treatment option. Individual treatment of ALS patients and retrospective evaluation was done after written informed consent. The ethics committee of the University of Regensburg approved a retrospective analysis (ethics approval: 15-101-0106 and 14-101-0011). The principles of the Declaration of Helsinki (World Medical Association, revised version 2013) were strictly adhered to. Survival was defined as the time between diagnosis and death from confirmed ALS-related complications, including suicide.

ALS patients were treated with subcutaneous injections of recombinant human G-CSF (Filgrastim) on an outpatient basis. Dose and application modes were adapted individually upon initiation and over time (**Figure 1**; **Table S1**). Adaption was made with the intent to maximize patient wellbeing and safety in the presence of any emerging safety signals, and with the aim of increasing efficacy as monitored by levels of mobilized hematopoietic stem cells, a potential individual marker of biological activity of G-CSF. This resulted in heterogeneous treatment schemes. The intervention and evaluation was initiated in January 2010 and is still ongoing. The data were analyzed up to March 2017. The treatment was provided by the hospital and not funded by a pharmacological company or other external source. No external or internal funding sources were involved in patient selection, study design, data analysis or interpretation.

Patient safety was analyzed at baseline (initiation of treatment) followed by monthly control visits with clinical examinations, blood counts, cytokines, blood smears and estimation of bone marrow function. We conducted baseline spleen sonography with follow-ups upon dose escalation. Clinical ALS progression was monitored using the established ALSFRS-R (29). If patients were not able to continue visits and treatment, patient survival was monitored by phone calls to patients, their families and general practitioners.

Changes in pro- and anti-inflammatory immune profiles were evaluated at baseline, at 3 months, and then every 6 months throughout treatment by multiplex electrochemoluminescence with the panel assay V-PLEX Human Biomarker 40-Plex Kit (MesoScale Discovery®, Maryland, USA). This industry standard panel has been validated in different immune related and non-immune diseases (manufacture's information). In patients receiving G-CSF on five consecutive days, evaluations of cytokine levels in the peripheral blood were conducted twice a month, before (day 0) and after G-CSF application (day 7).

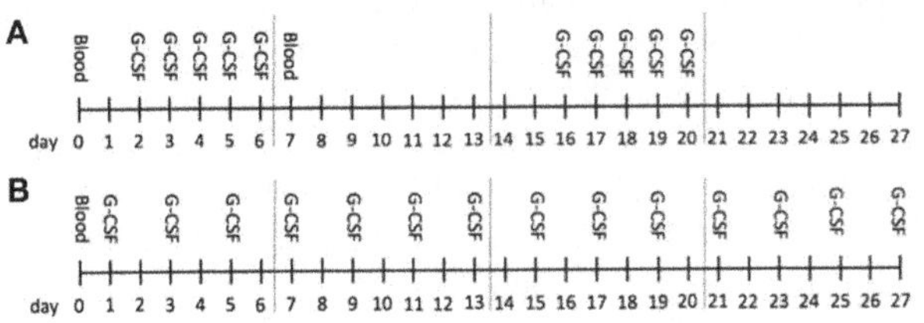

FIGURE 1 | Treatment course. The monthly protocol is illustrated; this schedule was repeated and individually adapted over the long-term treatment. G-CSF was administered subcutaneously. Mainly, patients received G-CSF either as a 5-day bolus **(A)** once (1st week) or twice (1st and 3rd week) or continuously **(B)** on single days up to every second day; G-CSF was administered in one or two doses á day. Blood was obtained before treatment onset at baseline (d0) and then once á month (d0) in patients receiving G-CSF continuously, and before (d0) as well as after a 5-day treatment (d7) in patients on bolus application. Cytokines were analyzed at d0 in both groups and at d7 in bolus treatment in the first month (baseline), then at the 3rd and 6th month during ongoing treatment.

In patients receiving G-CSF twice a week or every second day, analyses were conducted on a monthly basis 1 day after application. Peripheral blood serum was collected during regular visits at the hospital and immediately stored at −20°C for cytokine assays. For each assay, 25 μl of serum samples were used and test carried out in duplicates, according to the manufacturer's instructions.

We analyzed white blood cells including cell differentiation, platelet and red blood cell counts, and hemoglobin levels with an automatic cell counter (Sysmex®, Kobe, Japan). Peripheral blood smears were done on a 3-month basis by light microscopy. Peripheral blood $CD34^+$ and $CD34^+CD38^-$ hematopoietic stem and progenitor cells (HSPC) were analyzed by flow cytometry as earlier described by our group (25). In short, 1 ml donor blood was lysed in 9 ml NH_4Cl lysis buffer and cells were then stained for 30 min at 4°C with combinations of anti-CD45-FITC (clone HI30, BD Pharmingen, Franklin Lakes, NJ, USA), CD34-APC (clone 581, Biolegend, San Diego, CA, USA) and CD38-PE (clone HIT2, BioLegend) monoclonal antibodies. Analysis was performed on a Becton Dickinson CALIBUR flow cytometer (BD, East Rutherford, NJ, US).

Calculations and Statistics

Findings of immune parameters from three time points, baseline (initiation of treatment), 3 months and 6 months were selected for analysis. As patients did not always visit the outpatient clinic on the exact days of the given time points, the time points had to be defined as time periods. When assessing the ALSFRS-R at baseline, data from day of treatment initiation ±28 days were included. For baseline measures of blood counts, stem cell mobilization parameters and cytokines, only data obtained before the first G-CSF application were selected. The 3-month time point was defined as day 45–134 and the 6-month time point as ranging from day 135 to 224. If patients visited more than once during these time periods, the day closest to the intended time point was selected.

The immediate effects of G-CSF treatment on peripheral levels of cytokines, hematopoietic stem cells and blood counts were assessed by comparing respective levels 2 days before and 1 day after a 5-day treatment course with G-CSF. We then explored different patterns of immune responses depending on individual survival. Survival time was defined as time elapsed from day of diagnosis to day of death or day of last observation in the case of censoring. For this purpose, G-CSF treated patients were divided into two groups based on their survival being longer or shorter than 30 months from diagnosis, as this was a time point that separated the patients into two equal-sized groups. At the point of database closure, patients who were still alive were censored and included in the "long survival" group if they had been observed for over 30 months ($n = 7$). Patients who were alive and had not yet been observed for over 30 months were not considered for this analysis ($n = 3$). The same censoring was applied for correlation analysis. We then retrospectively analyzed baseline levels of cytokines, hematopoietic stem cells and blood counts in the long and short survivor groups and further correlated survival with cytokines upon treatment initiation.

R or GraphPad Prism 7 was employed for statistical analysis and graph design. Correlations were analyzed using two-tailed Pearson correlation and presented with correlation coefficient (r), coefficient of determination (R^2) and p-value. Comparisons were made with Mann-Whitney test and paired Wilcoxon test. Data were considered significant at $p \leq 0.05$. A trend was noted at $p \leq 0.1$. Comparisons were corrected for multiple testing by false discovery rate approach (FDR, two-stage step-up method of Benjamin, Krieger and Yekutieli with desired FDR (Q) at 10%) and considered a discovery at FDR-adjusted p-value (q) < 0.1. We used an Area Under the Curve (AUC) approach to estimate mobilization of hematopoietic stem cells after G-CSF treatment over time. Stem cell measurements before and after G-CSF dosing were available for patients on the 5-day treatment scheme. For better comparability regarding long and short survival times after diagnosis, we selected patients with ongoing 5-day treatment over the first 4 months. All patient measurements were used in the calculation. If patients had fewer data points, their mean AUC value calculated from all data points was applied (in the case of one patient). The AUC value was calculated with the *auc* function of the R-package "flux" (Jurasinski, Koebsch, Guenther and Beetz, 2014). The baseline value at day 0 or from any day prior to treatment start was used as threshold for the calculation.

RESULTS

Demographics, Intervention and Safety

36 caucasian ALS patients (25 male, 11 female, 28 limb onset, 8 bulbar onset, mean age 51.9 years, mean ALSFRS-R on initiation 38/48) were treated with G-CSF in addition to riluzole treatment. We here report on individual treatment on a named patient basis—consequently, treatment schemes were heterogeneous. Dose and application modes were adapted individually upon initiation and over time (**Table S1**). In summary, G-CSF was injected subcutaneously in a dose-range from 90 to 2160 Mio IU per month (900–21,600 μg/month), with a mean dose of 464 Mio IU/month (4,640 μg/month). Application modes ranged from once weekly to every second day in an ongoing individually tailored manner. The median duration of treatment was 13.7 months (mean 16.7 months; range from 2.7 to 73.8 months) (**Table 1**, **Figure 1**).

Long-term outpatient treatment with G-CSF was generally well tolerated in ALS patients and compliance was excellent. Minor adverse events were mild to moderate bone pain after G-CSF injection and leukocytosis. One patient experienced an episode with heat sensation, lightheadedness, and 15 min. of dyspnea on 1 day of drug application 39 months into G-CSF treatment. Due to the possibility of drug-related intolerance or mild allergic reaction, G-CSF was discontinued in this patient; antibodies against G-CSF were not detectable. This patient was switched from Filgrastim to Pegfilgrastim, a PEGylated form of recombinant human G-CSF, from his 46th to 53rd month after initiation, and then ended the off-label treatment without further adverse reactions. As expected, mild to moderate splenomegaly evolved during ongoing G-CSF treatment in most patients. Without any further symptoms or complications, the mean spleen width increased from 4.3 to 4.9 cm and length from 10.7 to 12.1 cm during treatment. There were no severe adverse events (SAE), and no signs for pre-malignant transformation in peripheral blood smears.

Baseline hematology showed no abnormalities in our patients. G-CSF mobilizes neutrophil leukocytes as well as $CD34^+$ and $CD34^+CD38^-$ hematopoietic stem and progenitor cells (HSPC) from the bone marrow into the peripheral blood. Leukocyte counts increased significantly in all treated patients, from an initial mean of $6.9 \times 10^3/\mu l$ to $48.2 \times 10^3/\mu l$ (range 8.3–118.7 $\times 10^3/\mu l$, $p < 0.0001$) after G-CSF application. A predicted increase in the average percentage of neutrophils (from 64.8 to 87.3%, $p < 0.0001$) was accompanied by a relative decrease in lymphocytes (from 24.1 to 7.0%, $p < 0.0001$), monocytes (from 8.8 to 4.7%, $p < 0.0001$) and eosinophils (from 1.8 to 0.7%, $p < 0.0001$) as well as a small decrease in red blood cell count (from 5.03 to $4.83 \times 10^3/\mu l$, $p < 0.0001$), hemoglobin level (from 14.9 to 14.4 g/dl, $p < 0.0001$) and hematocrit (from 44.2 to 43.6, $p = 0.0362$) during monitoring (all comparisons by paired t-test, two-tailed p-value. **Figure S1**). There were no significant changes in basophiles and platelet count during monitoring. The fold increase of $CD34^+$ and $CD34^+CD38^-$ HSP cells in peripheral blood served as an indicator of mobilization efficiency and was determined by comparing cells at baseline to cells after mobilization. The mobilization efficacy was heterogeneous with high intra- and inter-personal variability (data not shown).

G-CSF-Mediated Stem Cell Mobilization Was Associated With Survival of ALS Patients

Twenty-six of thirty-six G-CSF treated patients deceased between January 2010 and March 2017. 10 patients were alive, of which 6 were still treated with G-CSF. The patient who had suffered from a possible allergic reaction was regularly seen at the clinic. Three patients ended G-CSF treatment at days 82, 420 and 427, and were all lost to follow up. The overall median survival of *deceased* patients was 24.2 months from diagnosis (mean 25.5; range 3.9–56.6 months). For further analysis, patients were divided into two equally sized groups by survival being longer or shorter than 30 months from diagnosis. Patients, who were alive at the time of database closure, were considered for this analysis had they been observed for at least 30 months. The mean (median) survival differed in the two survival groups: 46.59 (39.55) months, SD 16.34 and 17.04 (18.30) months, SD 8.16 (two-tailed p-value $<$ 0.0001; Mann-Whitney t-test). The ALSFRS-R slope over time was significantly flatter in longer surviving patients (Wilcoxon test, $p = 0.00086$; **Figure 2**). Long survivors were younger (mean age 46.8 vs. 56.5 y, unpaired t-test, $p = 0.0163$) and had a longer latency between diagnosis and treatment onset (mean 333 vs. 163 days, unpaired t-test, $p = 0.0377$). Their clinical function upon treatment initiation was not significantly different (mean ALSFRS-R 38.6/48 vs. 37.3/48). Further, longer surviving patients were less frequently female (18.8 vs. 47.1%), but had similar occurrence of bulbar onset of disease (18.8 vs. 17.6%) (**Table 1**).

G-CSF is known to mobilize HSPC into the peripheral circulation. $CD34^+$ and $CD34^+CD38^-$ HSPC were evaluated in the sera of patients 2 days before (day 0) and 1 day after

TABLE 1 | Demographics and intervention in G-CSF treated ALS patients.

ALS patient	Age (years)	Gender	ALSFRS-R baseline	Site of onset	Time diagnosis to treatment (days)	Dose G-CSF (mean; range (MioIE/month))	Treatment duration (months)	Survival (months) from diagnosis
1	50	F	38	Limb	498	150 (150–150)	19	36.2
2	42	M	32	Limb	619	280 (150–300)	31	52.2
3	77	M	21	Limb	759	173 (150–240)	5	33.4
4	68	F	39	Bulbar	29	150 (150–150)	3	3.9
5	67	M	33	Limb	439	260 (150–300)	20	56.6
6	26	M	33	Limb	486	485 (150–1170)	74	89.7*
7	50	F	33	Limb	536	240 (240–240)	7	25.4
8	73	M	41	Limb	270	166 (150–240)	11	21.4
9	50	M	28	Limb	393	133 (90–150)	7	21.4
10	56	M	37	Limb	770	242 (150–300)	14	40.0
11	41	M	38	Limb	24	287 (150–300)	27	36.3
12	35	F	40	Bulbar	115	296 (240–300)	14	63.7*
13	48	F	46	Limb	38	216 (150–300)	14	29.7
14	43	M	44	Limb	61	561 (192–768)	45	47.3
15	65	F	32	Limb	81	192 (192–192)	14	18.3
16	51	F	42	Limb	101	225 (150–300)	3	6.4
17	60	F	38	Limb	21	192 (192–192)	9	11.5
18	58	M	44	Limb	45	311 (240–480)	25	25.4
19	46	M	46	Limb	249	150 (150–150)	26	34.7
20	50	M	-	Limb	1	198 (192–240)	8	8.0
21	27	M	44	Limb	53	301 (150–600)	39	71.3*
22	45	M	48	Limb	26	666 (240–1296)	37	39.1*
23	55	M	40	Bulbar	26	263 (150–300)	3	41.9*
24	61	M	44	Limb	66	375 (150–510)	5	9.2
25	60	M	40	Bulbar	135	602 (240–816)	19	23.0
26	65	F	30	Bulbar	122	563 (240–900)	7	11.3
27	43	F	41	Limb	338	628 (240–720)	14	35.7*
28	60	M	42	Limb	23	589 (480–720)	11	12.1
29	45	F	28	Limb	493	535 (150–720)	6	29.6
30	47	M	29	Limb	396	585 (450–720)	5	19.3
31	50	M	40	Limb	23	667 (240–720)	8	13.7
32	39	M	41	Bulbar	343	1015 (450–1170)	20	31.7*
33	56	M	42	Bulbar	525	744 (450–1056)	11	35.6
34	59	M	38	Bulbar	52	1044 (450–1440)	14	#
35	69	M	39	Limb	62	1344 (450–2160)	16	#
36	35	M	38	Limb	288	1141 (300–1440)	14	#
Mean (SD)	51.9 (12.2)	11 F 25 M	38/48 (6.1)	28 Limb 8 Bulbar	236.3 (231.4)	222.7 (104.1)	16.7 (14.4)	25.5 (14.3) in *deceased* patients

*Patients marked by # or * were alive upon closure of data admission. Patients who had been observed for less than 30 months at time of closure of data admission are marked by #. The sign * indicates patients, who at time of closure of data admission, had been observed more than 30 months from diagnosis. Baseline ALSFRS-R was not available in one patient, marked by -.*

(day 7) a 5-day treatment course with G-CSF at baseline, 3 months and 6 months. G-CSF led to a sustained increase of $CD34^+$ and $CD34^+CD38^-$ HSPC at all time points (**Figure 3**). In patients treated with ongoing 5-day courses of G-CSF *t*-tests displayed no significant reductions in mobilization of $CD34^+$ and $CD34^+CD38^-$ HSPC when comparing the respective levels after G-CSF treatment at baseline and after 3 and 6 months of treatment (mean number of $CD34^+$/ml at baseline 30307,

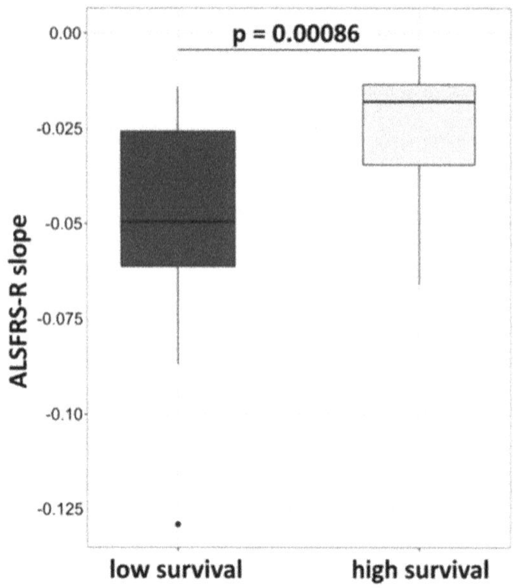

FIGURE 2 | ALSFRS-R decline is less rapid in patients who survive longer than 30 months. Patients were assigned to high survival group at survival longer or at 30 months, and to low survival group at survival below 30 months from diagnosis. The slope was calculated by robust calculation of the ALSFRS-R measurements. Median slope in the high survival group was −0.019 and −0.05 in the low survival group. Wilcoxon test, *p*-value 0.00086.

at 3 months 35250, at 6 months 22017; mean number of $CD34^+CD38^-$/ml at baseline 3092, at 3 months 2089, at 6 months 1632, all Wilcoxon paired *t*-test, all *p*-values not significant; **Figure S2**). However, we found a different capacity to mobilize hematopoietic stem cells in patients surviving longer or shorter than 30 months from diagnosis. This was analyzed by Area Under the Curve (AUC) approach to mobilized $CD34^+CD38^-$ cells within the first year of G-CSF treatment in 19 available patients, who all received ongoing 5-day treatment. Longer surviving patients displayed a significantly superior mobilization of $CD34^+CD38^-$ cells under G-CSF application at 1 year of treatment. At 4 months this difference was borderline significant (trend) (**Figure 4**).

Short and Long-Term Survivors Differed in Their Baseline Cytokine Levels

Survival in months from diagnosis was negatively correlated with baseline serum levels of the cytokine TNF-beta. MCP-1 and INF-gamma were, as a trend, negatively correlated with survival as well. IL-16 baseline levels displayed a positive correlation with survival. MDC, IL-8, IL-17A, and PIGF were, as a trend, positively correlated with survival (**Table 2**, **Figure 5**). We then dichotomized G-CSF treated patients according to their survival of either more or less than 30 months from diagnosis, and analyzed cytokines at baseline. Patients who survived longer than 30 months from diagnosis had significantly higher baseline levels of MDC and Tie-2. For IL-16, IL-17A, and PIGF we found similar trends. On the other hand, there were significantly higher baseline levels of TNF-beta and IL-7 in patients who survived less than 30 months from diagnosis. TNF-alpha and MCP-1 displayed similar trends. However, when correcting the cytokine comparisons in long and short survival for multiple testing, none of these findings remained significant [as assessed by the FDR-adjusted *p*-values (*q*-values) in **Table 2**].

G-CSF Treatment Modulated Serum Cytokine Levels of ALS Patients Over Time

The direct effects of G-CSF on cytokine levels were evaluated by comparing cytokine levels 2 days prior to and 1 day after ongoing 5-day G-CSF application in a subgroup of patients allowing this analysis. These immediate effects were determined at three different time points (baseline, 3 and 6 months after treatment initiation). Due to individual application modes, 5-day G-CSF applications with corresponding blood samples were available for 18 patients at baseline, for 17 patients at 3 months, and for 14 patients at 6 months of ongoing G-CSF treatment.

We found G-CSF to have an immediate effect on the level of various cytokines (**Table 3**, **Figure S3**). The serum level of IL-10 increased after 5 days of G-CSF treatment at baseline, 3 months and 6 months compared to its respective level before G-CSF application, however, at 3 months only as a trend. The levels of IL-16, Tie-2, TNF-alpha, MIP1-beta, IL-15, IP-10, VCAM, ICAM-1, and of Flt-1 were significantly increased after G-CSF treatment at all above-mentioned time points. The levels of TARC, IL-7, INF-gamma, and MCP-1 were decreased at all above-mentioned time points. There was an increase in SAA, IL-12/IL-23p40, CRP, and VEGF-A levels after G-CSF at baseline and 6 months, the latter at 6 months only as a trend. The levels of VEGF-C and PIGF were increased after G-CSF at 6 months, that of PIGF also at 3 months as a trend. There was a decrease of Eotaxin-1, Eotaxin-3 and VEGF-D after G-CSF application at baseline and 3 months. TNF-beta was decreased at baseline, at 6 months by a trend. MCP-4 was decreased at 6 months, at baseline by a trend. The level of bFGF was decreased after G-CSF application at 3 months and 6 months.

DISCUSSION

Our Main Findings

Long term and individually adapted off-label treatment with G-CSF in 36 ALS patients was well tolerated and safe. The number of G-CSF-mobilized hematopoietic stem cells, as measured by AUC, was associated with longer survival. Initial levels of serum cytokines, such as MDC, TNF-beta, IL-7, IL-16, and Tie-2 were significantly associated with survival, indicating the potential of prognostic application of these immune markers in G-CSF treated ALS patients. Continued application of G-CSF led to persistent alterations in various serum cytokines and ongoing measurements revealed the multifaceted effects of G-CSF.

ALS as a Neuroinflammatory Disease

ALS has been recognized as a multifactorial disease. Neurodegenerative processes trigger neuroinflammation

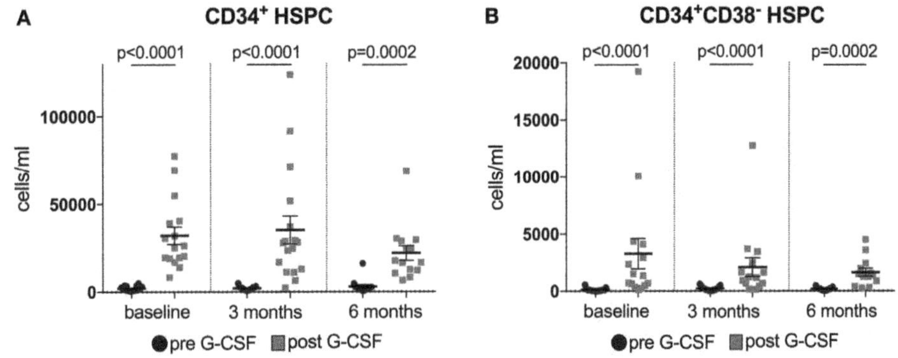

FIGURE 3 | (A,B) Mobilization of hematopoietic stem cells (HSPC) in G-CSF treated ALS patients. Plotted are $CD34^+$ (**Figure 2A**) and $CD34^+CD38^-$ HSPC (**Figure 2B**) in blood 2 days before (d0) and 1 day after (d7) daily application of G-CSF over 5 days in 16 (for $CD34^+$)/15 (for $CD34^+CD38^-$) patients at baseline, in 17 patients after 3 months, and in 14 (for $CD34^+$)/13 (for $CD34^+CD38^-$) patients after 6 months of treatment. Data are presented as scatter dot plot with mean + SEM. Paired Wilcoxon *t*-test, significance was taken at $p < 0.05$ (two-tailed). *T*-tests were corrected for multiple testing by FDR-adjusted *p*-values (*q*-values), discovery is indicated by $q < 0.1$. In $CD34^+$ and $CD34^+CD38^-$ HSPC at all time points: *q*-value = 0.0002.

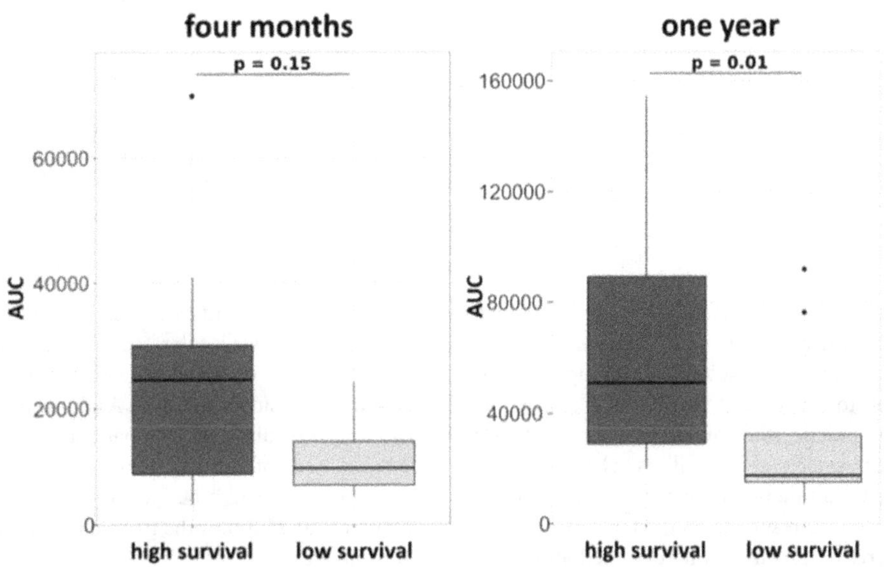

FIGURE 4 | Mobilization of $CD34^+CD38^-$ HSPC is associated with survival in ALS patients on a 5-day treatment scheme with G-CSF. Area under the curve (AUC) approach on blood HSPC over 4 months **(A)** and 1 year **(B)** in patients treated with 5-day application of G-CSF ($n = 20$). Patients were assigned survival groups dependent on survival being longer (high survival $n = 8$) or shorter (low survival) than 30 months from diagnosis.

and vice versa. Neuroinflammation with microglial activation, infiltration of peripheral immune cells into the CNS, and alterations in cytokine levels are pathological features in ALS. Cytokines are mediators of the immune communication that may cross the blood-brain barrier (BBB) and provide a mechanism by which the peripheral immune system may directly influence the CNS (30). In a recent study, we demonstrated a pro-inflammatory immune response with elevated inflammatory cytokines both in serum during disease and post-mortem in the CNS of ALS patients (31). However, immune response in ALS cannot be clearly dichotomized to a purely pro- or anti-inflammatory state, as cytokines are often pleiotropic, and their function may change over time and depend on concentration and specific disease context. Possibly, cytokine response in early ALS may be an attempt to restore homeostatic balance, whereas chronic exposure to pro-inflammatory cytokines might lead to cell destruction and loss of neuronal function. The latter supports a self-sustaining inflammatory process and possibly accelerates disease progression (7). Neuroinflammation and systemic inflammatory stimuli with their influence upon the CNS offer targets for therapeutic intervention in ALS (32). Analysis of peripheral blood is a feasible alternative for ongoing measurements of immune mediated and pathophysiological relevant parameters (33).

TABLE 2 | Cytokine levels at baseline in relation to survival.

Cytokine	Level in long survival	Correlation			Comparison (*t*-test)			
		r-value	R^2-value	*p*-value	Median long survival	Median short survival	*p*-value	*q*-value
ANTI-INFLAMMATORY								
MDC	↑	0.3269	0.1069	0.0726	939	227	**0.0494**	0.3088
PRO-INFLAMMATORY								
TNF-ß	↓	−0.4981	0.2481	**0.0043**	0.535	0.830	**0.0038**	0.1254
IL-7	↓	–	–	–	17	27	**0.0171**	0.2640
TNF-α	↓	–	–	–	2.5	3.0	0.0638	0.3088
MCP-1	↓	−0.3414	0.1166	0.0601	278	957	0.0544	0.3088
INF-γ	↓	−0.3264	0.1065	0.0731	–	–	–	–
IL-16	↑	0.4449	0.1979	**0.0122**	262	133	0.0655	0.3088
IL-8	↑	0.3492	0.1219	0.0542	–	–	–	–
IL-17A	↑	0.3749	0.1406	0.0710	2.58	0.68	0.0912	0.3421
ANGIOGENESIS								
Tie-2	↑	–	–	–	5762	4492	**0.0240**	0.2640
PIGF	↑	0.3277	0.1074	0.0719	33.8	31.7	0.0933	0.3421

Cytokine levels in pg/ml before first G-CSF application in ALS patients. Arrows indicate cytokine levels in patients with long compared to short survival. Then cytokine levels at baseline were correlated with survival. Next, Mann-Whitney test was calculated to assess differences in baseline cytokine levels in patients with survival longer or shorter than 30 months from diagnosis. Number of patients at baseline: 31 (16 long survival). Significance is indicated by bold marking when $p < 0.05$ (two-tailed p-value), trend when $p < 0.1$. T-tests were corrected for multiple testing by FDR-adjusted p-values (q-values), discovery is indicated by $q < 0.1$.

G-CSF in ALS

ALS is a multifactorial disease. Targeting common pathologic features such as neuro-inflammation and -degeneration may thus be beneficial for all ALS patients. Although G-CSF is an established, well-tolerated and safe growth factor for mobilization of hematopoietic stem and precursor cells (34), there is accumulating evidence that it is also a potent modulator of multiple CNS functions relevant to ALS (13). G-CSF modulates the immune response (35), it promotes anti-inflammatory and decreases pro-inflammatory mediators (36). Small clinical trials with G-CSF in ALS patients have delivered inconclusive results. Treatment with G-CSF was associated with a decrease in pro-inflammatory cytokine levels in serum and cerebrospinal fluid (CSF) of ALS patients (26), and minor benefits were detected by neuroimaging (27). But promising evidence for efficacy of G-CSF in ALS animal models has not yet been translated to ALS patients. It seems likely that a successful clinical translation requires higher dose, more frequent application and longer exposure to G-CSF as well as extended observation times (37). The latter is of crucial importance when aiming at structural and functional improvements or support of neurogenesis.

G-CSF Treatment in ALS Is Safe and Well Tolerated

Application of G-CSF in oncological indications is usually limited to treatment cycles, and the only clinical experience with life-long G-CSF therapy has accumulated with patients suffering from severe congenital neutropenia and cyclic neutropenia (38, 39). To our knowledge, we first reported on long-term G-CSF treatment in a CNS indication (25). We found G-CSF application to be generally well tolerated in ALS patients, with mild to moderate bone pain and leukocytosis after G-CSF applications as frequent minor adverse events. As this was off-label, experimental treatment of individual ALS patients, we had no control group for assessment of survival. If we only observe *deceased* patients and leave those still alive out, then the mean survival of these 26 patients at 25.5 months from diagnosis indicates no harm by G-CSF in ALS.

Stem Cell Mobilization Is Efficient and Associated With Longer Survival in G-CSF Treated ALS Patients

G-CSF is a well-known mobilizer of hematopoietic stem cells (8, 9). In all patients treated with G-CSF for five consecutive days, G-CSF increased mobilization of hematopoietic stem cells ($CD34^+$ and $CD34^+$ $CD38^-$) into the peripheral blood. Interestingly, we found an association between stem cell mobilization and survival. Patients who survived longer than 30 months from diagnosis mobilized more $CD34^+CD38^-$ hematopoietic stem cells than patients with shorter survival, as measured by Area Under the Curve after G-CSF treatment up to 1 year (**Figure 4**). Higher levels of circulating hematopoietic stem cells are associated with better clinical outcome and less structural damage after intracerebral hemorrhage in humans (40). The mechanism of how hematopoietic stem cells may contribute to neurodegenerative disease is yet unclear. Migration and

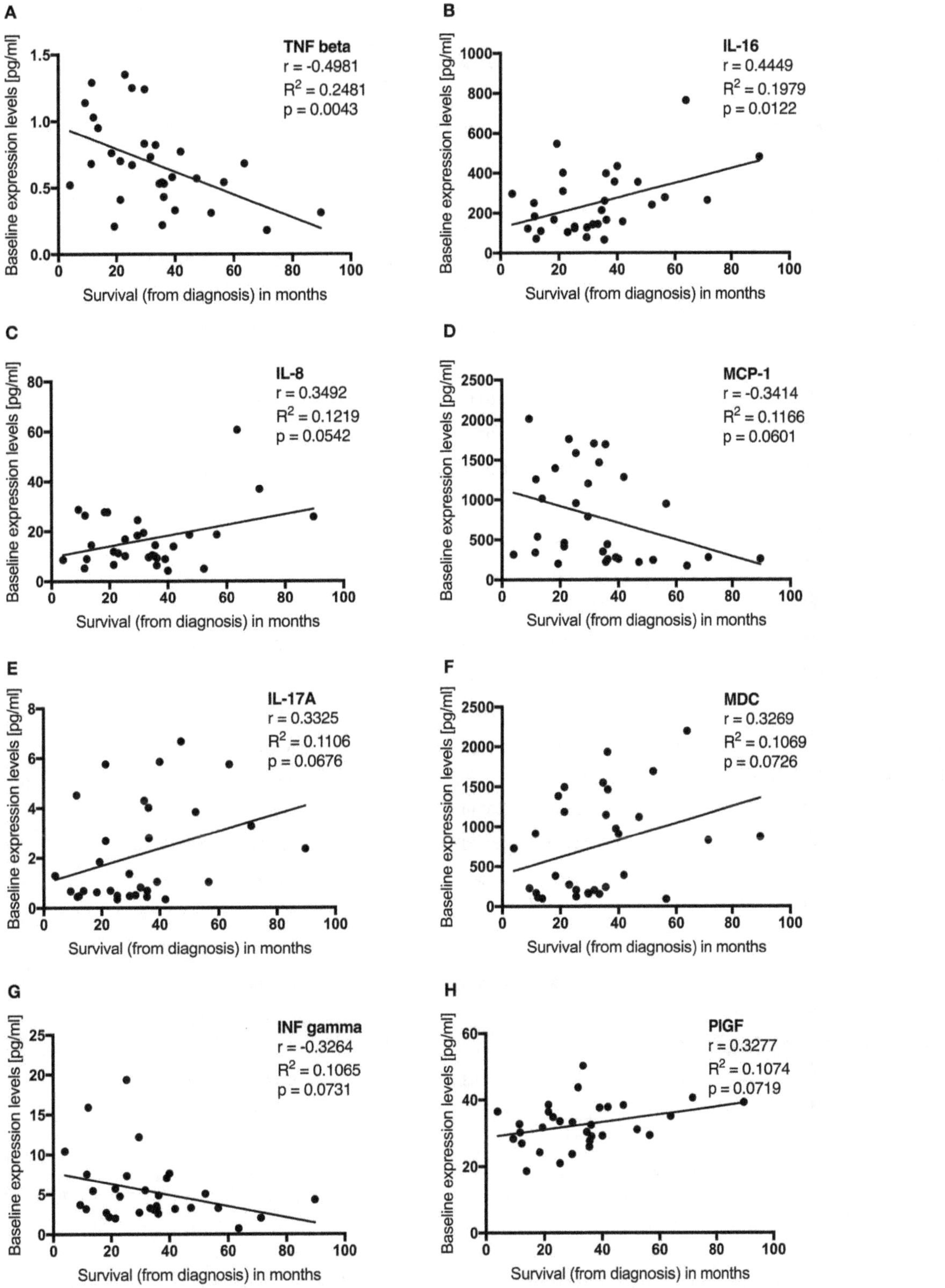

FIGURE 5 | (A–D) Baseline cytokine levels are associated with survival in G-CSF treated ALS patients. Plotted are initial cytokine levels of TNF beta **(A)**, IL-16 **(B)**, IL-8 **(C)**, MCP-1 **(D)**, IL-17A **(E)**, MDC **(F)**, ING gamma **(G)**, and PIGF **(H)** in pg/ml before first G-CSF application in 31 patients. Survival was assessed in months from diagnosis and censored upon data admission in living patients ($n = 7$). Displayed is Pearson r, the coefficient of determination (R^2), p-value (two-tailed) significant at $p < 0.05$, trend at $p < 0.1$.

TABLE 3 | Cytokine levels before and after G-CSF treatment at different time points.

Cytokine	Direction	Treatment start			3 months			6 months		
		Fold change d0-d7	*p*-value	*q*-value	Fold change d0-d7	*p*-value	*q*-value	Fold change d0-d7	*p*-value	*q*-value
ANTI-INFLAMMATORY										
IL-10	↑	1.95	**0.0016**	**0.0018**	1.24	0.0856	0.0371	2.02	**0.0004**	**0.0007**
PRO-INFLAMMATORY										
TNF-ß	↓	0.83	**0.0208**	**0.0112**	–	–	–	0.85	0.0591	0.0268
INF-γ	↓	0.81	**0.0214**	**0.0113**	0.78	**0.0182**	**0.0104**	0.62	**0.0009**	**0.0014**
IL-7	↓	0.66	**0.0003**	**0.0006**	0.80	**0.0011**	**0.0014**	0.80	**0.0107**	**0.0075**
MCP-1	↓	0.83	**0.0120**	**0.0080**	0.77	**0.0007**	**0.0012**	0.79	**0.0107**	**0.0075**
MCP-4	↓	0.94	0.0599	0.0268	0.92	**0.0150**	**0.0089**	–	–	–
TARC	↓	0.87	**0.0304**	**0.0148**	0.86	**0.0032**	**0.0030**	0.80	**0.0166**	**0.0097**
Eotaxin-1	↓	0.88	**0.0139**	**0.0085**	0.93	**0.0079**	**0.0059**	–	–	–
Eotaxin-3	↓	0.83	**0.0034**	**0.0030**	0.78	**0.0034**	**0.0030**	–	–	–
CRP	↑	4.45	**0.0010**	**0.0014**	–	–	–	3.99	**0.0085**	**0.0062**
SAA	↑	2.96	**0.0008**	**0.0013**	–	–	–	2.03	**0.0353**	**0.0168**
TNF-α	↑	1.77	**<0.0001**	**0.0003**	1.50	**0.0046**	**0.0038**	1.79	**0.0004**	**0.0007**
IP-10	↑	1.50	**0.0002**	**0.0004**	1.34	**0.0067**	**0.0052**	1.40	**0.0134**	**0.0085**
IL-15	↑	1.14	**0.0022**	**0.0022**	1.24	**0.0208**	**0.0112**	1.24	**0.0016**	**0.0018**
IL-12/IL-23p40	↑	1.24	**0.0047**	**0.0038**	–	–	–	1.19	**0.0052**	**0.0041**
IL-16	↑	3.14	**<0.0001**	**0.0003**	3.66	**0.0011**	**0.0014**	3.78	**0.0002**	**0.0004**
MIP1-ß	↑	3.38	**<0.0001**	**0.0003**	4.63	**0.0013**	**0.0015**	2.91	**0.0001**	**0.0003**
ANGIOGENESIS										
VEGF-A	↑	1.39	**0.0010**	**0.0014**	–	–	–	1.32	0.0580	0.0268
Tie-2	↑	1.27	**<0.0001**	**0.0003**	1.18	**0.0032**	**0.0030**	1.19	**0.0134**	**0.0085**
Flt-1	↑	1.45	**<0.0001**	**0.0003**	1.32	**0.0026**	**0.0026**	1.33	**0.0001**	**0.0003**
PIGF	↓	–	–	–	–	–	–	1.14	**0.0203**	**0.0112**
VEGF-C	↓	–	–	–		0.0984	0.0420	0.86	**0.0017**	**0.0017**
VEGF-D	↓	0.88	**0.0139**	**0.0085**	0.94	**0.0110**	**0.0075**	–	–	–
bFGF	↓	–	–	–	0.72	**0.0232**	**0.0121**	0.81	**0.0040**	**0.0035**
VASCULAR INJURY										
VCAM	↑	1.40	**<0.0001**	**0.0003**	1.28	**0.0267**	**0.0134**	1.41	**0.0001**	**0.0003**
ICAM-1	↑	1.30	**<0.0001**	**0.0003**	1.23	**0.0305**	**0.0148**	1.31	**0.0001**	**0.0003**

Paired Wilcoxon t-test. Arrows indicate direction, and fold change gives effect size of cytokine modulation when comparing respective levels 2 days before (d0) and 1 day after (d7) daily application of G-CSF over 5 days. Number of evaluable patients at baseline: 18, at 3 months: 17, and at 6 months: 14. Significance is indicated by bold marking when $p < 0.05$ (two-tailed p-value), trend when $p < 0.1$. T-tests were corrected for multiple testing by FDR-adjusted p-values (q-values), discovery is indicated by $q < 0.1$. Non-significant and non-trend findings are marked by -.

subsequent trans-differentiation of bone marrow derived cells within the CNS is controversially discussed (18). However, G-CSF increases the number of hematopoietic stem cells translocated to the damaged CNS (16, 17). There, hematopoietic stem cells modulate the immune system, they may interact with local cells, and produce neurotrophic factors, which promote growth of neural progenitors and survival (17, 18). A recent study in mice exposed to cranial irradiation demonstrated that G-CSF augments neurogenesis; bone marrow derived G-CSF-responsive cells migrate to the CNS, where they express macrophage and microglia phenotypes. The authors found that G-CSF treatment led to an improved functional outcome, thus arguing for the neuroprotective mechanisms of G-CSF on brain repair (15). Human studies have demonstrated G-CSF to directly affect monocytes and to modulate monocyte cytokine secretion toward an anti-inflammatory polarization (41). A recent study applying G-CSF in healthy humans described expansion of a mature variant monocyte subtype displaying strong immunosuppressive properties (42). Next to neural cells, also neural stem cells have G-CSF receptors and G-CSF treatment induces a neural phenotype of these cells (12). Effects of G-CSF on hematopoietic stem cells may therefore serve as a proxy for biological cellular activity of G-CSF on neural cells.

Cytokine Levels Are Associated to Survival and Affected by G-CSF

Neuroinflammation contributes to the pathogenesis of ALS (3). Apart from CNS inflammation, peripheral cytokines and other inflammatory markers are affected in ALS, and cytokine levels may serve as biomarkers (43). We found that different cytokines at baseline were correlated with survival (**Table 2**, **Figure 5**). When dichotomizing patients depending on individual survival being longer or shorter than 30 months from diagnosis, we detected different peripheral cytokine levels at baseline (**Table 2**). In general, five-day treatment courses with G-CSF exerted immediate effects on cytokine levels and were able to partly counteract the harmful immune response in ALS (**Table 3**, **Figure S3**).

The initial levels of 11 cytokines were associated with survival, of which 8 were altered by G-CSF application. However, the correlation models, as indicated by the rather low R^2-values, could only explain smaller parts of the variance. Even though the cytokine comparisons in long and short survival did not withstand correction for multiple testing, we decided to explore the findings because they might help to generate hypotheses for further studies and show biologically important findings in spite of the small number of patients tested. Moreover, G-CSF led to change in many inflammatory cytokines, as well as cytokines involved in angiogenesis and vascular injury, of which all significant changes remained so after testing for multiple comparison (**Tables 2, 3**).

Initial TNF-beta (LTA, lymphotoxin-alpha) levels negatively correlated with survival and were found at higher levels in shorter surviving ALS patients upon treatment initiation. G-CSF application led to reduction in TNF-beta, a pro-inflammatory cytokine and common cell death effector found to be increased in ALS sera (31). TNF-alpha was borderline increased in patients with shorter survival (trend) and G-CSF led to an increase in its serum levels. TNF-alpha is elevated in ALS (31, 43–46) and correlates with disease duration (47). But its role in ALS in unclear and the two TNF-alpha receptors, either associated with inflammation or neuroprotection, have opposing effects concerning survival in ALS (48). Dependent on subtype and context, activation can lead to neuroprotection and neurogenesis (49), reduced oxidative stress (50) and glutamate excitotoxicity (51). An increased occurrence of ALS after long-term use of TNF-alpha inhibitors in rheumatic arthritis, is suggested to be a consequence of deficient TNF-alpha mediated neuronal protection (52). Higher initial levels of IL-7 were associated with shorter survival, and reduced after ongoing treatment with G-CSF. IL-7 is considered a pro-inflammatory cytokine, and is increased in CSF (53) and serum (31) of ALS patients. MCP-1 (CCL2) was borderline correlated (trend) with shorter survival of ALS patients. We confirmed a reduction of MCP-1 levels in ALS after treatment with G-CSF (26). MCP-1 is a prominent pro-inflammatory cytokine that can enhance microglial recruitment to the CNS after injury, which may exacerbate ALS progression (54). MCP-1 correlates with faster disease progression (55) and ALS patients have elevated MCP-1 serum levels (31, 55, 56) and increased protein expression within spinal cord (31). INF-gamma was borderline negatively correlated with survival in our patients (trend). As known from healthy donors (57), INF-gamma levels were decreased by G-CSF. As a hallmark of proinflammatory cells, INF-gamma is proposed to contribute to motor neuron death in ALS (58). ALS patients have higher INF-gamma serum levels (47, 55, 59), that correlate with disease progression (47, 59) and shorter survival (55).

On the other hand, the pro-inflammatory marker IL-16 was positively correlated with survival and increased after G-CSF application. IL-16 also holds an immunomodulatory role by expansion of regulatory T cells (Treg) (60), that at lower levels in ALS, are associated with rapid disease progression and shorter survival (61). Thus, G-CSF related increase in IL-16 might be beneficial for ALS patients. Another pro-inflammatory cytokine, IL-17A, was borderline correlated with longer survival (trend) but not altered by G-CSF treatment. IL-17A has been reported elevated in serum (55, 62, 63) and CSF (64) of ALS patients. After G-CSF treatment, Chió et al. found a reduction of IL-17A in the CSF, but not in serum of ALS patients (26). IL-8 was borderline correlated with longer survival (trend), and not altered by G-CSF treatment. IL-8 is produced by several cells in response to inflammation, and higher plasma (44) and CSF levels (65) are known in ALS. MDC (CCL22) was associated with longer survival, however, not modulated by G-CSF treatment. MDC is an anti-inflammatory cytokine, and consistent with a proposed protective effect, ALS patients have lower MDC protein expression in the spinal cord (31). Further, angiogenic factors, such as Tie-2 and PIGF were associated with survival. Tie-2 was elevated in longer surviving patients and G-CSF led to an increase in it's serum levels. Angiogenesis is mediated by the angiopoietin-1/Tie-2 system (66), and stimulation of angiogenesis by another pro-angiogenic factor, VEGF, is found to increase neurogenesis (19). G-CSF treatment led to an increase in PIGF, and PIGF was as a trend both correlated with survival and elevated in longer surviving patients. PIGF supports angiogenesis (67), and may be a marker for the angiogenic niche.

The following 18 cytokines were significantly altered by G-CSF, however, not associated with survival. As known from healthy donors (68), IL-10 was markedly increased after G-CSF treatment. This anti-inflammatory cytokine is elevated in ALS-patients with mild symptoms or slow progression (53). G-CSF application led to reduced systemic levels of the pro-inflammatory cytokines MCP-4 (CCL13), TARC, Eotaxin-1 (CCL11), and Eotaxin-3 (CCL26). MCP-4 (31, 65), TARC (31) and Eotaxin-1 (65) are elevated in ALS serum. The latter is further associated with Alzheimer's dementia (69), aging and inhibition of neurogenesis in mice (70). We also noticed increase in levels of the pro-inflammatory cytokines CRP, SAA, IP-10 (CXCL10), IL-15, IL-12/IL-23p40, and MIP1-beta after G-CSF application. The acute-phase proteins CRP and SAA have been described as elevated in ALS patients (31, 71). IP-10 is negatively correlated with disease progression rate (72) and increase after G-CSF treatment has been described (26). IL-15 (31, 55, 73) and MIP1-beta (31) are elevated in serum of ALS patients. MIP1-beta shares receptor (CCR5) with MIP-alpha, which is elevated and considered neuroprotective in ALS (74). MIP-1 beta is negatively correlated with disease severity and progression rate, and thus might exert neuroprotective effects in ALS (72). IL-12/IL-23p40 describes the p40 subunit shared by the cytokines IL-12 and IL-23, and is considered a pro-inflammatory marker. However, we noted no increase in cytokines induced by IL-12/IL-23p40, such as INF-gamma and IL-17A, after G-CSF treatment. Aside from neuroinflammation, impaired neurotrophic support is a hallmark of ALS. Levels of VEGF-A and Flt-1 were increased, whereas VEGF-C, VEGF-D, and bFGF levels were decreased after G-CSF application. VEGF-A and bFGF, two common neurotrophic and possibly protective factors in ALS (55), are both increased in ALS CSF (64). Further, VEGF-A supports neurogenesis and neural development and is an attractant for HSPC that has been associated with longer survival in ALS (55). We found an increase in ICAM-1 and VCAM-1 after G-CSF treatment. At the vascular endothelium these cellular adhesion molecules are involved in leukocyte transport (75), but their role in ALS is unclear.

In ALS, a short time delay for diagnosis is associated with inferior prognosis as these patients are likely to have a more aggressive disease (76). Accordingly, we observed a briefer latency between diagnosis and treatment initiation in patients with shorter survival, which might reflect a more rapid progression of disease in these patients. Hence, longer surviving patients presumably initiated treatment at a later pathophysiological stage of their disease. This might offer an explanation for the fact that levels of some pro-inflammatory cytokines such as IL-16, IL-17A, and IL-8 were associated with longer survival. However, the role of inflammatory markers in ALS is unclear and our findings may also indicate that inflammation does not only negatively impact the disease (71). The remaining relation between cytokines and survival seen in our cohort highlights the importance of these markers in predicting individual survival. Thus, different cytokines may be used as biomarkers for initial patient stratification, predicting later clinical course, monitoring treatment response and progression of disease.

Possible direct effects of G-CSF upon the CNS were not assessed, as we did not obtain post-mortem analysis of deceased patients. Neuroimaging studies conducted on our G-CSF treated patient cohort (77) did not directly address possible G-CSF related structural effects—we also had no patient control group without G-CSF treatment. One indirect mode of action by which G-CSF exerts neuroprotective effects may be through polarization of the immune system toward an anti-inflammatory state (13). We observed an increase in anti-inflammatory cytokines and neurotrophic factors as well as a decrease in pro-inflammatory cytokines. However, we also captured an increase in some pro-inflammatory cytokines, which might be due to the pleiotropic effects of G-CSF and possibly reflect an unspecific cytokine reaction after application. Overall, the effects of G-CSF on peripheral cytokine levels and ALS appear to be versatile and should be assessed in a prospective clinical study.

Strengths and Limitations

This retrospective analysis has several limitations. Firstly, we have not conducted a controlled clinical trial and thus, there was no placebo-arm. Rather, the aim of the intervention was to offer individual ALS patients a potentially beneficial off-label treatment with G-CSF. Evaluation of respiratory function was driven by clinical indication and not systematically assessed. Hence, we did not regularly screen for respiratory deficits upon treatment initiation. The same applied to assessment of cognitive function. In addition, we did not systematically analyze for ALS-specific gene mutations. Such factors have predictive value concerning prognosis (78), the lack of initial screening of respiratory and cognitive function as well as genetic background might impede interpretation of the data. Given the objective of evaluating safety of G-CSF and the absence of a control group, in this paper we assessed survival from time of diagnosis, and not from treatment initiation. The latency between symptom onset and diagnosis was not assessed in this report. This is a limitation, as quantification of diagnostic delay - being associated with longer survival (78), could have offered prognostic implications. During the experimental treatment, patients were routinely seen on an outpatient basis to monitor safety and blood samples were regularly obtained. This enabled a dynamic observation of alterations in neuroinflammation due to ALS disease and treatment with G-CSF over time. However, with only 36 G-CSF treated patients caution should be applied in trying to generalize our findings. Moreover, application and dosing schemes for G-CSF treatment were decided upon on an individual patient level and thus complicated the establishment of dose-effect relationships. When we analyze cytokine levels upon treatment initiation in our patient cohort retrospectively, we have to take into account that these patients differ concerning covariant factors such as age, gender, bulbar vs. spinal-onset, and functional status (ALSFRS-R). Given the small number of patients treated with G-CSF, a statistical evaluation of the predictive value of these subpopulations was not reasonable. There was also great heterogeneity in the latency between time of diagnosis and treatment initiation. Cytokine levels alter during progression of disease. Altogether, these aspects lead to a reduced statistical power, which may also provide an explanation for the variation and modest correlation seen between initial cytokine levels and survival. Moreover, we found that cytokine comparisons in long and short surviving patients did not withstand correction for multiple testing. These signals may be of biological relevance, as they were detected in spite of a small number of patients and great disease heterogeneity, and thus may assist in hypothesis generation for future studies.

CONCLUSION

Altogether, we found that long term G-CSF treatment is feasible and safe for ALS patients. G-CSF efficiently mobilized hematopoietic stem cell into peripheral blood, and the amount of mobilized stem cells was associated with longer survival. Thus, stem cell mobilization could be a potential biomarker to monitor treatment response to G-CSF. Peripheral cytokines are relevant in the course of disease in ALS. We identified TNF-beta, MDC, IL-16, IL-7, and Tie-2 as cytokines whose baseline levels may predict G-CSF treatment response and survival. Additionally, long term G-CSF treatment led to sustained alterations of multiple cytokines in peripheral blood. Thus, cytokines represent potential biomarkers for survival prediction and for early monitoring of G-CSF treatment in ALS, all of which need further validation in a prospective controlled randomized trial.

AUTHOR CONTRIBUTIONS

SJ care for ALS patients, conception of intervention, analysis, interpretation, wrote the manuscript. UB clinical responsibility for intervention. UB, WS-M, and VS care for ALS patients, conception of intervention and analysis, revision of the manuscript. T-HB conception of intervention and analysis, revision of the manuscript. BB contribution to analysis, revision of the manuscript. A-LM care for ALS patients, revision of the manuscript. TK organization of care and disposition of patient material. SP and EW performed cytokine experiments, revision of the manuscript. SI and JG performed and analyzed HSPC experiments, revision of the manuscript. AS and WH revision of the manuscript.

FUNDING

Biomarker analysis was funded by BMBF grant GO-Bio CampoNeuro, and BayMWiT grant CrossTalk.

ACKNOWLEDGMENTS

The authors are grateful to all participating patients and their families. The authors are thankful to Andrei Khomenko (MD), Dobri Baldaranov (MD), Jenni Rösl (MD) and Ohnmar Hsam (MD) for sustained treatment of patients, and to Ines Kobor (MS) for assistance in maintenance of the database.

REFERENCES

1. Hardiman O, van den Berg LH, Kiernan MC. Clinical diagnosis and management of amyotrophic lateral sclerosis. *Nature Rev Neurol.* (2011) 7:639–49. doi: 10.1038/nrneurol.2011.153
2. Alonso A, Logroscino G, Jick SS, Hernán MA. Incidence and lifetime risk of motor neuron disease in the United Kingdom: a population-based study. *Eur J Neurol.* (2009) 16:745–51. doi: 10.1111/j.1468-1331.2009.02586.x
3. Hardiman O, Al-Chalabi A, Chiò A, Corr EM, Logroscino G, Robberecht W, et al. Amyotrophic lateral sclerosis. *Nat Rev Dis Primers.* (2017) 3:17071–19. doi: 10.1038/nrdp.2017.71
4. Traxinger K, Kelly C, Johnson BA, Lyles RH, Glass JD. Prognosis and epidemiology of amyotrophic lateral sclerosis: Analysis of a clinic population, 1997-2011. *Neurology* (2013) 3:313–20. doi: 10.1212/CPJ.0b013e3182a1b8ab
5. Lacomblez L, Bensimon G, Leigh PN, Guillet P, Meininger V. Dose-ranging study of riluzole in amyotrophic lateral sclerosis. Amyotrophic Lateral Sclerosis/Riluzole Study Group II. *Lancet* (1996) 347:1425–31. doi: 10.1016/S0140-6736(96)91680-3
6. Abe K, Aoki M, Tsuji S, Itoyama Y, Sobue G, Togo M, et al. Safety and efficacy of edaravone in well defined patients with amyotrophic lateral sclerosis: a randomised, double-blind, placebo-controlled trial. *Lancet Neurol.* (2017) 16:505–12. doi: 10.1016/S1474-4422(17)30115-1
7. Becher B, Spath S, Goverman J. Cytokine networks in neuroinflammation. *Nature Publishing Group* (2017) 17:49–59. doi: 10.1038/nri.2016.123
8. Demetri GD, Griffin JD. Granulocyte colony-stimulating factor and its receptor. *Blood.* (1991) 78:2791–808.
9. Welte K, Platzer E, Lu L, Gabrilove JL, Levi E, Mertelsmann R, et al. Purification and biochemical characterization of human pluripotent hematopoietic colony-stimulating factor. *Proc Natl Acad Sci USA.* (1985) 82:1526–30. doi: 10.1073/pnas.82.5.1526
10. Hartung T. Anti-inflammatory effects of granulocyte colony-stimulating factor. *Curr Opin Hematol.* (1998) 5:221–5. doi: 10.1097/00062752-199805000-00013
11. Root RK, Dale DC. Granulocyte colony-stimulating factor and granulocyte-macrophage colony-stimulating factor: comparisons and potential for use in the treatment of infections in nonneutropenic patients. *J Infect Dis.* (1999) 179 (Suppl 2):S342–52. doi: 10.1086/513857
12. Schneider A, Krüger C, Steigleder T, Weber D, Pitzer C, Laage R, et al. The hematopoietic factor G-CSF is a neuronal ligand that counteracts programmed cell death and drives neurogenesis. *J Clin Invest.* (2005) 115:2083–98. doi: 10.1172/JCI23559
13. Wallner S, Peters S, Pitzer C, Resch H, Bogdahn U, Schneider A. The Granulocyte-colony stimulating factor has a dual role in neuronal and vascular plasticity. *Front Cell Dev Biol.* (2015) 3:1–13. doi: 10.3389/fcell.2015.00048
14. Henriques A, Pitzer C, Dupuis L, Schneider A. G-CSF protects motoneurons against axotomy-induced apoptotic death in neonatal mice. *BMC Neurosci.* (2010) 11:25. doi: 10.1186/1471-2202-11-25
15. Dietrich J, Baryawno N, Nayyar N, Valtis YK, Yang B, Ly I, et al. Bone marrow drives central nervous system regeneration after radiation injury. *J Clin Invest.* (2018) 128:281–93. doi: 10.1172/JCI90647
16. Koda M, Nishio Y, Kamada T, Someya Y, Okawa A, Mori C, et al. Granulocyte colony-stimulating factor (G-CSF) mobilizes bone marrow-derived cells into injured spinal cord and promotes functional recovery after compression-induced spinal cord injury in mice. *Brain Research.* (2007) 1149:223–31. doi: 10.1016/j.brainres.2007.02.058
17. Xiao B-G, Lu C-Z, Link H. Cell biology and clinical promise of G-CSF: immunomodulation and neuroprotection. *J Cell Mol Med.* (2007) 11:1272–90. doi: 10.1111/j.1582-4934.2007.00101.x
18. Schneider A, Kuhn H-G, Schäbitz W-R. A role for G-CSF (granulocyte-colony stimulating factor) in the central nervous system. *Cell Cycle.* (2005) 4:1753–7. doi: 10.4161/cc.4.12.2213
19. Schanzer A, Wachs FP, Wilhelm D, Acker T, Cooper-Kuhn C, Beck H, et al. Direct stimulation of adult neural stem cells in vitro and neurogenesis in vivo by vascular endothelial growth factor. *Brain Pathol.* (2004) 14:237–48. doi: 10.1111/j.1750-3639.2004.tb00060.x
20. Henriques A, Pitzer C, Dittgen T, Klugmann M, Dupuis L, Schneider A. CNS-targeted viral delivery of G-CSF in an animal model for ALS: improved efficacy and preservation of the neuromuscular unit. *Mol Ther.* (2011) 19:284–92. doi: 10.1038/mt.2010.271

21. Schneider A, Pitzer C, Henriques A, Kruger C, Plaas C, Kirsch F, et al. Granulocyte-colony stimulating factor improves outcome in a mouse model of amyotrophic lateral sclerosis. *Brain* (2008) 131:3335–47. doi: 10.1093/brain/awn243
22. Pollari E, Savchenko E, Jaronen M, Kanninen K, Malm T, Wojciechowski S, et al. Granulocyte colony stimulating factor attenuatesinflammation in a mouse model of amyotrophiclateral sclerosis. *J Neuroinflam.* (2011) 8:74. doi: 10.1186/1742-2094-8-74
23. Zhang Y, Wang L, Fu Y, Song H, Zhao H, Deng M, et al. Preliminary investigation of effect of granulocyte colony stimulating factor on amyotrophic lateral sclerosis. *Amyotroph Lateral Scler.* (2009) 10:430–1. doi: 10.3109/17482960802588059
24. Nefussy B, Artamonov I, Deutsch V, Naparstek E, Nagler A, Drory VE. Recombinant human granulocyte-colony stimulating factor administration for treating amyotrophic lateral sclerosis: a pilot study. *Amyotroph Lateral Scler.* (2010) 11:187–93. doi: 10.3109/17482960902933809
25. Grassinger J, Khomenko A, Hart C, Baldaranov D, Johannesen S, Mueller G, et al. Safety and feasibility of long term administration of recombinant human granulocyte-colony stimulating factor in patients with amyotrophic lateral sclerosis. *Cytokine* (2014) 67:21–8. doi: 10.1016/j.cyto.2014.02.003
26. Chiò A, Mora G, Bella VL, Caponnetto C, Mancardi G, Sabatelli M, et al. Repeated courses of granulocyte colony-stimulating factor in amyotrophic lateral sclerosis: clinical and biological results from a prospective multicenter study. *Muscle Nerve* (2011) 43:189–95. doi: 10.1002/mus.21851
27. Duning T, Schiffbauer H, Warnecke T, Mohammadi S, Floel A, Kolpatzik K, et al. G-CSF Prevents the progression of structural disintegration of white matter tracts in amyotrophic lateral sclerosis: a pilot trial. *PLoS ONE* (2011) 6:e17770. doi: 10.1371/journal.pone.0017770
28. Brooks BR, Miller RG, Swash M, Munsat TL, World Federation of Neurology Research Group on Motor Neuron Diseases. El Escorial revisited: revised criteria for the diagnosis of amyotrophic lateral sclerosis. *Amyotroph Lateral Scler Other Motor Neuron Disord.* (2000) 1:293–9. doi: 10.1080/146608200300079536
29. Cedarbaum JM, Stambler N, Malta E, Fuller C, Hilt D, Thurmond B, et al. The ALSFRS-R: a revised ALS functional rating scale that incorporates assessments of respiratory function. *J Neurol Sci.* (1999) 169:13–21. doi: 10.1016/S0022-510X(99)00210-5
30. Banks WA. The blood-brain barrier in neuroimmunology: tales of separation and assimilation. *Brain Behav Immun.* (2015) 44:1–8. doi: 10.1016/j.bbi.2014.08.007
31. Peters S, Zitzelsperger E, Kuespert S, Iberl S, Heydn R, Johannesen SW, et al. The TGF-β System As a Potential Pathogenic Player in Disease Modulation of Amyotrophic Lateral Sclerosis. *Front Neurol.* (2017) 8:181–20. doi: 10.3389/fneur.2017.00669
32. Ransohoff RM. How neuroinflammation contributes to neurodegeneration. *Science* (2016) 353:777–83. doi: 10.1126/science.aag2590
33. Vu LT, Bowser R. Fluid-based biomarkers for amyotrophic lateral sclerosis. *Neurotherapeutics* (2017) 14:119–34. doi: 10.1007/s13311-016-0503-x
34. Roberts AW. G-CSF: A key regulator of neutrophil production, but that's not all! *Growth Factors* (2005) 23:33–41. doi: 10.1080/08977190500055836
35. Martins A, Han J, Kim SO. The multifaceted effects of granulocyte colony-stimulating factor in immunomodulation and potential roles in intestinal immune homeostasis. *IUBMB Life* (2010) 62:611–7. doi: 10.1002/iub.361
36. Hartung T, Döcke WD, Gantner F, Krieger G, Sauer A, Stevens P, et al. Effect of granulocyte colony-stimulating factor treatment on ex vivo blood cytokine response in human volunteers. *Blood.* (1995) 85:2482–9. Available online at: http://www.bloodjournal.org/content/85/9/2482
37. Henriques A, Pitzer C, Schneider A. Neurotrophic growth factors for the treatment of amyotrophic lateral sclerosis: where do we stand? *Front Neurosci.* (2010) 4:32. doi: 10.3389/fnins.2010.00032
38. Skokowa J, Dale DC, Touw IP, Zeidler C, Welte K. Severe congenital neutropenias. *Nat Rev Dis Primers* (2017) 3:17032. doi: 10.1038/nrdp.2017.32
39. Dale DC, Bolyard A, Marrero T, Makaryan V, Bonilla M, Link DC, et al. Long-term effects of G-CSF therapy in cyclic neutropenia. *N Engl J Med.* (2017) 377:2290–2. doi: 10.1056/NEJMc1709258
40. Sobrino T, Arias S, Pérez-Mato M, Agulla J, Brea D, Rodríguez-Yáñez M, et al. $Cd34^+$progenitor cells likely are involved in the good functional recovery after intracerebral hemorrhage in humans. *J Neurosci Res.* (2011) 89:979–85. doi: 10.1002/jnr.22627
41. Saito M, Kiyokawa N, Taguchi T, Suzuki K, Sekino T, Mimori K, et al. Granulocyte colony-stimulating factor directly affects human monocytes and modulates cytokine secretion. *Exp Hematol.* (2002) 30:1115–23. doi: 10.1016/S0301-472X(02)00889-5
42. D'Aveni M, Rossignol J, Coman T, Sivakumaran S, Henderson S, Manzo T, et al. G-CSF mobilizes $CD34^+$ regulatory monocytes that inhibit graft-versus-host disease. *Sci Transl Med.* (2015) 7:281ra42–2. doi: 10.1126/scitranslmed.3010435
43. Hu Y, Cao C, Qin X-Y, Yu Y, Yuan J, Zhao Y, et al. Increased peripheral blood inflammatory cytokine levels in amyotrophic lateral sclerosis: a meta-analysis study. *Sci Rep.* (2017) 7:9094. doi: 10.1038/s41598-017-09097-1
44. Lu C-H, Allen K, Oei F, Leoni E, Kuhle J, Tree T, et al. Systemic inflammatory response and neuromuscular involvement in amyotrophic lateral sclerosis. *Neurol Neuroimmunol Neuroinflamm.* (2016) 3:e244–11. doi: 10.1212/NXI.0000000000000244
45. Poloni M, Facchetti D, Mai R, Micheli A, Agnoletti L, Francolini G, et al. Circulating levels of tumour necrosis factor-alpha and its soluble receptors are increased in the blood of patients with amyotrophic lateral sclerosis. *Neurosci Lett.* (2000) 287:211–4. doi: 10.1016/S0304-3940(00)01177-0
46. Cereda C, Baiocchi C, Bongioanni P, Cova E, Guareschi S, Metelli MR, et al. TNF and sTNFR1/2 plasma levels in ALS patients. *J Neuroimmunol.* (2008) 194:123–31. doi: 10.1016/j.jneuroim.2007.10.028
47. Babu GN, Kumar A, Chandra R, Puri SK, Kalita J, Misra UK. Elevated inflammatory markers in a group of amyotrophic lateral sclerosis patients from Northern India. *Neurochem Res.* (2008) 33:1145–9. doi: 10.1007/s11064-007-9564-x
48. Tortarolo M, Coco Lo D, Veglianese P, Vallarola A, Giordana MT, Marcon G, et al. Review articleamyotrophic lateral sclerosis, a multisystem pathology: insights into the role of TNF. *Mediators Inflamm.* (2017) 2017:2985051. doi: 10.1155/2017/2985051
49. Figiel I. Pro-inflammatory cytokine TNF-alpha as a neuroprotective agent in the brain. *Acta Neurobiol Exp.* (2008) 68:526–34.
50. Fischer R, Maier O, Siegemund M, Wajant H, Scheurich P, Pfizenmaier K. A TNF receptor 2 selective agonist rescues human neurons from oxidative stress-induced cell death. *PLoS ONE* (2011) 6:e27621–11. doi: 10.1371/journal.pone.0027621
51. Dolga AM, Granic I, Blank T, Knaus H-G, Spiess J, Luiten PGM, et al. TNF-α mediates neuroprotection against glutamate-induced excitotoxicity via NF-κB-dependent up-regulation of K Ca2.2 channels. *J Neurochem.* (2008) 107:1158–67. doi: 10.1111/j.1471-4159.2008.05701.x
52. Börjesson A, Grundmark B, Olaisson H, Waldenlind L. Is there a link between amyotrophic lateral sclerosis and treatment with TNF-alpha inhibitors? *Ups J Med Sci.* (2013) 118:199–200. doi: 10.3109/03009734.2013.785999
53. Furukawa T, Matsui N, Fujita K, Nodera H, Shimizu F, Miyamoto K, et al. CSF cytokine profile distinguishes multifocal motor neuropathy from progressive muscular atrophy. *Neurol Neuroimmunol Neuroinflamm.* (2015) 2:e138. doi: 10.1212/NXI.0000000000000138
54. Henkel JS, Engelhardt JI, Siklós L, Simpson EP, Kim SH, Pan T, et al. Presence of dendritic cells, MCP-1, and activated microglia/macrophages in amyotrophic lateral sclerosis spinal cord tissue. *Ann Neurol.* (2004) 55:221–35. doi: 10.1002/ana.10805
55. Guo J, Yang X, Gao L, Zang D. Evaluating the levels of CSF and serum factors in ALS. *Brain Behav.* (2017) 7:e00637–8. doi: 10.1002/brb3.637
56. Baron P, Bussini S, Cardin V, Corbo M, Conti G, Galimberti D, et al. Production of monocyte chemoattractant protein-1 in amyotrophic lateral sclerosis. *Muscle Nerve.* (2005) 32:541–4. doi: 10.1002/mus.20376
57. Rodríguez-Cortés O, Vela-Ojeda J, López-Santiago R, Montiel-Cervantes L, Reyes-Maldonado E, Estrada-García I, et al. Granulocyte colony-stimulating factor produces a decrease in IFNgamma and increase in IL-4 when administrated to healthy donors. *J Clin Apher.* (2010) 25:181–7. doi: 10.1002/jca.20234
58. Aebischer J, Cassina P, Otsmane B, Moumen A, Seilhean D, Meininger V, et al. IFNγ triggers a LIGHT-dependent selective death of motoneurons contributing to the non-cell-autonomous effects of mutant SOD1. *Cell Death Differ.* (2011) 18:754–68. doi: 10.1038/cdd.2010.143

59. Liu J, Gao L, Zang D. Elevated levels of IFN-γ in CSF and Serum of patients with amyotrophic lateral sclerosis. *PLoS ONE* (2015) 10:e0136937. doi: 10.1371/journal.pone.0136937
60. McFadden C, Morgan R, Rahangdale S, Green D, Yamasaki H, Center D, et al. Preferential migration of T regulatory cells induced by IL-16. *J Immunol.* (2007) 179:6439–45. doi: 10.4049/jimmunol.179.10.6439
61. Henkel JS, Beers DR, Wen S, Rivera AL, Toennis KM, Appel JE, et al. Regulatory T-lymphocytes mediate amyotrophic lateral sclerosis progression and survival. *EMBO Mol Med.* (2013) 5:64–79. doi: 10.1002/emmm.201201544
62. Fiala M, Chattopadhay M, La Cava A, Tse E, Liu G, Lourenco E, et al. IL-17A is increased in the serum and in spinal cord CD8 and mast cells of ALS patients. *J Neuroinflam.* (2010) 7:76. doi: 10.1186/1742-2094-7-76
63. Rentzos M, Rombos A, Nikolaou C, Zoga M, Zouvelou V, Dimitrakopoulos A, et al. Interleukin-17 and interleukin-23 are elevated in serum and cerebrospinal fluid of patients with ALS: a reflection of Th17 cells activation? *Acta Neurol Scand.* (2010) 122:425–9. doi: 10.1111/j.1600-0404.2010.01333.x
64. Mitchell RM, Freeman WM, Randazzo WT, Stephens HE, Beard JL, Simmons Z, et al. A CSF biomarker panel for identification of patients with amyotrophic lateral sclerosis. *Neurology* (2009) 72:14–9. doi: 10.1212/01.wnl.0000333251.36681.a5
65. Kuhle J, Lindberg RLP, Regeniter A, Mehling M, Steck AJ, Kappos L, et al. Increased levels of inflammatory chemokines in amyotrophic lateral sclerosis. *Eur J Neurol.* (2009) 16:771–4. doi: 10.1111/j.1468-1331.2009.02560.x
66. Zacharek A, Chen J, Li A, Cui X, Li Y, Roberts C, et al. Angiopoietin1/TIE2 and VEGF/FLK1 induced by MSC treatment amplifies angiogenesis and vascular stabilization after stroke. *J Cereb Blood Flow Metab.* (2007) 27:1684–91. doi: 10.1038/sj.jcbfm.9600475
67. Takahashi H, Shibuya M. The vascular endothelial growth factor (VEGF)/VEGF receptor system and its role under physiological and pathological conditions. *Clin Sci.* (2005) 109:227–41. doi: 10.1042/CS20040370
68. Fidyk W, Mitrus I, Ciomber A, Smagur A, Chwieduk A, Głowala-Kosinska M, et al. Evaluation of proinflammatory and immunosuppressive cytokines in blood and bone marrow of healthy hematopoietic stem cell donors. *Cytokine.* (2017) 102:181–6. doi: 10.1016/j.cyto.2017.09.001
69. Bettcher BM, Fitch R, Wynn MJ, Lalli MA, Elofson J, Jastrzab L, et al. MCP-1 and eotaxin-1 selectively and negatively associate with memory in MCI and Alzheimer's disease dementia phenotypes. *Alzheim Dement.* (2016) 3:91–7. doi: 10.1016/j.dadm.2016.05.004
70. Villeda SA, Luo J, Mosher KI, Zou B, Britschgi M, Bieri G, et al. The ageing systemic milieu negatively regulates neurogenesis and cognitive function. *Nature* (2011) 477:90–4. doi: 10.1038/nature10357
71. Lunetta C, Lizio A, Maestri E, Sansone VA, Mora G, Miller RG, et al. Serum C-Reactive protein as a prognostic biomarker in amyotrophic lateral sclerosis. *JAMA Neurol.* (2017) 74:660–7. doi: 10.1001/jamaneurol.2016.6179
72. Tateishi T, Yamasaki R, Tanaka M, Matsushita T, Kikuchi H, Isobe N, et al. CSF chemokine alterations related to the clinical course of amyotrophic lateral sclerosis. *J Neuroimmunol.* (2010) 222:76–81. doi: 10.1016/j.jneuroim.2010.03.004
73. Rentzos M, Rombos A, Nikolaou C, Zoga M, Zouvelou V, Dimitrakopoulos A, et al. Interleukin-15 and interleukin-12 are elevated in serum and cerebrospinal fluid of patients with amyotrophic lateral sclerosis. *Eur Neurol.* (2010) 63:285–90. doi: 10.1159/000287582
74. Yang X, Gao L, Wu X, Zhang Y, Zang D. Increased levels of MIP-1 αin CSF and serum of ALS. *Acta Neurol Scand.* (2015) 134:94–100. doi: 10.1111/ane.12513
75. Haraldsen G, Kvale D, Lien B, Farstad IN, Brandtzaeg P. Cytokine-regulated expression of E-selectin, intercellular adhesion molecule-1 (ICAM-1), and vascular cell adhesion molecule-1 (VCAM-1) in human microvascular endothelial cells. *J Immunol.* (1996) 156:2558–65. Available online at: http://www.jimmunol.org/content/156/7/2558.long
76. Chiò A, Logroscino G, Hardiman O, Swingler R, Mitchell D, Beghi E, et al. Prognostic factors in ALS: a critical review. *Amyotroph Lateral Scler.* (2009) 10:310–23. doi: 10.3109/17482960802566824
77. Wirth AM, Khomenko A, Baldaranov D, Kobor I, Hsam O, Grimm T, et al. Combinatory biomarker use of cortical thickness, MUNIX, and ALSFRS-R at baseline and in longitudinal courses of individual patients with amyotrophic lateral sclerosis. *Front Neurol.* (2018) 9:614. doi: 10.3389/fneur.2018.00614
78. Westeneng H-J, Debray TPA, Visser AE, van Eijk RPA, Rooney JPK, Calvo A, et al. Prognosis for patients with amyotrophic lateral sclerosis: development and validation of a personalised prediction model. *Lancet Neurol.* (2018) 17:423–33. doi: 10.1016/S1474-4422(18)30089-9

5

An Overview of MicroRNAs as Biomarkers of ALS

Greig Joilin[1*], *P. Nigel Leigh*[2], *Sarah F. Newbury*[2] *and Majid Hafezparast*[1*]

[1] School of Life Sciences, University of Sussex, Brighton, United Kingdom,

[2] Brighton and Sussex Medical School, University of Sussex, Brighton, United Kingdom

***Correspondence:**
Greig Joilin
g.joilin@sussex.ac.uk
Majid Hafezparast
m.hafezparast@sussex.ac.uk

Amyotrophic lateral sclerosis (ALS; MND, motor neuron disease) is a debilitating neurodegenerative disease affecting 4.5 per 100,000 people per year around the world. There is currently no cure for this disease, and its causes are relatively unknown. Diagnosis is based on a battery of clinical tests up to a year after symptom onset, with no robust markers of diagnosis or disease progression currently identified. A major thrust of current research is to identify potential non-invasive markers ("biomarkers") in body fluids such as blood and/or cerebrospinal fluid (CSF) to use for diagnostic or prognostic purposes. Non-coding RNAs (ncRNAs), including microRNAs (miRNAs), are found at detectable and stable levels in blood and other bodily fluids. Specific ncRNAs can vary in levels between ALS patients and non-ALS controls without the disease. In this review, we will provide an overview of early findings, demonstrate the potential of this new class as biomarkers, and discuss future challenges and opportunities taking this forward to help patients with ALS.

Keywords: amyotrophic lateral sclerosis, motor neuron disease, biomarkers, non-coding RNA, microRNA

INTRODUCTION

Amyotrophic lateral sclerosis (ALS) is the most prevalent adult onset form of motor neuron disease. As a result of progressive death of motor neurons in the primary motor cortex, brainstem and spinal cord, there is atrophy of the muscles that are innervated by these neurons. This results in muscle weakness and paralysis with death usually occurring within 3–5 years. Over the last decade, significant progress has been made in identifying the genes responsible for familial cases of ALS (fALS). Of these, the most frequently mutated genes are chromosome 9 open reading frame 72 (*C9orf72*), superoxide dismutase 1 (*SOD1*), TAR DNA-binding protein 43 (*TARDBP*; TDP-43), and FUS RNA binding protein (*FUS*), accounting for over 70% of fALS cases (1). Nevertheless, fALS constitutes approximately 10% of all cases, with the genetic underpinnings of sporadic ALS (sALS) mostly unknown, though *C9orf72* is known to account for 5% of sALS cases.

The lack of a common cause has resulted in difficulties not only in timely disease diagnosis resulting in delay of treatment, but in developing drugs and treatments for the disease. Thus, identifying useful biomarkers as tools for early diagnosis, for determining subgroups in relation to pathogenesis and/or phenotype, and as indicators of treatment response, are urgently required. Development of biomarkers that are minimally invasive to obtain, simple to undertake, and time efficient are key and those derived from biofluids, such as blood, are well suited for this. Further, it is not necessary for the biomarkers to underlie the pathology of the disease if it correlates strongly and specifically to the disease. Indeed, this is more difficult to assess in diseases such as ALS where the underlying molecular causes of pathology is unknown or unclear.

One class of molecules increasingly investigated as potential biomarkers are short ncRNA species (those under 100 nucleotides long), which include tRNA, rRNA, piwi-RNA (piRNA), and microRNA (miRNA). MiRNA have been the main focus of most studies to date, driven by a good understanding of their biogenesis and function, an ease in profiling their expression with a range of techniques including microarray, RNA-seq, and RT-qPCR, a relatively simple structure, increased stability from RNase degradation and freeze-thaw cycles, and a presence in a range of biofluids including blood, cerebrospinal fluid (CSF), and urine (2, 3). To date, a number of studies have shown that miRNAs are differentially expressed in ALS patients when compared to controls in a variety of biofluids, including CSF, and in the blood-derived components plasma and serum (4–18) (summarized in **Table 1**). This review will aim to present recent work identifying miRNA-based biomarkers in biofluids, the possibility of using other ncRNA as biomarkers, and the next steps required to move this into a clinical setting.

EXISTING CIRCULATING RNA BIOMARKERS FOR ALS

Serum-Based Biomarkers

Freischmidt and colleagues have undertaken a number of studies to identify potential miRNA-based biomarkers in the ALS patient serum (4, 6, 8). Their first study selected ten miRNAs previously identified to regulate the ALS-related gene *TARDPB* and found five miRNAs were differentially expressed in serum of sALS patients (4). Their later study focused on miRNA expression in serum from fALS patients using Affymetrix miRNA array chips, and found downregulation of a set of 30 potential miRNA biomarkers for the disease [**Table 1**; 3]. Four miRNA were selected based on their false discovery rate (FDR)-adjusted *p*-value (MIR1915-3p, MIR3665, MIR4530, MIR4745-5p) and their downregulation validated with RT-qPCR in the fALS patients, and all but MIR1915-3p were further observed to be downregulated in sALS patients. While increased variability was observed in sALS patients, this suggested that there may be similarities in the miRNA profile between the two groups. Curiously, these three miRNAs (MIR3665, MIR4530, MIR4745-5p) were found not to be differentially expressed in their most recent study using sALS patients, which described only MIR1234-3p and MIR1825 as being downregulated (8). An interesting aspect of their 2014 study was investigating miRNA expression in non-symptomatic patients who had ALS-related genetic mutations, but predicted to present disease symptoms within the next 20 years. These predicted pre-symptomatic carriers shared 91.7% of the downregulated miRNA of symptomatic patients, although to a lesser dysregulation. This suggests that these biomarkers may be present before symptoms and could be used to identify potential ALS cases. Furthermore, considering there were differences between pre-symptomatic and symptomatic patients in the degree of dysregulation, this may suggest that these biomarkers could change with time. However, further work would be needed to determine this and if it would apply to sALS cases along with whether these biomarkers are specific to ALS itself.

Other studies have also identified potential biomarkers that may be differentially expressed in serum from ALS patients. The upregulation of MIR143-3p and MIR206, and the downregulation of MIR374B-5p were observed in 23 sALS patients and were further validated in an additional 27 sALS patients (13). Of these, 22 samples were in a longitudinal study and MIR143-3p and MIR374B-5p both became more dysregulated, suggesting a link to disease progression, though MIR206 remained stable for at least 3 months later. Another study using patient serum also found MIR206 upregulation in ALS patients along with MIR106b, differences that were reflected in a SOD1-G93A mouse model of ALS (7). MIR206, described as a myoMiR due to its high abundance in skeletal muscle tissue, is one of the few miRNA biomarkers identified across multiple studies, including those described below in serum and plasma (11, 12). The working hypothesis has been that as a result of muscle death, MIR206 is released from the muscle fibers and into the blood stream as a waste product (19). However, MIR206 has been identified as a blood-based biomarker for other muscle-related diseases and therefore not specific to ALS (20, 21). Nonetheless, it could play an important role in helping to identify ALS patients if used in conjunction with other biomarkers to help distinguish from ALS-like conditions. Lastly, one study has investigated the exosomes present in serum, and investigated a single miRNA (MIR27A-3p) based on the research group's previous work with myoblast exosomes (18). However, the normalization to MIR16-5p may limit the interpretation of this data as it has been shown to be dysregulated in ALS (15, 22) and no evidence was shown that MIR16-5p was stable. Nonetheless, with a fuller investigation, identifying dysregulated miRNA present in exosomes in ALS may provide clues as to the source, destination, and thus function of circulating miRNA in ALS.

Plasma-Based Biomarkers

Two studies have investigated biomarkers in sALS patients using plasma; the portion of blood which contains clotting factors. Using microarray analysis followed by RT-qPCR, Takahashi et al. (9) found significant upregulation of MIR4649-5p and downregulation of MIR4299 in ALS patients compared to healthy controls. Interestingly, this study incorporated a follow up analysis of the expression of miRNAs in seven of the patients, including one patient 24 months later. However, no significant change in the expression of any of the miRNAs were found, although there was a trend for an increase of MIR663b over time. Similarly, in another study, while MIR424 and MIR206 were found to be overexpressed in plasma of sALS patients, they did not show significant changes over 6 and 12 months in a cohort of sALS patients (11). This lack of change in MIR206 over time is consistent with the above results of Waller et al. (13). This suggests that for these miRNA, their expression levels are not correlated with disease progression and changes in the patient condition. This may mean that they may only be suitable as diagnostic markers and not useful in tracking treatment responses in disease.

TABLE 1 | Circulating miRNA-based biomarkers found to be differentially expressed in biofluids.

	Authors	ALS type	*n*	Validated changes		Controls	RNA extraction	Profiling technique	RT-qPCR validation	RT-qPCR Normalization
				Increase	Decrease					
Serum	Freischmidt et al. (4)	Sporadic	22	–	MIR132-5p MIR132-3p **MIR143-5p** **MIR143-3p** LET7B-5p	Age-matched healthy controls	miRNeasy Mini	–	Ncode VILO EXPRESS SYBR GreenER	Spiked in cel-MIR39-3p
	De Felice et al. (5)	Sporadic	72	MIR338-3p	–	Age-matched healthy controls	Trizol	–	miScript RT-qPCR	LET7A
	Freischmidt et al. (6)	Familial	22	–	MIR1825 MIR1915-3p MIR3665 MIR4530 MIR4745-5p	Age-matched healthy controls	QIAzol and miRNeasy Mini	Affymetrix GeneChip 3.0 Array	miScript RT-qPCR	Spiked in cel-MIR39-3p
		Sporadic	14	–	MIR3665 MIR4530 MIR4745-5p					
	Toivonen et al. (7)	–	12	**MIR106B** MIR206	–	Age-matched healthy controls	Norgen Total RNA	Affymetrix GeneChip 2.0 Array	TaqMan miRNA RT-qPCR	Spiked in cel-MIR39-3p
	Freischmidt et al. (8)	Sporadic	18	–	MIR1234-3p MIR1825	Age-matched healthy controls/ Alzheimer's/ Huntington's	QIAzol and miRNeasy Mini	Affymetrix GeneChip 3.0 Array	miScript RT-qPCR	Spiked in cel-MIR39-3p
	Waller et al. (13)	Sporadic	50	**MIR143-3p** MIR206	MIR374B-5p	Age-matched healthy controls/ disease mimics	Norgen Circulating Nucleic Acid Isolation	TaqMan Low Density RT-qPCR arrays	miScript RT-qPCR	MIR17-5p MIR24 MIR223-3p
	Matamala et al. (16)	Sporadic	20	MIR142-3p	MIR1249-3p	Age-matched healthy controls	Trizol LS and miRNeasy Serum/ Plasma	Illumina TruSeq Small RNA on Illumina MiSeq	TaqMan miRNA RT-qPCR	Spiked in cel-MIR39-3p

(Continued)

TABLE 1 | Continued

	Authors	ALS type	*n*	Validated changes		Controls	RNA extraction	Profiling technique	RT-qPCR validation	RT-qPCR Normalization
				Increase	Decrease					
	Raheja et al. (17)	Sporadic/ Familial	23	Screen only	Screen only	Healthy controls	miRcury	miRNA LNA RT- qPCR arrays	–	–
	Xu et al. (18)	–	10	–	MIR27A-3p	Healthy controls	Trizol or miRNeasy Micro	–	miDETECT A Track miRNA RT-qPCR or TaqMan miRNA RT-qPCR	MIR16-5p
Plasma	Takahashi et al. (9)	Sporadic	48	MIR4649-5p	MIR4299	Age-matched healthy controls	miRNeasy Serum/ Plasma	3D-Gene Human miRNA oligo chip	miScript RT-qPCR	MIR4516
	de Andrade et al. (11)	Sporadic	39	MIR424 MIR206	–	Aged match healthy control	miRVana PARIS	Affymetrix GeneChip array (on muscle)	TaqMan miRNA RT-qPCR	MIR16-5p
	Sheinerman et al. (12)	–	50	MIR206/MIR338-3p MIR9/MIR129-3p MIR335-5p/MIR338-3p		Age-matched healthy controls	Trizol and Ambion Glass fiber Columns	Literature search	TaqMan miRNA RT–qPCR	–
Cerebrospinal Fluid	Freischmidt et al. (4)	Sporadic	22	**MIR143-5p** MIR574-5p	MIR132-5p MIR132-3p **MIR143-3p**	Age-matched healthy controls	miRNeasy Mini	–	Ncode VILO EXPRESS SYBR GreenER	Spiked in cel-MIR39-3p
	De Felice et al. (5)	Sporadic	72	MIR338-3p	–	Age-matched healthy controls	Trizol	–	miScript RT-qPCR	MIR24
	Benigni et al. (10)	Sporadic	24	MIR181A-5p	LET7A-5p LET7B-5p LET7F-5p MIR15b-5p MIR21-5p MIR195-5p MIR148A-3p	Age-matched healthy controls	miRNeasy Mini	Human miFinder 384HC miRNA PCR array	SYBR Green RT-qPCR	Spiked in cel-MIR39-3p MIR608 MIR328-3p
	Waller et al. (14)	Sporadic	32	Screen only	Screen only	Age-matched healthy controls/disease mimics	miRVana PARIS	Illumina TruSeq Small RNA on Illumina HiScanSq	miScript II RT-qPCR	Spiked in cel-MIR39-3p MIR30A-5p

(Continued)

TABLE 1 | Continued

	Authors	ALS type	*n*	Validated changes		Controls	RNA extraction	Profiling technique	RT-qPCR validation	RT-qPCR Normalization
				Increase	Decrease					
Whole Blood	Liguori et al. (15)	Sporadic	56	-	LET7A-5p LET7D-5p LET7F-5p LET7G-5p LET7I-5p MIR15A-5p MIR15B-5p MIR151A-5p MIR151B MIR16-5p MIR22-3p MIR23A-3p MIR26A-5p MIR26B-5p MIR27B-3p MIR28-3p MIR30B-5p MIR30C-5p MIR93-5p MIR103A-3p **MIR106B-3p** MIR128-3p MIR130A-3p MIR130B-3p MIR144-5p MIR148A-3p MIR148B-3p MIR182-5p MIR183-5p MIR186-5p MIR221-3p MIR223-3p MIR342-3p MIR425-5p MIR451A MIR532-5p MIR550A-3p MIR584-5p	Age-matched healthy controls	PAXgene Blood RNA	Illumina TruSeq Small RNA on Illumina HiSeq2500	TaqMan Advanced miRNA RT-qPCR	MIR484

Those miRNA underlined show consistent directional changes between control and ALS cases while those in bold show contrasting directional changes between control and ALS cases.

Cerebrospinal Fluid-Based Biomarkers

In addition to serum and plasma, differential expression of ncRNA has also been investigated in CSF. Although CSF is not as easily obtainable as blood, changes in expression may potentially be more insightful due to its close proximity to the central nervous system. Using RT-qPCR, De Felice et al. (5) not only found MIR338-3p to be over-expressed in serum, but also in CSF, blood leukocytes, and spinal cord tissue in ALS patients compared to controls and other patient groups (including patients with Alzheimer's and Parkinson's disease). *In situ* hybridization staining of spinal cord tissue post mortem found that MIR338-3p was localized in the dorsal root gray matter and overexpressed in ALS patients, suggesting a potential source of the miRNA. In contrast, Freischmidt et al. (4) used the biomarkers identified in their serum work to find out if there were similar changes in the CSF. While four of those miRNAs were dysregulated, only MIR143-3p showed a significant correlative relationship between the serum and CSF, suggesting there is low correlation in miRNA expression between these two biofluids. Combined with generally higher concentrations of miRNA in the serum, the authors concluded that there might be separate regulatory mechanisms underlying the levels of miRNAs in these two body compartments. This is supported by other papers looking into CSF which have shown very little overlap with other serum studies, but studies that have looked at both within the same sample groups are limited.

EMERGING THEMES IN ALS BIOMARKER DISCOVERY

Recently, two main themes are starting to emerge in biomarker discovery, including in those for ALS. Firstly, it is becoming evident that seeking to identify singular biomarkers for disease is unlikely, underscored by the minimal overlap demonstrated by the above studies. In a study to identify miRNA biomarkers in CSF, using ratios between the expression of two miRNA as determined by RT-qPCR increased sensitivity and specificity in identifying sALS cases compared to using a single miRNA (10). The study pointed out that the use of more than one miRNA as a "biomarker signature" is preferable as it reduces the dependency on variation between individuals. The pairing of the upregulated MIR181A-5p, with either of their two downregulated miRNA, MIR21-5p and MIR15B-5p, increased both the sensitivity and the specificity, with MIR15B-5p increased by 15% on average. Another study has also used this concept for miRNA present in serum, using a number of pairs to identify not only patients with ALS, but other neurological disorders such as Alzheimer's disease, frontotemporal dementia, and Parkinson's disease (12). Having identified 37 brain- or inflammation-enriched miRNA, they found the combination of the three pairs of miRNAs (MIR206/MIR338-3p, MIR9/MIR129-3p, and MIR335-5p/MIR338-3p) were able to clearly distinguish between ALS and control patients in their cohort with a sensitivity of 84% and a specificity of 82%. Furthermore, other paired combinations were able to differentiate between other neurodegenerative diseases and ALS. Sheinerman et al. (12) found an 8-fold increase in MIR206 levels in the plasma of ALS patients when compared to the controls and this was enough to distinguish ALS patients from controls by itself. Therefore, on the whole, pairs of miRNA were able to distinguish between the various diseases and controls with higher accuracy than could be achieved by an individual miRNA.

Secondly, recent advances have improved the generation of high quality libraries from small amounts of starting RNA, allowing unbiased screening of potential ncRNA biomarkers by the RNA-seq technique. In one of the first studies, following on from their work with serum, Waller et al. (14) used RNA-seq to profile miRNA expression in the CSF of ALS patients. While they were able to successfully sequence the miRNA and identify potential candidates, they were unable to confirm those with RT-qPCR because of technical issues. Nonetheless, it supports the conclusion of the above studies that differences in miRNA can be detected in CSF and that CSF could be a source of biomarkers.

More recently, one study has used total blood to screen for miRNA biomarkers in ALS using RNA-seq (15). Following identification of 42 differentially expressed miRNA in the discovery cohort, 38 were validated using RT-qPCR, most of which have been previously reported in other papers. Interestingly, seven of the miRNAs (MIR30B-5p, MIR30C-5p, MIR106B-3p, MIR128-3p, MIR148B-3p, MIR186-5p, MIR342-3p) were able to distinguish between spinal and bulbar onset, with decreased expression present for those with spinal onset. Furthermore, this study also carried out RNA-seq on mRNAs in the same samples to help identify targets that could be regulated by the miRNA. The use of total blood, however, limits the interpretation of these results due to the presence of red blood cells in the samples and the possibility of variable numbers of different types of white blood cells between patient and control groups.

Matamala et al. (16) also utilized RNA-seq for the identification of ALS biomarkers, but started by profiling serum samples from transgenic mouse models of ALS, followed by RT-qPCR validation in human samples. While a number of miRNAs were found to change in levels between the ALS model and controls, there was limited cross-validation when this was taken forward to the human studies. Two miRNA that did show differences between ALS patients and controls in the human studies were MIR142-3p and MIR1249-3p. The authors found that MIR142-3p seemed to correlate negatively with a decline in clinical disability scale ALSFRS-R in patients, thus suggesting that this could be used to measure the effect of any disease-slowing treatment. Further, it was found to potentially target the expression of the ALS genes *TARDBP* and *C9orf72*. Interestingly, Matamala et al. (16) also briefly described the detection of non-miRNA ncRNA with their RNA-seq, but did not state if they were differentially expressed or whether they were investigated further. As such, there may be a range of potential biomarkers that have not yet been identified. Indeed, several other ncRNA species have been detected in serum including rRNA and tRNA (23–25). These have also been highlighted as potential biomarkers in diseases other than ALS in blood (26–29) and other tissues (24, 30–32). To this end, we are currently using RNA-seq to identify potential biomarkers in

ALS within the full cohort of ncRNA species, and early results suggest that we have potential candidates, which include miRNA, piRNA, and tRNA.

CHALLENGES AND OPPORTUNITIES

Across these studies, there is very little overlap in the miRNA species as potential biomarkers in the biofluids (see **Table 1**), and there are multiple potential reasons for this. Firstly, as these are mostly from elderly human patients, some of these patients could have other conditions which could alter the miRNA composition of the biofluids themselves, thus confound the detection of ALS-specific biomarkers; careful screening of patients therefore is required. Further, some of these studies do not include patients from ALS disease mimics to help identify ALS-specific markers. This is important as some biomarkers identified such as MIR206 are not specific to ALS as described above. Additionally, most of these studies have been carried out on samples from one population group. As differences may exist between different populations with the disease, the lack of cross-validation of changes in miRNA expression between studies may be reflective of differences in the patient population, whether that be mediated genetically and/or environmentally. The number of patients also differ, from 12 to 72 ALS patients, and so the statistical power for some of these biomarkers is limited.

Alternatively, the causes could be related to the methodology of the study, from the extraction of the biofluids and RNA, through to the screening and validation of the miRNA biomarkers. As seen in **Table 1** and **Figure 1**, a range of different workflows have been undertaken across all the studies, all of which may contribute to differences in the changes that are detected. In addition, some of these factors potentially could affect the strength of some of these studies. For example, how the samples were collected and processed may vary. Some of the studies did not describe their collection procedures, and it is well known that differences in the centrifugation time post-collection, speed of centrifugation, and temperature can all affect the quality and quantity of RNA in the samples (33, 34).

Further, techniques used to normalize the RT-qPCR could be considered questionable in a number of studies. Due to the minimal and varied amount of RNA in biofluids, and the resultant difficulty in quantifying the RNA concentration, most miRNA RT-qPCR kits used fixed sample volumes instead of fixed total RNA amounts. Therefore, miRNA RT-qPCR normalization must control for input RNA, not just for technical variation, by crucially using a reliable target as a normalizer. However, no universal normalizer for biomarker work exists, and identification of a suitable normalizer is a problem across

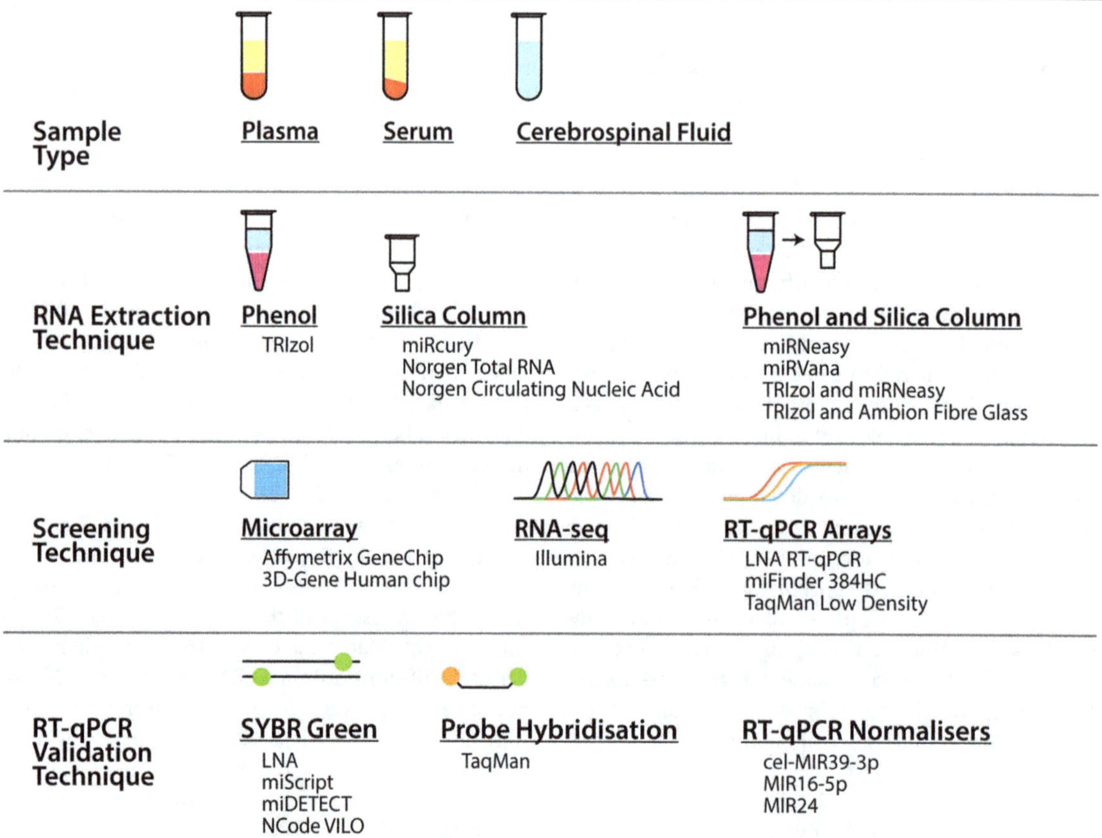

FIGURE 1 | Summary of the different sample types, techniques, and tools that were used to profile miRNA biomarkers in ALS in the studies presented in this review. As can be seen alongside **Table 1**, numerous different combinations of these sample types and tools across the techniques were employed across a number of studies.

all biofluid biomarker studies (35, 36). Normalizers should be selected per study from those ncRNA with the most stable expression in their screen and then validated. Instead, a number of the above studies have used the synthetic spike-in cel-MIR39B, but this would only control for technical variation introduced from RNA extraction onwards, not for the total RNA amount in the starting volume. Others have used miRNA recommended as normalizers such as MIR16-5p, but as described above, it has been shown to be regulated in ALS (15, 22), and also in stress and in red blood cells (37, 38). Indeed, as some studies did not check for hemolysis in their samples, the observed changes may be due to released miRNA from the lysed red blood cells. Taken together, this underlies why there may be limited cross-validation between studies and thus careful consideration of identifying objective normalizers are required.

One question is how do these miRNA-based biomarkers compare to other biomarkers for ALS? While the properties of miRNA as biomarkers as described above are ideal, there are other molecules such as DNA, RNA, protein, and metabolites that could also be used. One of the most commonly used biomarkers in ALS is the neurofilament proteins, which form part of the cytoskeleton of neurons and has been found to be present in both CSF and serum. Studies have shown that neurofilaments are able to help with identification of ALS cases but like MIR206 are not specific to ALS, and rather a measure of axonal death. As such, it is likely that singular miRNA or neurofilaments by themselves will not be able to help with ALS diagnosis or prognosis, but they could form part of any potential biomarker signature. Therefore, it is likely that an integrative approach is required, using data on the levels of a number of ncRNA biomarkers, as has been shown for other diseases (39). Such approaches include utilizing multiple biomarkers, including both miRNA and non-miRNA based biomarkers, and integrating them into a signature model such as a discriminant model, or by using ratios of miRNA expression and using them to help with classification of the disease state, and a number of the above studies have done this. Together, this may help allow ALS patients to be specifically identified, not only from healthy controls but from disease mimics. Therefore, taking this work forward into larger cohorts of patients is vital to test integrating these biomarkers together.

Indeed, opportunities from well-designed studies to validate their biomarkers in separate and larger cohorts could allow for these biomarkers to be used clinically. Further, these studies have been designed first and foremost to find biomarkers for ALS with little attempt to determine the biology underlying these changes, as presence alone does not infer function. Nonetheless, considering the wide and varied biological roles of miRNAs, determining their biological function will be important. Future studies need to include their source and destination, potentially by investigating exosomes and their contents and function. These studies would provide new insights into the mechanisms that may underlie ALS. Therefore, not only do larger cohorts need to be screened but proper experimental design needs to be undertaken to ensure that results are valid and can be used to progress the field further.

What is ultimately being sought is a set of biomarkers that are able to help with the diagnosis and prognosis of ALS patients. Diagnosis and prognosis of patients based on an ncRNA biomarker could assist with the development of tailored and targeted treatments to extend or improve patients' quality of life. As such, these studies have shown that there is potential here for ncRNA-based biomarkers to be identified, and with careful consideration, future work will help to further refine this to progress this to the clinical setting.

AUTHOR CONTRIBUTIONS

GJ wrote and edited the manuscript. MH, PL, and SN critically reviewed and edited the manuscript.

ACKNOWLEDGMENTS

The work was supported during Motor Neurone Disease Association project grants awarded to MH, PL, and SN (Hafezparast/Apr15/836-791 and Hafezparast/Apr18/861-791) and a Biotechnology and Biological Sciences Research Council project grant (BB/P021042/1) to SN.

REFERENCES

1. Martin S, Al Khleifat A, Al-Chalabi A. What causes amyotrophic lateral sclerosis? *F1000Res.* (2017) 6:371. doi: 10.12688/f1000research.10476.1
2. Chen X, Ba Y, Ma L, Cai X, Yin Y, Wang K, et al. Characterization of microRNAs in serum: a novel class of biomarkers for diagnosis of cancer and other diseases. *Cell Res.* (2008) 18:997–1006. doi: 10.1038/cr.2008.282
3. Jin XF, Wu N, Wang L, Li J. Circulating microRNAs: a novel class of potential biomarkers for diagnosing and prognosing central nervous system diseases. *Cell Mol Neurobiol.* (2013) 33:601–13. doi: 10.1007/s10571-013-9940-9
4. Freischmidt A, Muller K, Ludolph AC, Weishaupt JH. Systemic dysregulation of TDP-43 binding microRNAs in amyotrophic lateral sclerosis. *Acta Neuropathol Commun.* (2013) 1:42. doi: 10.1186/2051-5960-1-42
5. De Felice B, Annunziata A, Fiorentino G, Borra M, Biffali E, Coppola C, et al. miR-338-3p is over-expressed in blood, CFS, serum and spinal cord from sporadic amyotrophic lateral sclerosis patients. *Neurogenetics.* (2014) 15:243–53. doi: 10.1007/s10048-014-0420-2
6. Freischmidt A, Muller K, Zondler L, Weydt P, Volk AE, Bozic AL, et al. Serum microRNAs in patients with genetic amyotrophic lateral sclerosis and pre-manifest mutation carriers. *Brain.* (2014) 137(Pt 11):2938–50. doi: 10.1093/brain/awu249
7. Toivonen JM, Manzano R, Olivan S, Zaragoza P, Garcia-Redondo A, Osta R. MicroRNA-206: a potential circulating biomarker candidate for amyotrophic lateral sclerosis. *PLoS ONE.* (2014) 9:e89065. doi: 10.1371/journal.pone.0089065
8. Freischmidt A, Muller K, Zondler L, Weydt P, Mayer B, von Arnim CA, et al. Serum microRNAs in sporadic amyotrophic lateral sclerosis. *Neurobiol Aging.* (2015) 36:2660.e2615–e2620. doi: 10.1016/j.neurobiolaging.2015.06.003
9. Takahashi I, Hama Y, Matsushima M, Hirotani M, Kano T, Hohzen H, et al. Identification of plasma microRNAs as a biomarker of sporadic Amyotrophic Lateral Sclerosis. *Mol Brain.* (2015) 8:67. doi: 10.1186/s13041-015-0161-7
10. Benigni M, Ricci C, Jones AR, Giannini F, Al-Chalabi A, Battistini S. Identification of miRNAs as potential biomarkers in cerebrospinal fluid from

amyotrophic lateral sclerosis patients. *Neuromolecular Med.* (2016) 18:551–60. doi: 10.1007/s12017-016-8396-8

11. de Andrade HM, de Albuquerque M, Avansini SH, de SRC, Dogini DB, Nucci A, et al. MicroRNAs-424 and 206 are potential prognostic markers in spinal onset amyotrophic lateral sclerosis. *J Neurol Sci.* (2016) 368:19–24. doi: 10.1016/j.jns.2016.06.046
12. Sheinerman KS, Toledo JB, Tsivinsky VG, Irwin D, Grossman M, Weintraub D, et al. Circulating brain-enriched microRNAs as novel biomarkers for detection and differentiation of neurodegenerative diseases. *Alzheimers Res Ther.* (2017) 9:89. doi: 10.1186/s13195-017-0316-0
13. Waller R, Goodall EF, Milo M, Cooper-Knock J, Da Costa M, Hobson E, et al. Serum miRNAs miR-206, 143-3p and 374b-5p as potential biomarkers for amyotrophic lateral sclerosis (ALS). *Neurobiol Aging.* (2017) 55:123–31. doi: 10.1016/j.neurobiolaging.2017.03.027
14. Waller R, Wyles M, Heath PR, Kazoka M, Wollff H, Shaw PJ, et al. Small RNA sequencing of sporadic amyotrophic lateral sclerosis cerebrospinal fluid reveals differentially expressed miRNAs related to neural and glial activity. *Front Neurosci.* (2017) 11:731. doi: 10.3389/fnins.2017.00731
15. Liguori M, Nuzziello N, Introna A, Consiglio A, Licciulli F, D'Errico E, et al. Dysregulation of microRNAs and target genes networks in peripheral blood of patients with sporadic amyotrophic lateral sclerosis. *Front Mol Neurosci.* (2018) 11:288. doi: 10.3389/fnmol.2018.00288
16. Matamala JM, Arias-Carrasco R, Sanchez C, Uhrig M, Bargsted L, Matus S, et al. Genome-wide circulating microRNA expression profiling reveals potential biomarkers for amyotrophic lateral sclerosis. *Neurobiol Aging.* (2018) 64:123–38. doi: 10.1016/j.neurobiolaging.2017.12.020
17. Raheja R, Regev K, Healy BC, Mazzola MA, Beynon V, Von Glehn F, et al. Correlating serum micrornas and clinical parameters in amyotrophic lateral sclerosis. *Muscle Nerve.* (2018) 58:261–9. doi: 10.1002/mus.26106
18. Xu Q, Zhao Y, Zhou X, Luan J, Cui Y, Han J. Comparison of the extraction and determination of serum exosome and miRNA in serum and the detection of miR-27a-3p in serum exosome of ALS patients. *Intractable Rare Dis Res.* (2018) 7:13–8. doi: 10.5582/irdr.2017.01091
19. Wang F, Wang J, He J, Li W, Li J, Chen S, et al. Serum miRNAs miR-23a, 206, and 499 as potential biomarkers for skeletal muscle atrophy. *Biomed Res Int.* (2017) 2017:8361237. doi: 10.1155/2017/8361237
20. Matsuzaka Y, Kishi S, Aoki Y, Komaki H, Oya Y, Takeda S, et al. Three novel serum biomarkers, miR-1, miR-133a, and miR-206 for Limb-girdle muscular dystrophy, Facioscapulohumeral muscular dystrophy, and Becker muscular dystrophy. *Environ Health Prev Med.* (2014) 19:452–8. doi: 10.1007/s12199-014-0405-7
21. Coenen-Stass AML, Wood MJA, Roberts TC. Biomarker potential of extracellular miRNAs in duchenne muscular dystrophy. *Trends Mol Med.* (2017) 23:989–1001. doi: 10.1016/j.molmed.2017.09.002
22. Si Y, Cui X, Crossman DK, Hao J, Kazamel M, Kwon Y, et al. Muscle microRNA signatures as biomarkers of disease progression in amyotrophic lateral sclerosis. *Neurobiol Dis.* (2018) 114:85–94. doi: 10.1016/j.nbd.2018.02.009
23. Cheng L, Sharples RA, Scicluna BJ, Hill AF. Exosomes provide a protective and enriched source of miRNA for biomarker profiling compared to intracellular and cell-free blood. *J Extracell Vesicles.* (2014) 3:23743. doi: 10.3402/jev.v3.23743
24. Lopez JP, Diallo A, Cruceanu C, Fiori LM, Laboissiere S, Guillet I, et al. Biomarker discovery: quantification of microRNAs and other small non-coding RNAs using next generation sequencing. *BMC Med Genomics.* (2015) 8:35. doi: 10.1186/s12920-015-0109-x
25. Umu SU, Langseth H, Bucher-Johannessen C, Fromm B, Keller A, Meese E, et al. A comprehensive profile of circulating RNAs in human serum. *RNA Biol.* (2018) 15:242–50. doi: 10.1080/15476286.2017.1403003
26. Zhang L, Yang M, Marks P, White LM, Hurtig M, Mi QS, et al. Serum non-coding RNAs as biomarkers for osteoarthritis progression after ACL injury. *Osteoarthr Cartil.* (2012) 20:1631–7. doi: 10.1016/j.joca.2012.08.016
27. Iliev R, Fedorko M, Machackova T, Mlcochova H, Svoboda M, Pacik D, et al. Expression levels of PIWI-interacting RNA, piR-823, are deregulated in tumor tissue, blood serum and urine of patients with renal cell carcinoma. *Anticancer Res.* (2016) 36:6419–23. doi: 10.21873/anticanres.11239
28. Steinbusch MM, Fang Y, Milner PI, Clegg PD, Young DA, Welting TJ, et al. Serum snoRNAs as biomarkers for joint ageing and post traumatic osteoarthritis. *Sci Rep.* (2017) 7:43558. doi: 10.1038/srep43558
29. Yoffe L, Gilam A, Yaron O, Polsky A, Farberov L, Syngelaki A, et al. Early detection of preeclampsia using circulating small non-coding RNA. *Sci Rep.* (2018) 8:3401. doi: 10.1038/s41598-018-21604-6
30. Liao J, Yu L, Mei Y, Guarnera M, Shen J, Li R, et al. Small nucleolar RNA signatures as biomarkers for non-small-cell lung cancer. *Mol Cancer.* (2010) 9:198. doi: 10.1186/1476-4598-9-198
31. Su Y, Guarnera MA, Fang H, Jiang F. Small non-coding RNA biomarkers in sputum for lung cancer diagnosis. *Mol Cancer.* (2016) 15:36. doi: 10.1186/s12943-016-0520-8
32. Khurana R, Ranches G, Schafferer S, Lukasser M, Rudnicki M, Mayer G, et al. Identification of urinary exosomal noncoding *RNAs* as novel biomarkers in chronic kidney disease. *RNA.* (2017) 23:142–52. doi: 10.1261/rna.058834.116
33. McDonald JS, Milosevic D, Reddi HV, Grebe SK, Algeciras-Schimnich A. Analysis of circulating microRNA: preanalytical and analytical challenges. *Clin Chem.* (2011) 57:833–40. doi: 10.1373/clinchem.2010.157198
34. Kirschner MB, Edelman JJ, Kao SC, Vallely MP, van Zandwijk N, Reid G. The impact of hemolysis on cell-free microRNA biomarkers. *Front Genet.* (2013) 4:94. doi: 10.3389/fgene.2013.00094
35. Moldovan L, Batte KE, Trgovcich J, Wisler J, Marsh CB, Piper M. Methodological challenges in utilizing miRNAs as circulating biomarkers. *J Cell Mol Med.* (2014) 18:371–90. doi: 10.1111/jcmm.12236
36. Mumford SL, Towler BP, Pashler AL, Gilleard O, Martin Y, Newbury SF. Circulating microRNA biomarkers in melanoma: tools and challenges in personalised medicine. *Biomolecules.* (2018) 8:21. doi: 10.3390/biom8020021
37. Katsuura S, Kuwano Y, Yamagishi N, Kurokawa K, Kajita K, Akaike Y, et al. MicroRNAs miR-144/144* and miR-16 in peripheral blood are potential biomarkers for naturalistic stress in healthy Japanese medical students. *Neurosci Lett.* (2012) 516:79–84. doi: 10.1016/j.neulet.2012.03.062
38. Pritchard CC, Kroh E, Wood B, Arroyo JD, Dougherty KJ, Miyaji MM, et al. Blood cell origin of circulating microRNAs: a cautionary note for cancer biomarker studies. *Cancer Prev Res.* (2012) 5:492–7. doi: 10.1158/1940-6207.CAPR-11-0370
39. Caserta S, Kern F, Cohen J, Drage S, Newbury SF, Llewelyn MJ. Circulating plasma microRNAs can differentiate human sepsis and Systemic Inflammatory Response Syndrome (SIRS). *Sci Rep.* (2016) 6:28006. doi: 10.1038/srep28006

6

Metabolomics Biomarkers: A Strategy Toward Therapeutics Improvement in ALS

*Débora Lanznaster[1], Denis Reis de Assis[1], Philippe Corcia[1,2,3], Pierre-François Pradat[4,5,6] and Hélène Blasco[1,7]**

[1] Université de Tours, Inserm U1253, Tours, France, [2] Centre Constitutif SLA, CHRU Bretonneau, Tours, France, [3] Federation des centres SLA de Tours et Limoges, LITORALS, Tours, France, [4] Département des Maladies du Système Nerveux, Centre Référent Maladie Rare SLA, Hôpital de la Pitié-Salpêtrière, Paris, France, [5] Laboratoire d'Imagerie Biomédicale, Sorbonne Université, CNRS, INSERM, Paris, France, [6] Northern Ireland Centre for Stratified Medicine, Biomedical Sciences Research Institute Ulster University, C-TRIC, Altnagelvin Hospital, Londonderry, United Kingdom, [7] Service de Biochimie et Biologie Moléculaire, CHRU de Tours, Tours, France

***Correspondence:**
Hélène Blasco
helene.blasco@univ-tours.fr

Biomarkers research in amyotrophic lateral sclerosis (ALS) holds the promise of improving ALS diagnosis, follow-up of patients, and clinical trials outcomes. Metabolomics have a big impact on biomarkers identification. In this mini-review, we provide the main findings of metabolomics studies in ALS and discuss the most relevant therapeutics attempts that targeted some prominent alterations found in ALS, like glutamate excitotoxicity, oxidative stress, alterations in energetic metabolism, and creatinine levels. Metabolomics studies have reported putative diagnosis or prognosis biomarkers, but discrepancies among these studies did not allow validation of metabolic biomarkers for clinical use in ALS. In this context, we wonder whether metabolomics knowledge could improve ALS therapeutics. As metabolomics identify specific metabolic pathways modified by disease progression and/or treatment, we support that adjuvant or combined treatment should be used to rescue these pathways, creating a new perspective for ALS treatment. Some ongoing clinical trials are already trying to target these pathways. As clinical trials in ALS have been disappointing and considering the heterogeneity of the disease presentation, we support the application of a pharmacometabolomic approach to evaluate the individual response to drug treatments and their side effects, enabling the development of personalized treatments for ALS. We suggest that the best strategy to apply metabolomics for ALS therapeutics progress is to establish a metabolic signature for ALS patients in order to improve the knowledge of patient metabotypes, to choose the most adequate pharmacological treatment, and to follow the drug response and side effects, based on metabolomics biomarkers.

Keywords: ALS, metabolomics, pharmacometabolomics, therapeutic, creatinine

INTRODUCTION

Amyotrophic lateral sclerosis (ALS) is the most common adult-onset motor neuron disease, which ultimately leads to death due to respiratory failure usually 3–5 years after the appearance of first symptoms. ALS wandering diagnosis spreads ~12 months after symptoms onset—this long delay being partly related to the lack of specific diagnostic tests. Today, only two pharmacological treatments are approved for ALS: riluzole and edaravone, which only show small effects on survival and decline of functional impairment, respectively. Numerous clinical trials have been conducted on the identification of new therapies for ALS, but their findings are disappointing. One of the reasons of these failures could be the use of inappropriate methodology in the clinical studies, like poor design or lack of appropriate cohort enrichment strategies (1). Early diagnosis could also increase recruitment of patients in earlier stages of the disease to clinical trials (2). Moreover, the functional scales used to assess motor function in ALS patients (ALS Functional Rating Scale-Revised; ALSFRS-R, forced vital capacity, and muscular testing) may be insensitive to subtly follow drug response. Thus, the search and identification of reliable biomarkers for ALS diagnosis and prognosis is of utmost importance, as biomarkers follow-up could help in the identification of drug-response phenotypes, improving evaluation of treatment efficacy.

"Omics" research comprise systemic analyses (including transcriptomics, genomics, proteomics, lipidomics, and metabolomics) that advanced immensely in the field of biomarkers. For example, proteomics research identified a structural neuronal protein, the neurofilament, as a putative biomarker for ALS, especially for ALS diagnosis regarding its sensitivity and specificity (3). Neurofilaments also showed promising results in the field of prognostic prediction factors (4–6), but its application was not yet validated in the clinical practice.

Metabolomics studies identified several metabolites related to pathways implicated in the pathophysiology of ALS, both in animal models and in ALS patients, thus improving our knowledge about the disease mechanisms (7, 8). These metabolites could represent ALS biomarkers alone or in combination, by composing a metabolic signature for ALS. Furthermore, as identified metabolites are related to pathways that are modified in the disease, adjuvant therapy could target these pathways, and compensate their dysfunction. Identification of metabolic signatures also enables a personalized therapy and the direct follow up of drug effect in each patient—a proposition of a new field called pharmacometabolomics. In this review, we provide the main findings of metabolomics studies in ALS for biomarkers identification or for understanding ALS pathophysiology. Furthermore, we summarize recent evidence that support metabolomics applications in the clinical practice, as improvement of therapeutics and treatment follow-up. Here, we shed a light into other applications of metabolomics knowledge through the extension of its interest beyond the biomarkers research.

WHAT CAN METABOLOMICS ANALYSES TELL US?

Metabolomics is based on the global search for metabolites, defined as small molecules that represent the downstream products of ongoing biological processes in cells, tissues, and other biological samples (9). A particular metabolic profile—or "metabotype"—of a systemic biofluid (such as blood or the cerebrospinal fluid, CSF) reflects directly the metabolic status of different organs and tissues because of continuous exchanges of metabolites between tissues and fluids (7). To design a metabolic profile, metabolites are selected according to their polarity, mass, and concentrations using high-throughput techniques (10). After data pre-treatment, metabolites are analyzed by univariate analysis and multivariate analysis to identify the most important contributors to the discrimination between samples (11, 12).

Metabolomics research identified several individual metabolites and metabolic signatures (with or without identification of each metabolite composing such signature) that can discriminate ALS from non-ALS cases (10, 13–16). Metabolomics can also determine metabolic signatures that identify distinct subgroups of ALS patients according to their clinical characteristics or disease evolution (17–19). Altogether, the main objectives of metabolomics studies performed in ALS have been punctually reached. However, its application in the clinical routine or its extension to other aims (for example, for following drug responses) will depend on the ability to overcome several limitations of the method—for example, the differences in samples treatment, data analysis, and lack of external validation for many of these identified signatures.

METABOLOMICS STUDIES IDENTIFIED METABOLITES RELATED WITH PATHOPHYSIOLOGICAL MECHANISMS IN ALS

Although the exact mechanism that initiate ALS pathogenesis remain partially unknown, glutamatergic excitotoxicity, oxidative stress, and mitochondrial dysfunction have been reported as key contributors to the motor neuron degeneration (20). Metabolomics may provide a new light to evaluate these pathophysiological pathways by identifying metabolites directly associated with these pathways (8). Here we summarize the main findings of metabolomics studies linked with the most prominent pathophysiological alterations observed in ALS patients. Interestingly, these alterations were also observed in ALS models.

Glutamate

Glutamate plays a key role in ALS, as it is not only involved in excitotoxicity, but also in other mechanisms such as oxidative stress and metabolism disturbance (21). The only treatment approved that counteract the glutamatergic hyperactivation in ALS is riluzole, a non-competitive blocker of glutamatergic transmission (22–24). Glutamate remains the most cited metabolite increased in blood samples (12, 25, 26) and CSF (25, 27–29) from ALS patients, as reported by independent research groups. Recently, a metabolomics study proposed glutamic acid as a potential biomarker for ALS, after validating it in a healthy cohort (30). The increase of glutamate in CSF could be linked with the decrease in astrocytic glutamate transporter (GLT)-1 expression in motor cortex and spinal cord observed in ALS patients (17, 31, 32). Interestingly, ALS animal models also present alterations in glutamate levels (33–35). Rats expressing the ALS-linked familial mutation Super Oxide Dismutase-1 (SOD1)-G93A showed a decrease in the astrocytic glutamate transporter expression in the spinal cord (36), as reported in ALS patients. Is important to note that astrocytes have been pointed as key elements in the pathophysiology of ALS, as is for their role in mediating glutamatergic activation or as for their metabolic support to neurons (37).

Antioxidants

Oxidative stress is also a well-known mechanism involved in ALS and is directly linked with glutamatergic toxicity that increases the production of reactive oxygen species (ROS) (38, 39). Astrocytes release ascorbic acid (an endogenous antioxidant) after glutamatergic stimulation, and the elevated level of ascorbate in the CSF of ALS patients may reflect a compensatory mechanism (11, 40). Another antioxidant metabolite, uric acid, was shown to be involved in ALS pathophysiology. Increased levels of uric acid were suggested to be associated with a slow progression of ALS (41, 42). Homocysteine, another endogenous antioxidant, was also pointed by metabolomics studies as a potential biomarker for ALS (30, 39).

Lipids

ALS patients usually present compromised energy homeostasis, including basal hypermetabolism, body weight loss, and abnormal metabolism of glucose and lipids (43, 44). In agreement with that, ALS patients present a 10-fold increase in the cholesterol esters C16:0 and C18:0 in the spinal cord, while in a mice model of ALS these substances are increased by 4- and 10-fold in the lower spinal cord during the presymptomatic and symptomatic phases, respectively (45). *Postmortem* analyses show that the spinal cord tissue from ALS patients presents a remarkable decrease in docosahexaenoic acid (DHA) levels and in n-3 polyunsaturated fatty acids (PUFA), in sharp contrast with the increase of DHA content found in the brain cortex (46).

Creatinine

Reduced levels of creatinine in the CSF or blood from ALS patients were reported from different research groups, including metabolomics studies (42, 47–49). Creatinine reflects skeletal muscle production and reduced levels of this metabolite are directly related to amyotrophy, a cardinal ALS symptom. Use of plasma creatinine levels as a biomarker in ALS was suggested for monitoring disease progression in clinical trials (50), and creatinine was the first metabolite already used to evaluate drug therapy response to dexpramipexole in a clinical trial (51).

Findings regarding metabolomics are promising but disappointing, as, to date, no biomarker was approved for diagnosis or prognosis use (10). To go further with this approach, well-designed and large cohorts studies would be essential for biomarker validation (52), and the improvement of analytical and statistical steps may improve the robustness of the strategy (16, 19). Importantly, all metabolomics studies published so far have identified metabolites linked to the same pathophysiological pathways, thus reinforcing the potential of metabolomics to explain pathophysiological mechanisms underlying ALS. In this context, we suggest that metabolomics analyses may be useful for other applications than identifying diagnostic or prognostic biomarkers, such as for example, monitoring disease course and identifying treatment outcomes and side effects in clinical trials.

METABOLOMICS-IDENTIFIED ALTERATIONS AS TARGETS FOR NEW THERAPEUTIC STRATEGIES

Disturbed pathways identified through metabolomics studies in cellular and animal models, as well as in ALS patients, hold the potential to be used for the discovery of new therapies in ALS (48). The application of metabolomics findings in preclinical and clinical studies to target glutamatergic toxicity (21) and energy metabolism dysfunction (44) were already reviewed. Thus, here we will summarize the ongoing therapeutics attempts that target alterations identified by metabolomics studies and with beneficial effects in ALS preclinical tests (**Table 1**).

As mentioned before, metabolomics and non-metabolomics studies demonstrated alterations in glutamate levels in CFS and blood of ALS patients. Several clinical trials tried to demonstrate the effect of anti-glutamatergic drugs—already approved for the treatment of other neurological diseases—for the treatment of ALS, but failed to show any improvements. This is the case for lamotrigine, topiramate, gabapentin, and talampanel (21). Current active clinical trials investigate the potential effect of memantine and perampanel in ALS, drugs used for Alzheimer's disease and epilepsy treatment, respectively (21).

Focusing on oxidative stress (as edaravone, the recent drug approved by the FDA for ALS treatment that is a ROS scavenger), a clinical trial is investigating the effect of inosine treatment for

TABLE 1 | Ongoing clinical trials with therapeutics interventions focused in alterations identified by metabolomics studies.

Target	Intervention	Clinical trials for ALS
Glutamatergic overactivation	Perampanel	Phase II, NCT03377309 (Lebanon); NCT03019419 (Japan); NCT03020797 (Unites States).
	Memantine	Ongoing (phase II, NCT02118727, Unites States). [No effect observed in phase II-III; (53)].
Oxidative stress	Inosine	Phase I, NCT02288091 (United States).
	CC100	Phase I, NCT03049046 (United States).
Hypermetabolism	Triheptanoin	Phase I-II, NCT03506425 (United States).
	High caloric fatty diet	NCT02306590 (Germany).
	Oral nutritional supplementation (high fat and protein)	NCT02152449 (France).

Information available in clinicaltrials.gov.

ALS. Inosine is a precursor of uric acid, an antioxidant molecule that is found altered in ALS patients. Furthermore, this clinical trial will follow therapy response by analyzing uric acid levels in treated individuals, applying metabolomics approaches both at treatment strategy and follow-up. CC100 (a synthetic form of the caffeic acid phenethyl ester) is another molecule with antioxidant properties that is currently being investigated in a Phase I clinical trial. The caffeic acid phenethyl ester is a natural compound with effects on lipid peroxidation and lipid metabolism (54).

Considering that energy metabolism is also altered in ALS patients, several studies focused in providing additional fuel to increase energy uptake (44). While preclinical studies successfully showed the beneficial effects of these treatments, clinical trials failed to show the same results. In the case of dexpramipexole (an improver of oxidative phosphorylation and thus of ATP synthesis), a Phase II clinical trial showed prevention of functional decline of ALS patients following a 12-month treatment (55). However, Phase III failed to show improvements (56). A Phase II clinical trial performed between 2009 and 2012 analyzed the beneficial effects of two hypercaloric (one high-fat and other high-carbohydrate) diets in ALS patients receiving enteral nutrition. Patients receiving a high-carbohydrate enteral formula presented less adverse effects compared to control subjects. They found that both diets were safe and tolerable, although they did not modify disease progression (57). Currently, ongoing clinical trials investigate the effect of high caloric fatty supplementation (Calogen®) and high caloric protein/fat supplementation (Fortimel®) in ALS patients.

Novel therapeutic strategies may focus on creatinine as a marker to identify the efficacy of drugs and follow-up of treatments aiming the inhibition of the muscular loss observed in ALS, or even in treatments aiming the increase of muscle mass in the patients. For example, in ALS animal models, inhibition of myostatin (a negative regulator of muscle growth) improved muscular mass and strength. Although myostatin treatment did not change the disease onset and progression, it improved the muscular function, especially in the diaphragm of the animals (58). If translated for the human disease, it could improve the quality of life of ALS patients during disease progression.

METABOLOMICS-DRIVEN THERAPEUTICS MANAGEMENT: THE ADVENT OF PHARMACOMETABOLOMICS

Metabotype information can be used to identify alterations in biochemical pathways in ALS patients that are modified or not by treatment. This new field, called pharmacometabolomics, allows clinicians to identify a metabolic state at baseline and after drug therapy, increasing information about treatment outcomes, especially drug-response phenotype (59).

Different studies revealed the potential of pharmacometabolomics to assess drug therapy response and identify distinct signatures of metabolites before and after treatment exposure in diverse pathologies, from cancer to cardiovascular diseases. For ALS, one study analyzed metabolites and lipids composition of plasma samples from individuals enrolled in a phase III clinical trial for Olexosime. This study identified a metabolic profile that distinguished the placebo from the Olexosime group, characterized mainly by alterations in the levels of glycine, citrulline/arginine, and kynurenine. Furthermore, clinical progression of ALS correlated with amino acids, lipids, and spermidine levels in the Olexosime group, and with glutamine levels in the placebo group (19). It is noteworthy to highlight that these metabolites are linked with some of the pathological pathways involved in ALS pathology (glutamatergic alteration and energy metabolism dysfunction), as described before.

In practice, pharmacometabolomics findings may improve the strategy of drug administration scheme, as a complementary tool of pharmacokinetics, and may provide new light on drug-response effect and downstream signaling pathways (60). This information may provide details on biochemical pathways involved in disease and in treatment effect in ALS patients in a narrowly controlled process.

METABOLOMICS RESEARCH IN ALS SHOULD IMPROVE THERAPEUTICS—CONCLUDING REMARKS

Metabolomics represent a new approach that is increasingly gaining importance as it helps to identify biomarkers and unravels pathways that contribute to the pathophysiology of ALS. Significant therapeutic advances are based on a deep knowledge of ALS pathogenesis and metabolomics holds great potential to play a key role in this objective. However, despite the efforts made by metabolomics researchers to identify biomarkers for ALS,

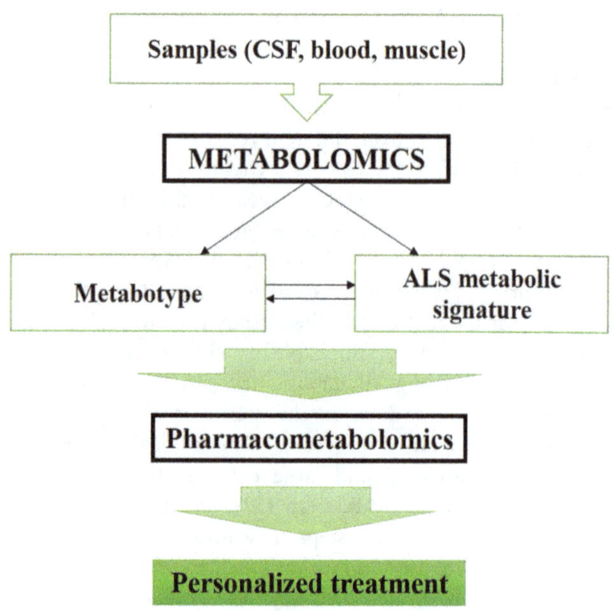

FIGURE 1 | Metabolomics applicability enhance ALS therapeutic management and allows a personalized medicine.

no biomarker was validated yet. Metabolomics studies should rather focus in identifying metabolic signatures then individual biomarkers for ALS. This would be a revolutionary step toward developing efficient strategies to evaluate not only disease progression, but also treatment responses to drug therapies (19).

This also point out the urgent need of metabolomics research to combine analysis and information (1) of different tissues in ALS patients, as CSF, blood and muscle samples; and (2) by combining different approaches (proteomics, transcriptomics, lipidomics, etc.) (52). Combination of "omics" approaches with clinical evaluation (for example, ALSFRS-R) could be the best practice for an early diagnosis of ALS (10). Importantly, omics analysis should be standardized between different research centers together with refinement of statistical analysis tools to analyze better the results obtained. Altogether, these efforts should readily improve metabolomics application in the daily clinical practice.

Metabolomics can also be applied to identify outcomes of pharmacological treatment. Usual parameters and endpoints used in clinical trials to evaluate drug efficacy are probably not enough sensitive to observe a slight effect. In this regard, metabolomics could identify biomarkers that are sensitive enough to detect even small effects of drugs tested in Phase II clinical trials, allowing them to be investigated into Phase III. Furthermore, pharmacometabolomics approaches provide help in evaluating drug effect as a primary or additional parameter. Metabolome may provide longitudinal, reproducible, and objective data that are crucial criteria to evaluate drug effect. Besides, adjuvant therapy based on metabolomics findings could compensate the identified altered pathways in a subtype of patients, allowing a personalized therapeutic strategy targeting specifically these pathways. Ongoing trials using this strategy are presented in **Table 1**. However, no study yet tried to approach several pathways at once, using a combined therapeutic strategy. This approach should be more relevant than focusing only on one altered pathway.

Metabolomics applied early in ALS management should improve therapeutic strategy and development. The major interest of metabolomics at disease onset is to build homogeneous subgroups of patients in order to apply a personalized therapeutic approach (**Figure 1**). Metabolomics complement data obtained from genomics, transcriptomics and proteomics, and combined with pharmacometabolomics approaches, they add the final piece of information to the study of disease pathophysiology and drug response (60). We propose to combine omics and clinical data to improve our comprehension about the specific metabolic pathways affected in each individual patient. Stratification of patients based on all these findings would considerably improve trials methodology and care management, as well as therapeutics strategies by providing a mean to a personalized medicine. To our knowledge, this review is the first to present diagnosis and prognosis biomarkers as an initial step to develop therapeutics. This new light on metabolomics application is promising for complex and heterogeneous diseases, like ALS, characterized by successive therapeutics failures.

AUTHOR CONTRIBUTIONS

DL and HB wrote the manuscript. DL, DRA, PC, PFP and HB critically revised the manuscript for important intellectual content. All authors read and approved the submitted version.

ACKNOWLEDGMENTS

Authors would like to thank the Region Centre-Val de Loire and the program ARD2020 Biopharmaceuticals.

REFERENCES

1. Atassi N. When a negative trial in ALS has a positive effect on research. *Lancet Neurol.* (2018) 17:653–5. doi: 10.1016/S1474-4422(18)30210-2
2. Ryberg H, Bowser R. Protein biomarkers for amyotrophic lateral sclerosis. *Expert Rev Proteomics* (2008) 5:249–62. doi: 10.1586/14789450.5.2.249
3. Goncalves M, Tillack L, de Carvalho M, Pinto S, Conradt HS, Costa J. Phosphoneurofilament heavy chain and N-glycomics from the cerebrospinal fluid in amyotrophic lateral sclerosis. *Clin Chim Acta* (2015) 438:342–9. doi: 10.1016/j.cca.2014.09.011
4. Boylan KB, Glass JD, Crook JE, Yang C, Thomas CS, Desaro P, et al. Phosphorylated neurofilament heavy subunit (pNF-H) in peripheral blood and CSF as a potential prognostic biomarker in amyotrophic lateral sclerosis. *J Neurol Neurosurg Psychiatry* (2013) 84:467–72. doi: 10.1136/jnnp-2012-303768
5. Ganesalingam J, An J, Bowser R, Andersen PM, Shaw CE. pNfH is a promising biomarker for ALS. *Amyotroph Lateral Scler Frontotemporal Degener.* (2013) 14:146–9. doi: 10.3109/21678421.2012.729596
6. Lehnert S, Costa J, de Carvalho M, Kirby J, Kuzma-Kozakiewicz M, Morelli C, et al. Multicentre quality control evaluation of different biomarker candidates for amyotrophic lateral sclerosis. *Amyotroph Lateral Scler Frontotemporal Degener.* (2014) 15:344–50. doi: 10.3109/21678421.2014.884592
7. Kumar A, Ghosh D, Singh RL. Amyotrophic lateral sclerosis and metabolomics: clinical implication and therapeutic approach. *J Biomark.* (2013) 2013:538765. doi: 10.1155/2013/538765
8. Blasco H, Vourc'h P, Pradat PF, Gordon PH, Andres CR, Corcia P. Further development of biomarkers in amyotrophic lateral sclerosis. *Expert Rev Mol Diagn.* (2016) 16:853–68. doi: 10.1080/14737159.2016.1199277
9. Forsberg EM, Huan T, Rinehart D, Benton HP, Warth B, Hilmers B, et al. Data processing, multi-omic pathway mapping, and metabolite activity analysis using XCMS Online. *Nat Protoc.* (2018) 13:633–51. doi: 10.1038/nprot.2017.151
10. Blasco H, Nadal-Desbarats L, Pradat PF, Gordon PH, Madji Hounoum B, Patin F, et al. Biomarkers in amyotrophic lateral sclerosis: combining metabolomic and clinical parameters to define disease progression. *Eur J Neurol.* (2016) 23:346–53. doi: 10.1111/ene.12851
11. Blasco HCorcia P, Moreau C, Veau S, Fournier C, Vourc'h P, et al. 1H-NMR-based metabolomic profiling of CSF in early amyotrophic lateral sclerosis. *PLoS ONE* (2010) 5:e13223. doi: 10.1371/journal.pone.0013223
12. Kumar A, Bala L, Kalita J, Misra UK, Singh RL, Khetrapal CL, et al. Metabolomic analysis of serum by (1) H NMR spectroscopy in amyotrophic lateral sclerosis. *Clin Chim Acta* (2010) 411:563–7. doi: 10.1016/j.cca.2010.01.016
13. Sussmuth SD, Brettschneider J, Ludolph AC, Tumani H. Biochemical markers in CSF of ALS patients. *Curr Med Chem.* (2008) 15:1788–801. doi: 10.2174/092986708785133031

14. Tumani H, Teunissen C, Sussmuth S, Otto M, Ludolph AC, Brettschneider J. Cerebrospinal fluid biomarkers of neurodegeneration in chronic neurological diseases. *Expert Rev Mol Diagn.* (2008) 8:479–94. doi: 10.1586/14737159.8.4.479
15. Mitchell RM, Freeman WM, Randazzo WT, Stephens HE, Beard JL, Simmons Z, et al. A CSF biomarker panel for identification of patients with amyotrophic lateral sclerosis. *Neurology* (2009) 72:14–9. doi: 10.1212/01.wnl.0000333251.36681.a5
16. Blasco H, Corcia P, Pradat PF, Bocca C, Gordon PH, Veyrat-Durebex C, et al. Metabolomics in cerebrospinal fluid of patients with amyotrophic lateral sclerosis: an untargeted approach via high-resolution mass spectrometry. *J Proteome Res.* (2013) 12:3746–54. doi: 10.1021/pr400376e
17. Wuolikainen A, Moritz T, Marklund SL, Antti H, Andersen PM. Disease-related changes in the cerebrospinal fluid metabolome in amyotrophic lateral sclerosis detected by GC/TOFMS. *PLoS ONE* (2011) 6:e17947. doi: 10.1371/journal.pone.0017947
18. Wuolikainen A, Andersen PM, Moritz T, Marklund SL, Antti H. ALS patients with mutations in the SOD1 gene have an unique metabolomic profile in the cerebrospinal fluid compared with ALS patients without mutations. *Mol Genet Metab.* (2012) 105:472–8. doi: 10.1016/j.ymgme.2011.11.201
19. Blasco H, Patin F, Descat A, Garcon G, Corcia P, Gele P, et al. A pharmaco-metabolomics approach in a clinical trial of ALS: identification of predictive markers of progression. *PLoS ONE* (2018) 13:e0198116. doi: 10.1371/journal.pone.0198116
20. Vucic S, Kiernan MC. Pathophysiology of neurodegeneration in familial amyotrophic lateral sclerosis. *Curr Mol Med.* (2009) 9:255–72. doi: 10.2174/156652409787847173
21. Blasco H, Mavel S, Corcia P, Gordon PH. The glutamate hypothesis in ALS: pathophysiology and drug development. *Curr Med Chem.* (2014) 21:3551–75. doi: 10.2174/0929867321666140916120118
22. Doble A. The pharmacology and mechanism of action of riluzole. *Neurology* (1996) 47(6 Suppl. 4):S233–S241.
23. Zarate CA, Manji HK. Riluzole in psychiatry: a systematic review of the literature. *Expert Opin Drug Metab Toxicol.* (2008) 4:1223–34. doi: 10.1517/17425255.4.9.1223
24. Menon P, Kiernan MC, Vucic S. Biomarkers and future targets for development in amyotrophic lateral sclerosis. *Curr Med Chem.* (2014) 21:3535–50. doi: 10.2174/0929867321666140601161148
25. Spreux-Varoquaux O, Bensimon G, Lacomblez L, Salachas F, Pradat PF, Le Forestier N, et al. Glutamate levels in cerebrospinal fluid in amyotrophic lateral sclerosis: a reappraisal using a new HPLC method with coulometric detection in a large cohort of patients. *J Neurol Sci.* (2002) 193:73–8. doi: 10.1016/S0022-510X(01)00661-X
26. Andreadou E, Kapaki E, Kokotis P, Paraskevas GP, Katsaros N, Libitaki G, et al. Plasma glutamate and glycine levels in patients with amyotrophic lateral sclerosis: the effect of riluzole treatment. *Clin Neurol Neurosurg.* (2008) 110:222–6. doi: 10.1016/j.clineuro.2007.10.018
27. Niebroj-Dobosz I, Jamrozik Z, Janik P, Hausmanowa-Petrusewicz I, Kwiecinski H. Anti-neural antibodies in serum and cerebrospinal fluid of amyotrophic lateral sclerosis (ALS) patients. *Acta Neurol Scand.* (1999) 100:238–43.
28. Zhao W, Xie W, Le W, Beers DR, He Y, Henkel JS, et al. Activated microglia initiate motor neuron injury by a nitric oxide and glutamate-mediated mechanism. *J Neuropathol Exp Neurol.* (2004) 63:964–77. doi: 10.1093/jnen/63.9.964
29. Fiszman ML, Ricart KC, Latini A, Rodriguez G, Sica RE. *In vitro* neurotoxic properties and excitatory aminoacids concentration in the cerebrospinal fluid of amyotrophic lateral sclerosis patients. Relationship with the degree of certainty of disease diagnoses. *Acta Neurol Scand.* (2010) 121:120–6. doi: 10.1111/j.1600-0404.2009.01200.x
30. Cieslarova Z, Lopes FS, do Lago CL, Franca MC Jr, Colnaghi Simionato AV. Capillary electrophoresis tandem mass spectrometry determination of glutamic acid and homocysteine's metabolites: potential biomarkers of amyotrophic lateral sclerosis. *Talanta* (2017) 170:63–8. doi: 10.1016/j.talanta.2017.03.103
31. Rothstein JD, Tsai G, Kuncl RW, Clawson L, Cornblath DR, Drachman DB, et al. Abnormal excitatory amino acid metabolism in amyotrophic lateral sclerosis. *Ann Neurol.* (1990) 28:18–25. doi: 10.1002/ana.410280106
32. Rothstein JD, Van Kammen M, Levey AI, Martin LJ, Kuncl RW. Selective loss of glial glutamate transporter GLT-1 in amyotrophic lateral sclerosis. *Ann Neurol.* (1995) 38:73–84. doi: 10.1002/ana.410380114
33. Ghoddoussi F, Galloway MP, Jambekar A, Bame M, Needleman R, Brusilow WS. Methionine sulfoximine, an inhibitor of glutamine synthetase, lowers brain glutamine and glutamate in a mouse model of ALS. *J Neurol Sci.* (2010) 290:41–7. doi: 10.1016/j.jns.2009.11.013
34. Valbuena GN, Rizzardini M, Cimini S, Siskos AP, Bendotti C, Cantoni L, et al. Metabolomic analysis reveals increased aerobic glycolysis and amino acid deficit in a cellular model of amyotrophic lateral sclerosis. *Mol Neurobiol.* (2016) 53:2222–40. doi: 10.1007/s12035-015-9165-7
35. Madji Hounoum B, Blasco H, Coque E, Vourc'h P, Emond P, Corcia P, et al. The metabolic disturbances of motoneurons exposed to glutamate. *Mol Neurobiol.* (2018) 55:7669–76. doi: 10.1007/s12035-018-0945-8
36. Howland DS, Liu J, She Y, Goad B, Maragakis NJ, Kim B, et al. Focal loss of the glutamate transporter EAAT2 in a transgenic rat model of SOD1 mutant-mediated amyotrophic lateral sclerosis (ALS). *Proc Natl Acad Sci USA.* (2002) 99:1604–9. doi: 10.1073/pnas.032539299
37. Lee J, Hyeon SJ, Im H, Ryu H, Kim Y. Astrocytes and microglia as non-cell autonomous players in the pathogenesis of ALS. *Exp Neurobiol.* (2016) 25:233–40. doi: 10.5607/en.2016.25.5.233
38. Barber SC, Shaw PJ. Oxidative stress in ALS: key role in motor neuron injury and therapeutic target. *Free Radic Biol Med.* (2010) 48:629–41. doi: 10.1016/j.freeradbiomed.2009.11.018
39. Blasco H, Garcon G, Patin F, Veyrat-Durebex C, Boyer J, Devos D, et al. Panel of oxidative stress and inflammatory biomarkers in ALS: a pilot study. *Can J Neurol Sci.* (2017) 44:90–5. doi: 10.1017/cjn.2016.284
40. Ihara Y, Nobukuni K, Takata H, Hayabara T. Oxidative stress and metal content in blood and cerebrospinal fluid of amyotrophic lateral sclerosis patients with and without a Cu, Zn-superoxide dismutase mutation. *Neurol Res.* (2005) 27:105–8. doi: 10.1179/016164105X18430
41. Ikeda K, Hirayama T, Takazawa T, Kawabe K, Iwasaki Y. Relationships between disease progression and serum levels of lipid, urate, creatinine and ferritin in Japanese patients with amyotrophic lateral sclerosis: a cross-sectional study. *Intern Med.* (2012) 51:1501–8. doi: 10.2169/internalmedicine.51.7465
42. Atassi N, Berry J, Shui A, Zach N, Sherman A, Sinani E, et al. The PRO-ACT database: design, initial analyses, and predictive features. *Neurology* (2014) 83:1719–25. doi: 10.1212/WNL.0000000000000951
43. Dupuis L, Pradat PF, Ludolph AC, Loeffler JP. Energy metabolism in amyotrophic lateral sclerosis. *Lancet Neurol.* (2011) 10:75–82. doi: 10.1016/S1474-4422(10)70224-6
44. Tefera TW, Borges K. Metabolic dysfunctions in amyotrophic lateral sclerosis pathogenesis and potential metabolic treatments. *Front Neurosci.* (2016) 10:611. doi: 10.3389/fnins.2016.00611
45. Cutler RG, Pedersen WA, Camandola S, Rothstein JD, Mattson MP. Evidence that accumulation of ceramides and cholesterol esters mediates oxidative stress–induced death of motor neurons in amyotrophic lateral sclerosis. *Ann Neurol.* (2002) 52:448–57. doi: 10.1002/ana.10312
46. Ilieva EV, Ayala V, Jové M, Dalfó E, Cacabelos D, Povedano M, et al. Oxidative and endoplasmic reticulum stress interplay in sporadic amyotrophic lateral sclerosis. *Brain* (2007) 130:3111–23. doi: 10.1093/brain/awm190
47. Lawton KA, Brown MV, Alexander D, Li Z, Wulff JE, Lawson R, et al. Plasma metabolomic biomarker panel to distinguish patients with amyotrophic lateral sclerosis from disease mimics. *Amyotroph Lateral Scler Frontotemporal Degener.* (2014) 15:362–70. doi: 10.3109/21678421.2014.908311
48. Kori M, Aydin B, Unal S, Arga KY, Kazan D. Metabolic biomarkers and neurodegeneration: a pathway enrichment analysis of Alzheimer's disease, Parkinson's disease, and amyotrophic lateral sclerosis. *OMICS* (2016) 20:645–61. doi: 10.1089/omi.2016.0106
49. Wuolikainen A, Jonsson P, Ahnlund M, Antti H, Marklund SL, Moritz T, et al. Multi-platform mass spectrometry analysis of the CSF and plasma metabolomes of rigorously matched amyotrophic lateral sclerosis, Parkinson's disease and control subjects. *Mol Biosyst.* (2016) 12:1287–98. doi: 10.1039/c5mb00711a
50. van Eijk RPA, Eijkemans MJC, Ferguson TA, Nikolakopoulos S, Veldink JH, van den Berg LH. Monitoring disease progression with plasma creatinine

in amyotrophic lateral sclerosis clinical trials. *J Neurol Neurosurg Psychiatry* (2018) 89:156–61. doi: 10.1136/jnnp-2017-317077

51. Bozik ME, Mitsumoto H, Brooks BR, Rudnicki SA, Moore DH, Zhang B, et al. A *post hoc* analysis of subgroup outcomes and creatinine in the phase III clinical trial (EMPOWER) of dexpramipexole in ALS. *Amyotroph Lateral Scler Frontotemporal Degener.* (2014) 15:406–13. doi: 10.3109/21678421.2014.943672
52. Mitropoulos K, Katsila T, Patrinos GP, Pampalakis G. Multi-omics for biomarker discovery and target validation in biofluids for amyotrophic lateral sclerosis diagnosis. *OMICS* (2018) 22:52–64. doi: 10.1089/omi.2017.0183
53. de Carvalho M, Pinto S, Costa J, Evangelista T, Ohana B, Pinto A. A randomized, placebo-controlled trial of memantine for functional disability in amyotrophic lateral sclerosis. *Amyotroph Lateral Scler.* (2010) 11:456–60. doi: 10.3109/17482968.2010.498521
54. Gong P, Chang X, Chen X, Bai X, Wen H, Pi S, et al. Metabolomics study of cadmium-induced diabetic nephropathy and protective effect of caffeic acid phenethyl ester using UPLC-Q-TOF-MS combined with pattern recognition. *Environ Toxicol Pharmacol.* (2017) 54:80–92. doi: 10.1016/j.etap.2017.06.021
55. Cudkowicz M, Bozik ME, Ingersoll EW, Miller R, Mitsumoto H, Shefner J, et al. The effects of dexpramipexole (KNS-760704) in individuals with amyotrophic lateral sclerosis. *Nat Med.* (2011) 17:1652–6. doi: 10.1038/nm.2579
56. Cudkowicz ME, van den Berg LH, Shefner JM, Mitsumoto H, Mora JS, Ludolph A, et al. Dexpramipexole versus placebo for patients with amyotrophic lateral sclerosis (EMPOWER): a randomised, double-blind, phase 3 trial. *Lancet Neurol.* (2013) 12:1059–67. doi: 10.1016/S1474-4422(13)70221-7
57. Wills AM, Hubbard J, Macklin EA, Glass J, Tandan R, Simpson EP, et al. Hypercaloric enteral nutrition in patients with amyotrophic lateral sclerosis: a randomised, double-blind, placebo-controlled phase 2 trial. *Lancet* (2014) 383:2065–72. doi: 10.1016/S0140-6736(14)60222-1
58. Holzbaur EL, Howland DS, Weber N, Wallace K, She Y, Kwak S, et al. Myostatin inhibition slows muscle atrophy in rodent models of amyotrophic lateral sclerosis. *Neurobiol Dis.* (2006) 23:697–707. doi: 10.1016/j.nbd.2006.05.009
59. Balashova EE, Maslov DL, Lokhov PG. A metabolomics approach to pharmacotherapy personalization. *J Pers Med.* (2018) 8:3. doi: 10.3390/jpm8030028
60. Kaddurah-Daouk R, Weinshilboum RM. Pharmacometabolomics: implications for clinical pharmacology and systems pharmacology. *Clin Pharmacol Ther.* (2014) 95:154–67. doi: 10.1038/clpt.2013.217

7

Biological Significance of microRNA Biomarkers in ALS—Innocent Bystanders or Disease Culprits?

*Sophie Foggin, Raquel Mesquita-Ribeiro, Federico Dajas-Bailador and Rob Layfield**

School of Life Sciences, University of Nottingham Medical School, Nottingham, United Kingdom

Correspondence:
Rob Layfield
robert.layfield@nottingham.ac.uk

MicroRNAs (miRNAs) represent potential biomarkers for neurodegenerative disorders including amyotrophic lateral sclerosis (ALS). However, whether expression changes of individual miRNAs are simply an indication of cellular dysfunction and degeneration, or actually promote functional changes in target gene expression relevant to disease pathogenesis, is unclear. Here we used bioinformatics to test the hypothesis that ALS-associated miRNAs exert their effects through targeting genes implicated in disease etiology. We documented deregulated miRNAs identified in studies of ALS patients, noting variations in participants, tissue samples, miRNA detection or quantification methods used, and functional or bioinformatic assessments (if performed). Despite lack of experimental standardization, overlap of many deregulated miRNAs between studies was noted; however, direction of reported expression changes did not always concur. The use of *in silico* predictions of target genes for the most commonly deregulated miRNAs, cross-referenced to a selection of previously identified ALS genes, did not support our hypothesis. Specifically, although deregulated miRNAs were predicted to commonly target ALS genes, random miRNAs gave similar predictions. To further investigate biological patterns in the deregulated miRNAs, we grouped them by tissue source in which they were identified, indicating that for a core of frequently detected miRNAs, blood/plasma/serum may be useful for future profiling experiments. We conclude that *in silico* predictions of gene targets of deregulated ALS miRNAs, at least using currently available algorithms, are unlikely to be sufficient in informing disease pathomechanisms. We advocate experimental functional testing of candidate miRNAs and their predicted targets, propose miRNAs to prioritise, and suggest a concerted move towards protocol standardization for biomarker identification.

Keywords: microRNA, amyotrophic lateral sclerosis, ALS, MND, biomarker, ALS genes, bioinformatics, neurodegeneration

INTRODUCTION

MicroRNAs (miRNAs) are small non-coding RNAs, typically 20–22 nucleotides (nt) long, which act as post-transcriptional regulators of gene expression (1). MiRNA seed sequences provide specificity for the 3′ untranslated region (UTR) of target mRNA, leading to mRNA degradation or translational inhibition (2). Around a third of human gene products are regulated by miRNAs (3), being present in both intracellular and extracellular environments and in almost all biological fluids (4, 5). Extracellularly, miRNAs are detected within membrane vesicles and also freely, forming complexes with other macromolecules (6).

Amyotrophic lateral sclerosis (ALS) is characterized by the progressive loss of upper and lower motor neurons in the spinal cord, cerebral cortex, and brainstem, resulting in muscle weakness and wasting (7, 8). Life expectancy is 2–5 years after onset (9). Approximately 5% of ALS patients develop frontotemporal dementia (FTD) and the ALS-FTD spectrum is hereafter referred to as ALS (10). Around 90% of ALS cases are sporadic (sALS) and 10% are familial (fALS), being associated with inherited mutations. Multiple genes have been linked with ALS (11). Interestingly, some ALS-associated genes, including *TARDBP* and *FUS*, encode RNA-binding proteins which are involved in miRNA processing (12), and indirectly implicate miRNAs in ALS pathophysiology. However in addition to RNA metabolism, ALS-associated genes show diverse functions, with roles in intracellular transport, proteostasis, axonal outgrowth, and glutamatergic signaling (7).

MiRNAs are unusually well-preserved in a range of biological samples, including blood plasma, serum, and cerebrospinal fluid, and are measurable with greater sensitivity and stability than proteins (5, 13). As a result, the last decade has seen a drive to identify specific miRNA biomarkers for ALS, in order to potentiate more rapid and accurate diagnosis, disease stratification and monitoring. Numerous studies have demonstrated deregulation of miRNAs in ALS patients, most aiming to identify clinically-relevant biomarkers.

Relevant to the ALS context, CSF miRNAs are potentially good representatives of central nervous system (CNS) disorders, since a blood-CSF barrier would prevent CNS miRNA dilution in the wider circulation (14). However, it is possible for miRNAs to transfer across this barrier, such that blood miRNAs may provide a window on nervous system dysfunction (15). Although the functional significance of circulating miRNAs is less clear, it has been demonstrated that cells can transfer functional miRNAs between one another in an exosome-mediated manner (16). It has been proposed cells can select the miRNAs to be released (17), although cells also shed material when degenerating. Thus, extracellular vesicles (EVs) may reflect the cells of origin, and some of these circulating miRNAs potentially mirror ALS pathophysiology.

Despite considerable efforts, no specific, robust diagnostic molecular biomarker set has been identified for ALS (18). Recently, Dardiotis et al. (19) reviewed the results of 24 studies, from 2010 to 2017, documenting miRNAs reported in ALS biomarker studies, aiming to clarify those most appropriate for future evaluation. In this same Frontiers issue, Joilin et al. (20) review recent attempts to define a "biomarker-relevant" signature of miRNAs, discussing their great potential and the challenges once the field moves toward clinical validation. However, beyond the key importance of biomarker identification, most studies so far do not attempt systematic bioinformatic or experimental functional interpretation of transcripts targeted by ALS-relevant miRNAs. Consequently, whether changes in miRNA expression simply reflect cellular dysfunction and degeneration, or are active participants in the functional changes of target genes relevant to disease pathogenesis, is unknown.

Here, we also focus on miRNA profiling studies comparing expression levels of miRNAs from ALS patients and controls, over the 2013–2018 period. Our approach aims to evaluate various strategies that can be used to analyse these deregulated miRNAs: *number of reported studies for a given miRNA*, *predicted functional targets*, and *tissue distribution* (i.e., where detected). We document the overlap between miRNAs reported as deregulated in these studies; and for these miRNAs, propose a series of *in silico* methods to identify those predicted to target known ALS genes, evaluating current limitations of such predictions in informing disease pathogenesis. Finally, we consider the source of patient tissue samples used for miRNA profiling, highlighting overlap of given miRNAs and revealing the importance of sample analyzed.

RESULTS AND DISCUSSION

Literature Analysis

To define relevant studies we performed a PubMed literature search with the MeSH terms "microRNA" AND "amyotrophic lateral sclerosis" from 1/1/2013-31/12/2018. We identified 27 peer-reviewed studies fulfilling our selection criteria, which specifically included those recording and comparing levels of multiple miRNAs directly from ALS patients and controls (**Table S1**). Of these studies, 15 were previously considered by Dardiotis and colleagues, whilst Joilin et al. (20) in this same issue considered 11 of the studies presented here.

Detailed observation noted a large degree of variation between the studies, from sample source (serum, plasma, whole blood, CSF, spinal cord, muscle etc.), numbers and clinical characteristics of patient participants (both sALS and fALS) and controls (healthy and other diseases), to the methods used for sample preparation, miRNA profiling and analysis. Additionally, we identified the need for reporting specific arms of mature miRNAs, since in ambiguous cases we could only assume the dominant strand as that reported/detected (miRBase release 22.1: 2018).

In those few studies that investigate functional implications potentially derived from miRNA changes, a wide variety of bioinformatic approaches were used to identify possible mRNA targets of deregulated miRNAs, including different versions of TargetScan, Pictar, miRanda, DIANA-Tarbase, and miRtarbase. Further attempts to identify those gene/signaling networks targeted, built on protein-protein interaction (PPI) networks, gene ontology and pathway analysis, generating a variety of outcomes (21, 22).

Most Commonly Deregulated microRNAs

As a first approach to select potentially pathologically relevant miRNAs, we ranked them according to the number of times they were reported as deregulated in different studies. In the 27 miRNA profiling studies, a total of 559 miRNAs were shown as deregulated. Among these, nine miRNAs were reported six or more times, compared to 38 reported in five or more studies, directing the threshold selected for our analysis. Those nine most frequently reported ($\geq$6) are shown in **Table 1A**. Since any miRNA deregulation could have deleterious effects on gene targets, initial selection did not discriminate between up- vs. down-regulation. Indeed, for many miRNAs, the reported direction of deregulation was inconsistent between studies, which may be accounted for by differences in the analytical protocol and/or miRNA profiling technique.

Of the most frequently reported miRNAs, hsa-miR-133a-3p was found deregulated in 9/27 studies. The high ranking of hsa-miR-133a-3p may be explained by the fact it is a known myomiR, enriched in muscle tissue (24) and several of the analyzed studies focused on expression levels of myomiRs alone, potentially introducing tissue bias (25–29) (**Table S1**). However despite its myomiR label, hsa-miR-133a-3p has also been suggested as motor neuron enriched (30).

Frequently Deregulated microRNAs and Target Prediction of ALS Genes

To connect biomarker reporting and potential functional relevance we have outlined an *in silico* method to determine whether these commonly reported miRNAs preferentially target selected known ALS-associated genes (http://alsod.iop.kcl.ac.uk/ [last updated 2015], an ALS bioinformatics repository online database) (31). The 37 ALS genes considered were (in alphabetical order):

ALS2, ANG, ARHGEF28, ATXN2, C9orf72, CHCHD10, CHGB, CHMP2B, CRYM, DAO, DCTN1, ERBB4, FIG4, FUS, GLE1, LUM, MATR3, NEFH, OPTN, PARK7, PFN1, PLEKHG5, SETX, SIGMAR1, SOD1, SPG11, SQSTM1, SS18L1, SYNE, TAF15, TARDBP, TBK1, TRPM7, TUBA4A, UBQLN2, VAPB, and *VCP*.

Although not updated since 2015, this database provides information regarding the ALS patients harboring mutations in these genes, such as patient numbers (fALS and sALS), gender and mean onset age as well as site of disease (bulbar/limb). Additionally, all ALS genes reviewed by Kirby et al. (10) except *hnRNPA1* are included in this list. For the prediction analysis we used DIANA-microT-CDS v5.0 (32, 33). As reviewed by Riffo-Campos et al. (34), the DIANA-microT attempts to apply a more balanced predictive approach, displaying TargetScan, and miRanda comparisons in its analysis.

From the *in silico* analysis, 8/9 most frequently deregulated miRNAs were predicted to target at least one of these ALS genes (**Table 1A**), with hsa-miR-9-5p, predicted to target 4/37 of the genes. There appeared to be no obvious relationship between the total number of ALS genes the individual miRNAs were predicted to target and the number of studies reporting these miRNAs as deregulated. The most frequently predicted ALS targeted genes were *ARHGEF28, CHMP2B,* and *MATR3* (2/9 miRNAs). The total count of predicted ALS target genes for the combined nine miRNAs was 18, and overall, 15/37 ALS genes were predicted as targets of at least one of the nine miRNAs. Whilst this approach highlights the potential of *in silico* predictive methods, evaluation of comparable analyses with less frequently reported deregulated miRNAs is also merited.

Other Deregulated microRNAs and Target Prediction of ALS Genes

To determine if the most commonly identified ALS miRNAs are the most relevant, the same analysis must be performed with an identical number (nine) of randomly selected miRNAs, which although reported to be deregulated in the 27 ALS studies, appeared in fewer than six reports. Randomization was achieved by selecting from all deregulated miRNAs, without duplicates, using a Microsoft Excel randomization function. The results of this preliminary analysis are shown in **Table 1B**. Of the nine miRNAs, deregulation was reported in between 1 and 5 (of 27) studies. 7/9 of these randomly selected miRNAs were predicted to target at least one of the 37 ALS genes. Further, one of the miRNAs, hsa-miR-766-3p (deregulated in 2/27 studies) was predicted to target 4/37 ALS genes. The most frequently predicted ALS targeted gene was *ERBB4* (4/9 miRNAs). The total count of predicted ALS target genes for the combined nine miRNAs was 16, comparable to that of the nine most commonly deregulated miRNAs (18, **Table 1A**). Overall, 10/37 ALS genes were predicted as targets of at least one of the nine miRNAs. Although this second analysis could indicate all deregulated miRNAs are equally important in their capacity to potentially target ALS relevant genes, a further *in silico* step requires comparison with a group of miRNAs not deregulated in biomarker studies.

Analysis of Randomly Selected and Non-deregulated microRNAs

To investigate if predicted gene targets for deregulated ALS miRNAs reflected an enrichment compared to non-deregulated miRNAs, we performed an example test with nine randomly selected mature miRNAs not reported as deregulated in any of the 27 studies and performed the same analysis (**Table 1C**). We selected from all *Homo sapien* mature miRNA sequences recorded on miRBase release 22.1: October 2018 (35). One of the random miRNAs, hsa-miR-603-3p, was predicted to target 6/37 of the ALS genes, including *ERBB4*. The major ALS gene, *TARDBP*, was predicted most frequently (3/9 miRNAs).

Compared to the nine most frequently reported (**Table 1A**) or not frequently reported deregulated miRNAs (**Table 1B**), this random miRNA selection gave a total count of 13 predicted ALS target genes (**Table 1C**), representing only 8/37 of the ALS genes. Notably, 5/9 of these random miRNAs were predicted to target at least one of the 37 ALS genes. Further selections of different sets of nine random miRNAs showed similar results (not shown).

The systematic approach outlined above would potentially allow the use of statistical analysis (i.e., binomial test) to indicate whether deregulated miRNAs from ALS patient studies more frequently target ALS genes (at least based on *in silico* predictions) than randomly selected miRNAs, but we suggest greater numbers of miRNAs would need to be considered. This analysis would not be trivial and is outside the scope of this article, which seeks to propose a workflow. Further, consideration of additional (to the 37 used here) ALS genes is likely merited, again expanding the complexity of the analysis. Current ALS genes also relate to different signaling networks, and more specific gene pathways may be required for target enrichment. In summary, we have defined a systematic *in silico* analysis that should be extended in the future to investigate functional links between deregulated miRNAs and ALS pathological processes.

TABLE 1 | The ALS genes predicted by DIANA-microT-CDS v5.0 to be targets of (A) the nine most frequently reported miRNAs from the studies, (B) nine deregulated miRNAs randomly selected from all ALS studies, and (C) nine randomly selected miRNAs not reported to be deregulated in the ALS studies.

	miRNAs	Number of Studies deregulated (out of 27)	Direction of deregulation (up, down or both)	ALS genes predicted by DIANA-T-CDS						
(A) Most Frequently Reported miRNAs	hsa-miR-133a-3p	9	Both	*TUBA4A*	*VAPB*					**MiRNA hits (8/9)**
	hsa-let-7a-5p	7	Both	*ARHGEF28*						**Genes (15/37)**
	hsa-miR-127-3p	6	Both							**Total (18)**
	hsa-miR-155-5p	6	Both	*TBK1*	***UBQLN2***					
	hsa-miR-206-3p	6	Both	*ATXN2*	***MATR3***					
	hsa-miR-26a-5p	6	Both	*ARHGEF28*	*ERBB4*	*MATR3*				
	hsa-miR-455-3p	6	Both	*TARDBP*						
	hsa-miR-9-5p	6	Both	***CHMP2B***	*CRYM*	*NEFH*	***TRPM7***			
	hsa-miR-124-3p	6	Both	***CHMP2B***	*SIGMAR1*	*SQSTM1*				
(B) Random miRNAs from ALS studies	hsa-let-7b-5p	5	Down	*ARHGEF28*						**MiRNA hits (7/9)**
	hsa-let-7c-5p	4	Down	*ARHGEF28*						**Genes (10/37)**
	hsa-miR-204-3p	1	Down	*ERBB4*	*VAPB*					**Total (16)**
	hsa-miR-766-3p	2	Both	***DAO***	*DCTN1*	*SIGMAR1*	*VAPB*			
	hsa-miR-212-3p	2	Down	*C9orf72*	*ERBB4*	*FIG4*				
	hsa-miR-329-3p	2	Down							
	hsa-miR-876-3p	1	Down	*ERBB4*	*MATR3*	*TUBA4A*				
	hsa-miR-302a-5p	1	Down	***ARHGEF28***	*ERBB4*					
	hsa-miR-154-5p	3	Down							
(C) Random miRNAs absent from ALS studies	hsa-miR-3168-5p			*TARDPB*						**MiRNA hits (5/9)**
	hsa-miR-875-5p									**Genes (8/37)**
	hsa-miR-611-5p									**Total (13)**
	hsa-miR-603-3p			*ATXN2*	*ERBB4*	*MATR3*	*OPTN*	*TARDBP*	***VAPB***	
	hsa-miR-500b-5p			*DCTN1*	*ERBB4*					
	hsa-miR-325-5p									
	hsa-miR-764-5p									
	hsa-miR-665-3p			*DCTN1*						
	hsa-miR-4277-5p			*DAO*	*TARDPB*	*VAPB*				

Note that we report mature miRNAs; where specific miRNAs were not reported we considered dominant strands as reported on miRBase release 22.1: October 2018. For (A), all miRNAs deregulated in at least six studies were considered. For (B) nine miRNAs were randomly selected from those reported by <6 of the 27 studies. Further analysis regarding strand specificity was also performed on this group and on the nine miRNAs not found deregulated in the studies (C). MiRNAs in bold have confirmed interactions with the target experimentally, using miRTarBase v7.0 (23).

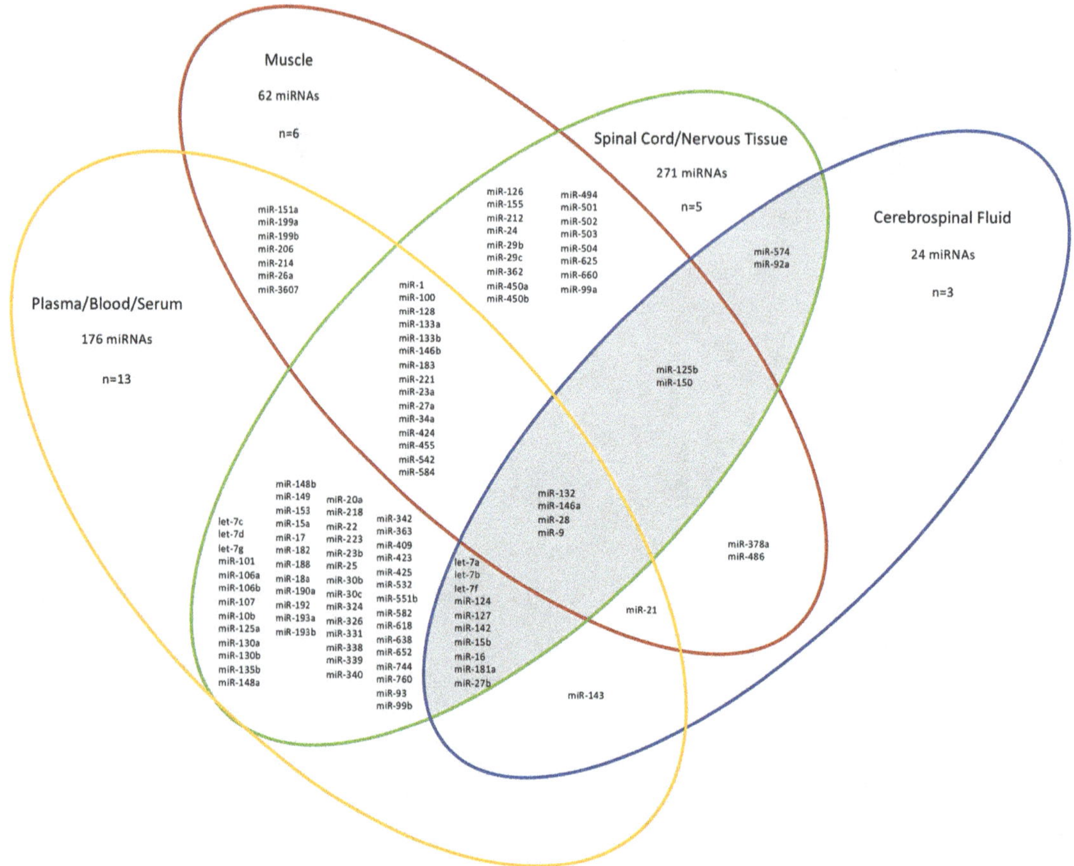

FIGURE 1 | Different tissue sources and overlap of miRNAs identified from ALS patients in 26/27 studies. n=the number of papers examined in each compartment. For simplicity, specific miRNA arms are not shown. The CSF-spinal cord/nervous tissue overlap is shaded. The miRNAs deregulated between patient neuromuscular junction and control blood and deregulated miRNAs from sALS patient fibroblasts are not included since they do not belong in any of the distinct source group compartments used here (21, 36). The total miRNAs present in each group are given. MiRNAs within a single compartment are not shown.

Tissue Distribution of Deregulated miRNAs

Next, we considered the different tissue sources of the ALS-relevant miRNAs identified in 26/27 studies ($n = 410$ unique miRNAs, for exclusions see **Figure 1** legend), and grouped the miRNAs based on four "compartments": CSF, spinal cord/nervous tissue, muscle, and plasma/blood/serum. **Figure 1** shows the overlap between studies after mapping the deregulated miRNAs to the compartment (tissue) they were determined in. 265/410 deregulated miRNAs were present in at least two different tissues. We noted considerable correspondence between miRNAs extracted from plasma/blood/serum with those from CSF (total of 16/24 miRNAs within the CSF group), supporting the notion that blood miRNAs can provide a window into CSF changes (15). Since ALS is a neurodegenerative disorder, those miRNAs deregulated in patient CSF and spinal cord/nervous tissue were of particular interest and these 18 miRNAs are shown in a shaded region in **Figure 1**. Of these 18 miRNAs, two are exclusive to only these two sources (hsa-miR-92a-5p/3p and hsa-miR-574-5p/3p). Notably, of the nine most frequently reported miRNAs found to be deregulated in the 27 studies (**Table 1A**), four overlapped with these 18 miRNAs.

Most Frequently Deregulated miRNAs Within the CSF-Spinal Cord/Nervous Tissue Overlap

As noted above, four miRNAs in the CSF-spinal cord/nervous tissue overlap are also amongst the most frequently reported deregulated miRNAs (**Table 1A**; hsa-miR-124-3p, hsa-miR-127-3p, hsa-let-7a-5p, and hsa-miR-9-5p). The latter is discussed in the section MicroRNAs Present in all Tissue Sources.

Hsa-miR-124-3p was reported down-regulated in ALS patients in five studies (21, 37–40), with only one study finding it upregulated (41). Despite the caveats to the predictive approach highlighted above, it is notable that the predicted targets of this miRNA are *CHMP2B*, *SQSTM1*, and *SIGMAR1*. Hsa-miR-124-3p has been shown to be deregulated in the spinal cord and brainstem of *SOD1* transgenic mice and has been linked to astrocyte differentiation and neurogenesis in the mouse brain (42, 43). Further, hsa-miR-124-3p is found to be expressed almost exclusively in the brain and spinal cord (44).

Hsa-miR-127-3p was not predicted to target any of the ALS genes and was found almost consistently down-regulated in ALS patients (22, 37, 39, 45, 46) with only one study reporting its upregulation (41). Whilst little is reported in relation to ALS, hsa-miR-127-3p has been found deregulated in FTD patients compared to control groups and Alzheimer's disease patients (47). This result is consistent with hsa-miR-127-3p predominantly being expressed in brain tissue (44).

Hsa-let-7a-5p, most highly expressed in the cerebellum, is predicted to target *ARHGEF28* (**Table 1A**) (44). Let-7a-5p has been found downregulated in the plasma of Parkinson's disease patients compared to healthy controls, showing it may not be useful as an ALS specific biomarker (48).

MicroRNAs Unique to the CSF-Spinal Cord/Nervous Tissue Overlap

The two miRNAs unique to the CSF-spinal cord/nervous tissue group are hsa-miR-92a-5p/3p and hsa-miR-574-5p/3p. Hsa-miR-92a-5p/3p's predicted targets are *CHCHD10, TARDBP, PLEKHG5,* and *NEFH* and hsa-miR-574-5p/3p's are *VAPB* and *SIGMAR1*. According to a miRNA tissue atlas, both miRNAs show neither specific tissue specificity nor ubiquitous expression (44). Despite this, deregulation of these miRNAs in ALS could be tissue specific.

MicroRNAs Present in all Tissue Sources

Hsa-miR-132-5p/3p, hsa-miR-146a-5p/3p, hsa-miR-28-5p/3p, and hsa-miR-9-5p/3p were deregulated in all tissue samples (**Figure 1**) and are all predicted to target at least one ALS gene. Hsa-miR-132-3p has been implicated in a range of neurodegenerative disorders including multiple sclerosis, Parkinson's disease and Alzheimer's disease, demonstrating wider relevance beyond ALS (49). This is consistent with the miRNA tissue atlas, where it is primarily expressed in the brain (44). Downregulation of miR-146a-5p in cortical aberrant astrocytes has been implicated in motor neuron degeneration in ALS, whereas its upregulation has been implicated in motor neuron loss in spinal muscular atrophy (50, 51). No links between miR-28-5p/3p and ALS have yet been made, consistent with it being predicted to target just one ALS-associated gene (*SETX*). Mutations in *TARDBP* have been reported to cause deregulation of miR-9-5p and miR-9-5p/3p has been shown to be upregulated in mutant *SOD1* mice (52, 53). MiR-9-5p has been implicated in axon extension and branching *via* targeting of *Map1b* (54). It is also predominantly expressed in the brain and spinal cord (44).

CONCLUSIONS

We have shown that miRNAs found deregulated in published studies investigating ALS patients have limited overlap, likely due to the wide variation in tissue extraction and miRNA detection methods. Future emphasis should therefore be on standardizing tissue extraction and miRNA profiling methods.

However, we identified nine miRNAs repeatedly reported as deregulated in the 27 studies. Despite these miRNAs being commonly predicted to target ALS-associated genes, the randomly selected miRNAs not found deregulated in ALS patients, showed similar predictions. Therefore, our *in silico* analysis provided no clear correlation between deregulated miRNAs and the collection of ALS-linked genes analyzed. This indicates that whilst the ability to predict thousands of candidate genes with *in silico* methods remains informative, they should be used with caution and in combination with other methods, of which experimental functional testing is recommended. Although limitations of the bioinformatics approach may explain our observations, the currently identified ALS-associated genes may offer a limited view on the pathological pathways altered during disease progression. It is thus tempting to suggest *in silico* analyses are currently underpowered. In the future it would be interesting to perform this bioinformatics approach using ALS genes grouped by their relation to specific functional pathways, for example proteostasis or RNA metabolism.

We have additionally shown the source can influence the miRNAs detected, since only four deregulated miRNAs appeared in all tissue sources analyzed. Importantly, we have shown the four miRNAs reported most frequently deregulated appear in CSF, spinal cord/nervous tissue and blood/plasma/serum. This suggests miRNAs may indeed "travel" between CSF and blood, the latter potentially providing a clinically accessible source which may mirror ALS pathology in the CNS. We therefore propose four miRNAs—hsa-miR-124-3p, hsa-miR-127-3p, hsa-let-7a-5p, and hsa-miR-9-5p—as good candidates for further study and suggest blood, serum or plasma as a clinically accessible source.

Overall we have demonstrated the need for a multifaceted approach, utilizing patient data, bioinformatics, but most critically, experimental follow-up, to resolve the true biological significance of these implicated miRNAs and determine the real disease culprits of ALS.

Note Added After Submission

Whilst this manuscript was under review, Yao et al. (55) identified *SQSTM1* as a target of miR-124-3p. Notably our analysis had indicated that hsa-miR-124-3p, present in the CSF-spinal cord/nervous tissue overlap (**Figure 1**), was one of the most frequently reported deregulated miRNAs (6/27 studies) and was predicted to target *SQSTM1* (**Table 1A**).

AUTHOR CONTRIBUTIONS

SF wrote and edited the manuscript. RL, FD-B, and RM-R critically reviewed and edited the manuscript.

FUNDING

This work was funded by a Prize Studentship from the MND Association (SF, FD-B, and RL), reference Layfield/Oct16/887/792.

REFERENCES

1. Krol J, Loedige I, Filipowicz W. The widespread regulation of microRNA biogenesis, function and decay. *Nat Rev Genet.* (2010) 11:597–610. doi: 10.1038/nrg2843
2. He L, Hannon GJ. MicroRNAs: small RNAs with a big role in gene regulation. *Nat Rev Genet.* (2004) 5:522–31. doi: 10.1038/nrg1379
3. Hammond SM. An overview of microRNAs. *Adv Drug Deliv Rev.* (2015) 87:3–14. doi: 10.1016/j.addr.2015.05.001
4. Sang Q, Yao Z, Wang H, Feng R, Wang H, Zhao X, et al. Identification of MicroRNAs in human follicular fluid: characterization of microRNAs that govern steroidogenesis *in vitro* and are associated with polycystic ovary syndrome *in vivo*. *J Clin Endocrinol Metab.* (2013) 98:3068–79. doi: 10.1210/jc.2013-1715
5. Weber JA, Baxter DH, Zhang S, Huang DY, Huang KH, Lee MJ, et al. The microRNA spectrum in 12 body fluids. *Clin Chem.* (2010) 56:1733–41. doi: 10.1373/clinchem.2010.147405
6. Turchinovich A, Samatov TR, Tonevitsky AG, Burwinkel B. Circulating miRNAs: cell-cell communication function? *Front Genet.* (2013) 4:119. doi: 10.3389/fgene.2013.00119
7. Morgan S, Orrell RW. Pathogenesis of amyotrophic lateral sclerosis. *Br Med Bull.* (2016) 119:87–98. doi: 10.1093/bmb/ldw026
8. Tao Q-Q, Wei Q, Wu Z-Y. Sensory nerve disturbance in amyotrophic lateral sclerosis. *Life Sci.* (2018) 203:242–5. doi: 10.1016/J.LFS.2018.04.052
9. Thomsen GM, Gowing G, Svendsen S, Svendsen CN. The past, present and future of stem cell clinical trials for ALS. *Exp Neurol.* (2014) 262:127–37. doi: 10.1016/J.EXPNEUROL.2014.02.021
10. Kirby J, Al Sultan A, Waller R, Heath P. The genetics of amyotrophic lateral sclerosis: current insights. *Degen Neurol Neuromusc Dis.* (2016) 6:49–64. doi: 10.2147/DNND.S84956
11. Nguyen HP, Van Broeckhoven C, van der Zee J. ALS Genes in the genomic era and their implications for FTD. *Trends Genet.* (2018) 34:404–23. doi: 10.1016/j.tig.2018.03.001
12. Kawahara Y, Mieda-Sato A. TDP-43 promotes microRNA biogenesis as a component of the Drosha and Dicer complexes. *Proc Natl Acad Sci USA.* (2012) 109:3347–52. doi: 10.1073/pnas.1112427109
13. Chen X, Ba Y, Ma L, Cai X, Yin Y, Wang K, et al. Characterization of microRNAs in serum: a novel class of biomarkers for diagnosis of cancer and other diseases. *Cell Res.* (2008) 18:997–1006. doi: 10.1038/cr.2008.282
14. Rao P, Benito E, Fischer A. MicroRNAs as biomarkers for CNS disease. *Front Mol Neurosci.* (2013) 6:39. doi: 10.3389/fnmol.2013.00039
15. Ricci C, Marzocchi C, Battistini S. MicroRNAs as biomarkers in amyotrophic lateral sclerosis. *Cells.* (2018) 7:219. doi: 10.3390/cells7110219
16. Valadi H, Ekström K, Bossios A, Sjöstrand M, Lee JJ, Lötvall JO. Exosome-mediated transfer of mRNAs and microRNAs is a novel mechanism of genetic exchange between cells. *Nat Cell Biol.* (2007) 9:654–9. doi: 10.1038/ncb1596
17. Sohel MH. Extracellular/circulating MicroRNAs: release mechanisms, functions and challenges. *Achiev Life Sci.* (2016) 10:175–86. doi: 10.1016/J.ALS.2016.11.007
18. Otake K, Kamiguchi H, Hirozane Y. Identification of biomarkers for amyotrophic lateral sclerosis by comprehensive analysis of exosomal mRNAs in human cerebrospinal fluid. *BMC Med Genomics.* (2019) 12:7. doi: 10.1186/s12920-019-0473-z
19. Dardiotis E, Aloizou A-M, Siokas V, Patrinos GP, Deretzi G, Mitsias P, et al. The role of microRNAs in patients with amyotrophic lateral sclerosis. *J Mol Neurosci.* (2018) 66:617–28. doi: 10.1007/s12031-018-1204-1
20. Joilin G, Leigh PN, Newbury SF, Hafezparast M. *An Overview of microRNAs as Biomarkers of ALS.* (2019). Retrieved from: www.frontiersin.org (accessed February 27, 2019).
21. De Felice B, Manfellotto F, Fiorentino G, Annunziata A, Biffali E, Pannone R, et al. Wide-ranging analysis of MicroRNA profiles in sporadic amyotrophic lateral sclerosis using next-generation sequencing. *Front Genet.* (2018) 9:310. doi: 10.3389/fgene.2018.00310
22. Saucier D, Wajnberg G, Roy J, Beauregard A-P, Chacko S, Crapoulet N, et al. Identification of a circulating miRNA signature in extracellular vesicles collected from amyotrophic lateral sclerosis patients. *Brain Research.* (2019) 1708:100–8. doi: 10.1016/J.BRAINRES.2018.12.016
23. Chou C-H, Shrestha S, Yang C-D, Chang N-W, Lin Y-L, Liao K-W, et al. miRTarBase update 2018: a resource for experimentally validated microRNA-target interactions. *Nucleic Acids Res.* (2018) 46:D296. doi: 10.1093/NAR/GKX1067
24. Siracusa J, Koulmann N, Banzet S. Circulating myomiRs: a new class of biomarkers to monitor skeletal muscle in physiology and medicine. *J Cachexia, Sarcopenia Muscle.* (2018) 9:20–7. doi: 10.1002/jcsm.12227
25. Jensen L, Jørgensen LH, Bech RD, Frandsen U, Schrøder HD. Skeletal muscle remodelling as a function of disease progression in amyotrophic lateral sclerosis. *BioMed Res Int.* (2016) 2016:5930621. doi: 10.1155/2016/5930621
26. Pegoraro V, Merico A, Angelini C. Micro-RNAs in ALS muscle: differences in gender, age at onset and disease duration. *J Neurol Sci.* (2017) 380:58–63. doi: 10.1016/J.JNS.2017.07.008
27. Di Pietro L, Baranzini M, Berardinelli MG, Lattanzi W, Monforte M, Tasca G, et al. Potential therapeutic targets for ALS: MIR206, MIR208b and MIR499 are modulated during disease progression in the skeletal muscle of patients. *Sci Rep.* (2017) 7:9538. doi: 10.1038/s41598-017-10161-z
28. Russell AP, Wada S, Vergani L, Hock MB, Lamon S, Léger B, et al. Disruption of skeletal muscle mitochondrial network genes and miRNAs in amyotrophic lateral sclerosis. *Neurobiol Dis.* (2013) 49:107–17. doi: 10.1016/J.NBD.2012.08.015
29. Tasca E, Pegoraro V, Merico A, Angelini C. Circulating microRNAs as biomarkers of muscle differentiation and atrophy in ALS. *Clin Neuropathol.* (2016) 35:22–30. doi: 10.5414/NP300889
30. Hoye ML, Koval ED, Wegener AJ, Hyman TS, Yang C, O'Brien DR, et al. MicroRNA profiling reveals marker of motor neuron disease in ALS models. *J Neurosci.* (2017) 37:5574–86. doi: 10.1523/JNEUROSCI.3582-16.2017
31. Abel O, Shatunov A, Jones AR, Andersen PM, Powell JF, Al-Chalabi A. Development of a Smartphone App for a genetics website: the amyotrophic lateral sclerosis online genetics database (ALSoD). *JMIR MHealth UHealth.* (2013) 1:18. doi: 10.2196/mhealth.2706
32. Paraskevopoulou MD, Georgakilas G, Kostoulas N, Vlachos IS, Vergoulis T, Reczko M, et al. DIANA-microT web server v5.0: service integration into miRNA functional analysis workflows. *Nucleic Acids Res.* (2013) 41:W169–73. doi: 10.1093/nar/gkt393
33. Reczko M, Maragkakis M, Alexiou P, Grosse I, Hatzigeorgiou AG. Functional microRNA targets in protein coding sequences. *Bioinformatics.* (2012) 28:771–6. doi: 10.1093/bioinformatics/bts043
34. Riffo-Campos ÁL, Riquelme I, Brebi-Mieville P. Tools for sequence-based miRNA target prediction: what to choose? *Int J Mol Sci.* (2016) 17:1987. doi: 10.3390/ijms17121987
35. Kozomara A, Griffiths-Jones S. miRBase: annotating high confidence microRNAs using deep sequencing data. *Nucleic Acids Res.* (2014) 42:D68–73. doi: 10.1093/nar/gkt1181
36. Raman R, Allen SP, Goodall EF, Kramer S, Ponger L-L, Heath PR, et al. Gene expression signatures in motor neurone disease fibroblasts reveal dysregulation of metabolism, hypoxia-response and RNA processing functions. *Neuropathol Appl Neurobiol.* (2015) 41:201–26. doi: 10.1111/nan.12147
37. Campos-Melo D, Droppelmann CA, He Z, Volkening K, Strong MJ. Altered microRNA expression profile in amyotrophic lateral sclerosis: a role in the regulation of NFL mRNA levels. *Molecular Brain.* (2013) 6:26. doi: 10.1186/1756-6606-6-26
38. Chen Y, Wei Q, Chen X, Li C, Cao B, Ou R, et al. Aberration of miRNAs expression in leukocytes from sporadic amyotrophic lateral sclerosis. *Front Mol Neurosci.* (2016) 9:69. doi: 10.3389/fnmol.2016.00069
39. D'Erchia AM, Gallo A, Manzari C, Raho S, Horner DS, Chiara M, et al. Massive transcriptome sequencing of human spinal cord tissues provides new insights into motor neuron degeneration in ALS. *Sci Rep.* (2017) 7:10046. doi: 10.1038/s41598-017-10488-7
40. Emde A, Eitan C, Liou L-L, Libby RT, Rivkin N, Magen I, et al. Dysregulated miRNA biogenesis downstream of cellular stress and ALS-causing mutations: a new mechanism for ALS. *EMBO J.* (2015) 34:2633–51. doi: 10.15252/embj.201490493
41. Waller R, Wyles M, Heath PR, Kazoka M, Wollff H, Shaw PJ, et al. Small RNA sequencing of sporadic amyotrophic lateral sclerosis cerebrospinal fluid reveals differentially expressed miRNAs related to neural and

glial activity. *Front Neurosci.* (2017) 11:731. doi: 10.3389/fnins.2017.00731

42. Cheng L-C, Pastrana E, Tavazoie M, Doetsch F. miR-124 regulates adult neurogenesis in the subventricular zone stem cell niche. *Nat Neurosci.* (2009) 12:399–408. doi: 10.1038/nn.2294
43. Zhou F, Zhang C, Guan Y, Chen Y, Lu Q, Jie L, et al. Screening the expression characteristics of several miRNAs in *G93A-SOD1* transgenic mouse: altered expression of miRNA-124 is associated with astrocyte differentiation by targeting Sox2 and Sox9. *J Neurochem.* (2018) 145:51–67. doi: 10.1111/jnc.14229
44. Ludwig N, Leidinger P, Becker K, Backes C, Fehlmann T, Pallasch C, et al. Distribution of miRNA expression across human tissues. *Nucleic Acids Res.* (2016) 44:3865–77. doi: 10.1093/nar/gkw116
45. De Felice B, Guida M, Guida M, Coppola C, De Mieri G, Cotrufo R. A miRNA signature in leukocytes from sporadic amyotrophic lateral sclerosis. *Gene.* (2012) 508:35–40. doi: 10.1016/J.GENE.2012.07.058
46. Figueroa-Romero C, Hur J, Lunn JS, Paez-Colasante X, Bender DE, Yung R, et al. Expression of microRNAs in human post-mortem amyotrophic lateral sclerosis spinal cords provides insight into disease mechanisms. *Mol Cell Neurosci.* (2016) 71:34–45. doi: 10.1016/j.mcn.2015.12.008
47. Piscopo P, Grasso M, Puopolo M, D'Acunto E, Talarico G, Crestini A, et al. Circulating miR-127-3p as a potential biomarker for differential diagnosis in frontotemporal dementia. *J Alzheimer's Dis.* (2018) 65:455–64. doi: 10.3233/JAD-180364
48. Chen L, Yang J, Lü J, Cao S, Zhao Q, Yu Z. Identification of aberrant circulating miRNAs in Parkinson's disease plasma samples. *Brain Behav.* (2018) 8:e00941. doi: 10.1002/brb3.941
49. Qian Y, Song J, Ouyang Y, Han Q, Chen W, Zhao X, et al. Advances in roles of miR-132 in the nervous system. *Front Pharmacol.* (2017) 8:770. doi: 10.3389/fphar.2017.00770
50. Gomes C, Cunha C, Nascimento F, Ribeiro JA, Vaz AR, Brites D. Cortical neurotoxic astrocytes with early ALS pathology and miR-146a deficit replicate gliosis markers of symptomatic SOD1G93A mouse model. *Mol Neurobiol.* (2018) 1–22. doi: 10.1007/s12035-018-1220-8
51. Sison SL, Patitucci TN, Seminary ER, Villalon E, Lorson CL, Ebert AD. Astrocyte-produced miR-146a as a mediator of motor neuron loss in spinal muscular atrophy. *Hum Mol Genet.* (2017) 26:3409–20. doi: 10.1093/hmg/ddx230
52. Zhang Z, Almeida S, Lu Y, Nishimura AL, Peng L, Sun D, et al. Downregulation of microRNA-9 in iPSC-derived neurons of FTD/ALS patients with TDP-43 mutations. *PLoS ONE.* (2013) 8:e76055. doi: 10.1371/journal.pone.0076055
53. Zhou F, Guan Y, Chen Y, Zhang C, Yu L, Gao H, et al. miRNA-9 expression is upregulated in the spinal cord of G93A-SOD1 transgenic mice. *Int J Clin Exp Pathol.* (2013) 6:1826–38.
54. Dajas-Bailador F, Bonev B, Garcez P, Stanley P, Guillemot F, Papalopulu N. microRNA-9 regulates axon extension and branching by targeting Map1b in mouse cortical neurons. *Nat Neurosci.* (2012) 15:697–9. doi: 10.1038/nn.3082
55. Yao L, Zhu Z, Wu J, Zhang Y, Zhang H, Sun X, et al. MicroRNA-124 regulates the expression of p62/p38 and promotes autophagy in the inflammatory pathogenesis of Parkinson's disease. *FASEB J.* (2019). doi: 10.1096/fj.201900363R

8

Diagnostic Challenge and Neuromuscular Junction Contribution to ALS Pathogenesis

Maria-Letizia Campanari [1,2†], Annis-Rayan Bourefis [1,2†] and Edor Kabashi [1,2*]*

[1] *Sorbonne Université, Université Pierre et Marie Curie, Université de Paris 06, Unité Mixte 75, Institut National de la Santé et de la Recherche Médicale (INSERM) Unité 1127, Centre National de la Recherche Scientifique, Unité Mixte de Recherche 7225 Institut du Cerveau et de la Moelle Épinière, Paris, France,* [2] *Imagine Institute, INSERM Unité 1163, Paris Descartes Université, Paris, France*

Correspondence:
Maria-Letizia Campanari
maria-letizia.campanari@institutimagine.org
Edor Kabashi
edor.kabashi@institutimagine.org

†These authors have contributed equally to this work

Amyotrophic lateral sclerosis (ALS) represents the major adult-onset motor neuron disease. Both human and animal studies reveal the critical implication of muscle and neuromuscular junctions (NMJs) in the initial phase of this disease. Despite the common efforts, ALS diagnosis remains particularly challenging since many other disorders can overlap yielding similar clinical phenotypic features. A combination of further research on the NMJ parameters that are specific for this disease and laboratory tests are crucial for the early determination of specific changes in the muscle, as well as in motor neuron and the prediction of ALS progression. Also, it could provide a powerful tool in the discrimination of particular ALS and ALS-mimic cases and increase the efficacy of therapeutic treatments.

Keywords: amyotrophic lateral sclerosis (ALS), axonopathy, neuromuscular junction (NMJ), dying back hypothesis, ALS-mimic diseases

AMYOTROPHIC LATERAL SCLEROSIS

Amyotrophic Lateral Sclerosis (ALS) is a disease characterized by a progressive degeneration of upper motor neurons (MNs) in the motor cortex and lower motor neurons in the brainstem and the spinal cord. The death of these neurons leads to spasticity, weakness, and atrophy of the muscles, progressing to paralysis. The incidence of ALS in Europe is 2–16 per 100,000 each year (1), with respiratory failure being the predominant mode of death in patients within 3 years of diagnosis (2). The onset of the disease occurs prevalently during adulthood (peak age of 58–63 years) (3), though with a small proportion of early-onset disease in certain patients (before 35 years of age). ALS also shares neuropathological and genetic features with another neurodegenerative disorder, frontotemporal dementia (FTD) (4, 5), with many ALS patients showing some cognitive or behavioral changes. This has led to consider ALS and FTD as the ends of the same spectrum of disease (6).

Although the majority of ALS cases occur sporadically (sALS), there is a Mendelian inheritance in about 10% of the cases (familial ALS, fALS), mainly in an autosomal, dominant fashion (7). The two are clinically indistinguishable and a variety of genetic defects in more than 20 genetic loci have been linked with the ALS phenotype (8), with new genes constantly being identified in subsets of ALS patients (9–11). Four major genes which mutations are known to cause ALS are the f ollowing: chromosome 9 open reading frame 72 (C9orf72), superoxide dismutase 1 (SOD1), transactive response DNA-binding protein (TARDBP) and fused in sarcoma (FUS) (12–15). C9orf72 has an important role in membrane trafficking and autophagy (16), and SOD1 primary function is thought to be as a cytosolic and mitochondrial antioxidant enzyme, converting superoxide to molecular oxygen and hydrogen peroxide (17). TARDBP and FUS encode nucleic acid-binding proteins that reside in the nucleus, and are involved in multiple aspects of RNA processing, such as transcription and splicing [reviewed in (18)].

NMJ INVOLVEMENT IN ALS

Despite the progress in our understanding of the molecular pathogenesis linked to these genes, it is still unclear where the motor neuron dysfunction begins and the extrinsic factors that accelerate motor neuron degeneration. This led to the consideration of ALS as either a *dying forward* process that proposes an anterograde degeneration of motor neurons by glutamate excitotoxicity from the cortex, or a *dying back* phenomenon in which motor neuron degeneration starts distally at the nerve terminal or at the neuromuscular junction (NMJ) and progresses toward the cell body (3, 19). The NMJ is a tripartite synapse composed by the presynaptic motor neuron, the postsynaptic muscle and the synapse-associated glial cells (terminal Schwann cells, TSC) and allows the transmission of action potentials from motor neurons to muscles [reviewed in (20)]. In this complex structure, besides motor neuron degeneration, glial cells, and muscle fibers play also a major role in ALS onset and progression.

The muscle contribution in ALS development, through NMJs disassembly, is still a matter of debate. Nonetheless, increasing evidence points to the critical role of NMJ defects in the early stage of the disease in ALS patients [reviewed in (21)] and a variety of animal models have permitted important advances into exploring this hypothesis.

The human SOD1^{G93A} transgenic mouse, the first and most studied ALS model, is the one that has yielded the majority of information about the muscular deficits in ALS (22). Spatiotemporal analysis of NMJs in SOD1^{G93A} mouse revealed end-plates denervation before the appearance of clinical symptoms and neuron cell body loss (23), with the fast-fatigable synapses being more vulnerable to denervation (24). Because of its high expression in ALS muscle biopsies, the neurite outgrowth inhibitor Nogo-A was proposed as a factor responsible for motor nerve terminals repulsion and destabilization at the NMJ at very early asymptomatic stages (25, 26). This hypothesis was then confirmed in SOD1^{G93A} mouse model, where genetic ablation of Nogo-A in muscle led to marked reduction of muscle denervation and prolonged survival (27). Morphological observation of NMJs in SOD1^{G93A} also contributed to reinforce the dying back hypothesis, showing more detailed NMJ alterations prior to functional symptom onset (28). A detailed overview of the findings concerning neuromuscular defects in the SOD1^{G93A} mouse model has been reviewed by Dupuis and colleagues (22).

Despite the predominant use of rodent models for studying pathomechanisms and potential therapeutic targets in ALS, the use of smaller animal models, like *Drosophila melanogaster* and zebrafish (*Danio rerio*), is continually increasing. Their advantages lie in their fast development allowing quick generation of lines, their availability and the ease in manipulating gene expression and in drug screening. In drosophila, studies showed locomotor defects, reduced life span, and anatomical defects at the NMJ, causing impairments in synaptic transmission, in loss and gain of function models of TARDBP (29, 30). Similar results were found for FUS. Gene deficiency and overexpression of FUS in Drosophila models caused decreased synaptic transmission, reduced number of presynaptic active zones, altered postsynaptic glutamate receptor subunit composition at the NMJ, motor neuron degeneration and impaired motor behavior (31, 32). Zebrafish studies have highlighted gain and loss of function mechanisms for TARDBP and FUS, demonstrating shorter axonal projections from motor neurons, premature and excessive branching, impaired synaptic transmission at the NMJ leading to swimming defects (33–35). C9orf72 gene has also been modeled in zebrafish in a loss-of-function model that displayed behavioral and cellular deficits related to locomotion (36).For more details about the different models, all the ALS gene mutations that have been modeled are summarized in a recent review by Van Damme et al. (37).

Altogether, fundamental research supports the crucial role that NMJ could play in ALS pathogenesis and its possible employment as efficient early marker of the disease.

ALS DIAGNOSTIC CHALLENGES

The difficulty to diagnose ALS resides mainly in the existence of several mimic syndromes, unrelated to ALS but which present similar clinical features (38, 39).

Motor neuron diseases (MNDs) are classified in four main groups in which ALS represents the most common form (**Table 1**). Although these diseases affect people in different ways, they share several symptoms due to motor neuron loss of function. All of them present progressive weakening of skeletal muscles, which eventually affects the ability to speak, swallow and breathe. ALS diagnosis is even more difficult if we add to the list other neurological conditions unrelated to MNDs which can mimic its early symptoms. Moreover, increasing evidences point to a possible direct implication of muscle in the early stage of the disease, adding myopathies to the list of ALS-mimic pathologies (**Table 1**).

Standard diagnostic criteria for ALS have been established in 1991 [El Escorial criteria [EEC] (40)] and were revised in 1997 [AirlieHouse criteria [AHC] or El Escorial Revisited (41)]. Even though the essential requirements for ALS diagnosis were defined by these criteria, many neurologists and neuromuscular clinicians were missing the diagnosis, proving the low clinical accuracy of these diagnostic roles (42).

In 2008, electrodiagnostic studies, known as the Awaji criteria (43), were included in the clinical procedure to allow earlier and more accurate assessment of ALS diagnosis. However, the

TABLE 1 | General overview of neuromuscular diseases and ALS-mimic pathologies.

MOTOR NEURON DISEASES (MND)	
Amyotrophic Lateral Sclerosis (ALS)	
Primary Lateral Scerosis (PLS)	
Progressive Muscular Atrophy (PMA)	
Progressive Bulbar Palsy (PBP)	
OTHER NEUROLOGICAL CONDITIONS THAT CAN MIMIC ALS	
Mithochondrial Disorder (MID)	
Psedobulbar Palsy	
Spinal Muscular atrophy (SMA)	
Primary lateral sclerosis (some subtupes not related to ALS)	
Progressive spinal muscular atrophy (some subtype not related to ALS)	
Spinobulbar muscular atrophy (SBMA or Kennedy's disease)	
Autoimmune Syndromes Monoclonal	
Myopathies	
Cachectic myopathy	
Polymyositis Sarcoid myositis	
Carcinoid myopathy	
Nemaline myopathy	
Inflammatory myopathies	Polymyositis (PM)
	Dermatomyositis
	Inclusion-body myositis (IBM)

Neuromuscular Disorders (NMD) implicate deficits and degeneration of nerves (motor and sensory neurons) and muscles (skeletal muscles) of the central and peripheral nervous system, leading to muscles weaken and waste away (atrophy). NMDs are classified in 4 categories, with Amyotrophic lateral sclerosis representing the main one. ALS-mimic pathologies is a vast group of diseases characterized by weakness and wasting away of muscle tissue, with or without the breakdown of nerve tissue, thus mimicking ALS symptoms. Currently, no cure exists for NMDs and the treatments aim to relieve the symptoms and delay disease progression.

application of those sets of defined features are still insufficient to rule out other similar and related diseases (44, 45).

Methods for Diagnosis

Although the main ALS evaluation remains the clinical one, laboratory testing, based on advanced techniques of electrodiagnosis, neuroimaging, immunobiochemistry, and neurogenetics, is required for accurate ALS diagnosis.

Tests to rule out other neuromuscular conditions may include:

Electromyogram (EMG)

The needle EMG is the most important study in determining diagnostic certainty of ALS (46). During this test, a needle electrode is inserted through the skin into various muscles, starting with the most severely involved limb (**Figure 1**). The examination then progresses through four anatomical region: bulbar, cervical, thoracic, and lumbar. At least three anatomical regions have to be positive to this test to define ALS. The fasciculation potential (FP) has been included in Awaji criteria as a hallmark of ALS muscular denervation. In general, a decreased number of motor unit recruitment, with long duration of the motor unit potential, and abnormal spontaneous activity, are measured at the EMG in ALS patients [reviewed in (47)].

Nerve Conduction Study (NCS)

This test measures how fast an electrical impulse moves through the nerve (**Figure 1**). During the test, one electrode placed on the skin stimulates the nerve of interest with a very mild electrical impulse. Variations in time spent to reach a second electrode can help in identifying a nerve damage. Whereas, EMG measures the electrical activity in the muscles, the nerve conduction study is specific for nerves and helps to localize the disorder among nerve, neuromuscular junction, and muscle. NCS is a powerful tool to discriminate ALS from axonal demyelination or conduction block impairments (48). NCS parameters are generally normal in ALS, albeit the presence of prolonged distal motor latency and slowed conduction velocity could be consistent with the diagnosis of ALS (49, 50). These changes suggest loss of large myelinated fibers, but also motor axons regeneration phenomena (50).

Magnetic Resonance Imaging (MRI)

This technique is able to produce detailed images of the brain and spinal cord, the latter with the advantage of simultaneously investigating the upper and lower motor neurons. During several years, its application was related to the exclusion of other disorders, as tumors or hernias that can display certain of the ALS-mimic symptoms (51). The evolution and improvement of this multimodal tool has recently become essential for the diagnosis of ALS. MRI scans can show cerebral degeneration and gray/white matter atrophy [reviewed in (52)], and also detect abnormalities in ALS muscle, likely due to denervation atrophy process (53).

Blood and Urine Tests

Testing hematological factors is helpful to exclude diseases that are capable of mimicking ALS symptoms. Recently, a population-based study, proposed serum albumin, creatinine levels, and lymphocyte count as markers for ALS, indicating muscle waste and inflammation respectively (54). Other markers potentially related to a better ALS outcome have been proposed: LDL/HDL levels, which are elevated in ALS plasma and represent a general unexplained hypermetabolism (55, 56); serum uric acid levels, which are decreased among ALS patients, further demonstrating the possible role of oxidative stress in the induction and propagation of the disease (57); serum ferritin levels which are elevated in ALS patients and could reflect perturbation in iron metabolism (58); concentrations of certain amino acids, which are decreased in ALS (59); levels of serum proinflammatory cytokines, such as IL-6, which are increased in ALS (60). Finally, high level of circulating AChE and metalloproteinases (MMP) have been reported in ALS plasma (61, 62) and although the exact source of these two classes of enzymes remains uncertain, it could in part reflect a disruption of extracellularly bound AChE at the NMJ and early change in the nerve-muscle integrity.

Spinal Tap (Lumbar Puncture)

Using this particular test, a small amount of cerebrospinal fluid (CSF) is taken from the lower back of the patient for laboratory

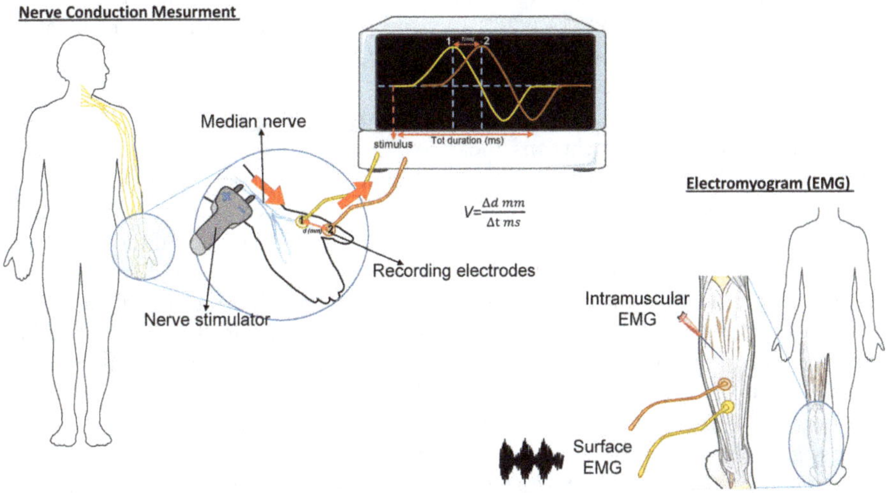

FIGURE 1 | Schematic representation of the nerve conduction and muscle contraction studies. *Nerve Conduction Velocity (NCV - left)* measures the velocity and the quality of conduction of the electrical signal in a nerve. During the test, your nerve is stimulated, with an electrode attached to your skin. One or two more electrodes patches are placed on the skin over your nerve. The electrical impulse of the stimulated nerve pass from the stimulator to the other receiving electrode. The time (in milliseconds) spent by the impulse to move from a point to another, on the order of millimeters, represent the Velocity. In ALS, the impulse conduction is slower respect with control cases and is worsened by the increase of axonal degeneration. The *electromyogram (EMG-right)* measures the electrical activity of the muscles at rest and during contraction. There are two kinds of EMG: surface EMG and intramuscular EMG. In the first one the muscle activity is recorded by one or more electrodes patched on the skin and it asses the contractile response of superficial muscles. This approach presents several limitation since the result signal is influenced by the depth of the subcutaneous tissue at the site of the recording and by the discharges of adjacent muscles. With the intramuscular EMG, specific deep muscle activity is recorded by using one needle electrode inserted into the muscle. EMG and NCV tests are often done together to give more complete information.

tests. Thanks to its proximity to the central nervous system, the CSF is considered one preferred tissue to search for ALS biomarkers [reviewed in (63)]. Several markers for ALS have been identified in CSF such as Tau, TDP43, Nefl, and MMP levels [reviewed in (64)]. In particular, MMPs with their ability to digest collagen, proteoglycan, and laminin (65), may reflect ongoing destruction of the matrix which wraps synapses (66) and pathological changes at the brain-blood barrier (62).

Muscle Biopsy

With this technique, a small portion of muscle is removed by needle biopsy and sent to a laboratory for histopathological analysis. Rarely performed because of its painful and invasive nature, this tool is useful when ALS diagnosis is in doubt. Generally, ALS muscles present signs of active denervation/reinnervation and an increased number of atrophic fibers (67).

Genetic Testing

People with familial ALS (fALS) background can get an efficient diagnosis through genetic testing (68, 69). This technique may help ALS patients to understand the basis of their condition, and improve the genotype-specific treatments (70). Unluckily, there is a lack of consensus among clinicians above the definition of fALS, since newly genes related to ALS are continuously found (71). Nowadays, genetic testing is not wildly used because of its high cost and the belief that ALS genetics is not well-enough understood to provide a better treatment plan, as reported in 2017 in a study which involved 167 clinicians from 21 different countries around the world (71).

EXAMPLES OF NMJ PATHOLOGIES ALS-MIMIC

Here we report some examples of ALS-mimic pathologies. The *Spinal muscular atrophy (SMA)* is an inherited MND that prevalently affects children. Its incidence is 1 per 11,000 live births (72). All forms of SMA are caused by the loss of SMN1, a gene implicated in axonal mRNA transport and snRNP biogenesis (73). Studies involving mice and fly mutants demonstrated that the probable origin of this pathology resides in the early loss of sensory information from proprioceptive neurons (74), which in turn causes degeneration of α motor neurons. In consequence, progressive muscle weakness, and, in severe cases, respiratory failure appear (75). Despite being considered a child's illness, the SMA type 4, that has an adult onset, overlaps with ALS diagnosis (76). Furthermore, like in ALS, several studies reveal the early implication of NMJs in SMA, with synaptic pathology prior to the appearance of clinical symptoms (77–81). However, the first evidence of neuromuscular pathology occurred at different time points of the disease progression, with presynaptic pathology preceding morphological changes at the endplate in ALS, and simultaneous pre and post-synaptic pathologies in SMA, suggesting the possibility to study this particular zone in diagnosis (81). Histochemical skin biopsy comparison was suggested as a powerful diagnostic tool in differentiating ALS and SMA, since the small collagen fibrils and the increased amount of amorphous material, which are characteristic of ALS, are not in SMA (82).

The *Spinobulbar muscular atrophy [(SBMA) Kennedy's disease]* is a X-linked hereditary lower motor neuron disease, where the expanded trinucleotide repeat (CAG > 37) in the androgen receptor gene (AR) causes its nuclear inclusions and impairment of its function (83, 84). The disease affects 1 per 200,000 males in Europe and Asia each year (85). In this pathology, degeneration of anterior horn cells of the spinal cord, where androgen receptors are widely expressed, is observed (86, 87). Although SBMA patients exhibit facial weakness as first sign of the disease, they progressively develop myopathic features, such as muscle atrophy and necrotic myofibers (88). Like ALS, SBMA disease reveals mixed pathological findings, with both myopathy and neurogenic atrophy features, which is the cause of misdiagnosis at the early stage of the disease.

Among the autoimmune syndromes, *myasthenia gravis (MG)* overlaps ALS syndrome. The annual incidence ranges from 3 to 30 per 1,000,000 people (89). In fact, the binding of autoantibodies to components of the NMJ in MG causes a characterized muscle weakness and fatigability (90). Even if acetylcholine receptor antibodies are considered to be highly specific for the diagnosis of MG, ALS patients can also present these autoantibodies at the blood test (91, 92). In these cases, it is very difficult to define the false positive cases and an experimental treatment with AChE inhibitors is necessary to differentiate MG from ALS (93).

The skeletal muscle disorders are represented with the term *Myopathies.* Myopathies hold a list of pathologies (**Table 1**) where muscle weakness can begin in the hands and feet (distal muscles) as well as in the muscles near the center of the body (proximal muscles) sometimes mimicking ALS features, confusing the diagnostic and the treatment decision. Among them, *Inclusion Body Myositis (IBM)* (94) is the most common ALS-mimic disease. It is the most common adult myopathy in 50 year-old persons and older, and its incidence is 3.5 per 100,000 (95). It is characterized by inflammatory cells surrounding and invading non-necrotic muscle fibers, rimmed vacuoles, congophilic inclusions, and protein aggregates in muscle (96, 97). In this case, the unique way to exclude ALS is the muscle biopsy combined with quantitative electromyographic analysis, especially in those patients where disease progression is slow and atypical (98).

CONCLUSION

Amyotrophic Lateral Sclerosis (ALS) and MNDs are not yet curable. However, accurate diagnosis is crucial to provide adequate counseling and information about the prognosis and disease course, and to avoid inappropriate therapy. Moreover, a good diagnosis could furnish a more equal stratification of cases and be important in the choice of additional medical support, as for example nutritional intervention strategies or physical therapy.

Currently, there is not a common consensus in the use of laboratory analysis for ALS diagnosis. Basically, clinicians decide for the application of certain techniques based on their experience, expertise and hospital practice. Progress in molecular genetics and identification of specific biomarkers is ongoing, which will translate to a refined diagnostic certitude. Therefore, there is the emerging need to establish a widely accepted protocol for laboratory tests to discriminate the majority of cases that present clinical features resembling ALS.

Increasing human and animal evidence proposed NMJ impairments as possible biomarkers for detection and discrimination of ALS and mimic diseases in an early, preclinical stage. However, further studies are needed to understand how these impairments could be monitored and specifically treated.

AUTHOR CONTRIBUTIONS

M-LC and A-RB contributed to conception and drafting. EK provided useful comments and reviewed the manuscript.

FUNDING

This study was funded by the ERC Consolidator Grant, ANR ToFU, E-rare ERA-NET program, ANR AFM, ARSLA, and the program Investissements d'avenir ANR-10-IAIHU-06 (EK).

REFERENCES

1. Logroscino, G, Traynor BJ, Hardiman O, Chiò A, Mitchell D, Swingler RJ, et al. Incidence of amyotrophic lateral sclerosis in Europe. *J Neurol Neurosurg Psychiatry* (2010) 81:385–90. doi: 10.1136/jnnp.2009.183525
2. Chiò, A, Logroscino G, Hardiman O, Swingler R, Mitchell D, Beghi E, et al. Prognostic factors in ALS: a critical review. *Amyotroph Lateral Scler.* (2009) 10:310–23. doi: 10.3109/17482960802566824
3. Kiernan MC[1], Vucic S, Cheah BC, Turner MR, Eisen A, Hardiman O, et al. Amyotrophic lateral sclerosis. *Lancet* (2011) 377:942–55. doi: 10.1016/S0140-6736(10)61156-7
4. Morita, M, Al-Chalabi A, Andersen PM, Hosler B, Sapp P, Englund E, et al. A locus on chromosome 9p confers susceptibility to ALS and frontotemporal dementia. *Neurology* (2006) 66:839–44. doi: 10.1212/01.wnl.0000200048.53766.b4
5. Vance, C, Al-Chalabi A, Ruddy D, Smith BN, Hu X, Sreedharan J, et al. Familial amyotrophic lateral sclerosis with frontotemporal dementia is linked to a locus on chromosome 9p13.2-21.3. *Brain* (2006) 129:868–76. doi: 10.1093/brain/awl030
6. Robberecht W, Philips T. The changing scene of amyotrophic lateral sclerosis. *Nat Rev Neurosci.* (2013) 14:248–64. doi: 10.1038/nrn3430
7. Strong MJ, Hudson AJ, Alvord WG. Familial amyotrophic lateral sclerosis, 1850-1989 : a statistical analysis of the world literature.*Can J Neurol Sci.* (1991) 18:45–58.
8. Brown RH, Al-Chalabi A. Amyotrophic lateral sclerosis. *N Engl J Med.* (2017) 377:162–72. doi: 10.1056/NEJMra1603471
9. Freischmidt, A, Wieland T, Richter B, Ruf W, Schaeffer V, Müller K, et al. Haploinsufficiency of TBK1 causes familial ALS and fronto-temporal dementia. *Nat Neurosci.* (2015) 18:631–6. doi: 10.1038/nn.4000

10. Brenner, D, Müller K, Wieland T, Weydt P, Böhm S, Lulé D, et al. NEK1 mutations in familial amyotrophic lateral sclerosis. *Brain* (2016) 139:e28. doi: 10.1093/brain/aww033
11. Mackenzie IR, Nicholson AM, Sarkar M, Messing J, Purice MD, Pottier C, et al. TIA1 mutations in amyotrophic lateral sclerosis and frontotemporal dementia promote phase separation and alter stress granule dynamics. *Neuron* (2017) 95:808–16.e9. doi: 10.1016/j.neuron.2017.07.025
12. Rosen DR, Siddique T, Patterson D, Figlewicz DA, Sapp P, Hentati A, et al. Mutations in Cu/Zn superoxide dismutase gene are associated with familial amyotrophic lateral sclerosis. *Nature* (1993) 362:59–62. doi: 10.1038/362059a0
13. Renton AE, Majounie E, Waite A, Simón-Sánchez J, Rollinson S, Gibbs JR, et al. A hexanucleotide repeat expansion in C9ORF72 is the cause of chromosome 9p21-linked ALS-FTD. *Neuron* (2011) 72:257–68. doi: 10.1016/j.neuron.2011.09.010
14. Sreedharan, J, Blair IP, Tripathi VB, Hu X, Vance C, Rogelj B, et al. TDP-43 mutations in familial and sporadic amyotrophic lateral sclerosis. *Science* (2008) 319:1668–72. doi: 10.1126/science.1154584
15. Kwiatkowski TJ, Bosco DA, Leclerc AL, Tamrazian E, Vanderburg CR, Russ C, et al. Mutations in the FUS/TLS gene on chromosome 16 cause familial amyotrophic lateral sclerosis. *Science* (2009) 547:1205–9. doi: 10.1126/science.1166066
16. Nassif M, Woehlbier U, Manque PA. The enigmatic role of C9ORF72 in autophagy. *Front Neurosci.* (2017) 11:442. doi: 10.3389/fnins.2017.00442
17. Bunton-Stasyshyn RKA, Saccon RA, Fratta P, Fisher EMC. SOD1 Function and its implications for amyotrophic lateral sclerosis pathology: new and renascent themes. *Neuroscientist* (2015) 21:519–29. doi: 10.1177/1073858414561795
18. Guerrero EN, Wang H, Mitra J, Hegde PM, Stowell SE, Liachko NF, et al. TDP-43/FUS in motor neuron disease: complexity and challenges. *Prog Neurobiol.* (2016) 145-6:78–97. doi: 10.1016/j.pneurobio.2016.09.004
19. Dadon-Nachum M, Melamed E, Offen D. The 'dying-back' phenomenon of motor neurons in ALS. *J Mol Neurosci.* (2011) 43:470–477. doi: 10.1007/s12031-010-9467-1
20. Campanari M-L, García-Ayllón M-S, Ciura S, Sáez-Valero J, Kabashi E. Neuromuscular junction impairment in amyotrophic lateral sclerosis: reassessing the role of acetylcholinesterase. *Front Mol Neurosci.* (2016) 9:160. doi: 10.3389/fnmol.2016.00160
21. Cappello V, Francolini M. Neuromuscular junction dismantling in amyotrophic lateral sclerosis. *Int J Mol Sci.* (2017) 18:E2092. doi: 10.3390/ijms18102092
22. Dupuis L, Loeffler J-P. Neuromuscular junction destruction during amyotrophic lateral sclerosis: insights from transgenic models. *Curr Opin Pharmacol.* (2009) 9:341–6. doi: 10.1016/j.coph.2009.03.007
23. Fischer LR, Culver DG, Tennant P, Davis AA, Wang M, Castellano-Sanchez A, et al. Amyotrophic lateral sclerosis is a distal axonopathy: evidence in mice and man. *Exp Neurol.* (2004) 185:232–40. doi: 10.1016/j.expneurol.2003.10.004
24. Frey D, Schneider C, Xu L, Borg J, Spooren W, Caroni P. Early and selective loss of neuromuscular synapse subtypes with low sprouting competence in motoneuron diseases. *J Neurosci.* (2000) 20:2534–42. doi: 10.1523/JNEUROSCI.20-07-02534.2000
25. Jokic N, Gonzalez de Aguilar JL, Pradat PF, Dupuis L, Echaniz-Laguna A, Muller A, et al. Nogo expression in muscle correlates with amyotrophic lateral sclerosis severity. *Ann Neurol.* (2005) 57:553–6. doi: 10.1002/ana.20420
26. Bruneteau G, Bauché S, Gonzalez de Aguilar JL, Brochier G, Mandjee N, Tanguy ML, et al. Endplate denervation correlates with Nogo-A muscle expression in amyotrophic lateral sclerosis patients. *Ann Clin Transl Neurol.* (2015) 2:362–72. doi: 10.1002/acn3.179
27. Jokic N, Gonzalez de Aguilar JL, Dimou L, Lin S, Fergani A, Ruegg MA, et al. The neurite outgrowth inhibitor Nogo-A promotes denervation in an amyotrophic lateral sclerosis model. *EMBO Rep.* (2006) 7:1162–7. doi: 10.1038/sj.embor.7400826
28. Clark JA, Southam KA, Blizzard CA, King AE, Dickson TC. Axonal degeneration, distal collateral branching and neuromuscular junction architecture alterations occur prior to symptom onset in the SOD1 G93A mouse model of amyotrophic lateral sclerosis. *J Chem Neuroanat.* (2016) 76(Pt A):35–47. doi: 10.1016/j.jchemneu.2016.03.003
29. Feiguin F, Godena VK, Romano G, D'Ambrogio A, Klima R, Baralle FE, et al. Depletion of TDP-43 affects Drosophila motoneurons terminal synapsis and locomotive behavior. *FEBS Lett.* (2009) 583:1586–92. doi: 10.1016/j.febslet.2009.04.019
30. Diaper DC, Adachi Y, Sutcliffe B, Humphrey DM, Elliott CJ, Stepto A, et al. Loss and gain of Drosophila TDP-43 impair synaptic efficacy and motor control leading to age-related neurodegeneration by loss-of-function phenotypes. *Hum Mol Genet.* (2013) 22:1539–57. doi: 10.1093/hmg/ddt005
31. Sasayama H, Shimamura M, Tokuda T, Azuma Y, Yoshida T, Mizuno T, et al. Knockdown of the Drosophila fused in sarcoma (FUS) homologue causes deficient locomotive behavior and shortening of motoneuron terminal branches. *PLoS ONE* (2012)7:e39483. doi: 10.1371/journal.pone.0039483
32. Machamer JB, Collins SE, Lloyd TE. The ALS gene FUS regulates synaptic transmission at the Drosophila neuromuscular junction. *Hum Mol Genet.* (2014) 23:3810–22. doi: 10.1093/hmg/ddu094
33. Kabashi E, Lin L, Tradewell ML, Dion PA, Bercier V, Bourgouin P, et al. Gain and loss of function of ALS-related mutations of TARDBP (TDP-43) cause motor deficits *in vivo*. *Hum Mol Genet.* (2009) 19:671–83. doi: 10.1093/hmg/ddp534
34. Kabashi E, Bercier V, Lissouba A, Liao M, Brustein E, Rouleau GA, et al. Fus and tardbp but not sod1 interact in genetic models of amyotrophic lateral sclerosis. *PLoS Genet.* (2011) 7:e1002214. doi: 10.1371/journal.pgen.1002214
35. Armstrong GAB, Drapeau P. Loss and gain of FUS function impair neuromuscular synaptic transmission in a genetic model of ALS. *Hum Mol Genet.* (2013) 22:4282–92. doi: 10.1093/hmg/ddt278
36. Ciura S, Lattante S, Le Ber I, Latouche M, Tostivint H, Brice A, et al. Loss of function of C9orf72 causes motor deficits in a zebrafish model of amyotrophic lateral sclerosis. *Ann Neurol.* (2013) 74:180–7 doi: 10.1002/ana.23946
37. Van Damme P, Robberecht W, Van Den Bosch L. Modelling amyotrophic lateral sclerosis: progress and possibilities. *Dis Model Mech.* (2017) 10:537–49. doi: 10.1242/dmm.029058
38. Ghasemi M. Amyotrophic lateral sclerosis mimic syndromes. *Iran J Neurol* (2016) 15:85–91.
39. Traynor BJ, Codd MB, Corr B, Forde C, Frost E, Hardiman O. Amyotrophic lateral sclerosis mimic syndromes. *Arch Neurol.* (2000) 57:109–13. doi: 10.1001/archneur.57.1.109
40. Brooks BR, Miller RG, Swash M, Munsat TL. El Escorial revisited: revised criteria for the diagnosis of amyotrophic lateral sclerosis. *Amyotroph Lateral Scler.* (2000) 1:293–9. doi: 10.1080/146608200300079536
41. Miller RG, Munsat TL, Swash M, Brooks BR. Consensus guidelines for the design and implementation of clinical trials in ALS. World Federation of Neurology committee on Research. *J Neurol Sci.* (1999) 169:2–12. doi: 10.1016/S0022-510X(99)00209-9
42. Traynor BJ, Codd MB, Corr B, Forde C, Frost E, Hardiman OM. Clinical features of amyotrophic lateral sclerosis according to the El Escorial and airlie house diagnostic criteria. *Arch. Neurol.* (2000) 57:1171–6. doi: 10.1001/archneur.57.8.1171
43. De Carvalho M, Swash M. Awaji diagnostic algorithm increases sensitivity of El Escorial criteria for ALS diagnosis. *Amyotroph Lateral Scler.* (2009) 10:53–57. doi: 10.1080/17482960802521126
44. Haverkamp LJ, Appel V, Appel SH. Natural history of amyotrophic lateral sclerosis in a database population. Validation of a scoring system and a model for survival prediction. *Brain* (1995) 118(Pt 3):707–19.
45. Davenport RJ, Swingler RJ, Chancellor AM, Warlow CP. Avoiding false positive diagnoses of motor neuron disease: lessons from the Scottish Motor Neuron Disease Register. *Neurol Neurosurg Psychiatry* (1996) 60:147–51.
46. Daube JR. Electrophysiologic studies in the diagnosis and prognosis of motor neuron diseases. *Neurol Clin.* (1985) 3:473–93. doi: 10.1016/S0733-8619(18)31017-X
47. Joyce NC, Carter GT. Electrodiagnosis in persons with amyotrophic lateral sclerosis. *PM R* (2013) 5:S89–95. doi: 10.1016/j.pmrj.2013.03.020
48. Duleep A, Shefner J. Electrodiagnosis of motor neuron disease. *Phys Med Rehabil Clin N Am.* (2013) 24:139–5. doi: 10.1016/j.pmr.2012.08.022
49. Argyriou AA, Polychronopoulos P, Talelli P, Chroni E. F wave study in amyotrophic lateral sclerosis: assessment of balance between upper and lower motor neuron involvement. *Clin Neurophysiol.* (2006) 117:1260–5. doi: 10.1016/j.clinph.2006.03.002
50. de Carvalho M, Swash, M. Nerve conduction studies in amyotrophic lateral sclerosis. *Muscle Nerve* (2000) 23:344–52. doi: 10.1002/(SICI)1097-4598(200003)23:3<344::AID-MUS5>3.0.CO;2-N

51. Filippi M, Agosta F, Abrahams S, Fazekas F, Grosskreutz J, Kalra S, et al. EFNS guidelines on the use of neuroimaging in the management of motor neuron diseases. *Eur J Neurol.* (2010) 17:526–e20. doi: 10.1111/j.1468-1331.2010.02951.x
52. Turner MR, Modo M. Advances in the application of MRI to amyotrophic lateral sclerosis. *Expert Opin Med Diagn.* (2010) 4:483–96. doi: 10.1517/17530059.2010.536836
53. Staff NP, Amrami KK, Howe BM. Magnetic resonance imaging abnormalities of peripheral nerve and muscle are common in amyotrophic lateral sclerosis and share features with multifocal motor neuropathy. *Muscle Nerve* (2015) 52:137–9. doi: 10.1002/mus.24630
54. Chiò A, Calvo A, Bovio G, Canosa A, Bertuzzo D, Galmozzi F, et al. Amyotrophic lateral sclerosis outcome measures and the role of albumin and creatinine. *JAMA Neurol.* (2014) 71:1134–42. doi: 10.1001/jamaneurol.2014.1129
55. Dupuis L, Corcia P, Fergani A, Gonzalez De Aguilar JL, Bonnefont-Rousselot D, Bittar R, et al. Dyslipidemia is a protective factor in amyotrophic lateral sclerosis. *Neurology* (2008) 70:1004–9. doi: 10.1212/01.wnl.0000285080.70324.27
56. Dorst J, Kühnlein P, Hendrich C, Kassubek J, Sperfeld AD, Ludolph AC. Patients with elevated triglyceride and cholesterol serum levels have a prolonged survival in amyotrophic lateral sclerosis. *J Neurol.* (2011) 258:613–7. doi: 10.1007/s00415-010-5805-z
57. Keizman D, Ish-Shalom M, Berliner S, Maimon N, Vered Y, Artamonov I, et al. Low uric acid levels in serum of patients with ALS: Further evidence for oxidative stress? *J Neurol Sci.* (2009) 285:95–9. doi: 10.1016/j.jns.2009.06.002
58. Qureshi M, Brown RH, Rogers JT, Cudkowicz ME. Serum ferritin and metal levels as risk factors for amyotrophic lateral sclerosis. *Open Neurol J.* (2008) 2:51–4. doi: 10.2174/1874205X00802010051
59. Ilzecka J, Stelmasiak Z, Solski J, Wawrzycki S, Szpetnar M. Plasma amino acids concentration in amyotrophic lateral sclerosis patients. *Amino Acids* (2003) 25:69–73. doi: 10.1007/s00726-002-0352-2
60. Ono S, Hu J, Shimizu N, Imai T, Nakagawa H. Increased interleukin-6 of skin and serum in amyotrophic lateral sclerosis. *J Neurol Sci.* (2001) 187:27–34. doi: 10.1016/S0022-510X(01)00514-7
61. Festoff BW, Fernandez HL. Plasma and red blood cell acetylcholinesterase in amyotrophic lateral sclerosis. *Muscle Nerve* (1981) 4:41–7. doi: 10.1002/mus.880040108
62. Niebroj-Dobosz I, Janik P, Sokołowska B, Kwiecinski H. Matrix metalloproteinases and their tissue inhibitors in serum and cerebrospinal fluid of patients with amyotrophic lateral sclerosis. *Eur J Neurol.* (2010) 17:226–31. doi: 10.1111/j.1468-1331.2009.02775.x
63. Barschke P, Oeckl P, Steinacker P, Ludolph A, Otto M. Proteomic studies in the discovery of cerebrospinal fluid biomarkers for amyotrophic lateral sclerosis. *Expert Rev Proteomics* (2017) 14:769–77. doi: 10.1080/14789450.2017.1365602
64. Shaw PJ, Williams R. Serum and cerebrospinal fluid biochemical markers of ALS. *Amyotroph Lateral Scler Other Motor Neuron Disord.* (2000) 1(Suppl. 2):S61–7. doi: 10.1080/14660820050515773-1
65. Vincenti MP, Brinckerhoff CE. Signal transduction and cell-type specific regulation of matrix metalloproteinase gene expression: can MMPs be good for you? *J Cell Physiol.* (2007) 213:355–64. doi: 10.1002/jcp.21208
66. Lim GP, Backstrom JR, Cullen MJ, Miller CA, Atkinson RD, Tökés ZA. Matrix metalloproteinases in the neocortex and spinal cord of amyotrophic lateral sclerosis patients. *J Neurochem.* (1996) 67:251–9. doi: 10.1046/j.1471-4159.1996.67010251.x
67. Jensen L, Jørgensen LH, Bech RD, Frandsen U, Schrøder HD. Skeletal muscle remodelling as a function of disease progression in amyotrophic lateral sclerosis. *Biomed Res Int.* (2016) 2016:5930621. doi: 10.1155/2016/5930621
68. Lattante S, Rouleau GA, Kabashi E. TARDBP and FUS mutations associated with amyotrophic lateral sclerosis: summary and update. *Hum Mutat.* (2013) 34:812–26. doi: 10.1002/humu.22319
69. Ciura S, Sellier C, Campanari M-L, Charlet-Berguerand N, Kabashi E. The most prevalent genetic cause of ALS-FTD, C9orf72 synergizes the toxicity of ATXN2 intermediate polyglutamine repeats through the autophagy pathway. *Autophagy* (2016) 12:1406–8. doi: 10.1080/15548627.2016.1189070
70. Roggenbuck J, Quick A, Kolb SJ. Genetic testing and genetic counseling for amyotrophic lateral sclerosis: an update for clinicians. *Genet Med.* (2017) 19:267–74. doi: 10.1038/gim.2016.107
71. Vajda A, McLaughlin RL, Heverin M, Thorpe O, Abrahams S, Al-Chalabi A, et al. Genetic testing in ALS: a survey of current practices. *Neurology* (2017) 88:991–9. doi: 10.1212/WNL.0000000000003686
72. Kolb SJ, Kissel JT. Spinal muscular atrophy. *Neurol Clin.* (2015) 33:831–46. doi: 10.1016/j.ncl.2015.07.004
73. Burghes AHM, Beattie CE. Spinal muscular atrophy: why do low levels of survival motor neuron protein make motor neurons sick? *Nat Rev Neurosci.* (2009) 10:597–609. doi: 10.1038/nrn2670
74. Fletcher EV, Mentis GZ. Motor circuit dysfunction in spinal muscular atrophy. *Spinal Muscular Atrophy.* (2017) 153–65. doi: 10.1016/B978-0-12-803685-3.00009-4
75. Crawford TO, Pardo CA. The Neurobiology of childhood spinal muscular atrophy. *Neurobiol Dis.* (1996) 3:97–110. doi: 10.1006/nbdi.1996.0010
76. Farrar MA, Kiernan MC. The genetics of spinal muscular atrophy: progress and challenges. *Neurotherapeutics* (2015) 12:290–302. doi: 10.1007/s13311-014-0314-x
77. Cifuentes-Diaz C, Nicole S, Velasco ME, Borra-Cebrian C, Panozzo C, Frugier T, et al. Neurofilament accumulation at the motor endplate and lack of axonal sprouting in a spinal muscular atrophy mouse model. *Hum Mol Genet.* (2002) 11:1439–47. doi: 10.1093/hmg/11.12.1439
78. Kariya S, Park GH, Maeno-Hikichi Y, Leykekhman O, Lutz C, Arkovitz MS, et al. Reduced SMN protein impairs maturation of the neuromuscular junctions in mouse models of spinal muscular atrophy. *Hum Mol Genet.* (2008) 17:2552–69. doi: 10.1093/hmg/ddn156
79. Murray LM, Comley LH, Thomson D, Parkinson N, Talbot K, Gillingwater TH. Selective vulnerability of motor neurons and dissociation of pre- and post-synaptic pathology at the neuromuscular junction in mouse models of spinal muscular atrophy. *Hum Mol Genet.* (2008) 17:949–62. doi: 10.1093/hmg/ddm367
80. Ling KKY, Gibbs RM, Feng Z, Ko C-P. Severe neuromuscular denervation of clinically relevant muscles in a mouse model of spinal muscular atrophy. *Hum Mol Genet.* (2012) 21:185–95. doi: 10.1093/hmg/ddr453
81. Comley LH, Nijssen J, Frost-Nylen J, Hedlund E. Cross-disease comparison of amyotrophic lateral sclerosis and spinal muscular atrophy reveals conservation of selective vulnerability but differential neuromuscular junction pathology. *J Comp Neurol.* (2016) 524:1424–42. doi: 10.1002/cne.23917
82. Ono S, Mannen T, Toyokura Y. Differential diagnosis between amyotrophic lateral sclerosis and spinal muscular atrophy by skin involvement. *J Neurol Sci.* (1989) 91:301–10. doi: 10.1016/0022-510X(89)90059-2
83. Li M, Miwa S, Kobayashi Y, Merry DE, Yamamoto M, Tanaka F, et al. Nuclear inclusions of the androgen receptor protein in spinal and bulbar muscular atrophy. *Ann Neurol.* (1998) 44:249–54. doi: 10.1002/ana.410440216
84. Takeyama K, Ito S, Yamamoto A, Tanimoto H, Furutani T, Kanuka H, et al. Androgen-dependent neurodegeneration by polyglutamine-expanded human androgen receptor in Drosophila. *Neuron* (2002) 35:855–64. doi: 10.1016/S0896-6273(02)00875-9
85. Fischbeck KH. Kennedy disease. *J Inherit Metab Dis.* (1997) 20:152–8. doi: 10.1023/A:1005344403603
86. Diaz-Abad M, Porter NC. Rapidly worsening bulbar symptoms in a patient with spinobulbar muscular atrophy. *Neurol Int.* (2013) 5:21. doi: 10.4081/ni.2013.e21
87. MacLean HE, Warne GL, Zajac JD. Spinal and bulbar muscular atrophy: androgen receptor dysfunction caused by a trinucleotide repeat expansion. *J Neurol Sci.* (1996) 135:149–57. doi: 10.1016/0022-510X(95)00284-9
88. Cortes CJ, Ling SC, Guo LT, Hung G, Tsunemi T, Ly L, et al. Muscle expression of mutant androgen receptor accounts for systemic and motor neuron disease phenotypes in spinal and bulbar muscular atrophy. *Neuron* (2014) 82:295–307. doi: 10.1016/j.neuron.2014.03.001
89. Casetta I, Groppo E, De Gennaro R, Cesnik E, Piccolo L, Volpato S, et al. Myasthenia gravis: a changing pattern of incidence. *J Neurol.* (2010) 257:2015–9. doi: 10.1007/s00415-010-5651-z
90. Tai H, Cui L, Guan Y, Liu M, Li X, Huang Y, et al. Amyotrophic lateral sclerosis and myasthenia gravis overlap syndrome: a review of two cases and the associated literature. *Front Neurol.* (2017) 8:218. doi: 10.3389/fneur.2017.00218
91. Abbott RJ, Holden D, Currie S. False positive anti-acetylcholine receptor antibodies in motorneurone disease. *Lancet* (1986) 1:906–7. doi: 10.1016/S0140-6736(86)91005-6

92. Ashizawa T. False positive anti-acetylcholine receptor antibodies in motorneurone disease. *Lancet* (1986) 1:1272. doi: 10.1016/S0140-6736(86)91408-X
93. Gold R, Hohlfeld R, Toyka KV. Progress in the treatment of myasthenia gravis. *Ther Adv Neurol Disord.* (2008) 1:36–51. doi: 10.1177/1756285608093888
94. Naddaf E, Barohn RJ, Dimachkie MM. Inclusion body myositis: update on pathogenesis and treatment. *Neurotherapeutics* (2018) 15:995–1005. doi: 10.1007/s13311-018-0658-8
95. Dimachkie MM, Barohn RJ. Inclusion body myositis. *Neurol Clin.* (2014) 32:629–46. doi: 10.1016/j.ncl.2014.04.001
96. Chahin N, Engel AG. Correlation of muscle biopsy, clinical course, and outcome in PM and sporadic IBM. *Neurology* (2008) 70:418–24. doi: 10.1212/01.wnl.0000277527.69388.fe
97. Chilingaryan A, Rison RA, Beydoun SR. Misdiagnosis of inclusion body myositis: two case reports and a retrospective chart review. *J Med Case Rep.* (2015) 9:169. doi: 10.1186/s13256-015-0647-z
98. Dabby R, Lange DJ, Trojaborg W, Hays AP, Lovelace RE, Brannagan TH, et al. Inclusion body myositis mimicking motor neuron disease. *Arch Neurol* (2001) 58:1253–6. doi: 10.1001/archneur.58.8.1253

9

Circadian Rhythm Dysfunction Accelerates Disease Progression in a Mouse Model with Amyotrophic Lateral Sclerosis

Zhilin Huang[1†], Qiang Liu[2†], Yu Peng[2], Jiaying Dai[3], Youna Xie[1], Weineng Chen[1], Simei Long[1], Zhong Pei[1], Huanxing Su[2] and Xiaoli Yao[1]**

[1] Department of Neurology, National Key Clinical Department and Key Discipline of Neurology, Guangdong Key Clinical Laboratory for Diagnosis and Treatment of Major Neurological Diseases, The First Affiliated Hospital, Sun Yat-sen University, Guangzhou, China, [2] State Key Laboratory of Quality Research in Chinese Medicine, Institute of Chinese Medical Sciences, University of Macau, Macao, China, [3] Comprehensive Department, Sun Yat-sen Memorial Hospital affiliated to Sun Yat-sen University, Guangzhou, China

***Correspondence:**
Huanxing Su
huanxingsu@umac.mo;
Xiaoli Yao
yaoxiaol@mail.sysu.edu.cn

[†]These authors have contributed equally to this article and should be considered co-first authors.*

Amyotrophic lateral sclerosis (ALS) is a fatal neurodegenerative disease caused by interactions between environmental factors and genetic susceptibility. Circadian rhythm dysfunction (CRD) is a significant contributor to neurodegenerative conditions such as Alzheimer's disease and Parkinson's disease. However, whether CRD contributes to the progression of ALS remains little known. We performed behavioral and physiological tests on SOD1G93A ALS model mice with and without artificially induced CRD, and on wild-type controls; we also analyzed spinal cord samples histologically for differences between groups. We found that CRD accelerated the disease onset and progression of ALS in model mice, as demonstrated by aggravated functional deficits and weight loss, as well as increased motor neuron loss, activated gliosis, and nuclear factor κB-mediated inflammation in the spinal cord. We also found an increasing abundance of enteric cyanobacteria in the ALS model mice shortly after disease onset that was further enhanced by CRD. Our study provides initial evidence on the CRD as a risk factor for ALS, and intestinal cyanobacteria may be involved.

Keywords: circadian rhythm dysfunction, amyotrophic lateral sclerosis, inflammation, NF-κB, cyanobacteria

INTRODUCTION

Amyotrophic lateral sclerosis (ALS) is a fatal neurodegenerative disease that impairs motor neurons (MNs) in the brain and spinal cord, normally causing death within 3–5 years of onset (1). Although the precise mechanisms remain unclear, the consensus is that ALS is the pathological outcome of a combination of genetic and environmental factors. So far, more than 180 potential genetic risk factors have been identified, including mutations in SOD1 (Cu/Zn superoxide dismutase 1), TDP-43 (TAR DNA-binding protein 43), FUS (fused in sarcoma/translated in liposarcoma), and an increased number of repeats in C9ORF72 (2). Numerous studies have sought to identify ALS-related environmental factors, such as excessive exercise, mercury and heavy metal toxicity, geographical clustering, electromagnetic fields, head injuries, and neurotoxins (3, 4). Specifically, sleep disorders including nocturnal hypoventilation, restless legs syndrome, mood disorders, sleep-disordered breathing, and circadian disturbances occur frequently in ALS patients (5, 6). Some studies suggest that circadian rhythm dysfunction (CRD) alters molecular, cellular, or physiologic functions that favor the development of neurodegenerative conditions (7–9).

The circadian system is considered to be a complex network of positive and negative feedback loops consisting of clock genes (clock and bmal1; per1-3 and cry1-2) and their transcriptional products (BMAL1-CLOCK complexes; PER1-3 and CRY1-2) and regulated by posttranslational events, such as phosphorylation and dephosphorylation (10, 11). The suprachiasmatic nucleus (SCN) is the core circadian clock, and is entrained by a zeitgeber ("time giver"), a signal such as the light–dark (diurnal) cycle transduced through the retinohypothalamic tract (12). Studies have shown that peripheral cells and tissues also have their own rhythmicity in the immune (13), cardiovascular (14), and digestive systems (15) with time. The SCN can synchronize both central nervous system rhythms and those of peripheral tissues through neural and humoral controls (16). Accumulating evidence demonstrates that CRD contributes to the progression of neurodegenerative diseases such as Alzheimer's disease (AD) and Parkinson's disease (PD) (7–9, 17, 18). Several mechanisms of functional impairment by abnormal circadian clocks have been proposed, including epigenetic signals, cellular metabolic changes, and inflammation (19). Gliosis play crucial roles in MN death *via* non-cell-autonomous mechanisms (20). A large body of evidence indicates that nuclear factor κB (NF-κB)-mediated signaling plays an important role in neuronal survival in many pathological conditions [for a review see Ref. (21)]. The p65 subunit is considered the most important NF-κB subunit in the nervous system, and the activation of NF-κB has been shown to involve the phosphorylation of p65 (p-p65) and IκB kinase (p-IKK) (22).

The gut and its microbiome are also regulated by the SCN circadian clock in a complex way. Although the digestive system cannot perceive illumination, the SCN, driven by the light zeitgeber, regulates digestive rhythms in a distinct way, by affecting the intestinal bacterial compositions of the host (23). However, other signals, such as feeding and drinking, were also found to act as zeitgebers for digestive clocks. Thus, it is quite possible for an enteric clock to be desynchronized from the SCN clock rhythm, an event that can result in broad-spectrum disorders like metabolic diseases (24). Indeed, a recent study has stated that the intestinal microbiome can regulate host transcriptomic oscillations through regulating rhythmic biogeography and the metabolome (25).

Increasing evidence suggests that disturbances in the gut microbiota contribute to the development of neurological diseases. For example, colonization with microbiota from patients with PD enhances motor impairments in animal models of PD (26). It has also been hypothesized that an unknown toxin produced by gut microbes causes ALS through the gut–microbe–brain axis (27, 28). Cyanobacteria (formerly known as blue-green algae) are common in water, cycads, and intestinal flora. Epidemiological studies suggest that the areas near rivers and lakes with cyanobacteria blooms, including Wisconsin, New Hampshire, and Southern France, had a higher incidence of ALS (29). Interestingly, cyanobacteria possess an internal clock system with a three-protein (Kai A/B/C) oscillator that maintains rhythmicity in certain biological activities, such as nitrogen fixation. Kai B folds into two different three-dimensional structures that can drive the internal transition between day and night (30). In addition, nitrogen starvation of cyanobacteria can trigger the production of β-*N*-methylamino-L-alanine (BMAA), a neurotoxin which inhibits MN growth (31). Very little information on the relationship between circadian rhythms, cyanobacteria, and ALS progression is available, particularly regarding alterations in gut microbiome compositions and the abundance of cyanobacteria at different stages in the progression of ALS. Therefore, the present study investigated whether CRD could alter either cyanobacteria abundance in gut microbiome compositions or disease progression in adult ALS model mice, or both.

MATERIALS AND METHODS

Animals and Circadian Dysfunction

Transgenic mice overexpressing human SOD1 were obtained from the Nanjing Biomedical Research Institute of Nanjing University, and the genotypes of their offspring were identified by polymerase chain reaction (PCR) using a standard protocol (32). Male transgenic [B6SJL-Tg (SOD1-G93A) 1GurJ] mice and their wild-type (WT) littermates were randomly divided into four groups: a SOD1G93A group with a light-induced CRD (ALS + CRD, $n = 19$), a SOD1G93A group with a normal light/dark cycle (ALS, $n = 18$), a WT group with a light-induced CRD (WT + CRD, $n = 20$), and a WT group with a normal light/dark cycle (WT, $n = 15$). All of the animals in CRD (altered rhythm) groups lived under a 20/4-h light/dark cycle from the age of 42 days until they were sacrificed; the animals in the other two groups lived under a normal 12/12-h light/dark cycle. Mice were sacrificed at the ages of 60, 90, or 120 days. All animals were provided *ad libitum* access to food and water in a temperature (25°C) and humidity (45–55%) -controlled environment. All experiments were performed according to the policies for the care and use of experimental animals and were approved by the Animal Ethical Committee at Sun Yat-Sen University, China. All animals were used only for one procedure and were humanely sacrificed under anesthesia after the completion of the experiment.

Body Weight and Motor Function Assessments

The mice were transferred to the new light/dark environments and adapted for 1 week before measurement of body weight and motor function. Body weight and motor function measurements were performed every 3 days from the age of 50 days to one of the above three time points by a trained observer blinded to the experimental conditions. The final time point was set at the age of 120 days because ALS mice begin to die at this age. Using the widely accepted 4-point evaluation system for motor deficits in SOD1G93A mice (33), we defined the day of disease onset as the day on which hind limb tremors were evident when suspending the mouse in the air by its tail. Impending terminal impairment was defined as the day on which a mouse was unable to right itself within 30 s, and survival rate was calculated as a percentage of mice that had not reached the terminal stage.

Fecal Bacteria Analysis

Gene sequencing of 16S ribosomal RNA (rRNA) was performed to characterize the distal gut microbiota (22,800 ± 35,017 trimmed sequences per sample). At each of the three time points, fresh fecal samples were collected in sterile 1.5-ml Eppendorf tubes at approximately 0900–1100 and immediately frozen in liquid nitrogen for 5 min. The fresh fecal samples were then transferred to −80°C until further processing. Microbial genomic DNA was extracted from stools, and the V4 region of the 16S rRNA gene was PCR-amplified using the following primers: 515F, GTGCCAGCMGCCGCGGTAA, and 806R, GGACTACHVGGGTWTCTAAT. The PCR products were sequenced on an Illumina Hiseq 2 × 300 bp platform (TinyGene Bio-Tech Co. Ltd.; Shanghai, China). The comparisons of relative abundance of bacterial taxa were performed based on the total number of classified reads for each sample.

Immunolabeling

At the end of each time point, the mice were deeply anesthetized and transcardially perfused with ice-cold normal saline and followed by 4% paraformaldehyde. Then the spinal cords were carefully extracted, fixed in 4% paraformaldehyde for 24 h, and successively cryoprotected by immersion in 20 and 30% sucrose overnight. The cervical and lumbar enlargements were cut into 20-μm sections on a cryostat. Selected slices were blocked with 10% normal donkey serum (Beyotime) for 1 h at room temperature, and then incubated with primary antibodies to detect MNs (anti-choline acetyltransferase [ChAT], 1:400, OmnimAbs), astrocytes [anti-glial fibrillary acidic protein (GFAP), 1:400, Sigma], and microglia [anti-ionized calcium binding adaptor molecule 1 (Iba1), 1:200, Millipore] overnight at 4°C. Species-specific secondary antibodies were then added to incubate the slices at 37°C for 1 h in the dark. Images were captured using a Leica SP5 confocal microscope. The anterior horns of labeled sections were visualized and imaged with a laser scanning confocal microscope (Leica TCS SP5MP).

Western Blotting

Mice were deeply anesthetized and transcardially perfused with ice-cold normal saline and the spinal cords were carefully removed. Total protein was extracted from each sample using the extraction protocol (Pierce). The extraction buffer contained protease and phosphatase inhibitors. Equal amounts of protein (10 μg) were loaded onto 8 or 10% sodium dodecyl sulfate polyacrylamide gel electrophoresis gel (SDS-PAGE) and separated. The proteins were transferred onto 0.22-μm polyvinylidene difluoride membranes (Millipore). Non-specific binding was blocked using 5% bovine serum albumin for 1 h at room temperature. The blots were subsequently incubated overnight at 4°C in primary antibodies with mild agitation. The primary antibodies used were rabbit anti-ChAT (1:1,000, OmnimAbs), rabbit anti-GFAP (1:1,000, Sigma), rabbit anti-Iba1 (1:1,000, Millipore), rabbit anti-p65 (1:1,000, CST), rabbit anti-p-p65 (1:1,000, CST), rabbit anti-p-Ikkα/β (1:1,000, CST), rabbit anti-β-actin (1:2,000, Sigma), and rabbit anti-GAPDH (1:2,000, Sigma). The membranes were washed three times for 10 min with Tris-buffered saline containing Tween-20 (TBS/T) and incubated with goat anti-rabbit secondary antibody (1:2,000, abcam) for 1 h at room temperature. The membranes were subsequently washed four times for 10 min with TBS/T. Immunoreactive proteins were visualized using the chemiluminescent horseradish peroxidase substrate (Pierce) and scanned using image analyzer software (Bio-Rad, Image lab 4.1).

Analysis of MN Survival and Inflammation Activation in the Spinal Cord

Previous reports indicate that MNs in the cervical and lumbar segments of ALS model mice have very similar characteristics. We, therefore, studied sections from the cervical segment as representative of the spinal cord in the ALS model mice. About five sections per mice were labeled, and five fields of the ventral horn per slice were randomly selected at 250× magnification. We counted the numbers of ChAT-positive cells in these sections to assess the survival of MNs in the cervical spinal cord. We only counted ChAT-expressing cells clearly displaying a nucleolus located in the ventral horns of spinal sections. The number of surviving ventral horn MNs was described quantitatively as a percentage of the number counted in the WT controls. The luminescence intensity values of western blot bands were calculated by integrating the signals using ImageJ software. The normalized value of p-p65 is represented by the ratio of p65. All expression levels of gliosis and NF-κB are shown as rates of values in the WT controls.

Statistical Analysis

All the data are presented as the means ± SEM. The comparisons of the relative abundances of microflora were analyzed using the Differentially Abundant Features program (Metastats, http://metastats.cbcb.umd.edu). A one-way of analysis of variance followed by Bonferroni's *post hoc* test for multiple comparisons was used to analyze MN survival and glial activation. The comparisons between two groups were made using GraphPad Prism 5 (GraphPad Prism; La Jolla, CA, USA). p-Values < 0.05 were considered significant.

RESULTS

CRD Accelerated Disease Onset and Progression in ALS Model Mice

As shown in **Figure 1A**, the 42-day-old ALS model and WT mice were housed in a 20/4-h light/dark (ALS + CRD and WT + CRD groups) and a regular 12/12-h light/dark cycle (ALS and WT groups). Body weight and behavioral assessments were acquired every 3 days until euthanasia at days 60, 90, and 120. Symptom onset, as assessed based on motor function tests, occurred at 74.00 ± 2.60 days of age in the ALS group ($n = 14$). The end stage occurred at 130.00 ± 3.662 days of age in the ALS model mice ($n = 7$). In contrast, symptom onset was significantly advanced in the ALS + CRD group, occurring 12 days earlier than in the ALS group (**Figure 1B**; ALS + CRD: 62.00 ± 0.78 days of age, $n = 15$, $p < 0.01$); CRD also significantly

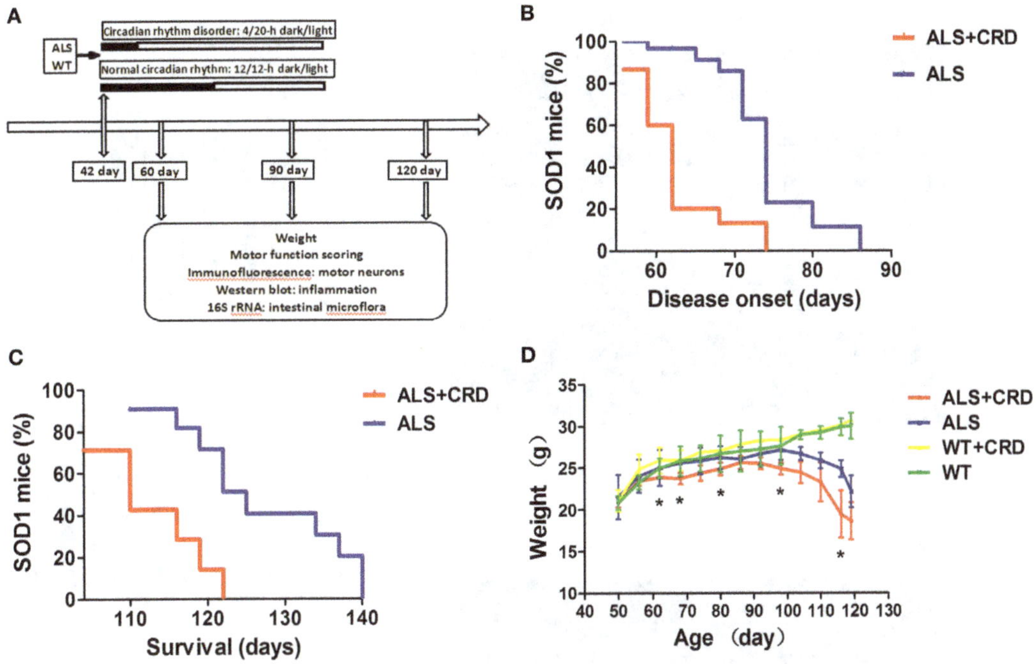

FIGURE 1 | Circadian rhythm dysfunction (CRD) accelerated disease onset and progression in *SOD1G93A* mice. **(A)** A schematic showing the experimental procedures. **(B,C)** Survival curves: disease onsets and disease progression in the ALS + CRD and the ALS group. **(D)** Body weights loss of four groups starting from the day 50 to the day 119. $N = 4$–6 animals per group, $^{*}p < 0.05$. Error bars represent SEM.

shortened the lifespan of ALS mice (**Figure 1C**; ALS + CRD: 116.00 ± 3.00 days of age, $n = 7$, $p < 0.05$). We measured the change in body weight of the mice over time because body weight is a reliable index of disease progression in ALS (33). All mice in both the ALS and ALS + CRD groups demonstrated weight loss over time. A rapid and significant drop in body weight was found in the ALS group at the age of 83 days compared to the WT group (**Figure 1D**, $p < 0.05$). Notably, CRD accelerated the body weight loss of the ALS model mice such that the weight loss in the ALS + CRD group was significantly worse than that in the ALS group beginning at about 62 days of age (**Figure 1D**, $p < 0.05$). In contrast, WT mice gained weight during the experimental period; CRD did not affect body weight in the WT mice (**Figure 1D**, $p > 0.05$). Taken together, these results suggested that CRD accelerated the onset and progression of the ALS in the model mice.

CRD Aggravated Neurodegeneration and Induced Inflammation in SOD1G93A Mice

The most typical pathological feature of ALS is the degeneration of spinal MNs. As shown in **Figure 2A**, there were no significant differences in the numbers of ChAT-positive cells at any time point between the WT + CRD group and WT groups, suggesting that chronic CRD did not lead to MN death in WT mice. In comparison, the percentage of remaining ChAT-positive cells in the ALS + CRD group was significantly lower than that of the ALS group at the 60-day time point (**Figures 2A–C**; $p < 0.01$) and the 90-day time point (**Figures 2A–C**; $p < 0.05$); the difference between the two groups at the 120-day time point was not significant because of the paucity of cells remaining in both the ALS + CRD and ALS groups at that time. Glial activation was assessed using both immunofluorescence and western blot measurements of GFAP and Iba1. Significantly more intense GFAP expression was detected in the ALS + CRD group relative to the ALS group at the 60- and 90-day time points (**Figures 2A,D,F**; $p < 0.05$). There were similar differences in Iba1 intensity between the ALS + CRD and ALS groups, although these differences were significant only at the 90-day and 120-day time points (**Figures 2B,E,F**; $p < 0.01$). The mice in the WT + CRD group also had a slight increase in GFAP and Iba1 expression when compared to those in the WT group. We measured the expression levels of p65, p-p65, and p-IKK, which are important constituents of the classical NF-κB inflammatory pathway. The expression levels of p-p65 and p-IKK were all slight increased in the ALS + CRD group when compared to the ALS group at each time point, but only had significance in p-p65 at days 90 and 120. A increase trend was observed in the WT + CRD group when compared to the WT group (**Figures 3A–C**, $p < 0.05$). All of the inflammatory markers assessed in the ALS group were increased significantly in association with disease progression. These data suggest that CRD exacerbated MNs loss and increased the numbers of gliosis and NF-κB inflammatory responses in the spinal anterior horn in transgenic ALS mice.

CRD Increased Enteric Cyanobacteria Abundance in SOD1G93A Mice

Ribosomal RNA analyses allowed for a phylum-level description of the intestinal flora in the different experimental groups.

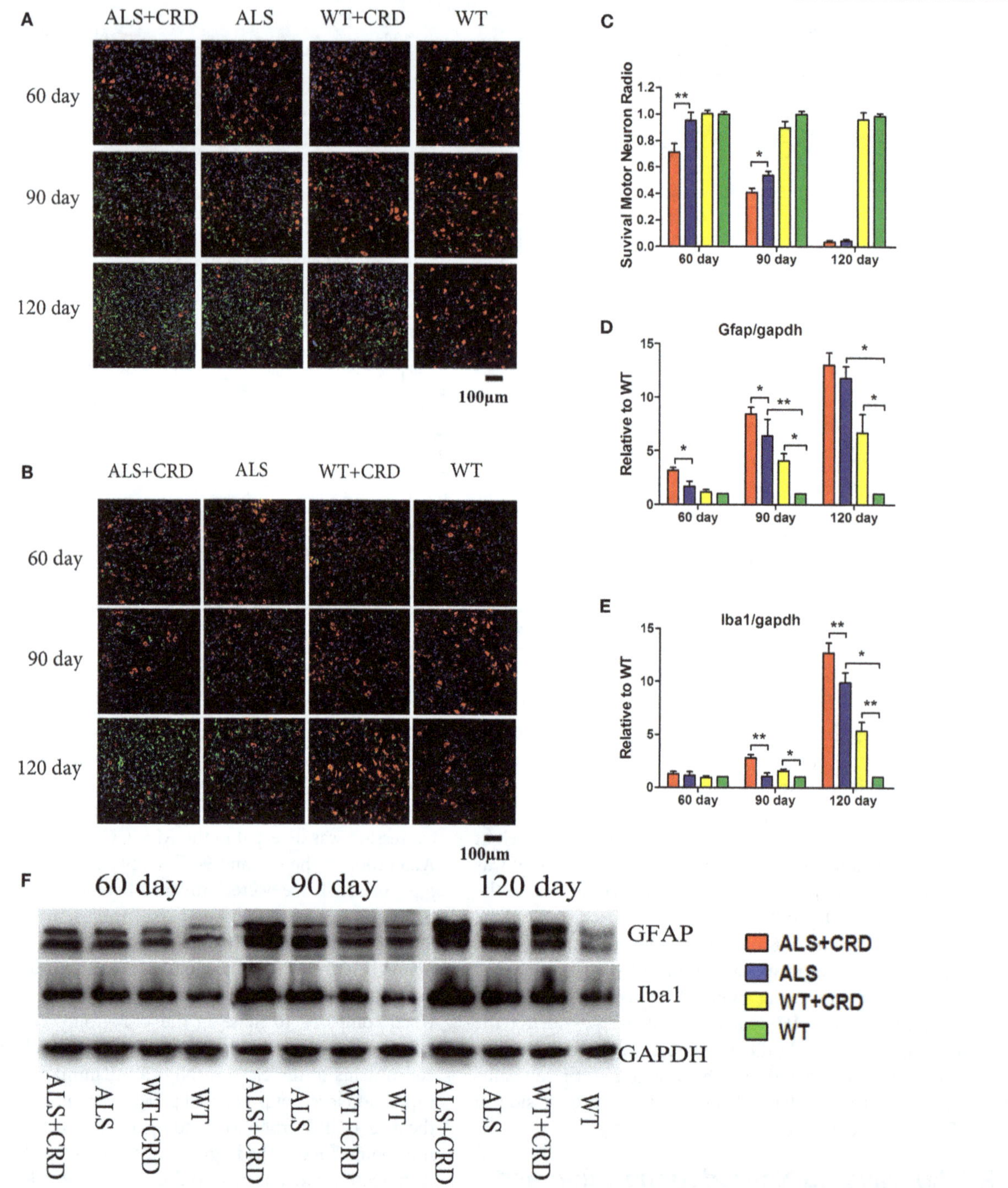

FIGURE 2 | Circadian rhythm dysfunction (CRD) aggravated motor neuron (MN) loss and activated glial cells in *SOD1G93A* mice. **(A)** MNs [choline acetyltransferase (ChAT)-positive cells, red] and astrocytes [glial fibrillary acidic protein (GFAP)-positive cells, green] expression in four groups for three stages. **(B)** MNs (ChAT-positive cells, red) and microcytes (Iba1-positive cells, green) expression in four groups for three stages. Scale bars represent 100 μm. **(C)** Statistical evaluation of surviving MNs radio by counting the number of ChAT-positive cells. $^{**}p < 0.01$; $^{*}p < 0.05$ (one-way ANOVA, n = 4–6 animals per group). **(D,E)** GFAP and Iba1 expression was quantified at three stages by western blotting (one-way ANOVA, n = 2–3 animals per group). **(F)** Expression of GFAP and Iba1 in the spinal cord. $^{**}p < 0.01$; $^{*}p < 0.05$. Error bars represent SEM.

The microbial gut compositions of the four groups at the three time points are presented in **Figure 4A**. The most abundant fecal microbes found in all four groups at all time points belonged to the phyla Bacteroidetes, Firmicutes, Proteobacteria, Verrucomicrobia, Deferribacteres, and Cyanobacteria (**Figure 4A**). Principle component analysis identified evident cluster differences

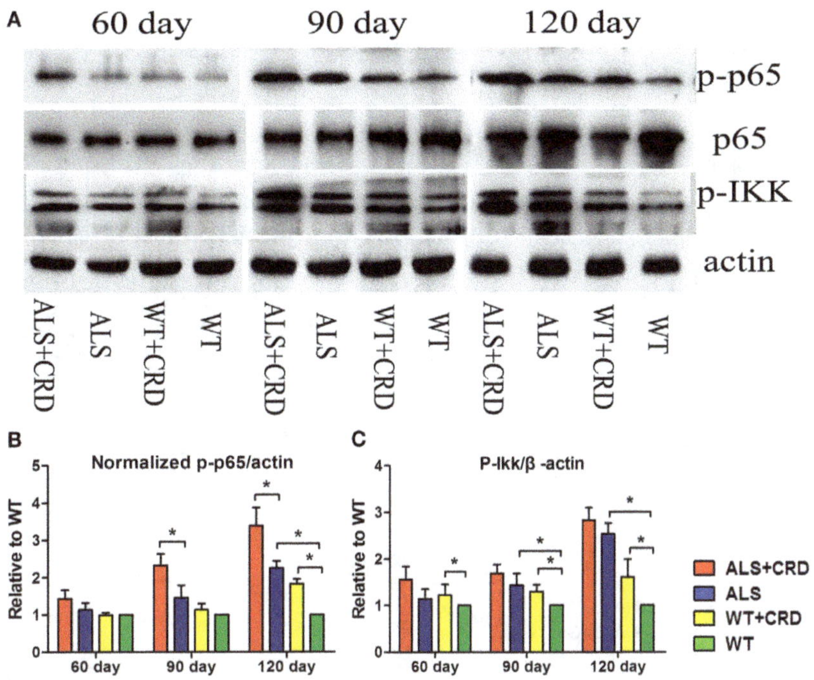

FIGURE 3 | Circadian rhythm dysfunction (CRD) aggravated nuclear factor κB-mediated inflammation in *SOD1G93A* mice. **(A)** Expression of p65, p-p65, and p-IKK in the spinal cord. **(B,C)** Expression of p-IKK and normalized p-p65 was quantified at three stages by western blotting (one-way ANOVA, $n = 2$–3 animals per group). $^{**}p < 0.01$; $^{*}p < 0.05$. Error bars represent SEM.

in the compositions of gut flora between the ALS + CRD and ALS groups at both the 60- and 90-day time points (**Figure 4B**). Because epidemiological studies suggest that an increased abundance of cyanobacteria is associated with a higher incidence of ALS (29). Therefore, we focused our attention on the possible relationship between CRD and the abundance of enteric cyanobacteria. A significant increase in the relative quantity of cyanobacteria in the ALS model mice vs. the WT mice was found at the 90-day time point (**Figure 4C**, 0.8807 ± 0.3429% reads in the ALS group vs. 0.1180 ± 0.0264% reads in the WT group, $p < 0.05$). CRD significantly increased the cyanobacteria abundance beyond that of the ALS group at the 60-day time point (**Figure 4C**; day 60: 0.3512 ± 0.0743% reads in the ALS + CRD group vs. 0.1471 ± 0.0406% reads in the ALS group, $p < 0.05$), but only a slight increase at day 90-day time point (**Figure 4C**; day 90: 1.886 ± 0.5680% reads in the ALS + CRD group vs. 0.8807 ± 0.3429% reads in the ALS group, $p > 0.05$). These data showed that CRD might enrich the proportion cyanobacteria in the gut of ALS model mice. CRD did not lead to significant changes in the cyanobacteria levels in the WT mice at any of the three time points (**Figure 4C**; day 60: 0.2222 ± 0.1624% reads in the WT + CRD group vs. 0.0898 ± 0.0086% reads in the WT group, $p > 0.05$; day 90: 1.1689 ± 0.6295% reads in the WT + CRD group vs. 0.118 ± 0.0264% reads in the WT group, $p > 0.05$; day 120: 0.1892 ± 0.0579% reads in the WT + CRD group vs. 0.3335 ± 0.1574% reads in the WT group, $p > 0.05$). Moreover, no significant difference in the cyanobacteria levels was found between the ALS + CRD group and the WT + CRD group at any of the three time points (**Figure 4C**; day 60: 0.3512 ± 0.0743% reads in the ALS + CRD group vs. 0.2222 ± 0.1624% reads in the WT + CRD group, $p > 0.05$; day 90: 1.8862 ± 0.5680% reads in the ALS + CRD group vs. 1.1689 ± 0.6295% reads in the WT + CRD group, $p > 0.05$; day 120: 0.2222 ± 0.0973% reads in the ALS + CRD group vs. 0.1892 ± 0.0579% reads in the WT + CRD group, $p > 0.05$).

DISCUSSION

Accumulating evidence suggests that disturbed circadian rhythms contribute to the progression of several neurodegenerative diseases such as AD and PD, and here, we provide evidence that CRD could contribute to ALS progression as well. We found that CRD exacerbated the degeneration of MNs in the spinal ventral horn, increased the numbers of glial cells, activated the NF-κB inflammatory pathway, increased the numbers of gut cyanobacteria, and accelerated both the onset and progression of the disease in the presence of an SOD1 mutation.

Disturbed circadian rhythms are comorbid with psychiatric abnormalities including stress, anxiety, depression, schizophrenia, and suicide (34). Transgenic animal models of clock disruptions such as PER1Brdm1−/−, CRY1−/−, and CRY2−/− mutant mice displayed evident depression or anxiety-like behaviors, as well as arrhythmic feeding behavior and impaired glucose tolerance (35). Interestingly, several of the above pathological states have been observed in patients and/or animals with ALS. Persistent exposure to intense stress led to more activation of astrocytes and

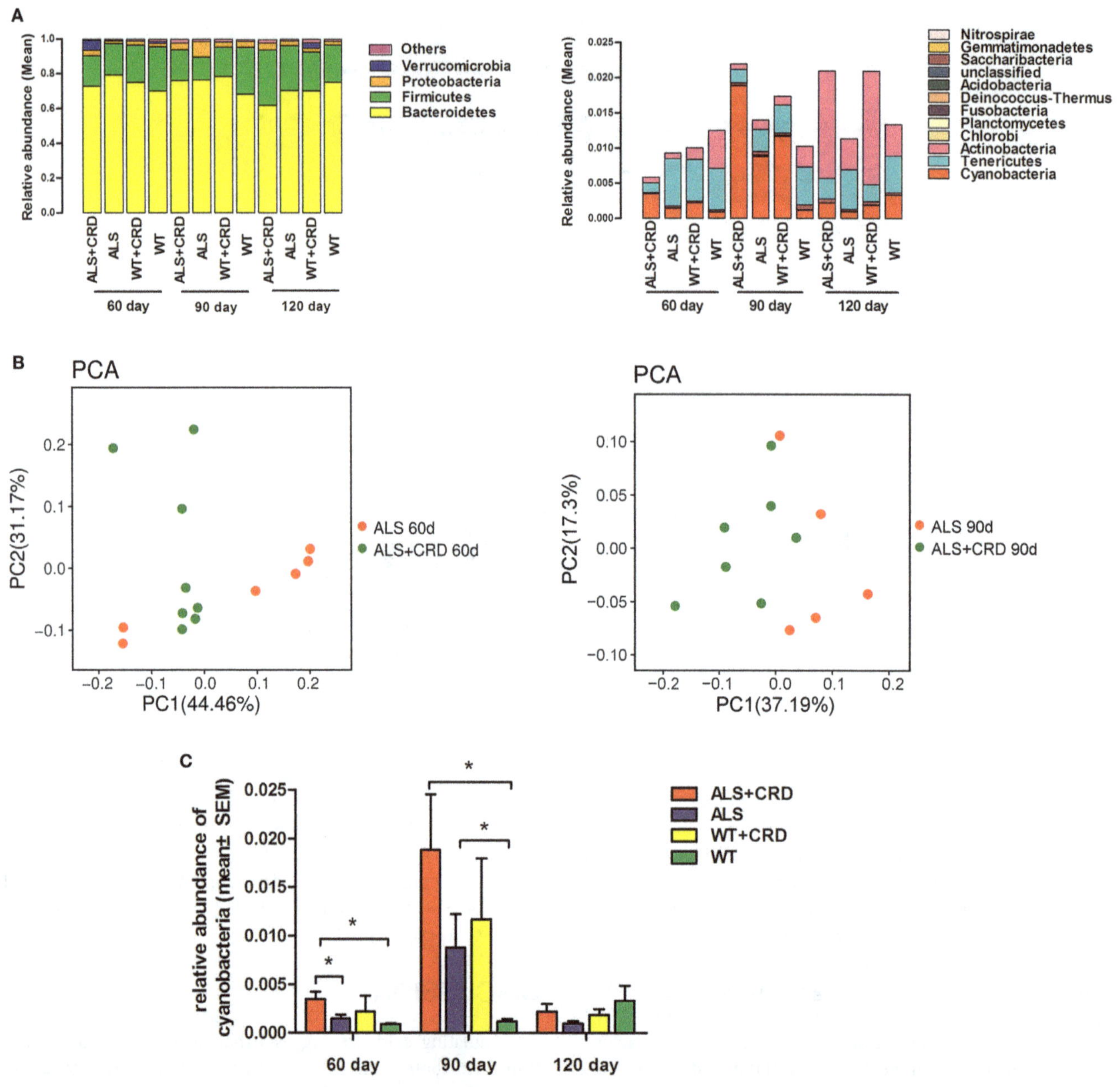

FIGURE 4 | Circadian rhythm dysfunction (CRD) increased enteric cyanobacteria abundance in *SOD1G93A* mice. **(A)** Intestinal bacterial abundance profiles at the level of phylum among the four groups at three time points using 16S high throughput sequencing. Flora were presented in the form of averages. Sample capacity of each group was 4–8. **(B)** Differences and distances of each sample between the amyotrophic lateral sclerosis (ALS) + CRD group and the ALS group at day 60 and 90, respectively, reflected by Principle Component Analysis (PCA). **(C)** Comparisons of relative abundances of cyanobacteria among the four groups at different disease stages. $N = 4–6$ per group per time point, $^*p < 0.05$. Error bars represent SEM.

microglia in the spinal cord, accelerated symptoms, and shortened the median survival period in mouse models with ALS (36). Disturbed eating behaviors and metabolic dysfunction worsened disease progression and prognosis of ALS (37). Additionally, the glial immune reactions that are crucial components of the process underlying ALS were found to follow a circadian variation in the mouse SCN, and could mediate peripheral signals being sent to the central circadian clock (38). Here, astrocytic and microglial activation in the spinal cord accompanying the disruption of circadian rhythmicity may support the role of glial immune reactions in ALS.

Many immunohistochemistry studies have shown that NF-κB is activated in glia in patients with familial and sporadic ALS and in animal models of the disease (39, 40). Consistent with these findings, we found a gradual increase in the activation of the constituents of the NF-κB pathway in the spinal cord in association with disease progress in SOD1G93A ALS mice. More direct evidence indicates that inappropriate NF-κB activation is the pathogenic mechanism underlying optineurin mutation-related ALS (41, 42). The circadian clock controls many physiological changes mediated by activation of the transcription factor NF-κB (43). In our study, activation of the NF-κB pathway in the spinal cord caused by circadian rhythm disorder further confirmed that NF-κB-induced inflammation mediates the connection between abnormal circadian rhythm and neuronal death in ALS model mice. Microglia, but not astrocytes, can induce MN death *via* the classical NF-κB pathway in ALS (44). Therefore, whether the effects of the abnormal circadian rhythm were mainly mediated by microglia or astrocytes requires further investigation, as both cell types were activated in our study. More intense inflammatory reactions were also seen in WT mice exposed to the unusual circadian rhythm, although such inflammatory changes were not sufficient to cause neuronal death in WT mice. We thus conclude that circadian rhythm disorder catalyzes pathological progress in individuals with ALS due to genetic mutations, although it is not a causative factor. If this is true, then prophylactic treatments to adjust the circadian rhythm might be required for patients with familiar ALS. Although our work defines CRD as a risk factor for ALS progression, the exact mechanisms linking the circadian clock and MNs, and the subsequent upregulation of inflammatory responses requires further in-depth studies.

The gut microbiome and the SCN circadian clock may interact reciprocally in complex ways (23–25). We, therefore, hypothesize that the negative effects of CRD on the progression of ALS result from multifaceted mechanisms involving the intestinal microbiota. The recent study regarding the colonization of microbiota from patients with PD cited in the Section "Introduction" demonstrates the importance of gut microbes in PD (26). Furthermore, constipation is a common and early non-motor symptom in patients with PD that can be improved by treatment with *Lactobacillus casei* Shirota (45). However, similar studies on the effects of gut microbes in ALS are rare, although gut health-related problems, such as eating difficulties, lower physical activity, and mood disorders, are common in patients with ALS (46). The use of 16S rRNA sequencing has improved the correlative analysis of gut microflora and disease. Recently, shifts in the intestinal microbiome and aberrant intestinal homeostasis were reported to be associated with ALS pathophysiology in SOD1G93A mice following 454 pyrosequencing (47). The oral administration of butyrate restored intestinal microbiota homeostasis, and thus delayed disease onset and progression in the SOD1G93A mice (47).

The prevalence of ALS is greater in areas with abundant cyanobacteria or high levels of BMAA (48, 49). We found a remarkable increase of the cyanobacteria abundance at day 90, shortly after disease onset in the ALS model mice, which hints a link between intestinal cyanobacteria and the onset and progression of ALS. Gut microflora are vulnerable to the changes of host diet, circadian clock, genotype, age, sex, medicine, and other conditions (50). In this study, the relative abundance of cyanobacteria was enriched by CRD in the ALS model mice at the day 60. However, there were no statistically significant differences in intestinal cyanobacteria in the terminal stages among the four groups. We suspect that this may be due to extremely disordered floral changes due to many different factors, such as an inability to eat or move at the end stages of the disease in ALS mice. Thus, it is tempting to conclude that CRD gradually desynchronizes the intestinal activity of cyanobacteria in the early stage of ALS progression. Cyanobacteria generate BMAA, which has been shown to be neurotoxic and correlated with the higher incidence of ALS-related neurodegenerative disease in Guam (48). Additionally, a recent study found that neonatal mice treated with BMAA had long-term learning impairments (51). Another study analyzing the gut in SOD1G93A mice demonstrated deficits in the tight junction protein zonula occludens-1 leading to increased gut permeability. The above report thus highlights a putative mechanism by which neurotoxins can move from the gut to the brain (52). Our results provide evidence that circadian rhythm disorders promote ALS disease onset and progression, possibly by increasing the abundance of gut cyanobacteria in the mice. However, assessments of the levels of BMAA and other cyanobacterial neurotoxins, such as saxitoxin and anatoxin (53–55), will be necessary in determining the mechanisms underlying the effects of gut cyanobacteria on disease onset and progression in ALS.

AUTHOR CONTRIBUTIONS

ZH, HS, and XY contributed to the conception and design of the study; ZH, QL, YP and SL organized the database; JD, YX and WC performed the statistical analysis; ZH, HS and XY wrote the first draft of the manuscript; QL and ZP wrote sections of the manuscript. All authors contributed to manuscript revision, read and approved the submitted final version.

FUNDING

This study was supported by the grants from Science and Technology Program of Guangzhou (No. 2014J4500031); Fundamental Research Funds for Central Universities (No.15ykcj15b); National Key Research and Development Program of China (No. 2017YFC0907703); National Key Research and Development Program of China (No. 2017YFA0105104); Guangdong Provincial Key Laboratory for Diagnosis and Treatment of Major Neurological Disease (No. 2014B030301035); The Southern China International Cooperation Base for Early Intervention and Functional Rehabilitation of Neurological Diseases (No. 2015B050501003); Guangzhou Clinical Research and Translational Center for Major Neurological Disease (No. 201604020010); and Guangdong Provincial Engineering Center for Major Neurological Disease Treatment.

REFERENCES

1. Gordon PH. Amyotrophic lateral sclerosis: an update for clinical features, pathophysiology, management and therapeutic trials. *Aging Dis* (2013) 4:295–310. doi:10.14336/AD.2013.0400295
2. Taylor JP, Brown RH, Cleveland DW. Decoding ALS: from genes to mechanism. *Nature* (2016) 539:197–206. doi:10.1038/nature20413
3. Al-Chalabi A, Hardiman O. The epidemiology of ALS: a conspiracy of genes, environment and time. *Nat Rev Neurol* (2013) 9:617–28. doi:10.1038/nrneurol.2013.203
4. Zufiría M, Gil-Bea FJ, Fernández-Torrón R, Poza JJ, Muñoz-Blanco JL, Rojas-García R, et al. ALS: a bucket of genes, environment, metabolism and unknown ingredients. *Prog Neurobiol* (2016) 142:104–29. doi:10.1016/j.pneurobio.2016.05.004
5. Ahmed RM, Newcombe RE, Piper AJ, Lewis SJ, Yee BJ, Kiernan MC, et al. Sleep disorders and respiratory function in amyotrophic lateral sclerosis. *Sleep Med Rev* (2016) 26:33–42. doi:10.1016/j.smrv.2015.05.007
6. Bourke SC, Shaw PJ, Gibson GJ. Respiratory function vs sleep-disordered breathing as predictors of QOL in ALS. *Neurology* (2001) 57:2040–2. doi:10.1212/WNL.57.11.2040
7. Musiek ES, Holtzman DM. Mechanisms linking circadian clocks, sleep, and neurodegeneration. *Science* (2016) 354:1004–8. doi:10.1126/science.aah4968
8. Roh JH, Huang YF, Bero AW, Kasten T, Stewart FR, Bateman RJ, et al. Disruption of the Sleep-Wake Cycle and Diurnal Fluctuation of Amyloid-β in Mice with Alzheimer's Disease Pathology. *Sci Transl Med* (2012) 4:122–50. doi:10.1126/scitranslmed.3004291
9. Breen DP, Vuono R, Nawarathna U, Fisher K, Shneerson JM, Reddy AB, et al. Sleep and circadian rhythm regulation in early Parkinson disease. *JAMA Neurol* (2014) 71:589–95. doi:10.1001/jamaneurol.2014.65
10. Gallego M, Virshup DM. Post-translational modifications regulate the ticking of the circadian clock. *Nature Rev Mol Cell Biol* (2007) 8:139–48. doi:10.1038/nrm2106
11. Welsh DK, Takahashi JS, Kay SA. Suprachiasmatic nucleus: cell autonomy and network properties. *Annu Rev Physiol* (2010) 72:551–77. doi:10.1146/annurev-physiol-021909-135919
12. Golombek DA, Rosenstein RE. Physiology of circadian entrainment. *Physiol Rev* (2009) 90:1063–102. doi:10.1152/physrev.00009.2009
13. Yu X, Rollins D, Ruhn KA, Stubblefield JJ, Green CB, Kashiwada M, et al. TH17 cell differentiation is regulated by the circadian clock. *Science* (2013) 342:727–30. doi:10.1126/science.1243884
14. Storch KF, Lipan O, Leykin I, Viswanathan N, Davis FC, Wong WH, et al. Extensive and divergent circadian gene expression in liver and heart. *Nature* (2002) 417:78–83. doi:10.1038/nature744
15. Scheving LA, Russell WE. It's about time: clock genes unveiled in the gut. *Gastroenterology* (2007) 133:1373–6. doi:10.1053/j.gastro.2007.08.068
16. Yamazaki S, Numano R, Abe M, Hida A, Takahashi R, Ueda M, et al. Resetting central and peripheral circadian oscillators in transgenic rats. *Science* (2000) 288:682–5. doi:10.1126/science.288.5466.682
17. Karatsoreos IN, Bhagat S, Bloss EB, Morrison JH, McEwen BS. Disruption of circadian clocks has ramifications for metabolism, brain, and behavior. *Proc Natl Acad Sci U S A* (2011) 108:1657–62. doi:10.1073/pnas.1018375108
18. Lauretti E, Di, Meco A, Merali S, Praticò D. Circadian rhythm dysfunction: a novel environmental risk factor for Parkinson's disease. *Mol Psychiatry* (2017) 22:280–6. doi:10.1038/mp.2016.47
19. Masri S, Sassone-Corsi P. The circadian clock: a framework linking metabolism, epigenetics and neuronal function. *Nat Rev Neurosci* (2013) 14:69–75. doi:10.1038/nrn3393
20. Clement AM, Nguyen MD, Roberts EA, Garcia ML, Boillée S, Rule M, et al. Wildtype nonneuronal cells extend survival of SOD1 mutant motor neurons in ALS mice. *Science* (2003) 302:113–7. doi:10.1126/science.1086071
21. Mincheva-Tasheva S, Soler RM. NF-κB signaling pathways: role in nervous system physiology and pathology. *Neuroscientist* (2013) 19:175–94. doi:10.1177/1073858412444007
22. Mattson MP, Meffert MK. Roles for NF-κB in nerve cell survival, plasticity, and disease. *Cell Death Differ* (2006) 13:852–60. doi:10.1038/sj.cdd.4401837
23. Liang X, Bushman FD, FitzGerald GA. Rhythmicity of the intestinal microbiota is regulated by gender and the host circadian clock. *Proc Natl Acad Sci U S A* (2015) 112:10479–84. doi:10.1073/pnas.1501305112
24. Landgraf D, Tsang AH, Leliavski A, Koch CE, Barclay JL, Drucker DJ, et al. Oxyntomodulin regulates resetting of the liver circadian clock by food. *Elife* (2015) 4:e06253. doi:10.7554/eLife.06253
25. Thaiss CA, Levy M, Korem T, Dohnalová L, Shapiro H, Jaitin DA, et al. Microbiota diurnal rhythmicity programs host transcriptome oscillations. *Cell* (2016) 167:1495–510. doi:10.1016/j.cell.2016.11.003
26. Sampson TR, Debelius JW, Thron T, Janssen S, Shastri GG, Ilhan ZE, et al. Gut microbiota regulate motor deficits and neuroinflammation in a model of Parkinson's disease. *Cell* (2016) 167:1469–80. doi:10.1016/j.cell.2016.11.018
27. Longstreth WT, Meschke JS, Davidson SK, Smoot LM, Smoot JC, Koepsell TD. Hypothesis: a motor neuron toxin produced by a clostridial species residing in gut causes ALS. *Med Hypotheses* (2005) 64:1153–6. doi:10.1016/j.mehy.2004.07.041
28. Kaneko K, Hachiya NS. Hypothesis: gut as source of motor neuron toxin in the development of ALS. *Med Hypotheses* (2006) 66:438–9. doi:10.1016/j.mehy.2005.09.012
29. Bradley WG, Borenstein AR, Nelson LM, Codd GA, Rosen BH, Stommel EW, et al. Is exposure to cyanobacteria an environmental risk factor for amyotrophic lateral sclerosis and other neurodegenerative diseases? *Amyotroph Lateral Scler Frontotemporal Degener* (2013) 14:325–33. doi:10.3109/21678421.2012.750364
30. Chang YG, Cohen SE, Phong C, Myers WK, Kim YI, Tseng R, et al. Circadian rhythms. A protein fold switch joins the circadian oscillator to clock output in cyanobacteria. *Science* (2015) 349:324–8. doi:10.1126/science.1260031
31. Downing S, Banack SA, Metcalf JS, Cox PA, Downing TG, et al. Nitrogen starvation of cyanobacteria results in the production of β-N-methylamino-L-alanine. *Toxicon* (2011) 58:187–94. doi:10.1016/j.toxicon.2011.05.017
32. Gurney ME, Pu H, Chiu AY, Dal Canto MC, Polchow CY, Alexander DD, et al. Motor neuron degeneration in mice that express a human Cu,Zn superoxide dismutase mutation. *Science* (1994) 264(5166):1772–5. doi:10.1126/science.8209258
33. Weydt P, Hong SY, Kliot M, Moller T. Assessing disease onset and progression in the *SOD1* mouse model of ALS. *Neuroreport* (2003) 14:1051–4. doi:10.1097/01.wnr.0000073685.00308.89
34. Lamont EW, Legault-Coutu D, Cermakian N, Boivin DB. The role of circadian clock genes in mental disorders. *Dialogues Clin Neurosci* (2007) 9:333–42.
35. Barandas R, Landgraf D, McCarthy MJ, Welsh DK. Circadian clocks as modulators of metabolic comorbidity in psychiatric disorders. *Curr Psychiatry Rep* (2015) 17:98. doi:10.1007/s11920-015-0637-2
36. Fidler JA, Treleaven CM, Frakes A, Tamsett TJ, McCrate M, Cheng SH, et al. Disease progression in a mouse model of amyotrophic lateral sclerosis: the influence of chronic stress and corticosterone. *FASEB J* (2011) 25:4369–77. doi:10.1096/fj.11-190819
37. Ahmed RM, Irish M, Piguet O, Halliday GM, Ittner LM, Farooqi S, et al. Amyotrophic lateral sclerosis and frontotemporal dementia: distinct and overlapping changes in eating behaviour and metabolism. *Lancet Neurol* (2016) 15:332–42. doi:10.1016/S1474-4422(15)00380-4
38. Leone MJ, Marpegan L, Bekinschtein TA, Costas MA, Golombek DA. Suprachiasmatic astrocytes as an interface for immune-circadian signalling. *J Neurosci Res* (2006) 84:1521–7. doi:10.1002/jnr.21042
39. Prell T, Lautenschlager J, Weidemann L, Ruhmer J, Witte OW, Grosskreutz J. Endoplasmic reticulum stress is accompanied by activation of NF-kappa B in amyotrophic lateral sclerosis. *J Neuroimmunol* (2014) 270:29–36.
40. Swarup V, Phaneuf D, Dupré N, Petri S, Strong M, Kriz J, et al. Deregulation of TDP-43 in amyotrophic lateral sclerosis triggers nuclear factor kB-mediated pathogenic pathways. *J Exp Med* (2011) 208:2429–47. doi:10.1084/jem.20111313
41. Maruyama H, Morino H, Ito H, Izumi Y, Kato H, Watanabe Y, et al. Mutations of optineurin in amyotrophic lateral sclerosis. *Nature* (2010) 465:223–6. doi:10.1038/nature08971
42. Akizuki M, Yamashita H, Uemura K, Maruyama H, Kawakami H, Ito H, et al. Optineurin suppression causes neuronal cell death via NF-κB pathway. *J Neurochem* (2013) 126:699–704. doi:10.1111/jnc.12326
43. Spenglera ML, Kuropatwinski KK, Comas K, Gasparian V, Fedtsova N, Gleiberman AS, et al. Core circadian protein CLOCK is a positive regulator of NF-κB–mediated transcription. *Proc Natl Acad Sci U S A* (2012) 109(37):E2457–65. doi:10.1073/pnas.1206274109
44. Frakes AE, Ferraiuolo L, Haidet-Phillips AM, Schmelzer L, Braun L, Miranda CJ, et al. Microglia induce motor neuron death via the classical NF-kB pathway in amyotrophic lateral sclerosis. *Neuron* (2014) 81:1009–23. doi:10.1016/j.neuron.2014.01.013

45. Cassani E, Privitera G, Pezzoli G, Pusani C, Madio C, Iorio L, et al. Use of probiotics for the treatment of constipation in Parkinson's disease patients. *Minerva Gastroenterol Dietol* (2011) 57:117–21.
46. Forshew DA, Bromberg MB. A survey of clinicians' practice in the symptomatic treatment of ALS. *Amyotroph Lateral Scler Other Motor Neuron Disord* (2003) 4:258–63. doi:10.1080/14660820310017344
47. Zhang YG, Wu SP, Yi JX, Xia YL, Jin DP, Zhou JS, et al. Target intestinal microbiota to alleviate disease progression in amyotrophic lateral sclerosis. *Clin Ther* (2017) 39:322–36. doi:10.1016/j.clinthera.2016.12.014
48. Cox PA, Banack SA, Murch SJ. Biomagnification of cyanobacterial neurotoxins and neurodegenerative disease among the Chamorro people of Guam. *Proc Natl Acad Sci U S A* (2003) 100:13380–3. doi:10.1073/pnas.2235808100
49. Kuzuhara S. Revisit to Kii ALS – the innovated concept of ALS-Parkinsonism-dementia complex, clinicopathological features, epidemiology and etiology. *Brain Nerve* (2007) 59:1065–74.
50. Maurice CF, Knowles SC, Ladau J, Pollard KS, Fenton A, Pedersen AB, et al. Marked seasonal variation in the wild mouse gut microbiota. *ISME J* (2015) 9:2423–34. doi:10.1038/ismej.2015.53
51. Karlsson O, Roman E, Brittebo EB. Long-term cognitive impairments in adult rats treated neonatally with beta-N-methylamino-L-alanine. *Toxicol Sci* (2009) 112:185–95. doi:10.1093/toxsci/kfp196
52. Wu SP, Yi JX, Zhang YG, Zhou JS, Sun J. Leaky intestine and impaired microbiome in an amyotrophic lateral sclerosis mouse model. *Physiol Rep* (2015) 3:e12356. doi:10.14814/phy2.12356
53. Kerrin ES, White RL, Quilliam MA. Quantitative determination of the neurotoxin β-N-methylamino-L-alanine (BMAA) by capillary electrophoresis-tandem mass spectrometry. *Anal Bioanal Chem* (2017) 409:1481–91. doi:10.1007/s00216-016-0091-y
54. Lajeunesse A, Segura PA, Gélinas M, Hudon C, Thomas K, Quilliam MA, et al. Detection and confirmation of saxitoxin analogues in freshwater benthic Lyngbya wollei algae collected in the St. Lawrence River (Canada) by liquid chromatography-tandem mass spectrometry. *J Chromatogr A* (2012) 6:93–103. doi:10.1016/j.chroma.2011.10.092
55. Dittmann E, Fewer DP, Neilan BA. Cyanobacterial toxins: biosynthetic routes and evolutionary roots. *FEMS Microbiol Rev* (2013) 37:23–43. doi:10.1111/j.1574-6976.2012.12000.x

10

Diaphragmatic Neurophysiology and Respiratory Markers in ALS

Mamede de Carvalho [1,2], Michael Swash [1,3] and Susana Pinto [1]*

[1] Instituto de Fisiologia-Instituto de Medicina Molecular, Faculdade de Medicina, Universidade de Lisboa, Lisbon, Portugal, [2] Department of Neurosciences and Mental Health, Hospital de Santa Maria-CHLN, Lisbon, Portugal, [3] Barts and the London School of Medicine, Queen Mary University of London, London, United Kingdom

***Correspondence:**
Mamede de Carvalho
mamedemg@mail.telepac.pt

The main reason for short survival in amyotrophic lateral sclerosis (ALS) is involvement of respiratory muscles. Severe compromise of diaphragmatic function due to marked loss of motor units causes poor inspiratory strength leading to symptomatic respiratory fatigue, and hypercapnia and hypoxemia, often firstly detected while sleeping supine. Weakness of expiratory muscles leads to cough weakness and poor bronchial clearance, increasing the risk of respiratory infection. Respiratory tests should therefore encompass inspiratory and expiratory function, and include measurements of blood gases during sleep. Non-volitional tests, such as phrenic nerve stimulation, are particularly convenient for investigating respiratory function in patients unable to perform standard respiratory function tests due to poor cooperation or facial weakness. However, SNIP is a sensitive test when patients with bulbar involvement are able to perform the necessary maneuvers. It is likely that central respiratory regulation is disturbed in some ALS patients, but its evaluation is more complex and not regularly implemented. Practical tests should incorporate tolerability, sensitivity, easy application for regular monitoring, and prognostic value. Impending respiratory failure can cause increased circulating inflammatory markers, but molecular assessment of respiratory distress requires further study. In future, home-monitoring of patients with accessible devices should be developed.

Keywords: amyotrophic lateral sclerosis, diaphragm physiology, progression, respiratory function tests, survival

INTRODUCTION

Respiratory insufficiency (RI) in ALS usually emerges in the late stage of disease progression, although it may sometimes be the presenting feature (1, 2). Respiratory complications, especially hypoventilation (2), reduced bronchial clearance and lung infection (3) account for the majority of deaths in ALS. Mild respiratory involvement causes fatigue in daily-life activities and disruption of sleep, with negative impact on quality of life (4, 5) and hypoxemia may impair cognitive function (6), especially important in a population with a lower cognitive reserve.

ALS affects both inspiratory and expiratory muscles, as well as upper airway muscles (7). Cough, an essential reflex for airway protection and clearance, depends on effective glottis closure and efficient expiratory muscle function. Bulbar muscle dysfunction impairs the former and, for this reason, cough effectiveness is not always correlated with expiratory muscle weakness (8). Weakness of pharyngeal and laryngeal muscles increases the risk of aspiration and lung infection. The latter is more critical when associated with marked cough deficiency. For active inspiration the diaphragm is the most important muscle, although other muscles function as accessory muscles of inspiration, e.g., sternocleidomastoid, scalenus, trapezius, external intercostal, pectoralis, and paraspinal muscles. These are particularly important when the diaphragm is weak and during exercise. Severe diaphragm weakness leads to hypoxemia and carbon dioxide retention, since the work capacity of these accessory muscles is not sufficient to compensate. Furthermore, these muscles are themselves progressively involved in the disease process (2). In ALS, the major reason for frank respiratory failure is involvement of the diaphragm (2). The phrenic nerve motor nuclei in the cervical spinal cord are located in a region early affected in ALS, shown by early morphometric changes in these neurons (9). Dyspnea in ALS is closely correlated with diaphragmatic dysfunction (10). Indeed, diaphragm weakness as assessed by the evoked response to transcutaneous phrenic nerve stimulation is predictive of hypoventilation (11) and survival (12). It is therefore relevant to assess the physiology of the diaphragm in people with ALS.

DIAPHRAGM PHYSIOLOGY

The diaphragm is the most important muscle of ventilation. It is a dome-shaped muscle that separates the thoracic and abdominal cavities. It has a musculo-fibrous structure, formed by a central non-contractile fibrous region, and contractile muscle fibers that radiate circumferentially from the central tendon to attach peripherally to the upper three lumbar vertebrae posteriorly (crural diaphragm) and onto the inner surface of the lower six ribs and costal cartilages antero-laterally (costal diaphragm). In humans, the diaphragm comprises approximately equal numbers of type I and type II fibers, but these muscle fibers are smaller than in the expiratory muscles. They have a rich capillary supply and are resistant to aging (13). Muscle spindles are present only in small numbers in the diaphragm (14), so muscle stretching does not much modulate phrenic neuronal excitability. Diaphragm is well adapted to the rhythmic continuous periodical inspiration of ventilation and to ocassional more forceful contractions, as in deep breaths and coughing. The mean diaphragm thickness at the point of functional residual capacity is 2.29 ± 0.4 mm, as measured by ultrasound (15) but is variable over its surface, and also dependent on body position. Diaphragmatic thickness can increase two-fold during full inspiration (16).

The motor innervation of the diaphragm is almost exclusively from the phrenic nerve (C3–5), which branches to innervate the entire muscle. Contraction of the diaphragm causes axial descent of the dome of the muscle, decreasing intrapleural pressure, and increassing intrabdominal pressure, thus exerting an expansive force on the lower thorax (17). This negative intrathoracic pressure causes an inflow of air to the lungs, promoting inspiration. The diaphragm is a very mobile muscle. With full inspiration it flattens, expanding the thorax down to the level of costal margin anteriorly, and during forced expiration it rises anteriorly to the level of the fourth or fifth intercostal space.

There is appreciable force reserve in the diaphragm. In humans the maximum transdiaphragmatic pressure is about 11 kPa, which more than 10 times the value measured during eupnea (18). Indeed, normal respiration activates fatigue-resistant slow-units (19). However, coughing and sneezing are demanding maneuvers requiring very strong diaphragmatic contraction, close to 50% of the maximum transdiaphragmatic pressure, which implies activation of fast-fatigable motor units (19).

During calm breathing at rest expiration, unlike inspiration, is a passive phenomenon resulting from the relaxation of the inspiratory muscles and reduction of lung compliance. However, active forced expiration relies on recruitment of expiratory muscles, namely the internal intercostals and the abdominal ventro-lateral muscles (20). Generation of an adequate expiratory flux is needed for coughing, sneezing or vomiting. This is only possible with strong inspiration, closure of the glottis, and a sudden increase of intra-abdominal and intra-thoracic pressures. Effective peak cough flow (PCF) in healthy subjects exceeds 360–400 L/min (21). Peak flow values >160–200 L/min are needed for effective mucus expectoration (22) and values above 250–270 L/min are required to prevent aspiration pneumonia in patients with neuromuscular disorders (23).

The inspiratory pace-maker is located in the pre-Bötzinger Complex in the medulla (24). Its activity, both during inspiration and expiration, is modulated by inhibitory pre-motor neurons and by the Bötzinger Complex (18). Although expiration is a passive movement, active expiration involves a rostral generator, the retrotrapezoid nucleus (25). Synaptic drive to phrenic nerve nuclei is derived from pre-motor neurons located in the ipsilateral ventrolateral and dorsomedial medullary tracts, which respond to central chemoreceptors, sensitive to hypercapnia, and peripheral chemoreceptors, especially the carotid bodies, that are sensitive to hypoxemia. These premotor neurons are also sensitive to sleep-wake state modulation (18). Spinal interneurons can modulate phrenic motoneuronal activity, in particular via intercostal muscle afferents signaling strain of the chest wall (26). Voluntary control of breathing depends on fast, direct corticospinal inputs, which are also critical for respiratory control during speech (18). This pathway can be investigated by magnetic stimulation of cortical areas.

ASSESSMENT OF RESPIRATORY DYSFUNCTION IN ALS

In ALS inspiratory and expiratory muscles, as well as upper airway muscles are progressively involved. Studies of a possible dysfunctional central respiratory drive are few, but it is likely this could be affected in some patients with ALS (27). As such, different tests are necessary to provide a global view of the respiratory function of diseased subjects. The American (28) and the European (29) guidelines agree that a first respiratory evaluation should be made at the baseline clinical assessment and then periodically thereafter. Nevertheless, this must be adjusted individually, according to the rate of progression of the disease and when there are intercurrent events, such as infection, that may affect respiratory function. A summary of the available tests, their utility and limitations is provided in **Table 1**.

Global Respiratory Evaluation

Forced vital capacity (FVC) is a non-invasive respiratory test that has long been used in ALS. It assesses both the inspiratory and expiratory loops, requiring expiration done forcefully after a maximal inspiration, as opposed to slow vital capacity (SVC). This test is sensitive to change and predictive of hypoventilation and survival in ALS (30). The change of FVC is an adequate test to follow ALS patients (30, 31), since its decline rate tends to be linear (~3.5/month), there is a high interpatient variability (32) but this rate is a strong predictor of survival (33). FVC can be an unreliable measure of ventilatory function in patients with bulbar involvement due to orofacial weakness, due to air leakage around the mouthpiece (2). FVC is more sensitive in detecting diaphragmatic weakness when performed in the supine position (34), but this position is often poorly tolerated due to secretions or to the extent of diaphragmatic weakness. In addition, it is not a very sensitive test to detect hypercapnia, since gas exchange is well maintained until FVC values are very low (35). SVC is easier to perform in patients with bulbar involvement, because the air is exhaled slowly, with less air-leakage around the mouthpiece. SVC has been preferred in a number of recent trials, as it is very strongly correlated with FVC (and with other respiratory tests such as Maximal Inspiratory Pressure and Maximal Expiratory Pressure), as well as with ALSFRS-R (36). It is a predictor of progression, the need for positive pressure ventilation, and survival in ALS (37, 38).

Maximal voluntary ventilation (MVV) assesses respiratory function on maintained efforts. The patient is asked to breathe in and out, through a mounthpiece, as deeply and quickly as possible during 12 s, for at least two trials (39). The value is extrapolated for 1 min. The test is demanding for ALS patients, due to their respiratory fatigue. It can be a sensitive measure of disease progression (30), but only in the early stages of the disease (39). This test is rarely performed in daily practice.

Nocturnal pulse oximetry (NPO) is a useful, non-invasive, inexpensive, and convenient method, which accesses respiratory function in a demanding state—when patients are lying and sleeping. It can be used individually or during polysonography, the latter allowing for clear characterization of possible central and/or peripheral apnea. NPO assesses percutaneous oxygen saturation (maximum, median, and minimum values), in relation with heart rate. Further, the pattern of the oxygen saturation curve overnight can be explored. NPO has been shown to be predictive of survival in ALS (40, 41). In addition, it can indicate central drive dysfunction in patients with normal respiratory muscles, a factor that is probably more common in spastic patients (42). NPO is a mandatory method to follow non-invasive ventilation adaptation in patients, which permits home-telemonitoring and distance alteration of ventilatory settings (43). Transcutaneous capnometry (PtcCO2) is a more modern approach to evaluate respiratory function in ALS and other neuromuscular disorders (44). PtcCO2 recordings show strong correlation with arterial measurements. A value higher than 49 mmHg during $\geq$10% of the total recording time indicates respiratory insufficiency (44). Transcutaneous capnography has been strongly recommended for detection of nocturnal hypoventilation in patients with ALS (45). In patients on non-invasive ventilation, PtcCO2 can be helpful to monitor a proper ventilation, in particular to differenciate between hypoventilation and hypoxemia related to other reasons like as ventilation/perfusion mismatch, as well as in detecting hyperventilation (46). Both techniques have some limitations, for example they cannot discriminate other causes of sleep disturbances, such as obstructive sleep apnea, drug-effect, or associated lung disorder. Nonetheless they are very convenient as a screening method.

Blood gas measurements provide information about CO_2 retention and hypoxemia when respiratory failure is severe. Because respiratory assessment is desiged to evaluate early changes, this test is not extensively used in ALS; however, it can provide relevant information for respiratory management in some patients.

Sleep studies have been investigated for a long time in ALS. In this disorder, reduction of the rapid eye movement (REM) sleep stage is typically observed, in particular when the diaphragm is markedly affected and accessory respiratory muscles are weak (47). It has been speculated that disturbed REM sleep might protect patients from hypoventilation (48). However, in patients with preserved diaphragmatic function, signs of sleep hypoventilation are observed as frequently in REM and non-REM phases (27), probably due to reduced respiratory drive (42). Arnulf et al. (48) found that ALS patients with upper motor neuron involvement to respiratory muscles tended to have abnormal REM sleep and poor prognosis. There is a strong link between severity of respiratory function impairment, poor quality of sleep, and daytime somnolence, in ALS (49).

Evaluation of Inspiration

Maximal inspiratory pressure (MIP) and nasal inspiratory pressure during a maximal *sniff* (SNIP) are inexpensive and non-invasive respiratory measures that access maximal inspiratory muscular strength, the first against a mouth occlusion and the second using a plug inserted in one nostril (50–52). In both, it is necessary to secure cooperation from patients to breath forcefully against a resistance. While 3 consistent measures are necessary to determine MIP (53), the number rises to 10 for SNIP, 5 in each nostril (53, 54), as the result improves with practice. Fatigue is a limiting factor for both techniques. MIP is more sensitive than FVC in detecting hypoventilation (55). However, its marked early decline (floor effect) limits its use in following patients and it is difficult to perform in patients with orofacial weakness (56) or with spasticity. SNIP is a sensitive tool especially suited for ALS patients with orofacial weakness. It is predictive of survival (57) and of the onset of significant hypoventilation in spinal-onset patients (5). There is some uncertainty about the best technical approach to test ALS patients in order to obtain reliable values (58). SNIP seems to depend more on diaphragm force and MIP

TABLE 1 | A summary of the most relevant respiratory tests in ALS.

	Tolerability	Simplicity	Reliability	Sensitivity	Rate of change	Technical difficulty	Cost*	Ease for monitoring**	Experience in trials
GLOBAL									
FVC	++	++	++	+	++	Volitional. Limited by orofacial paresis and dyscognition.	++	++	+++
SVC	++	+++	++	+	++	Volitional. Limited by orofacial paresis and dyscognition.	++	++	+++
MVV	+	+	+	+?	+?	Volitional. Needs motivation; Limited by orofacial paresis, fatigue, and dyscognition.	++	+?	0
NPO	+++	+++	+++	++	+	Limited by cold hands or poor sleep.	+	+++	0
TCP	+++	+++	+++	++	+?	Limited by cold hands and poor sleep.	++	+++	0
Sleep studies	+	0	+	+++	+	Limited by poor sleep.	+++	+	0
INSPIRATORY TESTS									
MIP	+	+	++	+++	+++	Volitional. Limited by orofacial paresis, fatigue, and dyscognition; early floor effect.	++	+	0
SNIP	++	++	++	++?	++	Volitional. Limited by orofacial paresis and dyscognition.	+	++	+++
Diaphragm US	+++	+++	+++	++?	++	Limited by dyscognition.	++	++	0
Phrenic stimulation	+	++	++	+	++	Limited by electrical stimulation intolerance.	++	++	
EXPIRATORY TESTS									
PEF	++	++	++	+?	++	Volitional. Limited by orofacial paresis and dyscognition.	++	++	0
PCF	++	+++	++	+?	++	Volitional. Limited by orofacial paresis and dyscognition.	+	++	0
MEP	+	+	++	+++	+++	Volitional. Limited by orofacial paresis, fatigue, and dyscognition; early floor effect.	++	+	0
CENTRAL DRIVE FUNCTION									
P01	++	+	+	+?	+?	Volitional. Limited by orofacial paresis, fatigue and dyscognition.	++	+	0

FVC, forced vital capacity; SCV, slow vital capacity; MVV, maximal voluntary ventilation; NPO, nocturnal percutaneous oximetry; TCP, percutaneous capography; MIP, maximal inspiratory pressure; US, ultrasound; PEF, peak-expiratory flow; PCF, peak-cough flow; MEP, maximal expiratory pressure; P01, mouth occlusion pressure (100 ms).

Cost (greater number of plus symbol means higher cost) was estimated taking into account equipament price and the requirement of a technician.

**Ease for monitoring was estimated considering patient confort and technical complexity.*

more on the sternocleidomastoid muscle power, making these tests complementary (59).

Transdiaphragmatic pressure (Pdi) can be assessed by inserting balloon catheters in the stomach and mid-esophagus and measuring the differential pressure during active maximal inspiration (60) or following stimulation of the phrenic nerve (61). This is an uncomfortable test that is not suited to clinical application.

Diaphragmatic ultrasound (US) is a non-invasive technique that assesses diaphramatic dynamics, and measures the muscle thickness at tidal volume and on maximal inspiration, as well as the ratio between baseline and maximal inspiration, useful measures to detect diaphragm involvement (62, 63). Significant correlations have been found between these measurements and FVC, SNIP, and the amplitude of the motor response of the phrenic nerve (62–64). However, ultrasound studies are less sensitive than phrenic nerve motor responses in assessing early deterioration of the diaphragm in ALS (65).

Phrenic nerve stimulation by percutaneous electrical or magnetic stimulation in the neck to elicit diaphragm motor responses is an objective, non-volitional test (66, 67) that can

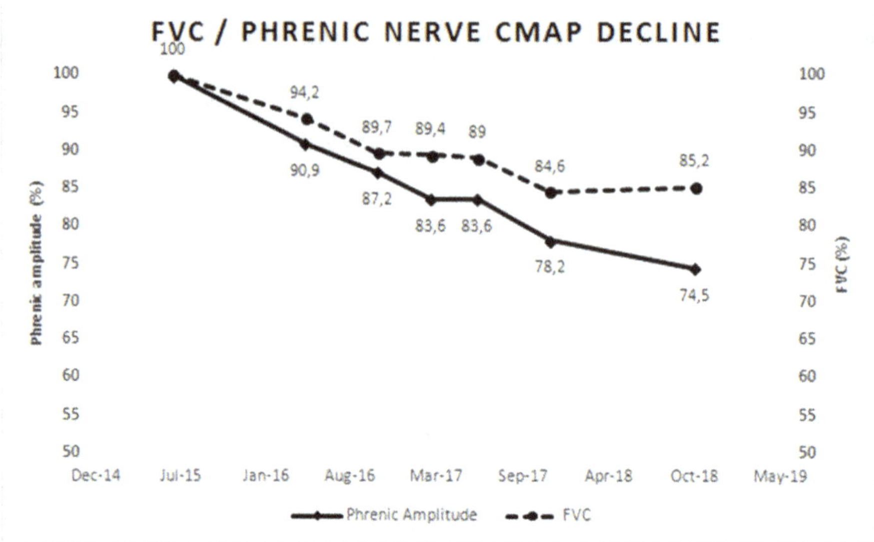

FIGURE 1 | Represents the progressive parallel decline of FVC and phrenic nerve compound muscle action potential amplitude in an ALS patient with slow progression. Values were normalized to 100% of normal at first assessment. This figure is simply for representative purposes and not intended to present research findings.

be used to assess the number of functional motor units in the diaphragm (68). Abnormal amplitude (or area) of the motor response has good predictive value for hypoventilation in both bulbar- and spinal-onset patients, and is correlated to FVC (11). This technique is useful in patients with marked facial weakness or in those unable to cooperate, for example those with fronto-temporal dementia. The amplitude of the motor response declines significantly over 3–6 months, and correlates with FVC and SNIP change (69); it is predictive of survival in ALS (12). **Figure 1** represents the progressive and parallel decline of FVC and phrenic nerve compound muscle action potential in an ALS patient.

Evaluation of Expiration

The efficiency of the expiratory muscles can be easily addressed by evaluating the peak expiratory flow (PEF) and the peak cough flow (PCF), and maximal expiratory pressure (MEP) evaluates the strength of these muscles. These three volitional tests are simple to perform, inexpensive, and non-invasive. Although they measure expiratory muscle function, they depend on central motor control as well as on the efficiency of the inspiratory muscles. Abnormally reduced values indicate inability to expel bronchial secretions, leading to a high risk of respiratory infections (39), leading to increased morbility and mortality (70). MEP values are measured by asking the patient to exhale forcefully against an ocluded mouthpiece. Abnormal values are common in ALS patients (8, 71), and correlate with inspiratory involvement. PEF and PCF use peak flow meters, coupled with a face mask for PCF testing, and assess the ability to exhale forcefully after a maximal inspiration (72, 73) and to cough after a submaximal inspiration (60). Coughing can also be assessed by the gastric pressure generated during a maximal cough, which is a sensitive method to assess expiratory muscle strength, but this is an invasive and poorly tolerated test (74).

Evaluation of the Central Respiratory Drive

Both NPO and sleep studies can detect respiratory center dysfunction, in particular in patients with normal respiratory muscles in whom nocturnal hypoventilation is detected without obstructive apnea (27). Inspiratory mouth occlusion pressure at 100 ms during quiet breathing (P0.1) is considered an indicator of respiratory drive. Spastic patients with normal diaphragm function tend to show abnormal P0.1/FVC values, associated with a poor prognosis for survival (42). P01 values are similar in bulbar and spinal-onset patients at presentation (56), suggesting that impaired central drive does not depend on the region of onset. The observation of "respiratory apraxia" in ALS patients highlights the complexity and importance of the cortical control of respiration and its potential involvement in ALS (75).

CONCLUSIONS

There are many tests available to evaluate different features of respiratory function in ALS. In general, most centers follow a conventional approach by evaluating SVC and FVC, which are are often applied in clinical trials. Patients may also be asked to undergo maximal pressure measurements, expiratory peak flows and nocturnal oximetry, sometimes associated with EEG recordings. Less commonly, diaphgram ultrasound or phenic nerve motor responses to percutaneous cervical electrical stimulation of the nerve are tested. Percutaneous capnography is emerging as a relevant technique. Disparity in patients'tolerability and technical limitations would recommend to apply more than one single test to assess respiratory function in ALS patients.

A future study combining most of these tests in a single set of ALS patients would provide more information about diagnostic accuracy, sensitivity, realibility, and convenience for monitoring disease progression. This would have major potential implications in clinical trials, since changing the rate of respiratory decline is critical for improving survival and functional capability.

The identification of a molecular marker of respiratory impairment in ALS would be a convenient and valuable test. Some research indicates that respiratory insufficiency can precipitate an inflammatory response (76, 77), and this is a new avenue yet to be fully explored. User-friendly devices for in-home respiratory evaluation is another future step. New tests to directly evaluate strength of respiratory muscles will require a better understanding of their physiology.

AUTHOR CONTRIBUTIONS

All authors listed have made a substantial, direct and intellectual contribution to the work, and approved it for publication.

FUNDING

This research was supported by UID/BIM/50005/2019, project funded by Fundação para a Ciência e a Tecnologia (FCT)/Ministério da Ciência, Tecnologia e Ensino Superior (MCTES) through Fundos do Orçamento de Estado.

ACKNOWLEDGMENTS

We are grateful to Mariana Pereira for preparing the figure.

REFERENCES

1. de Carvalho M, Matias T, Evangelista T, Pinto A, Sales Luís ML. Motor neuron disease presenting with respiratory failure. *J Neurol Sci.* (1996) 139:117–22. doi: 10.1016/0022-510X(96)00089-5
2. Pinto S, de Carvalho M. Breathing new life into treatment advances for respiratory failure in amyotrophic lateral sclerosis patients. *Neurodegener Dis Manag.* (2014) 4:83–102. doi: 10.2217/nmt.13.74
3. Corcia P, Pradat PF, Salachas F, Bruneteau G, Le Forestier N, Seilhean D, et al. Causes of death in a post-mortem series of ALS patients. *Amyotroph Lateral Scler.* (2008) 9:59–62. doi: 10.1080/17482960701656940
4. Lyall RA, Donaldson N, Fleming T, Wood C, Newsom-Davis I, Polkey MI, et al. A prospective study of quality of life in ALS patients treated with noninvasive ventilation. *Neurol* (2001) 57:153–6. doi: 10.1212/WNL.57.1.153
5. Lyall RA, Donaldson N, Polkey MI, Leigh PN, Moxham J. Respiratory muscle strength and ventilatory failure in amyotrophic lateral sclerosis. *Brain* (2001) 124:2000–13. doi: 10.1093/brain/124.10.2000
6. Newsom-Davis IC, Lyall RA, Leigh PN, Moxham J, Goldstein LH. The effect of non-invasive positive pressure ventilation (NIPPV) on cognitive function in amyotrophic lateral sclerosis (ALS): a prospective study. *J Neurol Neurosurg Psychiatry* (2001) 71:482–7. doi: 10.1136/jnnp.71.4.482
7. Benditt JO. Respiratory complications of amyotrophic lateral sclerosis. *Semin Repir Crit Care Med.* (2002) 23:239–47. doi: 10.1055/s-2002-33032
8. Polkey MI, Lyall RA, Green M, Leigh NP, Moxham J. Expiratory muscle function in amyotrophic lateral sclerosis. *Am J Respir Crit Care Med.* (1998) 158:734–41. doi: 10.1164/ajrccm.158.3.9710072
9. Bradley WG, Good P, Rasool CG, Adelman LS. Morphometric and biochemical studies of peripheral nerves in amyotrophic lateral sclerosis. *Ann Neurol.* (1983) 14:267–77. doi: 10.1002/ana.410140304
10. Similowski T, Attali V, Bensimon G, Salachas F, Mehiri S, Arnulf I, et al. Diaphragmatic dysfunction and dyspnoea in amyotrophic lateral sclerosis. *Eur Respir J.* (2000) 15:332–7. doi: 10.1034/j.1399-3003.2000.15b19.x
11. Pinto S, Geraldes R, Vaz N, Pinto A, de Carvalho M. Changes of the phrenic nerve motor response in amyotrophic lateral sclerosis: longitudinal study. *Clin Neurophysiol.* (2009) 120:2082–5. doi: 10.1016/j.clinph.2009.08.025
12. Pinto S, Pinto A, de Carvalho M. Phrenic nerve studies predict survival in amyotrophic lateral sclerosis. *Clin Neurophysiol.* (2012) 123:2454–9. doi: 10.1016/j.clinph.2012.05.012
13. Mizuno M. Human respiratory muscles: fibre morphology and capillary supply. *Eur Respir J.* (1991) 4:587–601.
14. Duron B, Jung-Caillol MC, Marlot D. Myelinated nerve fiber supply and muscle spindles in the respiratory muscles of cat: quantitative study. *Anat Embryol.* (1978) 152:171–92. doi: 10.1007/BF00315923
15. Dhungana A, Khilnani G, Hadda V, Guleria R. Reproducibility of diaphragm thickness measurements by ultrasonography in patients on mechanical ventilation. *World J Crit Care Med.* (2017) 6:185–9. doi: 10.5492/wjccm.v6.i4.185
16. Hellyer NJ, Andreas NM, Bernstetter AS, Cieslak KR, Donahue GF, Steiner EA, et al. Comparison of diaphragm thickness measurements among postures via ultrasound imaging. *PMR* (2017) 9:21–5. doi: 10.1016/j.pmrj.2016.06.001
17. Roussos C, Macklem PT. The respiratory muscles. *N Engl J Med.* (1982) 307:786–97. doi: 10.1056/NEJM198209233071304
18. Fogarty MJ, Mantilla CB, Sieck GC. Breathing: motor control of diaphragm muscle. *Physiology* (2018) 33:113–26. doi: 10.1152/physiol.00002.2018
19. Mantilla CB, Seven YB, Zhan WZ, Sieck GC. Diaphragm motor unit recruitment in rats. *Respir Physiol Neurobiol.* (2010) 173:153–6. doi: 10.1016/j.resp.2010.07.001
20. Ewing JM, Griscom NT, Wohl MEB. The effect of the absence of abdominal muscles on pulmonary function and exercise. *Am J Resp Crit Care Med.* (1996) 153:1314–21. doi: 10.1164/ajrccm.153.4.8616560
21. Gregg I, Nunn AJ. Peak expiratory flow in normal subjects. *Br Med J.* (1973) 3:282–4. doi: 10.1136/bmj.3.5874.282
22. Chatwin M, Ross E, Hart N, Nickol AH, Polkey MI, Simonds AK. Cough augmentation with mechanical insufflation/exsufflation in patients with neuromuscular weakness. *Eur Respir J.* (2003) 21:502–8. doi: 10.1183/09031936.03.00048102
23. Kang SW, Bach JR. Maximum insufflation capacity: vital capacity and cough flows in neuromuscular disease. *Am J Phys Med Rehabil.* (2000) 79:222–7. doi: 10.1097/00002060-200005000-00002
24. Richter DW. Generation and maintenance of the respiratory rhythm. *J Exp Biol.* (1982) 100:93–107.
25. Koizumi H, Koshiya N, Chia JX, Cao F, Nugent J, Zhang R, et al. Structural-functional properties of identified excitatory and inhibitory interneurons within pre-Botzinger complex respiratory microcircuits. *J Neurosci.* (2013) 33:2994–3009. doi: 10.1523/JNEUROSCI.4427-12.2013
26. Bellingham MC. Synaptic inhibition of cat phrenic motor neurons by internal intercostal nerve stimulation. *J Neurophysiol.* (1999) 82:1224–32. doi: 10.1152/jn.1999.82.3.1224
27. Atalaia A, de Carvalho M, Evangelista T, Pinto A. Sleep characteristics of amyotrophic lateral sclerosis in patients with preserved diaphragmatic function. *Amyotroph Lateral Scler.* (2007) 8:101–5. doi: 10.1080/17482960601029883
28. Miller RG, Jackson CE, Kasarskis EJ, England JD, Forshew D, Johnston W, et al. Practice parameter update: the care of the patient with amyotrophic lateral sclerosis: drug, nutritional, and respiratory therapies (an evidence-based review) Report of the Quality Standards Subcommittee of the American Academy of Neurology. *Neurology* (1999) 73:1218–26. doi: 10.1212/WNL.0b013e3181bc0141
29. Andersen PM, Abrahams S, Borasio GD, de Carvalho M, Chio A, Van Damme P, et al. EFNS guidelines on the clinical management of amyotrophic lateral sclerosis (MALS)-revised report of an EFNS Task Force on Diagnosis and

Management of Amyotrophic Lateral Sclerosis. *Eur J Neurol.* (2012) 19:360–75. doi: 10.1111/j.1468-1331.2011.03501.x

30. Fallat RJ, Jewitt B, Bass M, Kamm B, Norris F. Spirometry in amyotrophic lateral sclerosis. *Arch Neurol.* (1979) 36:74–80. doi: 10.1001/archneur.1979.00500380044004
31. Czaplinski A, Yen AA, Appel SH. Forced vital capacity (FVC) as an indicator of survival and disease progression in an ALS clinic population. *J Neurol Neurosurg Psychiatry* (2006) 77:390–2. doi: 10.1136/jnnp.2005.072660
32. Schiffman PL, Belsh JM. Pulmonary function at diagnosis of amyotrophic lateral sclerosis: rate of deterioration. *Chest* (1993) 103:508–13. doi: 10.1378/chest.103.2.508
33. Magnus T, Beck M, Giess R, Puls I, Naumann M, Toyka KV. Disease progression in amyotrophic lateral sclerosis: predictors of survival. *Muscle Nerve* (2002) 25:709–14. doi: 10.1002/mus.10090
34. Lechtzin N, Wiener CM, Shade DM, Clawson L, Diette GB. Spirometry in the supine position improves the detection of diaphragmatic weakness in patients with amyotrophic lateral sclerosis. *Chest* (2002) 121:436–42. doi: 10.1378/chest.121.2.436
35. Kaplan LM, Hollander D. Respiratory dysfunction in amyotrophic lateral sclerosis. *Clin Chest Med.* (1994) 15:675–81.
36. Pinto S, de Carvalho M. Correlation between Forced Vital Capacity and Slow Vital Capacity for the assessment of respiratory involvement in Amyotrophic Lateral Sclerosis: a prospective study. *Amyotroph Lateral Scler Frontotemporal Degener.* (2017) 18:86–91. doi: 10.1080/21678421.2016.1249486
37. Pinto S, de Carvalho M. Comparison of slow and forced vital capacities on ability to predict survival in ALS. *Amyotroph Lateral Scler Frontotemporal Degener.* (2017) 18:528–33. doi: 10.1080/21678421.2017.1354995
38. Andrews JA, Meng L, Kulke SF, Rudnicki SA, Wolff AA, Bozik ME, et al. Association between decline in slow vital capacity and respiratory insufficiency, use of assisted ventilation, tracheostomy, or death in patients with amyotrophic lateral sclerosis. *JAMA Neurol.* (2018) 75:58–64. doi: 10.1001/jamaneurol.2017.3339
39. Sherman MS, Paz HL. Review of respiratory care of the patient with amyotrophic lateral sclerosis. *Respiration* (1994) 61:61–7. doi: 10.1159/000196308
40. Velasco R, Salachas F, Munerati E, Pradat PF, Lacomblez L, Orvoen EF, et al. Nocturnal oxymetry in patients with amyotrophic lateral sclerosis: role in predicting survival. *Rev Neurol.* (2002) 158:575–8.
41. Pinto A, de Carvalho M, Evangelista T, Lopes A, Sales Luís ML. Nocturnal pulse oximetry: a new approach to establish the appropriate time for non-invasive ventilation in amyotrophic lateral sclerosis patients. *Amyotroph Lateral Scler.* (2003) 4:31–5. doi: 10.1080/14660820310006706
42. de Carvalho M, Costa J, Pinto S, Pinto A. Percutaneous nocturnal oximetry in amyotrophic lateral sclerosis: periodic desaturation. *Amyotroph Lateral Scler.* (2009) 10:154–61. doi: 10.1080/17482960802382305
43. Pinto A, Almeida JP, Pinto S, Pereira J, Oliveira AG, De Carvalho M. Home telemonitoring of non-invasive ventilation decreases healthcare utilisation in a prospective controlled trial of patients with amyotrophic lateral sclerosis. *J Neurol Neurosurg Psychiatry* (2010) 81:1238–42. doi: 10.1136/jnnp.2010.206680
44. Ogna A, Nardi J, Prigent H, Quera Salva MA, Chaffaut C, Lamothe L, et al. Prognostic value of initial assessment of residual hypoventilation using nocturnal capnography in mechanically ventilated neuromuscular patients: a 5-Year follow-up study. *Front Med.* (2016) 3:40. doi: 10.3389/fmed.2016.00040
45. Boentert M, Glatz CM, Helmle C, Okegwo AM, Young P. Prevalence of sleep apnoea and capnographic detection of nocturnal hypoventilation in amyotrophic lateral sclerosis. *J Neurol Neurosurg Psychiatry* (2018) 89:418–24. doi: 10.1136/jnnp-2017-316515
46. Janssens JP, Borel JC, Pépin JL, SomnoNIV Group. Nocturnal monitoring of home non-invasive ventilation: the contribution of simple tools such as pulse oximetry, capnography, built-in ventilator software and autonomic markers of sleep fragmentation. *Thorax* (2011) 66:438–45. doi: 10.1136/thx.2010.139782
47. Ferguson KA, Strong MJ, Ahmad D, George CF. Sleep disordered breathing in amyotrophic lateral sclerosis. *Chest* (1996) 110:664–9. doi: 10.1378/chest.110.3.664
48. Arnulf I, Similowski T, Salachas F, Garma L, Mehiri S, Attali V, et al. Sleep disorders and diaphragmatic function in patients with amyotrophic lateral sclerosis. *Am J Resp Crit Care Med.* (2000) 161:849–56. doi: 10.1164/ajrccm.161.3.9805008
49. Coco DL, Mattaliano P, Spataro R, Mattaliano A, La Bella V. Sleep-wake disturbances in patients with amyotrophic lateral sclerosis. *J Neurol Neurosurg Psychiatry* (2011) 82:899–842. doi: 10.1136/jnnp.2010.228007
50. Fitting JW. Sniff nasal inspiratory pressure: simple or too simple? *Eur Respir J.* (2006) 27:881–3. doi: 10.1183/09031936.06.00007906
51. Lechtzin N. Respiratory effects of amyotrophic lateral sclerosis: problems and solutions. *Respir Care* (2006) 51:871–81.
52. Caruso P, Albuquerque AL, Santana PV, Cardenas LZ, Ferreira JG, Prina E, et al. Diagnostic methods to assess inspiratory and expiratory muscle strength. *J Bras Pneumol.* (2015) 41:110–23. doi: 10.1590/S1806-37132015000004474
53. ATS/ERS Statement on Respiratory Muscle Testing. *Am J Respir Crit Care Med.* (2002) 166:518–624. doi: 10.1164/rccm.166.4.518
54. Uldry C, Janssens JP, de Muralt B, Fitting JW. Sniff nasal inspiratory pressure in patients with chronic obstructive pulmonary disease. *Eur Respir J.* (1997) 10:1292–6. doi: 10.1183/09031936.97.10061292
55. Jackson CE, Rosenfeld J, Moore DH, Bryan WW, Barohn RJ, Wrench M, et al. A preliminary evaluation of a prospective study of pulmonary function studies and symptoms of hypoventilation in ALS/MND patients. *J Neurol Sci.* (2001) 191:75–8. doi: 10.1016/S0022-510X(01)00617-7
56. Pinto S, Pinto A, de Carvalho M. Do bulbar-onset amyotrophic lateral sclerosis patients have an earlier respiratory involvement than spinal-onset amyotrophic lateral sclerosis patients? *Eura Medicoph.* (2007) 43:505–9.
57. Morgan RK, McNally S, Alexander M, Conroy R, Hardiman O, Costello RW. Use of sniff nasal inspiratory force to predict survival in amyotrophic lateral sclerosis. *Am J Respir Crit Care Med.* (2005) 171:269–74. doi: 10.1164/rccm.200403-314OC
58. Pinto S, de Carvalho M. Sniff nasal inspiratory pressure (SNIP) in amyotrophic lateral sclerosis: Relevance of the methodology for respiratory function evaluation. *Clin Neurol Neurosurg.* (2018) 171:42–5. doi: 10.1016/j.clineuro.2018.05.011
59. Pinto S, de Carvalho M. Motor responses of the sternocleidomastoid muscle in patients with amyotrophic lateral sclerosis. *Muscle Nerve* (2008) 38:1312–7. doi: 10.1002/mus.21109
60. Lechtzin N, Shade D, Clawson L, Wiener CM. Supramaximal inflation improves lung compliance in subjects with amyotrophic lateral sclerosis. *Chest* (2006) 129:1322–9. doi: 10.1378/chest.129.5.1322
61. Mills GH, Kyroussis D, Hamnegard CH, Wragg S, Moxham J, Green M. Unilateral magnetic stimulation of the phrenic nerve. *Thorax* (1995) 50:1162–672. doi: 10.1136/thx.50.11.1162
62. Pinto S, Alves P, Pimentel B, Swash M, de Carvalho M. Ultrasound for assessment of diaphragm in ALS. *Clin Neurophysiol.* (2016) 127:892–7. doi: 10.1016/j.clinph.2015.03.024
63. Fantini R, Mandrioli J, Zona S, Antenora F, Iattoni A, Monelli M, et al. Ultrasound assessment of diaphragmatic function in patients with amyotrophic lateral sclerosis. *Respirology* (2016) 21:932–8. doi: 10.1111/resp.12759
64. Noda Y, Sekiguchi K, Kohara N, Kanda F, Toda T. Ultrasonographic diaphragm thickness correlates with compound muscle action potential amplitude and forced vital capacity. *Muscle Nerve* (2016) 53:522–7. doi: 10.1002/mus.24902
65. Pinto S, Alves P, Swash M, de Carvalho M. Phrenic nerve stimulation is more sensitive than ultrasound measurement of diaphragm thickness in assessing early ALS progression. *Neurophysiol Clin.* (2017) 47:69–73. doi: 10.1016/j.neucli.2016.08.001
66. Similowski T, Fleury B, Launois S, Cathala HP, Bouche P, Derenne JP. Cervical magnetic stimulation: a new painless method for bilateral phrenic nerve stimulation in conscious humans. *J Appl Physiol.* (1989) 67:1311–8. doi: 10.1152/jappl.1989.67.4.1311
67. Evangelista T, de Carvalho M, Pinto A, Sales-Luis ML. Phrenic nerve conduction in amyotrophic lateral sclerosis. *J Neurol Sci.* (1995) 129:35–7. doi: 10.1016/0022-510X(95)00057-9
68. de Carvalho M, Pinto S, Swash M. Diaphragm motor responses to phrenic nerve stimulation in ALS: surface and needle recordings. *Clin Neurophysiol.* (2018) 129:349–53. doi: 10.1016/j.clinph.2017.11.019

69. Pinto S, Turkman A, Pinto A, Swash M, de Carvalho M. Predicting respiratory insufficiency in amyotrophic lateral sclerosis: the role of phrenic nerve studies. *Clin Neurophysiol.* (2009) 120:941–6. doi: 10.1016/j.clinph.2009.02.170
70. Bach JR. Amyotrophic lateral sclerosis: preditors for prolongation of life by noninvasive respiratory aids. *Arch Phys Med Rehabil.* (1995) 76:828–32. doi: 10.1016/S0003-9993(95)80547-8
71. Black LF, Hyatt RE. Maximal static respiratory pressures in generalized neuromuscular disease. *Am Rev Respir Dis.* (1971) 103:641–50.
72. Quanjer P, Lebowitz MD, Gregg I, Miller MR, Pedersen OF. Peak expiratory flow: conclusions and recommendations of a working party of the European Respiratory Society. *Eur Respir J.* (1997) 24:2S–8S.
73. Suárez AA, Pessolano FA, Monteiro SG, Ferreyra G, Capria ME, Mesa L, et al. Peak flow and peak cough flow in the evaluation of expiratory muscle weakness and bulbar impairment in patients with neuromuscular disease. *Am J Phys Med Rehabil.* (2002) 81:506–11. doi: 10.1097/00002060-200207000-00007
74. Chetta A, Aiello M, Tzani P, Olivieri D. Assessment and monitoring of ventilatory function and cough efficacy in patients with amyotrophic lateral sclerosis. *Monaldi Arch Chest Dis.* (2007) 67:43–52. doi: 10.4081/monaldi.2007.509
75. Pinto S, Pinto A, Atalaia A, Peralta R, de Carvalho M. Respiratory apraxia in amyotrophic lateral sclerosis. *Amyotroph Lateral Scler.* (2007) 8:180–4. doi: 10.1080/17482960701249340
76. Pronto-Laborinho AC, Gromicho M, Pereira M, Pinto S, Barros MdA, Swash M, et al. Plasma level of club-cell (CC-16) predicts outcome in amyotrophic lateral sclerosis. *Acta Neurol Scand.* (2018) 137:233–7. doi: 10.1111/ane.12851
77. Pronto-Laborinho A, Pinto S, Gromicho M, Pereira M, Swash M, de Carvalho M. Interleukin-6 and amyotrophic lateral sclerosis. *J Neurol Scii.* (2019) 398:50–3. doi: 10.1016/j.jns.2019.01.026

11

Positron Emission Tomography Molecular Imaging Biomarkers for Amyotrophic Lateral Sclerosis

Sheena Chew and Nazem Atassi*

Department of Neurology, Harvard Medical School, Neurological Clinical Research Institute, Massachusetts General Hospital, Boston, MA, United States

***Correspondence:**
Sheena Chew
schew1@partners.org

Amyotrophic lateral sclerosis (ALS) is a fatal neurodegenerative disorder with limited treatment options. Despite decades of therapeutic development, only two modestly efficacious disease-modifying drugs—riluzole and edaravone—are available to ALS patients. Biomarkers that can facilitate ALS diagnosis, aid in prognosis, and measure drug pharmacodynamics are needed to accelerate therapeutic development for patients with ALS. Positron emission tomography (PET) imaging has promise as a biomarker for ALS because it permits visualization of central nervous system (CNS) pathology in individuals living with ALS. The availability of PET radioligands that target a variety of potential pathophysiological mechanisms—including cerebral metabolism, neuroinflammation, neuronal dysfunction, and oxidative stress—has enabled dynamic interrogation of molecular changes in ALS, in both natural history studies and human clinical trials. PET imaging has potential as a diagnostic biomarker that can establish upper motor neuron (UMN) pathology in ALS patients without overt UMN symptoms, as a prognostic biomarker that might help stratify patients for clinical trials, and as a pharmacodynamic biomarker that measures the biological effect of investigational drugs in the brain and spinal cord. In this Review, we discuss progress made with 30 years of PET imaging studies in ALS and consider future research needed to establish PET imaging biomarkers for ALS therapeutic development.

Keywords: amyotrophic lateral sclerosis, neuroimaging, positron emission tomography, biomarker, diagnostic biomarker, pharmacodynamic biomarker, therapeutic development

INTRODUCTION

Amyotrophic lateral sclerosis (ALS) is a devastating disorder characterized by degeneration of motor neurons in the brain and spinal cord. It is clinically heterogeneous and shares clinical and pathological features with frontotemporal dementia (FTD). ALS invariably leads to weakness and death; ~70–80% of ALS patients die within 5 years of symptom onset (1).

Riluzole and edaravone are currently the only disease-modifying treatments for ALS. More efficacious therapy is urgently needed. Fortunately, the recent expansion of knowledge about genetics and pathophysiology of ALS (2) has generated a large pipeline of potential therapeutic agents to be tested in ALS. Biomarkers for ALS are now urgently needed to stratify patients for trial enrollment, to demonstrate biological drug effect, and to guide dose-selection and go-no-go decisions in early phase clinical trials.

Multiple types of biomarkers are being developed for use in ALS (3–5). Electrophysiological biomarkers of the upper motor neurons (UMNs) [transcranial magnetic stimulation (6)] and lower motor neurons (LMN) [motor unit number index (7) and electrical impedance myography (8)] directly quantify physiology of diseased tissues. Biological fluid-based biomarkers such as phosphorylated neurofilament heavy chain in cerebrospinal fluid (CSF) (9, 10), neurofilament light chain from CSF or serum (10–14), and urine p75 neurotrophin receptor extracellular domain (15) are being evaluated as markers of neuronal degeneration. Neuroimaging biomarkers using magnetic resonance imaging (MRI) or positron emission tomography (PET) techniques can objectively visualize changes associated with the disease processes and help to understand the mechanisms of neurodegeneration *in vivo* (16).

This Review will focus on development of PET molecular imaging biomarkers for ALS. References for this Review were identified by searching PubMed for the terms "amyotrophic lateral sclerosis" or "ALS" or "motor neuron disease" or "MND" AND "PET" or "positron emission tomography." As of October 11, 2018, 222 articles were identified. We excluded articles that were not focused on motor neuron diseases (17), were animal or post-mortem studies (18), were not focused on PET imaging (19), were not dedicated to brain or spinal cord (2), were not written in English (12), were inaccessible (7), studied fewer than 5 ALS or MND cases (20), or were literature reviews or guidelines (21), resulting in 48 papers.

THE DEVELOPMENT OF PET IMAGING IN ALS

PET imaging uses positron-emitting radioisotopes that are incorporated into molecules of interest ("tracers"), which are injected intravenously and enter the central nervous system (CNS). When positrons encounter electrons, they annihilate and emit pairs of gamma rays that travel away from one another at a 180° angle. The detection of gamma ray pairs by the PET camera enables localization of the annihilation event and subsequent three-dimensional reconstruction of radiotracer distribution in the tissue of interest (16). The development of PET tracers that permit visualization of glucose metabolism, cerebral blood flow, neurotransmitter metabolism, neuroreceptor binding, inflammation, and oxidative stress have permitted a deep investigation into the molecular pathophysiology of ALS *in vivo* (**Table 1**).

Glucose Metabolism and Cerebral Blood Flow

The first PET study in ALS, conducted in 1987, used the tracer ^{18}F-fluorodeoxyglucose ([^{18}F]-FDG) to demonstrate that ALS patients with UMN involvement had diffuse cortical hypometabolism compared to healthy controls (18). Subsequent [^{18}F]-FDG PET studies found variable cortical hypometabolism in ALS (22–24). PET studies using radiolabeled carbon dioxide (C[^{15}O]$_2$), which detects alterations in regional cerebral blood flow (40–42), revealed decreased cerebral blood flow to the prefrontal cortex (41–43) and thalamus (41, 43) that correlated with cognitive impairment in ALS. These early PET findings suggested that ALS pathology expanded outside the motor cortex, years before ALS was widely accepted as a disorder on the same spectrum as frontotemporal dementia (FTD).

The 2011 discovery that C9orf72 hexanucleotide repeat expansions cause both ALS and FTD (64–66) motivated new [^{18}F]-FDG PET studies that explored genotype-phenotype correlations and cognition in ALS. One study suggested that ALS patients with C9orf72 expansions had more widespread cortical hypometabolism than sporadic ALS patients (33), though this finding was not replicated (32). Other studies demonstrated frontal and prefrontal hypometabolism in patients with sporadic ALS-FTD compared to ALS patients without FTD (33–35).

In recent years, large cross-sectional [^{18}F]-FDG PET studies have established that sporadic ALS is associated with hypometabolism in the premotor and frontal cortices and hypermetabolism in the brainstem (28, 31, 32). There is now interest in spinal cord imaging: two [^{18}F]-FDG PET studies demonstrated hypermetabolism in the cervical cords of ALS patients (36, 38). These findings suggest potential differences between cortical vs. brainstem and spinal cord metabolism that warrant further exploration.

Neuroinflammation

Neuroinflammation, specifically microglial activation, is a pathological hallmark of ALS (67, 68) and is associated with rate of disease progression (69). The 18 kD translocator protein (TSPO) is highly expressed on activated microglia and astrocytes (70, 71). Radiotracers that bind to TSPO thus can visualize neuroinflammation and gliosis *in vivo*. Indeed, early PET studies of neuroinflammation in ALS used the first-generation TSPO ligands [^{11}C]-PK11195 (44) and [^{18}F]-DPA-714 (21) to demonstrate the presence of widespread glial activation in brains of ALS patients compared to healthy controls.

The second-generation TSPO tracer [^{11}C]-PBR28, which binds TSPO with an 80-fold higher specificity than [^{11}C]-PK11195 (72), has enabled more precise PET evaluation of glial activation. Several [^{11}C]-PBR28 PET studies demonstrated increased tracer uptake isolated to the motor cortices of ALS patients compared with controls (46, 47, 50). Areas of increased uptake correlated positively with Upper Motor Neuron Burden Scale and negatively with ALS Functional Rating Scale-Revised (ALSFRS-R) scores (46, 47, 50). Integrated [^{11}C]-PBR28 PET and MRI scans established that areas of increased uptake co-localize with areas of cortical thinning and reduced fractional anisotropy (47, 50).

[^{11}C]-PBR28 PET studies in patients with primary lateral sclerosis (PLS) found a pattern of glial activation similar to that seen in ALS patients, though tracer uptake was greatest in subcortical white matter in PLS patients and in cortical gray matter in ALS patients (48). The differences between ALS and PLS scans highlight the increased specificity of [^{11}C]-PBR28 tracer and merit further investigation into why such differences in glial activation might exist in these two conditions.

In the largest longitudinal ALS PET study to date, 10 patients underwent [^{11}C]-PBR28 PET scans twice over 6 months. Tracer uptake remained stable despite disease progression, as measured by a 3-point decrease in ALSFRS-R (50). This stability may mirror the pattern of beta-amyloid

TABLE 1 | PET studies in ALS.

References	Tracer	Target(s)	Cross sectional results	Longitudinal results	Clinical correlation
GLUCOSE METABOLISM					
Dalakas et al. (18)	^{18}F-FDG	Glucose metabolism	12 ALS vs. 11 HC: diffuse hypometabolism in cortex and basal ganglia of ALS patients with UMN involvement. Cerebellar metabolism similar between ALS and HC.	4 ALS with 2+ scans; variable changes in metabolism over time	No statistically significant difference in cortical metabolism between ALS patients without UMN signs and HC.
Hatazawa et al. (22)	^{18}F-FDG	Glucose metabolism	12 ALS vs. 11 HC: diffuse hypometabolism, greatest in motor-sensory cortex and putamen. No difference in metabolism in patients without UMN involvement	4 ALS with repeat studies showed reduction in metabolism over time	Cortical hypometabolism associated with disease duration at time of scan.
Ludolph et al. (23)	^{18}F-FDG	Glucose metabolism	18 ALS vs. 12 HC: diffuse hypometabolism in frontal regions not reaching statistical significance	None	Hypometabolism in frontal regions correlates with frontal dysfunction measured by neuropsychologic testing. No correlation between hypometabolism and disease duration at time of scan.
Hoffman et al. (24)	^{18}F-FDG	Glucose metabolism	7 ALS vs. 11 HC: no statistically significant difference when corrected for multiple comparisons	3 ALS with repeated scans after 1 year; no significant reduction in uptake despite clinical progression	Decreased motor strength correlated with hypometabolism in precentral gyri and hypermetabolism in middle frontal gyrus
Garraux et al. (25)	^{18}F-FDG	Glucose metabolism	3 ALS-FTD vs. 46 HC, 10 FTD vs. 46 HC: frontal and anterior temporal hypometabolism	None	No statistically significant differences in cortical hypometabolism between 3 ALS-FTD patients and 10 FTD patients when corrected for multiple comparisons
Jeong et al. (26)	^{18}F-FDG	Glucose metabolism	8 ALS-FTD vs. 11 HC: hypometabolism in bilateral frontal lobes, basal ganglia, thalamus	None	No statistically significant differences in cortical metabolism between 8 ALS-FTD and 29 FTD patients
Renard et al. (19)	^{18}F-FDG	Glucose metabolism	4 ALS-FTD vs. 6 ALS	None	ALS patients with FTD had hypometabolism in dorsolateral prefrontal, medial/lateral premotor cortices, insular cortices, anterior temporal lobes compared to ALS patients without FTD
Boeve et al. (27)	^{18}F-FDG	Glucose metabolism	5 C9 ALS: in 4 of 5, hypometabolism in anterior cingulate, frontal cortices compared to age-segmented normative database	1 ALS with second scan after 2 years showing more prominent cortical hypometabolism	Frontal cortical and anterior cingulate hypometabolism correlated with poor performance on neuropsychological measures of psychomotor speed, word fluency, sustained attention
Cistaro et al. (28)	^{18}F-FDG	Glucose metabolism	32 ALS vs. 22 HC: Hypermetabolism in amygdala, midbrain, pons, cerebellum.	None	13 bulbar onset vs. 19 spinal onset ALS: relative hypometabolism in bilateral frontal cortex, right insula, anterior cingulate, precuneus, interior parietal lobe. Bulbar onset patients with lower neuropsychological scores in verbal fluency
Lai et al. (29)	^{18}F-FDG	Glucose metabolism	10 spinobulbar muscular atrophy vs. 5 HC: hypometabolism in frontal areas	None	None reported
Clark et al. (30)	^{18}F-FDG	Glucose metabolism	9 Primary spastic dysarthria vs. HC: variable degrees of hypometabolism in premotor and motor cortices	None	Hypometabolism in premotor and motor cortices associated with symptom duration >2 years

(Continued)

TABLE 1 | Continued

References	Tracer	Target(s)	Cross sectional results	Longitudinal results	Clinical correlation
Pagani et al. (31)	^{18}F-FDG	Glucose metabolism	195 ALS vs. 40 HC: Hypometabolism in frontal, premotor, occipital cortices. Hypermetabolism in midbrain, temporal pole, hippocampus	None	Bulbar onset ALS patients had more rostral pattern of hypometabolism compared to spinal onset ALS patients. Analysis of Brodmann areas 6, 7, 9-11, 13, 17, 18, 21, 22, 24, 32, 37-40, 47 discriminated ALS from HC scans with 95.4% sensitivity and 82.5% specificity
Van Laere et al. (32)	^{18}F-FDG	Glucose metabolism	59 sALS vs. 20 HC: Hypometabolism in premotor and frontal cortices. Hypermetabolism in hippocampus, amygdala, brainstem, occipital, cerebellum. Similar pattern between 59 sALS, 7 PLS and 11 C9 ALS	None	Severe hypometabolism in frontotemporal regions correlated with shorter survival. Prefrontal hypometabolism is correlated with lower ALSFRS-R scores. Support vector machine analysis discriminated ALS from HC scans with 95.8% sensitivity, 80% specificity; PLS from HC with 57.1% sensitivity, 100% specificity.
Cistaro et al. (33)	^{18}F-FDG	Glucose metabolism	15 C9 ALS vs. 30 sALS: hypometabolism in cingulate, insula, caudate, thalamus, left frontal and superior temporal cortex. Hypermetabolism in midbrain, occipital cortex, globus pallidus, left inferior temporal cortex. 12 sALS-FTD vs. 30 sALS: hypometabolism in orbitofrontal, prefrontal, anterior cingulate, insula. Hypermetabolism in occipital, left precentral/postcentral, superior temporal cortices. 15 C9ALS vs. 12 sALS-FTD: hypometabolism in left temporal cortex.	None	Genotype-phenotype correlation: widespread cortical hypometabolism in C9 ALS more reminiscent of sALS-FTD than sALS, despite lack of FTD diagnosis in C9 patients.
Rajagopalan and Pioro (34)	^{18}F-FDG	Glucose metabolism	18 ALS-FTD vs. 15 HC: hypometabolism in frontotemporal lobes, cingulum, cerebellum, and motor cortex when normalized against pons and whole-brain. Most areas of hypometabolism corresponded with areas of gray matter atrophy.	None	None reported
Canosa et al. (35)	^{18}F-FDG	Glucose metabolism	20 ALS-FTD vs. 150 ALS (94 cognitively normal, 37 with cognitive impairment, 9 with behavioral impairment, 10 with nonspecific impairment): hypometabolism in frontal and prefrontal regions.	None	Continuum of frontal lobe hypometabolism correlates with continuum of cognitive impairment
Van Weehaeghe et al. (17)	^{18}F-FDG	Glucose metabolism	70 ALS (training set), 105 ALS (validation set) vs. 20 HC (used for both training and validation set): hypometabolism in frontal, premotor, inferolateral, parietal cortices. Hypermetabolism in primary visual cortex, cerebellum, upper brainstem, medial temporal cortex. 10 PLS vs. 20HC with similar pattern. Training and validation ALS cohorts had identical hypo- and hyper-metabolism patterns when compared to HC.	None	Frontotemporal hypometabolism predictive of shorter survival. Using volume of interest (VOI)-based discriminant analysis of training set: 88.8% accuracy in classifying ALS or PLS vs. HC in 105 prospective validation cases, if PMA scans excluded. Using voxel-based support vector machine (SVM) approach: 100% accuracy for classifying ALS or PLS vs. HC, if PMA scans excluded.
Marini et al. (36)	^{18}F-FDG	Glucose metabolism	30 ALS vs. 30 HC: hypermetabolism in spinal cord	None	Spinal hypermetabolism (>5th decile) associated with higher mortality rate at 3 years

(Continued)

TABLE 1 | Continued

References	Tracer	Target(s)	Cross sectional results	Longitudinal results	Clinical correlation
Matias-Guiu et al. (20)	^{18}F-FDG ^{18}F-florbetaben	Glucose metabolism, amyloid deposition	18 ALS vs. 24 HC: hypometabolism in frontal area, hypermetabolism in cerebellum. Concurrent use of tracer ^{18}F-florbetaben showed no significant difference in amyloid uptake between ALS and HC.	None	Cognitive impairment associated with decreased frontoparietal metabolism
Buhour et al. (37)	^{18}F-FDG	Glucose metabolism	37 ALS vs. 37 HC: hypometabolism in right paracentral lobule, left inferior parietal gyrus, bilateral thalamus, left superior medial frontal gyrus, cerebellar vermis. Hypermetabolism cerebellar lobules, medial temporal cortex, fusiform cortex.	None	Hypometabolism in hippocampus negatively correlated with changes in memory. Hypometabolism in left fusiform gyrus negatively correlated with theory of mind
Yamashita et al. (38)	^{18}F-FDG ^{11}C-flumazenil	Glucose metabolism, blood flow measured by early flumazenil binding	10 ALS vs. 10 HC: hypermetabolism in spinal cord ipsilateral to weakness at C5 and T1. No difference in flumazenil in spinal cord. Concurrent use of tracer ^{11}C-flumazenil showed no difference in spinal cord uptake between ALS and HC.	None	Cervical hypermetabolism associated with ipsilateral arm weakness
D'Hulst et al. (39)	^{18}F-FDG	Glucose metabolism	ALS (175 training scans from Belgium, 195 validation scans from Italy): minor differences in metabolism between ALS groups across two centers. HC (20 training scans from Belgium, 40 validation scans from Italy): prefrontal hypometabolism in Italian HC compared to Belgian HC cohort. Italian HC scans from patients with lung malignancy (no neurologic disease) who underwent oncologic surveillance PET scans	None	Using SVM analysis of training set, classified ALS or HC from validation set with 95% sensitivity, 12% specificity. Unable to reverse analysis using validation cohort as training cohort and vice versa. Diagnostic algorithm to classify ALS from control scans was unsuccessful when control scans came from patients with non-neurologic illness rather than healthy volunteers
CEREBRAL BLOOD FLOW					
Kew et al. (40)	$C^{15}O_2$	Regional CBF	12 ALS vs. 6 HC: At rest, decreased CBF in sensory and motor cortex, supplementary motor area, parietal regions. With joystick movement task, increased CBF in contralateral motor cortex and adjacent premotor and parietal areas	None	In ALS, poorer verbal fluency associated with decreased CBF in right parahippocampus, bilateral anterior thalamus, right anterior cingulate during joystick movement task No correlation between verbal fluency and resting CBF
Kew et al. (41)	$C^{15}O_2$	Regional CBF	10 ALS vs. 5 HC: decreased CBF during joystick movement task	None	In ALS, poorer verbal fluency associated with decreased CBF in right parahippocampus, anterior thalamus, anterior cingulate during task
Tanaka et al. (42)	$C^{15}O_2$ $^{15}O_2$	Regional CBF	9 ALS vs. 13 HC: non-significant reductions in CBF and oxygen metabolism. 4 ALS with dementia vs. 13 HC: decreased CBF and metabolism in anterior cerebral hemispheres and cerebellum	None	Comparison of CBF between ALS with and without clinical dementia not reported
Abrahams et al. (43)	$C^{15}O_2$	Regional CBF	6 ALS vs. 6 HC: decreased activation (smaller increase in CBF compared to CBF in control condition) during word generation task in right dorsal prefrontal, bilateral inferior parietal lobule, left middle/superior temporal gyri 6 ALS with cognitive impairment vs. 6 HC: decreased activation during word generation task in bilateral dorsolateral prefrontal cortex, medial pre-frontal, premotor, anterior thalamic, insular cortex	None	Poor verbal fluency associated with decreased activation in bilateral prefrontal, premotor, insular cortices, thalamus

(Continued)

TABLE 1 | Continued

References	Tracer	Target(s)	Cross sectional results	Longitudinal results	Clinical correlation
NEUROINFLAMMATION					
Turner et al. (44)	^{11}C-PK11195	TPSO	10 ALS vs. 14 HC: increased uptake in precentral gyri, pons, thalamus, dorsolateral prefrontal cortices	None	Increased uptake correlated with UMN-B. No correlation in ALSFRS-R or disease duration.
Johansson et al. (45)	^{11}C-L-deprenyl-D2	MAO-B—postulated nonspecific measure of astrocytosis	7 ALS vs. 7 HC: increased binding rate in white matter and pons, decreased binding rate in parietal and temporal cortices	2 ALS scans at 8 and 10 months, no change	No statistically significant correlation between binding and clinical characteristics
Corcia et al. (21)	^{18}F-DPA-713	TPSO	10 ALS vs. 8 HC: increased uptake in primary motor, supplementary motor, and temporal cortex. No increased activation in pons of bulbar-onset ALS patients.	None	No correlation between uptake and age, disease duration, or ALSFRS-R
Zurcher et al. (46)	^{11}C-PBR28	TPSO	10 ALS vs. 10 HC: increased uptake in motor cortices and corticospinal tracts	None	Increased uptake correlated negatively with ALSFRS-R, positively with UMN-B score.
Alshikho et al. (47)	^{11}C-PBR28	TSPO	10 ALS vs. 10 HC: increased uptake in left motor cortex correlates with decreased cortical thickness and fractional anisotropy	None	Increased uptake correlated positively with UMN-B score.
Paganoni et al. (48)	^{11}C-PBR28	TSPO	10 PLS vs. 10 HC: increased uptake in anatomically relevant motor regions co-localized with regional gray matter atrophy and decreased subcortical fractional anisotropy	None	No correlation between uptake and UMNB and ALSFRS-R
Albrecht et al. (49)	^{11}C-PBR28	TSPO	10 ALS, 10 HC, 10 low back pain. Occipital cortex may serve as pseudoreference region rather than whole brain for measuring PBR28 uptake.	None	None reported
Alshikho et al. (50)	^{11}C-PBR28	TSPO	53 ALS vs. 21 HC: increased uptake in precentral and paracentral gyri. 11 PLS vs. 21 HC: increased uptake in subcortical white matter of same regions. Increased uptake colocalizes with cortical thinning, reduced frational anisotropy, increased mean diffusivity.	10 scans 6 months apart, no significant change despite decrease in ALSFRS-R by 3 points	Increased uptake in regions of interest correlated positively with UMNB score. Uptake did not change significantly despite clinical decline
Ratai et al. (51)	^{11}C-PBR28	TSPO	40 ALS: PBR28 uptake correlates positively with mI/Cr and negatively with NAA/Cr in precentral gyri.	None	ALSFRS-R score correlated positively with NAA/Cr and negatively with mI/Cr. UMNB score correlated positively with PBR28 uptake and mI/Cr, negatively with NAA/Cr
GABAergic FUNCTION					
Lloyd et al. (52)	^{11}C-flumazenil	GABAa receptor	17 ALS vs. 17 HC: decreased uptake in bilateral prefrontal, parietal, visual association, left premotor/motor cortex.	None	No differences in uptake between ALS patients with or without pseudobulbar affect
Turner et al. (53, 54)	^{11}C-flumazenil	GABAa receptor	24 sALS vs. 24 HC: decreased uptake in premotor, motor, posterior association regions. 10 SOD1 D90A ALS vs. 24 HC: decreased uptake in left frontotemporal junction, anterior cingulate. 2 pre-symptomatic SOD1 D90A—decreased uptake in left frontotemporal junction. 4 PLS vs. HC: relative preservation of anterior and orbitofrontal binding compared to ALS.	None	In sALS, decreased uptake in dominant hemisphere correlated with higher UMN-B score. No correlation between uptake and ALSFRS-R. In SOD1 D90A ALS, uptake correlated positively with ALSFRS-R rather than UMNB.
Wicks et al. (55)	^{11}C-flumazenil	GABAa receptor	12 ALS with cognitive testing	None	Correlation between poorer performance in verbal fluency and reduced binding in right inferior frontal gyrus, superior temporal gyrus, anterior insula.

(Continued)

TABLE 1 | Continued

References	Tracer	Target(s)	Cross sectional results	Longitudinal results	Clinical correlation
Yabe et al. (56)	^{11}C-flumazenil	GABAa receptor	10 ALS with cognitive testing	None	Correlation between poorer confrontation naming and reduced binding in left inferior frontal gyrus/middle frontal gyrus. Correlation between writing errors and reduced binding in bilateral anterior cingulate gyrus
SEROTONERGIC FUNCTION					
Turner et al. (57)	^{11}C-WAY100635	5-HT1a receptor	21 ALS vs. 19 HC: marked decreased global cortical binding (21%). Regional decreased binding in frontotemporal regions, cingulate, lateral precentral, parahippocampal, and fusiform gyri	None	Greater decrease in cortical binding in ALS (21%) compared to historical data in depression (12%) and Parkinson's (15%). Trend toward greater reductions in binding in patients with bulbar involvement
Turner et al. (58)	^{11}C-WAY100635	5-HT1a receptor	11 SOD1 D90A ALS vs. 19 HC: decreased global cortical binding (12%), less dramatic when compared with reduction in binding in sporadic ALS vs. HC (21%)	None	Less reduction in cortical binding of D90A ALS compared to sporadic ALS, despite lower ALSFRS-R scores
DOPAMINERGIC FUNCTION					
Takahashi et al. (59)	^{18}F-6-fluorodopa	Levodopa metabolism	16 ALS vs. 13 HC: no difference in mean striatal uptake	None	Negative correlation between 6-fluorodopa uptake and duration of ALS symptoms. No correlation between uptake and severity of symptoms.
Przedborski et al. (60)	^{18}F-6-fluorodopa	Levodopa metabolism	7 SOD1 familial ALS, 7 non-SOD1 familial ALS, 14 HC. 5/14 familial ALS with reduced uptake in nigrostriatal region, more commonly seen in non-SOD1 patients.	None	No correlation between binding and duration of symptoms
Hideyama et al. (61)	^{18}F-6-fluorodopa, ^{11}C-N-methyl-spiperone	Levodopa metabolism and D2/D3 receptor antagonist	5 ALS with clinical parkinsonism: preganglionic and postganglionic striatonigral dopaminergic systems preserved	None	Parkinsonism in ALS patients not correlated with striatonigral dysfunction
Fu et al. (62)	^{18}F-fallypride	D2/D3 receptor antagonist	17 ALS vs. 11 HC: decreased binding in bilateral nucleus accumbens, frontal lobes, superior frontal gyri, left temporal lobe, left angular gyrus. No difference in striatum.	None	None reported
OXIDATIVE STRESS					
Ikawa et al. (63)	^{62}Cu-ATSM	Intracellular reductive state	12 ALS vs. 9 HC: increased uptake in bilateral pre- and post- central gyri and paracentral lobule, right superior parietal lobule.	None	Increased uptake negatively correlated with ALSFRS-R. No correlation between uptake and disease duration

ALS, amyotrophic lateral sclerosis; ALSFRS-R, ALS functional rating scale-Revised; C9, C9orf72 hexanucleotide repeat expansion; CBF, cerebral blood flow; FTD, frontotemporal dementia; HC, healthy control; mI/Cr, myoinositol/creatine ratio; NAA/Cr, N-acetylaspartate/creatine ratio; PMA, primary muscular atrophy; sALS, sporadic ALS; SOD1, superoxide dismutase 1; TSPO, translocator protein; UMN, upper motor neuron; UMN-B, Upper Motor Neuron Burden scale.

brain deposition in Alzheimer's disease, as measured by Pittsburg compound B (PiB) PET imaging: PiB uptake rises in patients developing mild cognitive impairment, then plateaus upon development of Alzheimer's dementia (73). Alternatively, it may reflect a bias toward recruitment of slowly-progressive patients into longitudinal neuroimaging studies. Longitudinal studies with larger sample sizes, rapidly progressing patients, and patients early in the disease course are needed to determine the natural history of glial activation in ALS.

GABAergic Function

Cortical excitability is altered in ALS (6). To evaluate whether loss of GABAergic inhibition contributes to cortical hyperexcitability in ALS, PET studies were conducted using the $GABA_A$ receptor ligand [^{11}C]-Flumazenil. These studies showed widespread reductions in binding in ALS patients compared to controls (52), and found that reduced binding in the frontal lobes (55) and anterior cingulate gyri (56) in ALS patients correlated with poorer performance on language tasks. Additionally, patients with slowly progressive ALS caused by SOD1 D90A mutations had smaller reductions in binding compared to sporadic ALS patients (53). Taken together, these findings could suggest that loss of GABAergic cortical inhibition is part of ALS pathogenesis, though it is also possible that it reflects generalized cortical neuronal loss rather than specific loss of GABAergic inhibition.

Serotonergic Function

The serotonin 5-hydroxytryptamine (5-HT1a) receptor is expressed widely in the cortex, including on layer III and V pyramidal neurons in the cortex (74). A PET imaging study using the 5-HT1a ligand [^{11}C]-WAY100635 demonstrated decreased tracer binding in the frontotemporal regions, precentral, cingulate, parahippocampal, and fusiform gyri in non-depressed ALS patients compared to healthy controls (57). A follow up study reported smaller reductions in [^{11}C]-WAY100635 uptake in patients with slowly progressive SOD1 D90A genetic ALS compared to sporadic ALS (58). Like the studies using $GABA_A$ ligands, these studies suggest widespread neuronal loss or dysfunction in ALS patients that is less apparent in slowly progressive disease.

Dopaminergic Function

Evidence of extramotor involvement in ALS has raised questions about its overlap with neurodegenerative disorders such as Parkinson's disease. Rare patients with ALS have parkinsonism, and post-mortem evaluation has revealed degeneration of the substantia nigra in ALS (75). To evaluate whether dopaminergic dysfunction plays a role in ALS pathogenesis, several PET studies were conducted using ligands that interrogate levodopa metabolism [[^{18}F]-fluorodopa (59, 61)], bind to dopamine receptors in the striatum [[^{11}C]-N-methylspiperone (61)], and bind to dopamine receptors in the cortex [[^{18}F]-fallypride (62)]. The [^{18}F]-fluorodopa and [^{11}C]-N-methylspiperone studies showed no significant difference in levodopa metabolism or dopamine receptor binding in the striatum of ALS vs. control subjects, even in patients with overt parkinsonism (59, 61). Conversely, the [^{18}F]-fallypride PET study showed decreased dopamine binding in the cortex of ALS patients (62), even though the patients were not noted to have clinical parkinsonism. One interpretation of these studies is that ALS is associated with cortical rather than striatal dopaminergic dysfunction. However, PET studies demonstrating decreased cortical binding of GABAergic, serotonergic, and now dopaminergic ligands in ALS patients argues against dopamine-specific pathogenesis of ALS and supports a generalized cortical neuronal loss or dysfunction in disease.

Oxidative Stress

Oxidative stress is considered one of the pathogenic mechanisms underlying neurodegeneration in ALS (76) and is the proposed target of edaravone, a free radical scavenger recently approved for treatment of ALS (77). The PET ligand [^{62}Cu]-ATSM is a copper-linked small molecule structurally similar to superoxide dismutase (78). It distributes to areas of hypoxia and oxidative stress in PET studies of patients with Parkinson's disease (79) and mitochondrial diseases (80). One [^{62}Cu]-ATSM PET study in ALS showed increased tracer accumulation in the motor cortices, paracentral lobules, and right superior parietal lobule in ALS patients compared to controls (63). Areas of increased uptake negatively correlated with ALSFRS-R score.

Notably, Cu-ATSM was selected as an investigational drug for ALS because human [^{62}Cu]-ATSM PET studies demonstrated effective penetration into the brain. Cu-ATSM's proposed mechanism of action is free radical scavenging and delivery of copper into the CNS (81). Cu-ATSM slowed disease progression in SOD^{G93A} mouse models of ALS (81, 82) and is now entering phase I human clinical trials for ALS (Clinicaltrials.gov NCT02870634).

CHALLENGES AND OPPORTUNITIES IN THE DEVELOPMENT OF MOLECULAR IMAGING BIOMARKERS FOR ALS

The FDA-NIH Biomarker Working Group defines a biomarker as a "characteristic that is measured as an indicator of normal biological processes, pathogenic processes, or responses to an exposure or intervention, including therapeutic interventions" (83). Because PET imaging can localize molecular changes in the brain, it has unique promise for use as a diagnostic, prognostic, and pharmacodynamic biomarker. Its advantages and disadvantages complement other biomarkers being developed for ALS (**Table 2**).

PET Imaging as a Diagnostic Biomarker

Mounting evidence of quantifiable PET imaging differences between ALS and control brains has generated interest in using PET as a diagnostic biomarker for ALS. Indeed, the sensitivity of PET makes it uniquely positioned to detect or confirm UMN dysfunction in suspected ALS patients, which has traditionally been difficult to measure.

Three successive studies recently assessed the diagnostic potential of [^{18}F]-FDG PET in ALS (17, 32, 39). In these studies, the authors used group differences in scans from ALS and control subjects to generate algorithms ("diagnostic algorithms") for classifying individual scans as ALS vs. control. Group-level differences in FDG uptake between ALS and control scans were consistent across time and between two imaging centers. Within one center, the diagnostic algorithm generated from a training cohort achieved high accuracy when classifying scans from a validation cohort (as ALS or control), though accuracy decreased when scans from PLS patients were included in the analysis (17). However, in a multicenter study, the diagnostic algorithm derived from one center's scans (training cohort) achieved 94.8% sensitivity but only 12.5% specificity in classifying scans from a second center (validation cohort) as ALS or control (39). The low specificity was attributed to relative frontal hypometabolism in the validation control scans, compared to training control scans. The validation control scans came from patients with non-neurologic malignancies undergoing surveillance

TABLE 2 | Advantages and disadvantages of potential biomarkers for ALS.

Biomarker type	Advantages	Disadvantages
Neuroimaging biomarkers: Positron emission tomography (PET)	Ability to interrogate disease mechanisms of interest using specific molecular ligands (e.g., energy metabolism, neuroinflammation, neuronal dysfunction, oxidative stress) Dynamic ligand binding enables visualization of treatment effect in central nervous system (CNS) Sensitive to early pathological changes Localizes pathology in CNS	Cost Limited scalability due to expertise and resources required (local cyclotron for production of radioisotopes) Small risk associated with repeated radiation Use may be limited by patient orthopnea
Neuroimaging biomarkers: Magnetic resonance imaging (MRI)	Widely available Advanced techniques permit evaluation of brain activation (functional MRI), white matter tracts (diffusion tensor imaging), and cellular metabolites (magnetic resonance spectroscopy) Free of radiation Localizes pathology in CNS	Large sample sizes required to demonstrate treatment effect limits pharmacodynamic potential (84) Use may be limited by patient orthopnea
Biological fluid-based biomarkers	Scalable Cost-effective Ease of collection Potential for standardization and centralization in core laboratory	Non-localizing
Electrophysiological biomarkers	Directly measures physiology of organs affected by disease Accepted use in diagnosis (electromyography) Sensitive to early pathological changes Good face value for monitoring disease progression	Reliability and reproducibility Sensitive to technical artifacts Potential patient discomfort (electromyography)

brain PET, whereas the training control scans came from healthy volunteers.

These studies highlight the challenges in translating population-level PET data into diagnostic criteria for individual patients. While progress is being made, PET is not yet a valid diagnostic biomarker for ALS. Validation will require longitudinal studies to determine whether prospectively collected scans of patients undergoing evaluation for ALS can distinguish UMN dysfunction before clinical signs emerge. The studies will also need to distinguish motor neuron disease not just from healthy volunteers, but also from disease mimics. If validated as a diagnostic biomarker, PET imaging could shorten the time from ALS symptom onset to diagnosis and facilitate earlier intervention in the neurodegenerative process.

PET Imaging as a Prognostic Biomarker

PET imaging has potential for prognostic use in ALS. Two studies in ALS patients found an association between mortality rate and presence of extensive frontotemporal hypometabolism on [^{18}F]-FDG PET scans (17, 32). Conversely, patients with spinal cord hypermetabolism in the top 20% of one study cohort had a significantly higher mortality rate compared to the rest of the cohort (36). Further longitudinal studies that evaluate whether PET imaging findings can predict the likelihood of future events (such as survival, development of cognitive impairment, or spread of disease from one anatomical region to another) are needed to establish valid prognostic PET biomarkers in ALS.

One intriguing potential use for prognostic PET imaging is in identifying when asymptomatic ALS gene carriers enter a high-risk period for developing clinical disease ("phenoconversion"). Rising levels of serum neurofilament light chain can detect neurodegeneration $\sim$1 year before phenoconversion in asymptomatic ALS gene mutation carriers (13). To evaluate whether PET imaging can detect also changes that predict phenoconversion, longitudinal [^{11}C]-PBR28 PET studies are being conducted in asymptomatic gene mutation carriers to look for neuroinflammation before disease onset. Prognostic biomarkers of phenoconversion may facilitate development of gene therapy trials designed to prevent ALS, which may be the best opportunity for treating or even curing certain genetic forms of ALS.

PET Imaging as a Pharmacodynamic Biomarker

PET imaging has value as a pharmacodynamic marker in ALS because it can rapidly measure and localize biological activity of investigational agents in the target tissue—the brain. The variety of available PET ligands may enable direct visualization of multiple pharmacologic targets. PET imaging's sensitivity to molecular changes can increase statistical power to detect a drug effect.

[^{11}C]-PBR28 PET is an appealing pharmacodynamic biomarker for ALS clinical trials because binding is dynamic and rapidly responsive to treatment: in Parkinson's disease (85) and traumatic brain injury (86) patients, anti-inflammatory treatment reduced cortical [^{11}C]-PBR28 binding in as little as 4 weeks (85). Additionally, the stability of [^{11}C]-PBR28 uptake in ALS over 6 months of disease progression permits a marked reduction in sample size needed to determine drug effect. A simulated sample size and power calculation using longitudinal [^{11}C]-PBR28 PET data found that 30 participants are needed in a single-arm ALS clinical trial to show a 2% change in [^{11}C]-PBR28 uptake after drug treatment, whereas hundreds of participants are needed to show a 30% reduction in ALSFRS-R slope (50). Currently, four ongoing clinical trials are using [^{11}C]-PBR28 PET as a pharmacodynamic biomarker to assess the biological activity of investigational treatments in ALS

(Clinicaltrials.gov NCT02714036, NCT02469896, NCT03127514, NCT03456882) (87).

In the future, PET imaging using an array of ligands will enable efficient evaluation of multiple pharmacologic targets. Pharmacodynamic data from PET studies may help confirm the biological activity of ALS drugs in the target tissue and inform dose selection based on biological activity. Data derived from these trials will enable deeper understanding of the role of different molecular mechanisms in disease pathogenesis.

CONCLUSIONS AND FUTURE DIRECTIONS

Thirty years of PET imaging has shed light on the pathophysiology of ALS and the expanding boundaries of cortical dysfunction in disease. Because PET imaging can localize molecular changes in the CNS *in vivo*, it has the potential to fill a critical gap in our armamentarium of diagnostic, prognostic, and pharmacodynamic biomarkers for ALS. To realize this potential, major limitations of the research to date will need to be addressed. First, most PET studies in ALS were small. Only 7 published studies enrolled more than 50 ALS patients (17, 31–33, 35, 39, 50), which raises concern for false positive and/or negative findings generated by studies with small sample sizes. Second, minimal longitudinal PET data exists in the ALS literature. A total of 24 ALS patients have had longitudinal PET scans in published studies (18, 22, 24, 27, 45, 50). Third, clinical-radiological correlations reported in the literature are insufficiently characterized and often contradictory. To address these limitations, we must conduct collaborative, multicenter longitudinal studies to collect PET imaging and clinical data in large patient cohorts. Moreover, to ascertain accurate clinical-radiologic correlations, clinical data should be captured by validated instruments that separate motor and cognitive deficits and reliably measure UMN dysfunction.

From a practical standpoint, the widespread use of PET imaging is presently limited by cost, need for expertise and local production of radioactive isotopes. Therefore, PET imaging currently is most useful as a pharmacodynamic biomarker for early clinical trials in ALS. Future multicenter longitudinal studies will allow us to establish the relationship between PET imaging findings and meaningful clinical outcomes, and thus develop and validate the PET imaging biomarkers that can accelerate drug development and advance care for people with ALS.

AUTHOR CONTRIBUTIONS

SC and NA drafted the manuscript. Both authors made a direct and intellectual contribution to the work and approved it for publication.

FUNDING

SC is supported by the Anne B. Young Neuroscience Translational Medicine Fellowship Award (Biogen MA, Inc.). NA is supported by The ALS Association (16-TACL-238), ALS Finding A Cure, ALS ONE, Muscular Dystrophy Association (511619), and the National Institute of Neurological Disorders and Stroke (K23NS083715). The content is of this work is solely the responsibility of the authors and does not necessarily represent the official views of these sponsors.

ACKNOWLEDGMENTS

We acknowledge the generosity of our patients and volunteers for participating in research studies.

REFERENCES

1. Traynor BJ, Codd MB, Corr B, Forde C, Frost E, Hardiman OM. Clinical features of amyotrophic lateral sclerosis according to the El Escorial and Airlie House diagnostic criteria: a population-based study. *Arch Neurol.* (2000) 57:1171–6. doi: 10.1001/archneur.57.8.1171
2. Taylor JP, Brown RH Jr, Cleveland DW. Decoding ALS: from genes to mechanism. *Nature.* (2016) 539:197–206. doi: 10.1038/nature20413
3. Turner MR, Kiernan MC, Leigh PN, Talbot K. Biomarkers in amyotrophic lateral sclerosis. *Lancet Neurol.* (2009) 8:94–109. doi: 10.1016/s1474-4422(08)70293-x
4. Chiò A, Pagani M, Agosta F, Calvo A, Cistaro A, Filippi M. Neuroimaging in amyotrophic lateral sclerosis: insights into structural and functional changes. *Lancet Neurol.* (2014) 13:1228–40. doi: 10.1016/s1474-4422(14)70167-x
5. Benatar M, Boylan K, Jeromin A, Rutkove SB, Berry J, Atassi N, et al. ALS biomarkers for therapy development: state of the field and future directions. *Muscle Nerve.* (2016) 53:169–82. doi: 10.1002/mus.24979
6. Vucic S, Ziemann U, Eisen A, Hallett M, Kiernan MC. Transcranial magnetic stimulation and amyotrophic lateral sclerosis: pathophysiological insights. *J Neurol Neurosurg Psychiatry.* (2013) 84:1161–70. doi: 10.1136/jnnp-2012-304019
7. Nandedkar SD, Nandedkar DS, Barkhaus PE, Stalberg EV. Motor unit number index (MUNIX). *IEEE Trans Biomed Eng.* (2004) 51:2209–11. doi: 10.1109/tbme.2004.834281
8. Rutkove SB, Caress JB, Cartwright MS, Burns TM, Warder J, David WS, et al. Electrical impedance myography correlates with standard measures of ALS severity. *Muscle Nerve.* (2014) 49:441–3. doi: 10.1002/mus.24128
9. Boylan KB, Glass JD, Crook JE, Yang C, Thomas CS, Desaro P, et al. Phosphorylated neurofilament heavy subunit (pNF-H) in peripheral blood and CSF as a potential prognostic biomarker in amyotrophic lateral sclerosis. *J Neurol Neurosurg Psychiatry.* (2013) 84:467–72. doi: 10.1136/jnnp-2012-303768
10. Feneberg E, Oeckl P, Steinacker P, Verde F, Barro C, Van Damme P, et al. Multicenter evaluation of neurofilaments in early symptom onset amyotrophic lateral sclerosis. *Neurology.* (2018) 90:e22–30. doi: 10.1212/WNL.0000000000004761
11. Gaiottino J, Norgren N, Dobson R, Topping J, Nissim A, Malaspina A, et al. Increased neurofilament light chain blood levels in neurodegenerative neurological diseases. *PLoS ONE.* (2013) 8:e75091. doi: 10.1371/journal.pone.0075091
12. Gaiani A, Martinelli I, Bello L, Querin G, Puthenparampil M, Ruggero S, et al. Diagnostic and prognostic biomarkers in amyotrophic lateral sclerosis:

neurofilament light chain levels in definite subtypes of disease. *JAMA Neurol.* (2017) 74:525–32. doi: 10.1001/jamaneurol.2016.5398

13. Benatar M, Wuu J, Andersen PM, Lombardi V, Malaspina A. Neurofilament light: a candidate biomarker of presymptomatic amyotrophic lateral sclerosis and phenoconversion. *Ann Neurol.* (2018) 84:130–9. doi: 10.1002/ana.25276
14. Khalil M, Teunissen CE, Otto M, Piehl F, Sormani MP, Gattringer T, et al. Neurofilaments as biomarkers in neurological disorders. *Nat Rev Neurol.* (2018) 14:577–89. doi: 10.1038/s41582-018-0058-z
15. Shepheard SR, Wuu J, Cardoso M, Wiklendt L, Dinning PG, Chataway T, et al. Urinary p75(ECD): a prognostic, disease progression, and pharmacodynamic biomarker in ALS. *Neurology.* (2017) 88:1137–43. doi: 10.1212/wnl.0000000000003741
16. Menke RA, Agosta F, Grosskreutz J, Filippi M, Turner MR. Neuroimaging endpoints in amyotrophic lateral sclerosis. *Neurotherapeutics.* (2017) 14:11–23. doi: 10.1007/s13311-016-0484-9
17. Van Weehaeghe D, Ceccarini J, Delva A, Robberecht W, Van Damme P, Van Laere K. Prospective validation of 18F-FDG brain PET discriminant analysis methods in the diagnosis of amyotrophic lateral sclerosis. *J Nucl Med.* (2016) 57:1238–43. doi: 10.2967/jnumed.115.166272
18. Dalakas MC, Hatazawa J, Brooks RA, Di Chiro G. Lowered cerebral glucose utilization in amyotrophic lateral sclerosis. *Ann Neurol.* (1987) 22:580–6. doi: 10.1002/ana.410220504
19. Renard D, Collombier L, Castelnovo G, Fourcade G, Kotzki PO, LaBauge P. Brain FDG-PET changes in ALS and ALS-FTD. *Acta Neurol Belg.* (2011) 111, 306–9.
20. Matias-Guiu JA, Pytel V, Cabrera-Martin MN, Galan L, Valles-Salgado M, Guerrero A, et al. Amyloid- and FDG-PET imaging in amyotrophic lateral sclerosis. *Eur J Nucl Med Mol Imaging.* (2016) 43:2050–60. doi: 10.1007/s00259-016-3434-1
21. Corcia P, Tauber C, Vercoullie J, Arlicot N, Prunier C, Praline J, et al. Molecular imaging of microglial activation in amyotrophic lateral sclerosis. *PLoS ONE.* (2012) 7:e52941. doi: 10.1371/journal.pone.0052941
22. Hatazawa J, Brooks RA, Dalakas MC, Mansi L, Di Chiro G. Cortical motor-sensory hypometabolism in amyotrophic lateral sclerosis: a PET study. *J Comput Assist Tomogr.* (1988) 12:630–6.
23. Ludolph AC, Langen KJ, Regard M, Herzog H, Kemper B, Kuwert T, et al. Frontal lobe function in amyotrophic lateral sclerosis: a neuropsychologic and positron emission tomography study. *Acta Neurol Scand.* (1992) 85, 81–9.
24. Hoffman JM, Mazziotta JC, Hawk TC, Sumida R. Cerebral glucose utilization in motor neuron disease. *Arch Neurol.* (1992) 49:849–54.
25. Garraux G, Salmon E, Degueldre C, Lemaire C, Franck G. Medial temporal lobe metabolic impairment in dementia associated with motor neuron disease. *J Neurol Sci.* (1999) 168:145–50.
26. Jeong Y, Park KC, Cho SS, Kim EJ, Kang SJ, Kim SE, et al. Pattern of glucose hypometabolism in frontotemporal dementia with motor neuron disease. *Neurology.* (2005) 64:734–6. doi: 10.1212/01.wnl.0000152047.58767.9d
27. Boeve BF, Boylan KB, Graff-Radford NR, DeJesus-Hernandez M, Knopman DS, Pedraza O, et al. Characterization of frontotemporal dementia and/or amyotrophic lateral sclerosis associated with the GGGGCC repeat expansion in C9ORF72. *Brain.* (2012) 135(Pt 3):765–83. doi: 10.1093/brain/aws004
28. Cistaro A, Valentini MC, Chio A, Nobili F, Calvo A, Moglia C, et al. Brain hypermetabolism in amyotrophic lateral sclerosis: a FDG PET study in ALS of spinal and bulbar onset. *Eur J Nucl Med Mol Imaging.* (2012) 39:251–9. doi: 10.1007/s00259-011-1979-6
29. Lai TH, Liu RS, Yang BH, Wang PS, Lin KP, Lee YC, et al. Cerebral involvement in spinal and bulbar muscular atrophy (Kennedy's disease): a pilot study of PET. *J Neurol Sci.* (2013) 335:139–44. doi: 10.1016/j.jns.2013.09.016
30. Clark HM, Duffy JR, Whitwell JL, Ahlskog JE, Sorenson EJ, Josephs KA. Clinical and imaging characterization of progressive spastic dysarthria. *Eur J Neurol.* (2014) 21:368–76. doi: 10.1111/ene.12271
31. Pagani M, Chio A, Valentini MC, Oberg J, Nobili F, Calvo A, et al. Functional pattern of brain FDG-PET in amyotrophic lateral sclerosis. *Neurology.* (2014) 83:1067–74. doi: 10.1212/wnl.0000000000000792
32. Van Laere K, Vanhee A, Verschueren J, De Coster L, Driesen A, Dupont P, et al. Value of 18fluorodeoxyglucose-positron-emission tomography in amyotrophic lateral sclerosis: a prospective study. *JAMA Neurol.* (2014) 71:553–61. doi: 10.1001/jamaneurol.2014.62
33. Cistaro A, Pagani M, Montuschi A, Calvo A, Moglia C, Canosa A, et al. The metabolic signature of C9ORF72-related ALS: FDG PET comparison with nonmutated patients. *Eur J Nucl Med Mol Imaging.* (2014) 41:844–52. doi: 10.1007/s00259-013-2667-5
34. Rajagopalan V, Pioro EP. Comparing brain structural MRI and metabolic FDG-PET changes in patients with ALS-FTD: 'the chicken or the egg?' question. *J Neurol Neurosurg Psychiatry.* (2015) 86:952–8. doi: 10.1136/jnnp-2014-308239
35. Canosa A, Pagani M, Cistaro A, Montuschi A, Iazzolino B, Fania P, et al. 18F-FDG-PET correlates of cognitive impairment in ALS. *Neurology.* (2016) 86:44–9. doi: 10.1212/wnl.0000000000002242
36. Marini C, Cistaro A, Campi C, Calvo A, Caponnetto C, Nobili FM, et al. A PET/CT approach to spinal cord metabolism in amyotrophic lateral sclerosis. *Eur J Nucl Med Mol Imaging.* (2016) 43:2061–71. doi: 10.1007/s00259-016-3440-3
37. Buhour MS, Doidy F, Mondou A, Pelerin A, Carluer L, Eustache F, et al. Voxel-based mapping of grey matter volume and glucose metabolism profiles in amyotrophic lateral sclerosis. *EJNMMI Res.* (2017) 7:21. doi: 10.1186/s13550-017-0267-2
38. Yamashita T, Hatakeyama T, Sato K, Fukui Y, Hishikawa N, Ohta Y, et al. Flow-metabolism uncoupling in the cervical spinal cord of ALS patients. *Neurol Sci.* (2017) 38:659–65. doi: 10.1007/s10072-017-2823-y
39. D'Hulst L, Van Weehaeghe D, Chio A, Calvo A, Moglia C, Canosa A, et al. Multicenter validation of [^{18}F]-FDG PET and support-vector machine discriminant analysis in automatically classifying patients with amyotrophic lateral sclerosis versus controls. *Amyotroph Lateral Scler Frontotemporal Degener.* (2018) 19:570–7. doi: 10.1080/21678421.2018.1476548
40. Kew JJ, Leigh PN, Playford ED, Passingham RE, Goldstein LH, Frackowiak RS, et al. Cortical function in amyotrophic lateral sclerosis. A positron emission tomography study. *Brain.* (1993) 116 (Pt 3):655–80.
41. Kew JJ, Goldstein LH, Leigh PN, Abrahams S, Cosgrave N, Passingham RE, et al. The relationship between abnormalities of cognitive function and cerebral activation in amyotrophic lateral sclerosis. A neuropsychological and positron emission tomography study. *Brain.* (1993) 116 (Pt 6):1399–423.
42. Tanaka M, Kondo S, Hirai S, Sun X, Yamagishi T, Okamoto K. Cerebral blood flow and oxygen metabolism in progressive dementia associated with amyotrophic lateral sclerosis. *J Neurol Sci.* (1993) 120:22–8.
43. Abrahams S, Goldstein LH, Kew JJ, Brooks DJ, Lloyd CM, Frith CD, et al. Frontal lobe dysfunction in amyotrophic lateral sclerosis. A PET study. *Brain.* (1996) 119 (Pt 6):2105–20.
44. Turner MR, Cagnin A, Turkheimer FE, Miller CC, Shaw CE, Brooks DJ, et al. Evidence of widespread cerebral microglial activation in amyotrophic lateral sclerosis: an [11C](R)-PK11195 positron emission tomography study. *Neurobiol Dis.* (2004) 15:601–9. doi: 10.1016/j.nbd.2003.12.012
45. Johansson A, Engler H, Blomquist G, Scott B, Wall A, Aquilonius SM, et al. Evidence for astrocytosis in ALS demonstrated by [11C](L)-deprenyl-D2 PET. *J Neurol Sci.* (2007) 255:17–22. doi: 10.1016/j.jns.2007.01.057
46. Zurcher NR, Loggia ML, Lawson R, Chonde DB, Izquierdo-Garcia D, Yasek JE, et al. Increased *in vivo* glial activation in patients with amyotrophic lateral sclerosis: assessed with [(11)C]-PBR28. *Neuroimage Clin.* (2015) 7:409–14. doi: 10.1016/j.nicl.2015.01.009
47. Alshikho MJ, Zurcher NR, Loggia ML, Cernasov P, Chonde DB, Izquierdo Garcia D, et al. Glial activation colocalizes with structural abnormalities in amyotrophic lateral sclerosis. *Neurology.* (2016) 87:2554–61. doi: 10.1212/wnl.0000000000003427
48. Paganoni S, Alshikho MJ, Zurcher NR, Cernasov P, Babu S, Loggia ML, et al. Imaging of glia activation in people with primary lateral sclerosis. *Neuroimage Clin.* (2018) 17:347–53. doi: 10.1016/j.nicl.2017.10.024
49. Albrecht DS, Normandin MD, Shcherbinin S, Wooten DW, Schwarz AJ, Zurcher NR, et al. Pseudoreference regions for glial imaging with (11)C-PBR28: investigation in 2 clinical cohorts. *J Nucl Med.* (2018) 59:107–14. doi: 10.2967/jnumed.116.178335
50. Alshikho MJ, Zurcher NR, Loggia ML, Cernasov P, Reynolds B, Pijanowski O, et al. Integrated magnetic resonance imaging and [(11) C]-PBR28 positron emission tomographic imaging in amyotrophic lateral sclerosis. *Ann Neurol.* (2018) 83:1186–97. doi: 10.1002/ana.25251

51. Ratai EM, Alshikho MJ, Zurcher NR, Loggia ML, Cebulla CL, Cernasov P, et al. Integrated imaging of [(11)C]-PBR28 PET, MR diffusion and magnetic resonance spectroscopy (1)H-MRS in amyotrophic lateral sclerosis. *Neuroimage Clin.* (2018) 20:357–64. doi: 10.1016/j.nicl.2018.08.007
52. Lloyd CM, Richardson MP, Brooks DJ, Al-Chalabi A, Leigh PN. Extramotor involvement in ALS: PET studies with the GABA(A) ligand [(11)C]flumazenil. *Brain.* (2000) 123 (Pt 11):2289–96. doi: 10.1093/brain/123.11.2289
53. Turner MR, Hammers A, Al-Chalabi A, Shaw CE, Andersen PM, Brooks DJ, et al. Distinct cerebral lesions in sporadic and 'D90A' SOD1 ALS: studies with [11C]flumazenil PET. *Brain.* (2005) 128(Pt 6):1323–9. doi: 10.1093/brain/awh509
54. Turner MR, Hammers A, Al-Chalabi A, Shaw CE, Andersen PM, Brooks DJ, et al. Cortical involvement in four cases of primary lateral sclerosis using [(11)C]-flumazenil PET. *J Neurol.* (2007) 254:1033–6. doi: 10.1007/s00415-006-0482-7
55. Wicks P, Turner MR, Abrahams S, Hammers A, Brooks DJ, Leigh PN, et al. Neuronal loss associated with cognitive performance in amyotrophic lateral sclerosis: an (11C)-flumazenil PET study. *Amyotroph Lateral Scler.* (2008) 9:43–9. doi: 10.1080/17482960701737716
56. Yabe I, Tsuji-Akimoto S, Shiga T, Hamada S, Hirata K, Otsuki M, et al. Writing errors in ALS related to loss of neuronal integrity in the anterior cingulate gyrus. *J Neurol Sci.* (2012) 315:55–9. doi: 10.1016/j.jns.2011.11.039
57. Turner MR, Rabiner EA, Hammers A, Al-Chalabi A, Grasby PM, Shaw CE, et al. [11C]-WAY100635 PET demonstrates marked 5-HT1A receptor changes in sporadic ALS. *Brain.* (2005) 128(Pt 4):896–905. doi: 10.1093/brain/awh428
58. Turner MR, Rabiner EA, Al-Chalabi A, Shaw CE, Brooks DJ, Leigh PN, et al. Cortical 5-HT1A receptor binding in patients with homozygous D90A SOD1 vs. sporadic. *ALS Neurol.* (2007) 68:1233–5. doi: 10.1212/01.wnl.0000259083.31837.64
59. Takahashi H, Snow BJ, Bhatt MH, Peppard R, Eisen A, Calne DB. Evidence for a dopaminergic deficit in sporadic amyotrophic lateral sclerosis on positron emission scanning. *Lancet.* (1993) 342:1016–8.
60. Przedborski S, Dhawan V, Donaldson DM, Murphy PL, McKenna-Yasek D, Mandel FS, et al. Nigrostriatal dopaminergic function in familial amyotrophic lateral sclerosis patients with and without copper/zinc superoxide dismutase mutations. *Neurology.* (1996) 47:1546–51.
61. Hideyama T, Momose T, Shimizu J, Tsuji S, Kwak S. A positron emission tomography study on the role of nigral lesions in parkinsonism in patients with amyotrophic lateral sclerosis. *Arch Neurol.* (2006) 63:1719–22. doi: 10.1001/archneur.63.12.1719
62. Fu X, Zhu W, Guo Z, Shu G, Cui F, Yang F, et al. (18)F-fallypride PET-CT of dopamine D2/D3 receptors in patients with sporadic amyotrophic lateral sclerosis. *J Neurol Sci.* (2017) 377:79–84. doi: 10.1016/j.jns.2017.03.013
63. Ikawa M, Okazawa H, Tsujikawa T, Matsunaga A, Yamamura O, Mori T, et al. Increased oxidative stress is related to disease severity in the ALS motor cortex: a PET study. *Neurology.* (2015) 84:2033–9. doi: 10.1212/wnl.0000000000001588
64. DeJesus-Hernandez M, Mackenzie IR, Boeve BF, Boxer AL, Baker M, Rutherford NJ, et al. Expanded GGGGCC hexanucleotide repeat in noncoding region of C9ORF72 causes chromosome 9p-linked FTD and ALS. *Neuron.* (2011) 72:245–56. doi: 10.1016/j.neuron.2011.09.011
65. Renton AE, Majounie E, Waite A, Simon-Sanchez J, Rollinson S, Gibbs JR, et al. A hexanucleotide repeat expansion in C9ORF72 is the cause of chromosome 9p21-linked ALS-FTD. *Neuron.* (2011) 72:257–68. doi: 10.1016/j.neuron.2011.09.010
66. Gijselinck I, Van Langenhove T, van der Zee J, Sleegers K, Philtjens S, Kleinberger G, et al. A C9orf72 promoter repeat expansion in a Flanders-Belgian cohort with disorders of the frontotemporal lobar degeneration-amyotrophic lateral sclerosis spectrum: a gene identification study. *Lancet Neurol.* (2012) 11:54–65. doi: 10.1016/s1474-4422(11)70261-7
67. Sargsyan SA, Monk PN, Shaw PJ. Microglia as potential contributors to motor neuron injury in amyotrophic lateral sclerosis. *Glia.* (2005) 51:241–53. doi: 10.1002/glia.20210
68. Boillee S, Yamanaka K, Lobsiger CS, Copeland NG, Jenkins NA, Kassiotis G, et al. Onset and progression in inherited ALS determined by motor neurons and microglia. *Science.* (2006) 312:1389–92. doi: 10.1126/science.1123511
69. Brettschneider J, Toledo JB, Van Deerlin VM, Elman L, McCluskey L, Lee VM, et al. Microglial activation correlates with disease progression and upper motor neuron clinical symptoms in amyotrophic lateral sclerosis. *PLoS ONE.* (2012) 7:e39216. doi: 10.1371/journal.pone.0039216
70. Brown AK, Fujita M, Fujimura Y, Liow JS, Stabin M, Ryu YH, et al. Radiation dosimetry and biodistribution in monkey and man of 11C-PBR28: a PET radioligand to image inflammation. *J Nucl Med.* (2007) 48:2072–9. doi: 10.2967/jnumed.107.044842
71. Lavisse S, Guillermier M, Herard AS, Petit F, Delahaye M, Van Camp N, et al. Reactive astrocytes overexpress TSPO and are detected by TSPO positron emission tomography imaging. *J Neurosci.* (2012) 32:10809–18. doi: 10.1523/jneurosci.1487-12.2012
72. Kreisl WC, Fujita M, Fujimura Y, Kimura N, Jenko KJ, Kannan P, et al. Comparison of [(11)C]-(R)-PK 11195 and [(11)C]PBR28, two radioligands for translocator protein (18 kDa) in human and monkey: implications for positron emission tomographic imaging of this inflammation biomarker. *Neuroimage.* (2010) 49:2924–32. doi: 10.1016/j.neuroimage.2009.11.056
73. Perrin RJ, Fagan AM, Holtzman DM. Multimodal techniques for diagnosis and prognosis of Alzheimer's disease. *Nature.* (2009) 461:916–22. doi: 10.1038/nature08538
74. Azmitia EC, Gannon PJ, Kheck NM, Whitaker-Azmitia PM. Cellular localization of the 5-HT1A receptor in primate brain neurons and glial cells. *Neuropsychopharmacology.* (1996) 14:35–46. doi: 10.1016/s0893-133x(96)80057-1
75. Williams TL, Shaw PJ, Lowe J, Bates D, Ince PG. Parkinsonism in motor neuron disease: case report and literature review. *Acta Neuropathol.* (1995) 89:275–83.
76. D'Amico E, Factor-Litvak P, Santella RM, Mitsumoto H. Clinical perspective on oxidative stress in sporadic amyotrophic lateral sclerosis. *Free Radic Biol Med.* (2013) 65:509–27. doi: 10.1016/j.freeradbiomed.2013.06.029
77. Takei K, Watanabe K, Yuki S, Akimoto M, Sakata T, Palumbo J. Edaravone and its clinical development for amyotrophic lateral sclerosis. *Amyotroph Lateral Scler Frontotemporal Degener.* (2017) 18:5–10. doi: 10.1080/21678421.2017.1353101
78. Wada K, Fujibayashi Y, Tajima N, Yokoyama A. Cu-ATSM, an intracellular-accessible superoxide dismutase (SOD)-like copper complex: evaluation in an ischemia-reperfusion injury model. *Biol Pharm Bull.* (1994) 17:701–4.
79. Ikawa M, Okazawa H, Kudo T, Kuriyama M, Fujibayashi Y, Yoneda M. Evaluation of striatal oxidative stress in patients with Parkinson's disease using [62Cu]ATSM PET. *Nucl Med Biol.* (2011) 38:945–51. doi: 10.1016/j.nucmedbio.2011.02.016
80. Ikawa M, Okazawa H, Arakawa K, Kudo T, Kimura H, Fujibayashi Y, et al. PET imaging of redox and energy states in stroke-like episodes of MELAS. *Mitochondrion.* (2009) 9:144–8. doi: 10.1016/j.mito.2009.01.011
81. Williams JR, Trias E, Beilby PR, Lopez NI, Labut EM, Bradford CS, et al. Copper delivery to the CNS by CuATSM effectively treats motor neuron disease in SOD(G93A) mice co-expressing the Copper-Chaperone-for-SOD. *Neurobiol Dis.* (2016) 89:1–9. doi: 10.1016/j.nbd.2016.01.020
82. Vieira FG, Hatzipetros T, Thompson K, Moreno AJ, Kidd JD, Tassinari VR, et al. CuATSM efficacy is independently replicated in a SOD1 mouse model of ALS while unmetallated ATSM therapy fails to reveal benefits. *IBRO Rep.* (2017) 2:47–53. doi: 10.1016/j.ibror.2017.03.001
83. FDA-NIH Biomarker Working Group. *BEST (Biomarkers, EndpointS, and other Tools) Resource [Internet].* Silver Spring, MD: Food and Drug Administration (US) (2016).
84. Zhang Y, Schuff N, Woolley SC, Chiang GC, Boreta L, Laxamana J, et al. Progression of white matter degeneration in amyotrophic lateral sclerosis: a diffusion tensor imaging study. *Amyotroph Lateral Scler.* (2011) 12:421–9. doi: 10.3109/17482968.2011.593036
85. Jucaite A, Svenningsson P, Rinne JO, Cselenyi Z, Varnas K, Johnstrom P, et al. Effect of the myeloperoxidase inhibitor AZD3241 on microglia: a PET study in Parkinson's disease. *Brain.* (2015) 138(Pt 9):2687–700. doi: 10.1093/brain/awv184
86. Scott G, Zetterberg H, Jolly A, Cole JH, De Simoni S, Jenkins PO, et al. Minocycline reduces chronic microglial activation after brain trauma but increases neurodegeneration. *Brain.* (2018) 141:459–71. doi: 10.1093/brain/awx339
87. Paganoni S, Alshikho MJ, Luppino S, Chan J, Pothier L, Schoenfeld D, et al. A pilot trial of RNS60 in amyotrophic lateral sclerosis. *Muscle Nerve.* (2018). doi: 10.1002/mus.26385. [Epub ahead of print].

12

Unbiased MRI Analyses Identify Micropathologic Differences Between Upper Motor Neuron-Predominant ALS Phenotypes

*Venkateswaran Rajagopalan[1,2] and Erik P. Pioro[3,4]**

[1] Department of Electrical and Electronics Engineering, Birla Institute of Technology and Science, Pilani, Hyderabad, India, [2] Department of Biomedical Engineering, ND2, Lerner Research Institute, Cleveland Clinic, Cleveland, OH, United States, [3] Department of Neurology, Neuromuscular Center, Neurological Institute, Cleveland Clinic, Cleveland, OH, United States, [4] Department of Neurosciences, Lerner Research Institute, Cleveland Clinic, Cleveland, OH, United States

***Correspondence:**
Erik P. Pioro
PIOROE@ccf.org

Amyotrophic lateral sclerosis (ALS) is an incurable and progressively fatal neurodegenerative disease that manifests with distinct clinical phenotypes, which are seen in neuroimaging, and clinical studies. T2- and proton density (PD)-weighted magnetic resonance imaging (MRI) displays hyperintense signal along the corticospinal tract (CST) in some ALS patients with upper motor neuron (UMN)-predominant signs. These patients tend to be younger and have significantly faster disease progression. We hypothesize that such ALS patients with CST hyperintensity (ALS-CST+) comprise a clinical subtype distinct from other ALS subtypes, namely patients with UMN-predominant ALS *without* CST hyperintensity, classic ALS, and ALS with frontotemporal dementia (FTD). Novel approaches such as fractal dimension analysis on conventional MRI (cMRI) and advanced MR techniques such as diffusion tensor imaging (DTI) reveal significant differences between ALS-CST+ and the aforementioned ALS subtypes. Our unbiased neuroimaging studies demonstrate that the ALS-CST+ group, which can be initially identified by T2-, PD-, and FLAIR-weighted cMRI, is distinctive and distinguishable from other ALS subtypes with possible differences in disease pathogenesis.

Keywords: MRI, UMN-predominant ALS, corticospinal tract hyperintensity, diffusion tensor imaging, micropathologic differences, fractal dimension, ALS phenotypes

INTRODUCTION

Etiology and site of origin of amyotrophic lateral sclerosis (ALS) within the central nervous system (CNS) are unknown (Mitsumoto et al., 1998). ALS diagnosis is based on motor neuron degeneration in both the CNS and peripheral nervous system (PNS), which include the upper motor neuron (UMN) and lower motor neuron (LMN), respectively. However, whether ALS begins in the CNS (Eisen et al., 1992) or PNS (Chou and Norris, 1993) is debated. Even if we consider a CNS origin, precisely where degeneration begins along the UMN pathway is unknown, as it can be anywhere along its rostrocaudal extent. If pathology originates in the corticomotoneuron within the cerebral cortex it would be considered a "neuronopathy"; if it originates somewhere along the axon in motor tracts (e.g., corticospinal and corticobulbar) within the subcortical white matter or spinal cord, it would be considered an "axonopathy." If ALS is an axonopathy, degeneration would begin distal to the neuronal cell body, and proceed retrogradely to affect it later; if it is a neuronopathy, the neuronal cell body would be affected first with subsequent loss of the entire axon because of wallerian degeneration.

In previous studies, we have evaluated brain MRI changes in patients with ALS based on their clinical phenotype and extent of UMN or cognitive impairment, including in those with UMN-predominant ALS, classic ALS [expressing relatively equal amounts of UMN and lower motor neuron (LMN) dysfunction], or ALS with frontotemporal dementia (ALS-FTD). Although an ALS diagnosis relies on the clinical presence of both UMN and LMN signs, a proportion of patients with ALS present with evidence of only UMN abnormalities and develop LMN signs later. A hyperintense signal is visible along both corticospinal tracts (CST's) on conventional T2-, proton density (PD)-, and FLAIR- weighted MRI in some patients with predominant or exclusive UMN signs (Mitsumoto et al., 1998), while others do not (Matte and Pioro, 2010), even though both patient groups have comparable degrees of clinical UMN dysfunction. A review of the literature revealed 17–67% (median 40%) of ALS patients with CST hyperintensity (Pioro, 2006), while a preliminary analysis at the Cleveland Clinic found this change in ~30% of ALS patients (Matte and Pioro, 2010). Although the precise cause of CST hyperintensities is unknown, an early radiologic-histopathologic study showed demyelination and wallerian degeneration in fibers of the tract (Yagishita et al., 1994). Even though ALS is primarily a motor neuron disorder, previous studies (Abrahams et al., 1996, 2005; Chang et al., 2005; Mezzapesa et al., 2007; Sage et al., 2007) have demonstrated involvement of extramotor regions subserving cognition and behavior, especially in ALS patients with dementia. Unlike Alzheimer's dementia, cognitive impairment in ALS patients with dementia predominantly affects frontotemporal regions of the brain and is termed frontotemporal dementia (FTD).

Unlike LMN abnormalities, which can be identified by routinely used electromyography (EMG), even if such signs are subclinical, objectively identifying UMN abnormalities (Brooks et al., 2000) is more challenging. Techniques applied to assess the latter such as transcranial magnetic stimulation and proton magnetic resonance spectroscopy are more labor intensive, and primarily used in research settings (Kaufmann et al., 2004). The neurologic examination remains the gold standard for detecting UMN abnormalities, but this is relatively subjective and dependent on the skill and acumen of the clinician. If in contrast, LMN changes like muscle atrophy, hypotonia, and hyporeflexia are very prominent, coexistent UMN signs can be masked, making diagnosis of ALS very difficult. Therefore, we evaluated conventional neuroimaging techniques used during routine clinical evaluation to provide non-invasive objective measures of UMN involvement.

The focus of this review is to summarize our previously published findings of how non-biased conventional MRI sequences acquired at 1.5T have identified differences between ALS patients with specific clinical phenotypes. Our goal was to demonstrate the utility of widely accessible routine clinical MRI in revealing unique macropathologic differences *in vivo* between such ALS patient groups and possibly to gain insights into disease pathogenesis and progression.

PATIENT DATA CONSIDERED

Groups of individuals evaluated by conventional clinical T2/PD/FLAIR-weighted MRI included: (1) UMN-predominant ALS patients *with* CST hyperintensity (ALS-CST+), (2) UMN-predominant ALS patients *without* CST hyperintensity (ALS-CST−), (3) patients with classic ALS (ALS-Cl), and (4) ALS patients with frontotemporal dementia (ALS-FTD), and (5) neurological controls. UMN-predominant ALS patients were defined as those with LMN signs that were either absent, or if present, were restricted to only one neuraxial level (bulbar, cervical, or lumbosacral) at time of MRI. UMN-predominant patients with CST hyperintensity were those in whom hyperintense signal was observed along the CST bilaterally in T2-, FLAIR-, and especially PD-weighted images. Patients with ALS-FTD displayed cognitive or behavioral impairment during clinical evaluation, as assessed by EP Pioro, including disturbances of language, executive function and impulse control. Such patients underwent bedside evaluation, including MoCA testing, extensive formal neuropsychometric testing by an experienced neuropsychologist, and usually both.

MRI STUDIES

After identifying CST hyperintensity on T2-, FLAIR-, and PD-weighted sequences in several ALS patients with UMN-predominant phenotype, we were puzzled when we observed other patients, relatively indistinguishable at initial clinical evaluation, who did *not* have CST hyperintensity. Since diffusion tensor imaging (DTI) could provide more insight with its diverse metrics (which are based on diffusion of water molecules), we studied the DTI metrics: fractional anisotropy (FA), axial diffusivity (AD), radial diffusivity (RD), and mean diffusivity (MD) along the CST in ALS patients of ALS-CST+ and ALS-CST− groups, compared to neurologic controls (Rajagopalan et al., 2011). Four levels along the rostrocaudal extent of the CST (identified by diffusion tensor tractographic reconstruction) in the white matter (WM) were examined: (1) subjacent to primary motor cortex (subPMC), (2) centrum semiovale at top of lateral ventricle (CSoLV), (3) posterior limb of internal capsule (IC), and (4) cerebral peduncle (CP), as shown in **Figure 1**. This allowed us to determine in our UMN-predominant ALS patients the level(s) where abnormalities in DTI metrics occur along the CST. Furthermore, it enabled us to determine whether quantitative differences exist corresponding to the qualitative presence or absence of CST hyperintensity.

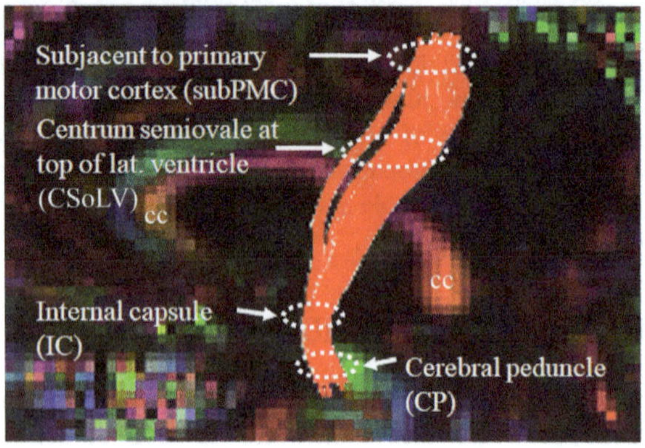

FIGURE 1 | Sagittal view of control subject brain with superimposed FA color map showing tractography-derived virtual CST fibers between subjacent to primary motor cortex (subPMC) rostrally and cerebral peduncle (CP) caudally. DTI metrics are also obtained at two intervening CST levels, including centrum semiovale at top of lateral ventricle (CSoLV) and posterior limb of the internal capsule (IC). cc corpus callosum.

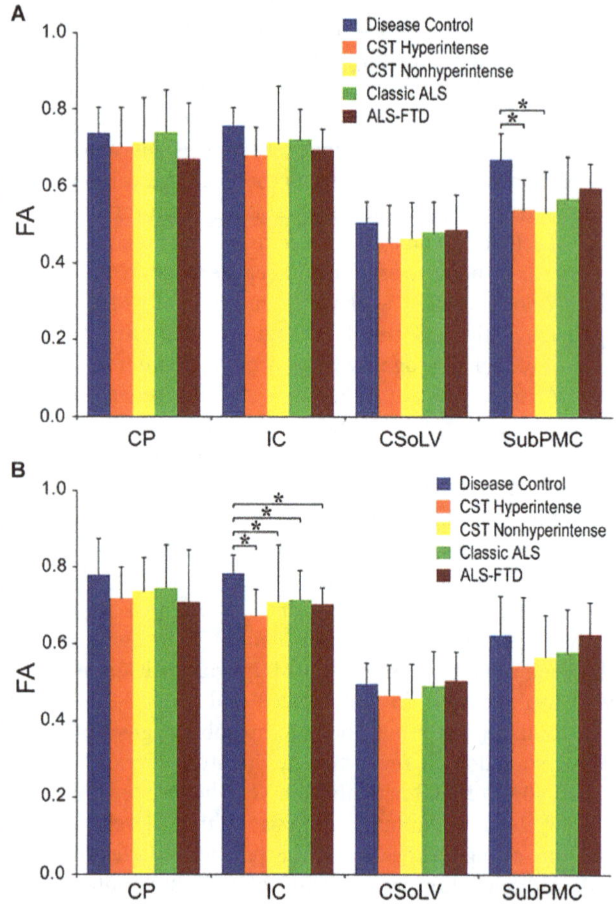

FIGURE 2 | Fractional anisotropy (FA) values at four CST levels in left **(A)** and right **(B)** hemispheres of ALS patients compared to controls showing significant differences as $^*P < 0.05$. CP, cerebral peduncle; IC, posterior limb of internal capsule; CSoLV, centrum semiovale at top of lateral ventricle; subPMC, subjacent to primary motor cortex. Reproduced with permission from Springer Nature.

Volumetric Studies in ALS-CST+ and ALS-CST− Patients

Our gray matter voxel based morphometry study (Rajagopalan and Pioro, 2014) revealed no significant difference in gray matter (GM) volume between ALS-CST+ and ALS-CST− groups in any brain region. Also, our brain parenchymal fraction (which includes GM and WM volume) study (Rajagopalan and Pioro, 2015) failed to reveal any significant difference in brain parenchymal fraction values between ALS-CST+ and ALS-CST− groups.

DTI Metrics Distinguish Between ALS-CST+ and Other ALS Patient Groups

Fractional anisotropy values were reduced in both ALS-CST+ and ALS-CST− groups when compared to controls. On the other hand, the AD and RD metrics showed significant differences at the internal capsule level only between controls and the ALS-CST+ group but not in the ALS-CST− group. It is in the posterior limb of the IC that hyperintensity is usually reported in the ALS literature (Yagishita et al., 1994; Ellis et al., 1999; Toosy et al., 2003; Pioro, 2006). Considering that AD and RD metrics reflect axonal and myelin integrity (Beaulieu, 2009), their abnormality in the ALS-CST+ group but not the ALS-CST− group suggests micropathologic differences along the CST. These results suggest that ALS patients with CST hyperintensity probably have different underling pathology from those who do not, which could arise from differing pathogenic mechanisms.

We further investigated whether neuroimaging, and specifically DTI metrics along the CST could objectively differentiate the ALS-CST+ group from the other ALS subtypes and neurologic controls (Rajagopalan et al., 2013b). In this study, we found that FA and AD values were lowest in the ALS-CST+ group when compared to controls and also when compared to the other ALS groups at rostral CST levels. When considering the CST separately in each hemisphere, significant FA differences were observed between controls and both ALS-CST+, and ALS-CST− groups (**Figure 2**). These findings, as well as significant differences in AD values between controls and patients in the ALS-CST+ group (but not between neurologic controls and those in ALS-CST− group) suggest differing micropathologies in the subcortical axons of the various ALS patient groups (**Figure 3**). Furthermore, AD, MD, and RD measures were significantly different between the ALS groups, distinguishing these values at IC and CSoLV levels of CST between patients in ALS-CST+ and ALS-FTD groups (**Figures 3–5**).

Diffusion Tensor Tractography Reveals Motor Fiber-Specific Truncation

The above studies demonstrated distinct pathological changes in regions of interest (ROIs) along the CST in the ALS-CST+

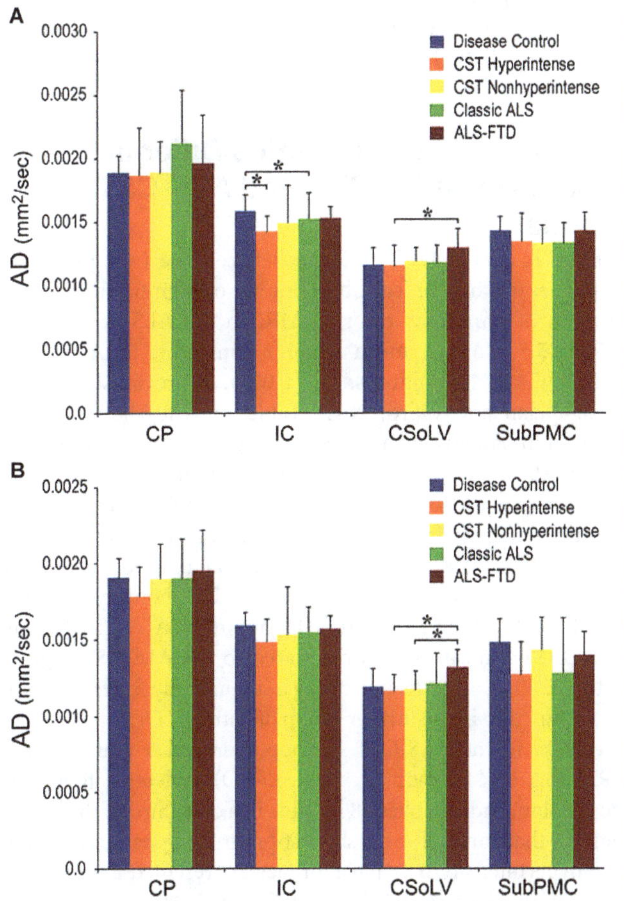

FIGURE 3 | AD values at four CST levels in left **(A)** and right **(B)** hemispheres of ALS patients compared to controls showing significant differences as $*P < 0.05$. CP, cerebral peduncle; IC, posterior limb of internal capsule; CSoLV, centrum semiovale at top of lateral ventricle; subPMC, subjacent to primary motor cortex. Reproduced with permission from Springer Nature.

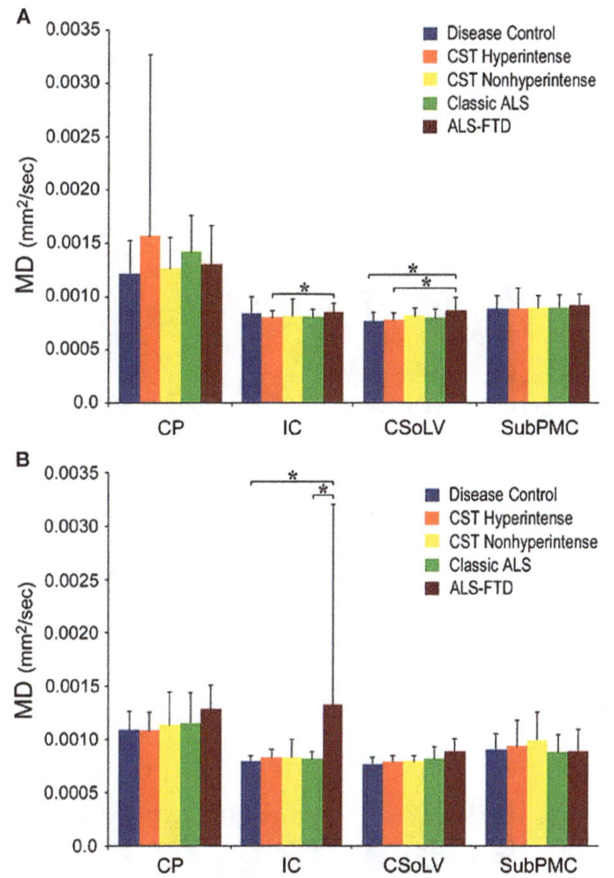

FIGURE 4 | Mean diffusivity (MD) values at four CST levels in left **(A)** and right **(B)** hemispheres of ALS patients compared to controls showing significant differences as $*P < 0.05$. CP, cerebral peduncle; IC, posterior limb of internal capsule; CSoLV, centrum semiovale at top of lateral ventricle; subPMC, subjacent to primary motor cortex. Reproduced with permission from Springer Nature.

group compared to other ALS groups and neurologic controls. However, the ROI approach is limited because of operator bias where voxels are placed, and evaluation of the CST only where voxels are placed, rather than along its entire length. In order to more accurately and objectively identify areas along the tract's entire length, we used diffusion tensor tractography (DTT) to reconstruct a "virtual" CST (Rajagopalan and Pioro, 2017). DTT identified virtual CST fibers between the CP and just beneath (Sub) the primary motor cortex (PMC) in ALS-CST+ patients, ALS-CST− patients, and neurologic controls. Surprisingly, we observed partial *absence* of virtual CST fibers in both groups of ALS patients but not in any controls. Specifically, these fibers were absent ("truncated") at the SubPMC level, which is between the PMC and CSoLV levels in several patients of both ALS-CST+ and ALS-CST− groups, as shown from a representative patient in **Figure 6**. Of note, no truncation was observed in any of the neurologic control subjects. CST truncation occurred primarily in ALS-CST+ patients (9 of 21, 42.8%) and less frequently in ALS-CST− patients (4 of 24, 16.6%; $P = 0.049$). Further, the frequency of virtual CST truncation was significantly ($P = 0.018$) higher in all ALS patients (both ALS-CST+ and ALS-CST− groups combined) than in the control group. To determine if this truncation was specific to descending motor fibers, we identified virtual non-motor fiber tracts connecting the primary sensory cortex (PSC) and subcortical white matter. Because most of these sensory fibers are afferents to the PSC, they should generally be unaffected by corticomotoneuron degeneration. In fact, truncation of such virtual non-motor (sensory) tracts occurred in only one subject from each of the ALS patient groups: 1 of 21 (4.7%) in ALS-CST+, and 1 of 24 (4.1%) in ALS-CST− groups. Our DTT findings of subcortical truncation of essentially only virtual motor (and not sensory) fibers, as shown from a representative patient in **Figure 6**, suggest microanatomic specificity of the underlying pathophysiologic process. This is in keeping with the notion that the sensory system remains relatively unaffected in ALS with the minority of patients reporting sensory symptoms.

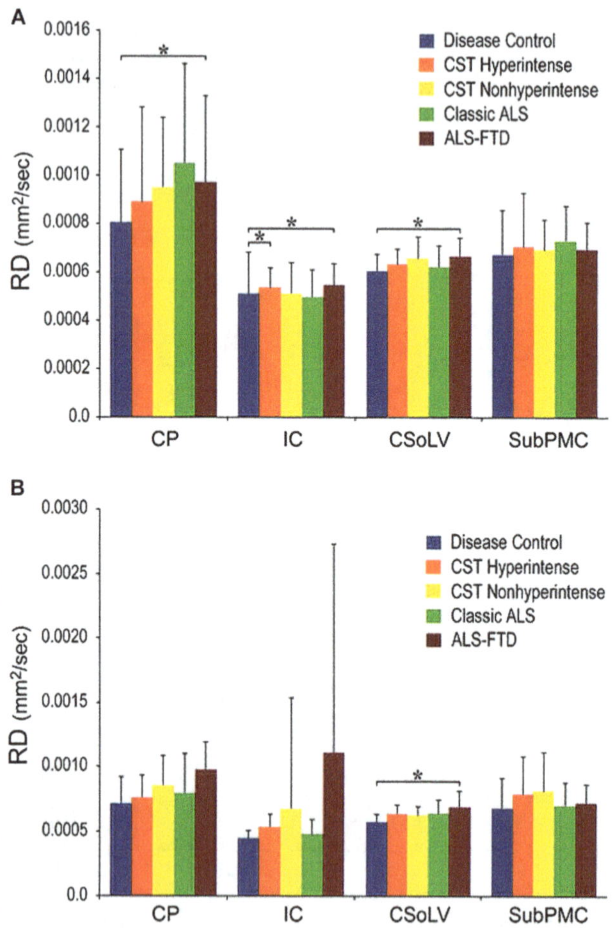

FIGURE 5 | Radial diffusivity (RD) values at four CST levels in right **(A)** and left **(B)** hemispheres of ALS patients compared to controls showing significant differences as *$P < 0.05$. CP, cerebral peduncle; IC, posterior limb of internal capsule; CSoLV, centrum semiovale at top of lateral ventricle; subPMC, subjacent to primary motor cortex. Reproduced with permission from Springer Nature.

Importantly, the truncation of motor fibers more frequently in one ALS phenotype than another, no truncation in neurologic controls, and differential involvement of motor but not sensory fibers all suggest that virtual CST truncation is and disease- and fiber-type specific. Therefore, these results further support unique pathologies along the CST in these two UMN-predominant ALS patient groups.

Disease Progression Rates Differ in Patients of ALS-CST+ and ALS-CST− Groups

Differences in the DTT findings between the two groups are supplemented by clinical observations of significantly shorter duration of symptoms prior to MRI in the ALS-CST+ group (9.6 ± 5.5 months, mean ± SD) compared to ALS-CST− group (36.4 ± 44.2 months, $P < 0.001$), as previously reported (Rajagopalan and Pioro, 2017; **Table 1**). The shorter disease duration in patients of the ALS-CST+ group compared to those of the ALS-CST− group translated into much faster disease progression in the former patients, even though both groups had essentially identical motor function scores of the revised ALS functional rating scale (ALSFRS-R) at time of MRI (34.6 ± 7.8, mean ± SD, vs. 34.1 ± 8.1, respectively). The monthly decline in ALSFRS-R (ΔFS) was three time higher in the ALS-CST+ group (1.38 ± 1.64, mean ± SD) compared to the ALS-CST− group (0.46 ± 0.43; $P = 0.001$), indicating a significantly faster decline of motor function in the former group of patients. Of note, duration of disease in the ALS-CST− group averaged 3 years prior to MRI (36.4 ± 44.2 months, mean ± SD), reflecting their slow progression, and was over 48 months in a one-third of them. This suggests that some of these slowest progressing patients without CST hyperintensity may have, in fact, represented a group with primary lateral sclerosis (PLS) (Gordon et al., 2006).

Fractal Dimension Analyses Reveal ALS Group Differences in White Matter Complexity

At a microscopic level, ALS pathology includes axonal swelling with neurofilament accumulation, dendritic attenuation, and wallerian degeneration of axons (Cluskey and Ramsden, 2001). Evidence of such micropathology, including axon degeneration and demyelination can be detected at a macroscopic level *in vivo* by certain MRI techniques (Metwalli et al., 2010). Neuronal degeneration with resultant loss of

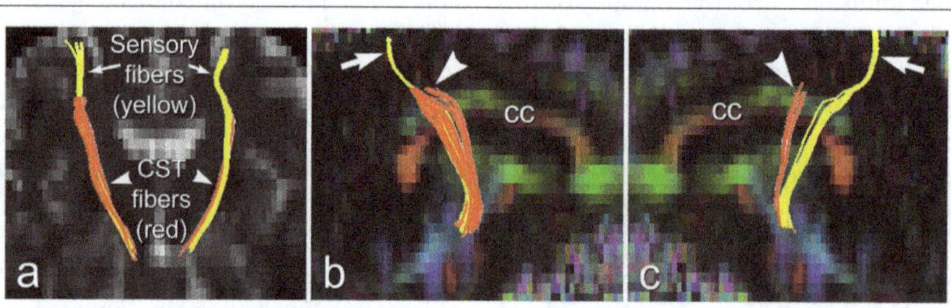

FIGURE 6 | Truncated virtual CST fibers arising from primary motor cortex (red, arrowheads) are contrasted with intact sensory fibers projecting to/from primary sensory cortex (yellow, arrows) in an UMN-predominant ALS patient with faster disease progression rate. Virtual tracts are projected on a coronal b0 image **(a)**, and on sagittal images of left **(b)**, and right **(c)** hemispheres. cc, corpus callosum. Reproduced with permission from Elsevier.

TABLE 1 | Clinical parameters of ALS patients.

Clinical measure/ALS subgroups	ALS-CST+ Mean ± SD	ALS-CST− Mean ± SD	P
n	21	24	NS
Age	52.3 ± 11.4	59.5 ± 12.1	< 0.05
Symptom duration prior to MRI (months)	9.6 ± 5.5	36.4 ± 44.2	< 0.001
ALSFRS-R score	34.6 ± 7.8	34.1 ± 8.1	NS
Disease progression rate	1.38 ± 1.64	0.46 ± 0.43	0.001

Key: SD, standard deviation. ALS-CST+, ALS patients with predominant upper motor neuron (UMN) signs and hyperintense signal along the corticospinal tract (CST) on conventional proton density (PD) and T2-weighted images and no clinical dementia. ALS-CST−, ALS patients with predominant UMN signs without CST hyperintensity and no clinical dementia (ALS-CST−). ALSFRS-R, ALS functional rating score-revised. NS, not significant.

dendrites and axons has been shown to reduce complexity of subcortical WM structure. Therefore, measuring WM structural complexity may reveal the effects of neuronal degeneration occurring in ALS.

Fractals are geometry objects that are self-similar at different scales, and were first proposed by Mandelbrot. The fractal dimension (FD) is a non-integer number that characterizes the morphometric variability of a complex and irregular shape. FD analysis can quantitatively measure the internal shape complexity of brain WM from MRI by characterizing multifractal behavior of different textures instead of using only pixel intensity values (Liu et al., 2003). Higher FD values reflect more WM complexity, as would be expected in healthy states, whereas lower values result with aging, and when WM becomes diseased more amorphous. In a study of patients with multiple sclerosis, reduced brain WM FD values were proposed to represent a more amorphous tissue state resulting from inflammation, decreased myelin content, and increased water content (Esteban et al., 2007).

We used FD analysis to evaluate WM structural degeneration in each of the four ALS patient groups: ALS-CST+, ALS-CST−, ALS-Cl, and ALS-FTD. In this study (Rajagopalan et al., 2013a), we estimated three quantitative measureable WM features using FD shape representations, including WM skeleton, GM/WM surface structure, and WM general structure. The skeleton captures the central line of the WM structure, which preserves the topological and geometric information of the WM, and represents its interior structure complexity. The surface structure comprised of voxels at the gray matter (GM)-WM interface, represents the shape of gyral and sulcal convolutions over the cortical surface. Finally, FD of general structure incorporates all WM voxels, including those at the GM/WM interface and skeleton in segmented images, and thereby represents brain volume. Because FD measures of skeleton, surface structure, and general structure represent different components of WM, they provided novel information about ALS-induced changes in brain WM structure and shape. General structure and skeleton FD values were significantly different between ALS-CST+ and ALS-FTD groups. Whole brain skeleton ($P = 0.001$) and general structure ($P = 0.02$) were significantly higher in ALS-CST+ patients compared to ALS-FTD patients, as shown in **Figure 7**. Although not significant, whole brain skeleton FD values in ALS-CST+ group patients trended higher than those in ALS-CST− ($P = 0.10$) and ALS-Cl ($P = 0.10$) groups. However, neurologic controls and ALS patients revealed no significant differences in FD values. These results indicate that shape complexity in the ALS-CST+ patient group was significantly greater than in the ALS-FTD group, and trended higher than in the other two patient subtypes. Although the significance of this higher FD in ALS-CST+ patients is unclear, it is likely related to differences in integrity of axons, myelin, and other changes within the neuropil, including inflammatory processes.

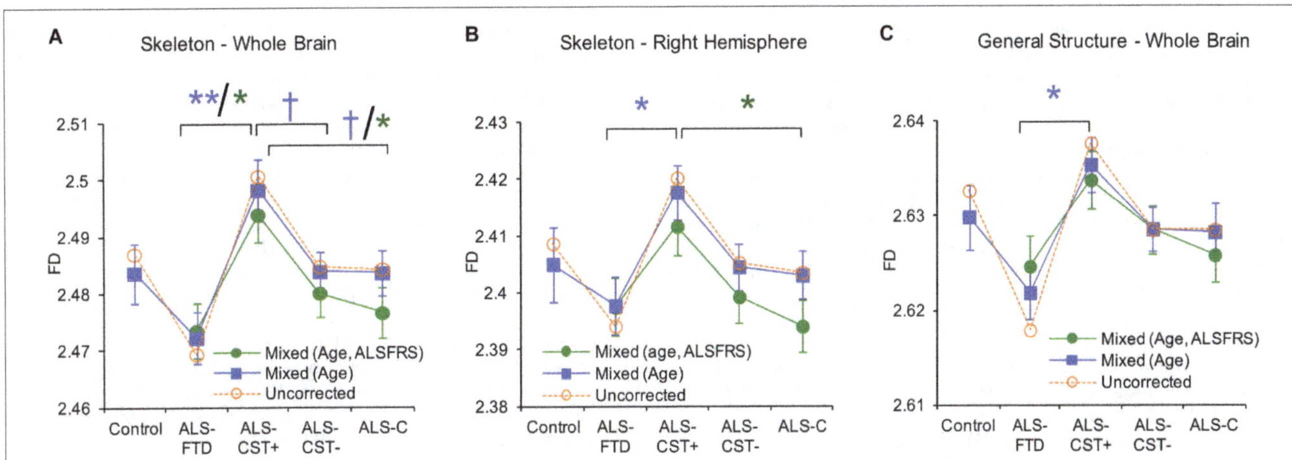

FIGURE 7 | Between group comparisons show significant differences in fractal dimension values of skeleton-whole brain **(A)**, skeleton right hemisphere **(B)**, and general structure whole brain **(C)**. Uncorrected means are represented as dashed lines and corrected means (mixed model) and standard error of the mean are shown as solid lines. Data for mixed models with gender, age as covariates are shown in blue or with gender, age, and ALSFRS-R as covariates are in green. Corrected mean comparisons between groups are performed using the Tukey multiple comparison method. $^{\dagger}p < 0.1$, $^{*}p < 0.05$, $^{**}p < 0.001$. Reproduced with permission from *PlosOne*.

Clinical Differences Between Patients in ALS-CST+ and Other Groups

Patients in the ALS-CST+ group were younger when compared to those in the ALS-CST− group ($P < 0.05$) (**Table 1**). In contrast, patients with ALS-FTD were significantly older than ALS-CST+ patients and neurologic controls. ALS-CST+ group revealed significantly shorter symptom duration compared to those in ALS-CST− ($p < 0.001$) and ALS-FTD groups ($p < 0.05$), indicating earlier neurologic evaluation after symptom onset. Also, disease progression rate was significantly faster in ALS-CST+ patients than in ALS-CST−, ALS-Cl, and ALS-FTD groups, as had been observed in a preliminary study of another group of ALS patients (Matte and Pioro, 2010). The revised ALSFRS-R score, which is a validated measure of physical function in ALS (Cedarbaum et al., 1999), was significantly lower (worse) in ALS-FTD patients compared to the ALS-Cl patients but essentially identical in ALS-CST+ and ALS-CST− patients at time of MRI.

CONCLUSION

The aforementioned brain MRI studies uniformly revealed objective differences in patients with the various ALS subtypes: UMN-predominant ALS with CST hyperintensity (ALS-CST+), UMN-predominant ALS without CST hyperintensity (ALS-CST−), classic ALS (ALS-Cl), and ALS with FTD (ALS-FTD). Specifically, patients in the ALS-CST+ group show distinctive and distinguishable changes from the others, including patients in the ALS-CST− group, which appear phenotypically similar, at least in relation to extent of UMN dysfunction. Coupled with the patients' distinct clinical characteristics, these neuroimaging abnormalities strongly suggest that CST hyperintensity, as revealed by conventional MRI (cMRI) T2/PD, and FLAIR sequences used during routine clinical evaluation, is not artefactual or non-specific but identifies a unique ALS patient group. *We hypothesize that ALS-CST+ patients comprise a distinct phenotype from ALS-CST−, ALS-Cl, and ALS-FTD with unique micropathology of the CST and potentially important differences in ALS pathogenesis.* Prescreening ALS patients for the presence of CST hyperintensity may be useful when enrolling or stratifying into clinical trials.

AUTHOR CONTRIBUTIONS

VR and EPP conceptualized the idea for the manuscript. VR wrote the manuscript. EPP made substantive revisions to the manuscript.

ACKNOWLEDGMENTS

We thank all the patients and their caregivers who participated in this study.

REFERENCES

1. Abrahams, S., Goldstein, L. H., Kew, J. J., Brooks, D. J., Lloyd, C. M., Frith, C. D., et al. (1996). Frontal lobe dysfunction in amyotrophic lateral sclerosis. A PET study. *Brain* 119(Pt 6), 2105–2120. doi: 10.1093/brain/119.6.2105
2. Abrahams, S., Goldstein, L. H., Suckling, J., Ng, V., Simmons, A., Chitnis, X., et al. (2005). Frontotemporal white matter changes in amyotrophic lateral sclerosis. *J. Neurol.* 252, 321–331. doi: 10.1007/s00415-005-0646-x
3. Beaulieu, C. (ed.) (2009). *Diffusion MRI: From Quantitative Measurement to In vivo Neuroanatomy.* San Diego, CA: Elsevier.
4. Brooks, B. R., Miller, R. G., Swash, M., and Munsat, T. L. (2000). El Escorial revisited: revised criteria for the diagnosis of amyotrophic lateral sclerosis. *Amyotroph. Lateral Scler. Other Motor Neuron Disord.* 1, 293–299. doi: 10.1080/146608200300079536
5. Cedarbaum, J. M., Stambler, N., Malta, E., Fuller, C., Hilt, D., Thurmond, B., et al. (1999). The ALSFRS-R: a revised ALS functional rating scale that incorporates assessments of respiratory function. BDNF ALS Study Group (Phase III). *J. Neurol. Sci.* 169, 13–21. doi: 10.1016/s0022-510x(99)00210-5
6. Chang, J. L., Lomen-Hoerth, C., Murphy, J., Henry, R. G., Kramer, J. H., Miller, B. L., et al. (2005). A voxel-based morphometry study of patterns of brain atrophy in ALS and ALS/FTLD. *Neurology* 65, 75–80. doi: 10.1212/01.wnl. 0000167602.38643.29
7. Chou, S. M., and Norris, F. H. (1993). Amyotrophic lateral sclerosis: lower motor neuron disease spreading to upper motor neurons. *Muscle Nerve* 16, 864–869. doi: 10.1002/mus.880160810
8. Cluskey, S., and Ramsden, D. B. (2001). Mechanisms of neurodegeneration in amyotrophic lateral sclerosis. *Mol. Pathol.* 54, 386–392.
9. Eisen, A., Kim, S., and Pant, B. (1992). Amyotrophic lateral sclerosis (ALS): a phylogenetic disease of the corticomotoneuron? *Muscle Nerve* 15, 219–224. doi: 10.1002/mus.880150215
10. Ellis, C. M., Simmons, A., Jones, D. K., Bland, J., Dawson, J. M., Horsfield, M. A., et al. (1999). Diffusion tensor MRI assesses corticospinal tract damage in ALS. *Neurology* 53, 1051–1058.
11. Esteban, F. J., Sepulcre, J., De Mendizabal, N. V., Goni, J., Navas, J., De Miras, J. R., et al. (2007). Fractal dimension and white matter changes in multiple sclerosis. *Neuroimage* 36, 543–549. doi: 10.1016/j.neuroimage.2007.03.057
12. Gordon, P. H., Cheng, B., Katz, I. B., Pinto, M., Hays, A. P., Mitsumoto, H., et al. (2006). The natural history of primary lateral sclerosis. *Neurology* 66, 647–653. doi: 10.1212/01.wnl.0000200962.94777.71
13. Kaufmann, P., Pullman, S. L., Shungu, D. C., Chan, S., Hays, A. P., Del Bene, M. L., et al. (2004). Objective tests for upper motor neuron involvement in amyotrophic lateral sclerosis (ALS). *Neurology* 62, 1753–1757.
14. Liu, J. Z., Zhang, L. D., and Yue, G. H. (2003). Fractal dimension in human cerebellum measured by magnetic resonance imaging. *Biophys. J.* 85, 4041–4046. doi: 10.1016/s0006-3495(03)74817-6
15. Matte, G. P., and Pioro, E. P. (2010). Clinical features and natural history in ALS patients with upper motor neuron abnormalities on conventional brain MRI. *Neurology* 74(Suppl. 2):A216.
16. Metwalli, N. S., Benatar, M., Nair, G., Usher, S., Hu, X., and Carew, J. D. (2010). Utility of axial and radial diffusivity from diffusion tensor MRI as markers of neurodegeneration in amyotrophic lateral sclerosis. *Brain Res.* 1348, 156–164. doi: 10.1016/j.brainres.2010.05.067
17. Mezzapesa, D. M., Ceccarelli, A., Dicuonzo, F., Carella, A., De Caro, M. F., Lopez, M., et al. (2007). Whole-brain and regional brain atrophy in amyotrophic lateral sclerosis. *AJNR Am. J. Neuroradiol.* 28, 255–259.
18. Mitsumoto, H., Chad, D. A., and Pioro, E. P. (1998). *Amyotrophic Lateral Sclerosis.* Philadelphia: F.A. Davis Company.
19. Pioro, E. P. (2006). "Neuroimaging in ALS and ALS with frontotemporal dementia," in *Dementia and Motor Neuron Disease*, ed. M. J. Strong (London: Informa Healthcare), 107–131. doi: 10.1201/b14376-11
20. Rajagopalan, V., Allexandre, D., Yue, G. H., and Pioro, E. P. (2011). Diffusion tensor imaging evaluation of corticospinal tract hyperintensity in upper motor neuron-predominant ALS patients. *J. Aging Res.* 2011:481745. doi: 10.4061/2011/481745
21. Rajagopalan, V., Liu, Z., Allexandre, D., Zhang, L., Wang, X. F., Pioro, E. P., et al. (2013a). Brain white matter shape changes in amyotrophic lateral sclerosis (ALS): a fractal dimension study. *PLoS One* 8:e73614. doi: 10.1371/journal.pone.0073614

22. Rajagopalan, V., Yue, G. H., and Pioro, E. P. (2013b). Brain white matter diffusion tensor metrics from clinical 1.5T MRI distinguish between ALS phenotypes. *J. Neurol.* 260, 2532–2540. doi: 10.1007/s00415-013-7012-1
23. Rajagopalan, V., and Pioro, E. P. (2014). Distinct patterns of cortical atrophy in ALS patients with or without dementia: an MRI VBM study. *Amyotroph. Lateral Scler. Frontotemporal. Degener.* 15, 216–225. doi: 10.3109/21678421. 2014.880179
24. Rajagopalan, V., and Pioro, E. P. (2015). Brain parenchymal fraction: a relatively simple mri measure to clinically distinguish ALS phenotypes. *Biomed. Res. Int.* 2015:693206. doi: 10.1155/2015/693206
25. Rajagopalan, V., and Pioro, E. P. (2017). Differential involvement of corticospinal tract (CST) fibers in UMN-predominant ALS patients with or without CST hyperintensity: a diffusion tensor tractography study. *Neuroimage Clin.* 14, 574–579. doi: 10.1016/j.nicl.2017.02.017
26. Sage, C. A., Peeters, R. R., Gorner, A., Robberecht, W., and Sunaert, S. (2007). Quantitative diffusion tensor imaging in amyotrophic lateral sclerosis. *Neuroimage* 34, 486–499. doi: 10.1016/j.neuroimage.2006.09.025
27. Toosy, A. T., Werring, D. J., Orrell, R. W., Howard, R. S., King, M. D., Barker, G. J., et al. (2003). Diffusion tensor imaging detects corticospinal tract involvement at multiple levels in amyotrophic lateral sclerosis. *J. Neurol. Neurosurg. Psychiatry* 74, 1250–1257. doi: 10.1136/jnnp.74.9.1250
28. Yagishita, A., Nakano, I., Oda, M., and Hirano, A. (1994). Location of the corticospinal tract in the internal capsule at MR imaging. *Radiology* 191, 455–460. doi: 10.1148/radiology.191.2.8153321

13

Tracking a Fast-Moving Disease: Longitudinal Markers, Monitoring, and Clinical Trial Endpoints in ALS

*Rangariroyashe Hannah Chipika, Eoin Finegan, Stacey Li Hi Shing, Orla Hardiman and Peter Bede**

Computational Neuroimaging Group, Biomedical Sciences Institute, Trinity College Dublin, Dublin, Ireland

***Correspondence:**
Peter Bede
bedep@tcd.ie

Amyotrophic lateral sclerosis (ALS) encompasses a heterogeneous group of phenotypes with different progression rates, varying degree of extra-motor involvement and divergent progression patterns. The natural history of ALS is increasingly evaluated by large, multi-time point longitudinal studies, many of which now incorporate presymptomatic and post-mortem assessments. These studies not only have the potential to characterize patterns of anatomical propagation, molecular mechanisms of disease spread, but also to identify pragmatic monitoring markers. Sensitive markers of progressive neurodegenerative change are indispensable for clinical trials and individualized patient care. Biofluid markers, neuroimaging indices, electrophysiological markers, rating scales, questionnaires, and other disease-specific instruments have divergent sensitivity profiles. The discussion of candidate monitoring markers in ALS has a dual academic and clinical relevance, and is particularly timely given the increasing number of pharmacological trials. The objective of this paper is to provide a comprehensive and critical review of longitudinal studies in ALS, focusing on the sensitivity profile of established and emerging monitoring markers.

Keywords: motor neuron disease, amyotrophic lateral sclerosis, biomarkers, magnetic resonance imaging, neuroimaging

INTRODUCTION

Amyotrophic lateral sclerosis (ALS) is a clinically, genetically, and pathologically heterogeneous neurodegenerative condition (1–3). Clinical heterogeneity in ALS is multidimensional owing to variations in upper motor neuron (UMN) and lower motor neuron (LMN) involvement, extra-motor symptoms, age of onset, survival, and progression-rates. Disease heterogeneity hinders biomarker development (3, 4) which in turn impedes the reliable assessment of candidate drugs in clinical trials (1). Current clinical trials recruit relatively heterogeneous cohorts of symptomatic patients, despite the notion that considerable pathological changes can already be detected at the time of diagnosis (5, 6). The considerable variability in progression rates in ALS is another confounding factor in clinical trial designs (1, 7–10). Imaging and electrophysiological markers have been repeatedly proposed as candidate monitoring markers (11, 12), but it is increasingly clear that a panel of several "wet" and "dry" biomarkers may be required to capture subtle changes over short periods of time (13, 14). The objective of this paper is the comprehensive and critical review of longitudinal studies in ALS, focusing on study designs, statistical power, clinical correlations, the sensitivity profile of proposed monitoring markers and their applicability to clinical trials.

METHODS

A formal literature search was performed on PubMed using the core search terms "amyotrophic lateral sclerosis" and "longitudinal" combined with each of the following keywords separately: "staging," "monitoring," "outcomes," "clinical," "clinical trials," "electrophysiology," "neurophysiology," "electromyography," "transcranial magnetic stimulation," "motor unit number estimation," "motor unit number index," "positon emission tomography," "single photon emission computed tomography," "magnetic resonance imaging," "neuroimaging," "imaging," "blood," "urine," "cerebrospinal fluid," "saliva," and "muscle." A supplementary search combined the core search terms with the following keywords: "presymptomatic," "asymptomatic," and "post-mortem." Inclusion criteria included longitudinal studies investigating imaging, neurophysiological, clinical, or biofluid biomarkers in ALS. Animal studies, review papers, opinion pieces, editorials, case reports, and case series were excluded. Only articles written in English and published between January 1980 and August 2018 were reviewed. Based on the above criteria a total of 118 original research papers were selected and reviewed in accordance with the Preferred Reporting Items for Systematic Reviews and Meta-Analyses (PRISMA) recommendations.

RESULTS

Neuroimaging

The sample size characteristics, study design features, follow-up intervals of longitudinal neuroimaging, neurophysiology, and clinical studies are summarized in **Table 1**. Whilst most longitudinal imaging studies in ALS evaluate cerebral alterations (10), a number of promising spinal studies have now also been published. Spinal imaging has gradually overcome the technical challenges of physiological motion, small cross-sectional dimensions and susceptibility gradients (19, 110–118). The majority of longitudinal studies in ALS are single-center studies eliminating the need for cross-platform MR sequence harmonization and inter-rater reliability tests. Given the low incidence of certain phenotypes such as primary lateral sclerosis (PLS), progressive muscular atrophy (PMA), and spinal and bulbar muscular atrophy (SBMA) however, multisite collaboration is often necessary (119). The infrastructure, funding and governance of such multicenter collaborations are now established via international consortia like the Neuroimaging Society in Amyotrophic Lateral Sclerosis (NISALS) or the Northeast ALS Consortium (NEALS) (16, 23, 120, 121). The need to include disease-controls in addition to healthy controls to describe ALS-specific changes

---

Abbreviations: 2D-DIGE, two-dimensional fluorescence difference gel electrophoresis; ABG, arterial blood gas; ACE-3, Addenbrookes Cognitive Examination - Third Edition; ACE-R, Addenbrooke's Cognitive Examination-revised; AD, axial diffusivity; ADM, abductor digiti minimi; ADQ, abductor digiti quinti; AGA, arterial gas analyses; AHB, abductor halluces brevis; ALS, amyotrophic lateral sclerosis; ALSAQ-40, ALS assessment questionnaire; ALS-CBS, ALS Cognitive Behavior Screen; ALS-CFB, ALS computerized frontal battery; ALS-FBI, ALS-Frontal Behavioral Inventory; ALSFRS-r, revised ALS functional rating scale; ALSS, ALS severity scale; ALSSQoL-R, revised ALS-specific Quality of Life questionnaire; APB, abductor pollicis brevis; ARSLA, Association pour la recherche sur la SLA; ATLIS, accurate test of limb isometric strength; BAI, body adiposity index; BMI, body mass index; CALR, Calreticulin; CALSNIC, Canadian ALS Neuroimaging Consortium; CHI3L1, chitinase-3-like protein 1; CHI3L2, chitinase-3-like protein 2; CHIT1, chitotriosidase-1; Cho, Choline; CIDP, chronic inflammatory demyelinating polyneuropathy; CIS20-R, checklist individual strength; CK, creatinine kinase; CLIC1, Chloride intracellular channel protein 1; CMAP, compound muscle action potential; CMCT, central motor conduction time; CMT, Charcot-Marie-Tooth disease; CNS-BFS, Center for Neurologic Study-Bulbar Function Scale; CNS-LS, Center for Neurologic Study-Lability Scale; COWAT, controlled oral word association test; Cr, creatinine; CSF, cerebrospinal fluid; CSP, cortical silence period; CypA, peptidyl-prolyl cis-trans isomerase A; DCMAP, distal compound muscle action potential; D-KEFS, Delis–Kaplan Executive Function System; DTI, diffusion tensor imaging; DWI, diffusion-weighted imaging; ECAS, Edinburgh Cognitive and Behavioral ALS Screen; ECL, electrochemiluminescence; EDB, extensor digitorum brevis; EMG, electromyography; ERp57, protein disulfide-isomerase A3; EURALS, European Registry of ALS Consortium; EUROMOTOR, European multidisciplinary ALS network identification to cure motor neurone degeneration; FA, fractional anisotropy; FAB, frontal assessment battery; FBI, frontal behavioral inventory; FD, fiber density; FEV1, forced expiratory volume; fibs-sw, fibrillation/sharp-waves; FM-ADP, fat mass air displacement plethysmography; FPs, fasciculation potentials; FSS, fatigue severity scale; FUBP1, far upstream element-binding protein 1; FVC, forced vital capacity; GM, gray matter; GSTO1, glutathione S-transferase omega-1; HADS, hospital anxiety and depression scale; HDAC4, histone deacetylase 4; HHD, handheld dynamometry; HSC70, heat shock cognate 71 kDa protein; IL, interleukin; IFN, interferon; IRAK4, Interleukin-1 receptor-associated kinase 4; JPND, EU Joint Programme for Neurodegenerative Disease Research; LGVF, letter guided verbal fluency; LMN, lower motor neuron; MAS, modified Ashworth scale; McDESPOT, multi-component driven equilibrium single pulse observation of T1/T2; MDRS-2, Mattis Dementia Rating scale-Second Edition; MEP, maximal static expiratory mouth pressure; MiND-B, motor neuron disease behavior scale; MIP, maximal inspiratory pressure; MiRNAs, micro-RNAs; MITOS, Milano-Torino staging system; MMSE, mini mental state examination; MMT, manual muscle testing; MND, Motor neuron disease; MoCA, Montreal Cognitive Assessment; MR, magnetic resonance; MRC, Medical Research Council Scale for muscle strength; MRCSS-LL, Medical Research Council sum score; MRI, magnetic resonance imaging; MRS, magnetic resonance spectroscopy; MS, multiple sclerosis; MU, motor unit; MUNE, motor unit number estimation; MUNIX, motor unit number index; MUPs, motor unit potentials; MUSIX, motor unit size index; NAA, N-acetylaspartate; NEALS, Northeast ALS Consortium; NF-L, neurofilament light chain; NI, neurophysiology index; NISALS, Neuroimaging Society in Amyotrophic Lateral Sclerosis; NMR, nuclear magnetic resonance; nUHPLC LC-MS, nano ultra-high performance liquid chromatography tandem mass spectrometry; p75ECD, neurotrophin receptor p75 extracellular domain; PA28a, proteasome activator complex subunit 1; PBA, pseudobulbar affect; PCR, polymerase chain reaction; PDI, protein disulfide-isomerase; PEFT, peak expiratory flow time; PET, positron emission tomography; PGGM, precentral gyruses gray matter; PGRN, progranulin; PLS, primary lateral sclerosis; PMA, progressive muscular atrophy; pNFH, Phosphorylated neurofilament heavy chain; PRDX2, peroxiredoxin-2; PRO-ACT, Pooled Resource Open-Access ALS Clinical Trials; QoL, quality of life; RD, radial diffusivity; RMN, Research Motor Neuron; ROA2, Heterogeneous nuclear ribonucleoproteins A2/B1; RSA, relative surface area; rsfMRI, resting state functional magnetic resonance imaging; SCA, spinocerebellar ataxia; SBMA, spinal and bulbar muscular atrophy; SEIQOL-DW, Schedule for the Evaluation of the Individual Quality of Life-Direct Weighting; SF-36, 36-Item short form health survey; SMA, spinal muscular atrophy; SMUAP, single motor unit action potential; SNIP, sniff nasal inspiratory pressure; SOD1, superoxide dismutase 1; SOP, Standard operating procedure; SPECT, single photon emission computed tomography; SPO2, peripheral capillary oxygen saturation; SVC, slow vital capacity; TA, tibialis anterior; TDP-43, TAR DNA-binding protein 43; TiM, Telehealth in Motor Neuron disease; TMS, transcranial magnetic stimulation; TNF, tumor necrosis factor; TUG, timed up and go test; Tw Pdi, twitch trans-diaphragmatic pressure; TWBC, total white blood cell count; UMN, upper motor neuron; VC, vital capacity; WALS, Western ALS Consortium; WVFI, Written Verbal Fluency Index.

TABLE 1 | Longitudinal "dry biomarker" studies in ALS: Neuroimaging, Neurophysiology and Clinical Studies.

Author(s) and year of publication	Follow-up interval (months)	Number of patients/Number or controls	Clinical assessment batteries/Functional rating scales	Imaging data	Main study findings
IMAGING STUDIES					
Floeter et al. (15)	6–18	28/28	ALSFRS-R, letter fluency, FBI, MMSE	DWI, structural (T2)	- progression and propagation detected (DTI measures) over 6 months - DTI measures correlated with ALSFRS-R, King's stage and cognitive measures
Kassubek et al. (16)	6	67/31	ALSFRS-R	DTI	- progression detected at group level and 27% of individual patients (DTI measures) - FA correlated with ALSFRS-R
Stampfli et al. (17)	3–6	21/13	ALSFRS-R	T1, DWI	-progression detected (FD values)
Baldaranov et al. (18)	26	6/6	ALSFRS-R	DTI	-progression detected (FA, AD/RD values) and correlated with progression on ALSFRS-R
Bede et al., 2017 (14)	4	32/69	ALSFRS-R	structural, DTI	-progression detected (GM)
de Albuquerque et al. (19)	8	27/27	ALSFRS-R, UMN scale	structural (T1, T2)	- progression detected (AD, MD) - correlation with ALSFRS-R change
Menke et al. (20)	24	16/0	ALSFRS-R, UMN score	T1, DTI, rs-Fmri	- progression detected - correlation with ALSFRS-R decline
Simon et al. (21)	3–6	21/13	ALSFRS-R, MRCSS-LL, MUNE	DTI, structural (T1)	- progression detected (FA values) - correlations with ALSFRS-R change, MUNE, functional disability and strength
Floeter et al. (22)	6	49/28	ALSFRS-R, FBI, MDRS-2, letter fluency, MMSE, D-KEFS	structural (T1)	-progression detected (ventricular volume)
Schulthess et al. (23)	6	135/56	ALSFRS-R	rs-Fmri, DTI	- progression detected (functional connectivity) - correlation with physical disability
McMillan et al. (24)	12	20/25	neuropsychology	structural (T1)	-hypermethylation protective against progression, correlation with protection of some components of neuropsychological assessment
Steinbach et al. (25)	3	16/16	ALSFRS-R, neuropsychology	DTI	-progression detected
Westeneng et al. (26)	5.5	112/60	ALSFRS-R	structural (T1)	- progression detected (volume measures) - correlation with ALSFRS-R
Menke et al. (4)	6	60/36	ALSFRS-R, ACE-R	structural (T1), DTI	-progression detected (GM)
Schuster et al. (27)	3–15	77/60	ALSFRS-R	structural (T1)	-progression detected (cortical thickness)
Stoppel et al. (28)	3	40/42	ALSFRS-R, MRC, neuropsychology	structural, Fmri	- progression detected - correlation with ALSFRS-R and MRC
Verstraete et al. (29)	5.5	24/19	ALSFRS-R	DTI, structural (T1)	- no progression detected - propagation detected
Ignjatovic et al. (30)	6	46/26	ALSFRS-R	structural (T1, T2, FLAIR)	-progression detected (hypointensities in PGGM)
Kwan et al. (31)	1.26–2.08 years	45/19	ALSFRS-R, finger tapping	T1, DTI	-progression detected (cortical thickness, GM volume)
Keil et al. (32)	6	24/24	ALSFRS-R, SF36, FAB, MMSE	DTI, structural (T1, T2)	- progression detected (FA values) - correlations with ALSFRS-R, physical and executive function
Menke et al. (33)	6	24/0	ALSFRS-R	DTI	-progression detected (AD)
Ichikawa et al. (34)	NA	6/NA	NA	NA	-progression detected, correlated to neuropsychology assessment
van der Graaff et al. (35)	NA	48/12	ALSFRS-R, finger tapping	DWI	-progression detected
Zhang et al. (36)	8	17/19	ALSFRS-R	structural (T1), DTI	- progression detected (FA)

(Continued)

TABLE 1 | Continued

Author(s) and year of publication	Follow-up interval (months)	Number of patients/Number or controls	Clinical assessment batteries/Functional rating scales	Imaging data	Main study findings
Agosta et al. (37)	9	16/10	ALSFRS	structural (T1)	- progression detected (GM)
Agosta et al. (38)	9	17/20	ALSFRS	DWI, structural	- progression detected (cord area, cord average FA)
Avants et al. (39)	5.3	4/4	0	structural (T1)	- progression detected (cortical atrophy)
Lule et al. (40)	6	25/15	ALSFRS-R	Fmri, structural (T1)	- progression detected (activity)
Unrath et al. (41)	6	11/0	ALSFRS	MRS, T1	- progression detected (NAA, NAA/Cr+Cho)
Suhy et al. (42)	Every 3 months	28/12	0	MRS, T1, T2	- progression detected (NAA, Cr, Cho)
Block et al. (43)	24	33/20	0	MRS	- progression detected
Irwin et al. (44)		143/0	MMSE, LGVF	structural VBM	- no progression on MRI reported
Kolind et al. (45)	42	30/12	ALSFRS-R, ACE,	mcDESPOT	- progression detected in PLS only
Verstraete et al. (46)	6	45/25	ALSFRS-R	structural (T1)	- no progression reported
Blain et al. (47)	6–12	23/25	ALSFRS-R, ALSS	structural (T2), DWI	- no significant progression detected (DTI measures)
Rule et al. (48)	3–12	45/17	0	MRS, structural (T1, T2)	- no clear pattern of progressive change over time (NAA rations)
Author(s) and year of publication	**Follow-up interval (months)**	**Total number of patients/Total number of controls**	**Neurophysiology modality**	**Target muscle**	**Key study findings**
NEUROPHYSIOLOGY STUDIES					
Escorcio-Bezerra et al. (49)	4.3	21/21	MUNIX	tibialis anterior (TA), abductor pollicis brevis (APB) and abductor digiti minimi (ADM) muscles	- progression detected (mean MUNIX)
de Carvalho et al. (50)	3–6	73/37	FPs, MUPs, fibs-sw, jitter- MU physiology	tibialis anterior	- progression detected
Boekestein et al. (51)	8	18/24	MUNIX, HD-MUNE, CMAP, MUSIX	thenar	- progression detected (MUNE, MUNIX)
Cheah et al. (52)	3	37/0	CMAP, axonal excitability	abductor pollicis brevis	- progression detected (CMAP)
Ahn et al. (53)	NA	135/NA	NA	NA	- asymmetric progression (MUNE)
Cheah et al. (54)	3	58/NA	NI, CMAP	abductor digiti minimi and ulnar nerve	- progression detected (NI)
de Carvalho et al. (55)	6	28/0	NI, CMAP, MUNE	abductor digiti minimi muscles	- progression detected (CSP)
Neuwirth et al. (56)	15	7/8	MUNIX, CMAP,	abductor pollicis brevis (APB), abductor digiti minimi (ADM), abductor halluces brevis (AHB), extensor digitorum brevis (EDB)	- progression detected (MUNIX)
Floyd et al. (57)	18	60/33	TMS, CMCT, MEP	abductor digiti minimi (ADM) and tibialis anterior (TA)	-linear progression detected (TMS threshold, CMCT, TMS amplitude corrected)
Gooch et al. (58)	NA	64/NA-1	TMS, MUNE,	NA	-progression detected (MUNE)
Liu et al. (59)	12	112/12	MUNE, CMAP	Abductor pollicis brevis (APB) and abductor digiti quinti (ADQ)	- progression detected (MUNE), correlated to ALSFRS descent
Albrecht et al. (60)	11.5	10/25	MUNE, S-MUAP	extensor digitorum brevis	- progression detected (MUNE)

(Continued)

TABLE 1 | Continued

Author(s) and year of publication	Follow-up interval (months)	Total number of patients/Total number of controls	Neurophysiology modality	Target muscle	Key study findings
Wang et al. (61)	12	20/70	MUNE, SMUP, CMAP, MU loss	thenar	- progression detected - (Thenar MUNE, CMAP)
Chan et al. (62)	24	NA	motor units	thenar	- progression detected
Felice et al. (63)	12	NA	MUNE	thenar	- progression detected (MUNE)
Yuen et al. (64)	6	NA	CMAP, MUNE	abductor digiti minimi	- progression detected (MUNE, fiber density)
Vucic et al. (65)	7–100 days	25/30, 35	cortical and axonal excitability- MEP, CMAP- TMS	abductor pollicus brevis	- aim to determine effect of riluzole
Aggarwal et al. (66)	36	31/57	MUNE	tibialis anterior, abductor pollicis brevis (APB), deltoid, and first dorsal interosseous muscles	- no progression reported
Arasaki et al. (67)	NA	NA	MUNE,	extensor digitorum brevis (EDB)	- no progression reported
de Carvalho et al. (68)	11.6	NA	CMAP, MEP, TMS	NA	- no progression detected
Swash et al. (69)	NA	14/NA	single fiber EMG	NA	- no definite progression detected

Author(s) and year publication	Follow-up interval (months)	Number of patients/Number of controls	Clinical assessment batteries/Functional rating scales	Summary of findings
CLINICAL STUDIES				
ALSFRS-R				
Thakore et al. (70)	NA	3367/0	ALSFRS-R, ALSFRS, bloods- creatinine, uric acid, CK, albumin, sodium bicarbonate, hematocrit, TWBC	- ALSFRS-R progression detected, pre-slope and post-slope have effects on survival
Rooney et al. (71)	NA	407/0	ALSFRS-R	- progression detected in ALSFRS-R subscores
*ACTS trial. (72)	NA	75/NA	ALSFRS	progression detected (ALSFRS-R), associated with motor and pulmonary function
Cognitive and behavior assessments				
Floeter et al. (73)	18	NA	ALSFRS-R, letter fluency, FBI	- progression detected (ALSFRS-R, FBI, letter fluency)
Elamin et al. (74)	NA	186/NA	cognitive testing	- progression detected (cognitive function)
Roberts-South et al. (75)	24	16/12	neuropsychology, language, discourse sampling, perfusion computerized transaxial tomography, pulmonary, clinical	- progression detected (cognitive language deficits)
*Duning et al. (76)	3	10/32	ALSFRS, clinical neuropsychological battery, imaging	- progression detected (DTI)
Poletti et al. (77)	24	168/0	ECAS	- no progression detected, ECAS scores improved over time
Xu et al. (78)	6	108/60	ACE-3, FAB, ECAS executive, MoCA, ALSFRS-R, ALS-FTD-Q, MiND-B	- no progression detected
Gillingham et al. (79)	9	20/36	ALS-CFB, ALSFRS-R	- no progression reported
Mioshi et al. (80)	6	79/53	MiND-B- apathy, disinhibition, stereotypical behavior, ACE-R, ALSFRS-R	- no progression reported
Quality of life assessments				
Jakobsson Larsson et al. (81)	24	36/0	SEIQoL-DW, ALSFRS-R, HADS	- anxiety decreased over time, depression correlated to QOL, QOL remained stable despite physical deterioration

(Continued)

TABLE 1 | Continued

Author(s) and year publication	Follow-up interval (months)	Number of patients/Number of controls	Clinical assessment batteries/Functional rating scales	Summary of findings
BMI and other clinical assessments				
Beck et al. (82)	6	78/39	skin water loss	- progression detected (skin water loss)
Garruto et al. (83)	NA	31/66	bone mass (wrist radiograph)	- progression detected (bone loss)
Ioannides et al. (84)	6	44/29	FM-ADP, BMI, BAI, ALSFRS-R	- BMI and BAI not accurate measures of fat mass in ALS
Peter et al. (85)	3	393/791	BMI, ALSFRS-R	- alterations in body weight present in ALS patients decades before manifestation of symptoms
Nunes et al. (86)	3	37/0	BMI, serum albumin, transferrin, total cholesterol	- no progression reported
Jablecki et al. (87)	NA	NA	clinical scores	- no progression reported
Respiratory and muscle assessments				
Andres et al. (88)	4–21	100/0	ATLIS, ALSFRS, VC	- ATLIS more sensitive to change than ALSFRS and VC
de Bie et al. (89)	12	10/0	RSA, ALSFRS-R, FVC	- progression detected(RSA and ALSFRS-R)
Shellikeri et al. (90)	NA	33/13	kinematic measures of tongue and jaw movement, speaking rate, intelligibility, ALSFRS-R	- progression detected (tongue movement size and speed)
Londral et al. (91)	2–20	19/26	typing activity, ALSFRS-R	- progression detected (typing activity)
Panitz et al. (92)	12	51/0	fatigue severity scale (FSS), CIS20-R-subjective fatigue experience, concentration, motivation, activity, ALSFRS-R, MRC, SVC	- progression detected (FSS, CIS20-R), correlated to ALSFRS-R, and ALSFRS-R progression
Atassi et al. (93)	NA	8635/0	ALSFRS-R, VC	- PRO-ACT database- progression detected (ALSFRS-R and VC)
Watanabe et al. (94)	1.7 years	451/0	ALSFRS-R, MRC, MMT	-progression detected (ALSRS-R)
Leonardis et al. (95)	every 3 months	NA/0	ALSFRS-R, Norris-r, AGA, FVC, MIP, MEP, SNIP	- progression detected (respiratory measures)
Mahajan et al. (96)	NA	362/0	VC	- progression detected (VC)
Pinto et al. (97)	4–6	49/0	Diaphragm amplitude, ALSFRS-R, MIP, FVC, SNIP, SPO2	- progression detected (Diaphragm amplitude, ALSFRS-R, respiratory measures)
Montes et al. (98)	6	31/0	TUG, ALSFRS-R, FVC, MMT	- linear progression detected (TUG) - associated with ALSFRS-R, MMT
Vender et al. (99)	NA	139/0	FVC	- progression detected (FVC)
Wilson et al. (100)	NA	55/NA	respiratory- FVC, FEV1, PEFT	- linear progression detected (PEFT)
Poloni et al. (101)	NA	NA	VC, Motley index, FEV1	- progression detected (respiratory measures)
Andersen et al. (102)	6–59	20/0	respiratory- SVC, cough peak flow, max inspiratory muscle strength, SNIP, max insufflation capacity	- no progression reported
Quaranta et al. (103)	NA	NA	respiratory function	- no progression reported
Proudfoot et al. (104)	24	61/39	eye tracking- anti saccadic, trail making, visual search tasks, ALSFRS-R, ACE-R, UMN, imaging)	- no progression detected
*Lenglet et al. (105)	18	512/0	ALSFRS-R, MMT, SVC	- clinical trial
Yamauchi et al. (106)	Every 6 months	43/30	ALSFRS-R, phrenic nerve conduction study (DCMAP), respiratory function tests (SNIP, FVC), nocturnal pulsed oximetry, MMT	- no progression reported
Mendoza et al. (107)	NA	161/0	MIP, FVC	- no progression reported
Marti-Fabregas et al. (108)	NA	NA	FVC	- no progression detected
Palmowski et al. (109)	NA	NA	electro-oculography	- not well-defined progression

Studies detecting progressive changes are listed first followed by studies not capturing longitudinal changes.
**indicates clinical trial.*

is increasingly recognized (30, 43, 44). With few exceptions (122–124), most ALS imaging studies use 3 Tesla platforms and 7 Tesla systems are more commonly used in post-mortem studies (125, 126). Disease progression has been detected across a range of MR imaging metrics including structural (22, 26), diffusion (16, 18), functional (28, 40), and spectroscopy (41, 42) measures. As the majority of studies have a two-timepoint design, it is often unclear if specific imaging metrics show linear or exponential changes. The few existing multi-timepoint studies suggest that pathological change is not linear (10). The revised ALS functional rating scale (ALSFRS-r) is the most commonly reported clinical measure (16, 18–20), with only few imaging studies reporting associations with staging (15) or neuropsychological performance (15, 24).

Neurophysiology

Most longitudinal neurophysiology studies are single center studies, reducing the risk of inter-rater and inter-center variability (127). As presented in **Table 1**, follow-up interval ranges between 7 days (65) and 3 years (66), and up to 7 follow-up time-points have been included in some studies (57, 60). Surprisingly few studies include disease controls such as peripheral neuropathy (60) or benign fasciculation syndrome (50). Clinical assessments performed in conjunction with neurophysiology typically include ALSFRS-r (51), forced vital capacity (FVC) (55), slow vital capacity (SVC) (56), grip strength (64), pinch strength (58), and manual muscle testing (MMT) (58), however, correlations between neurophysiological measures and clinical assessments are seldom reported. The majority of longitudinal neurophysiological studies focus on upper limb muscles, e.g., abductor pollicis brevis, deltoid, first dorsal interrosseus, extensor digitorum brevis, abductor digiti minimi (51, 52, 55, 60, 61) with relatively few studies evaluating lower limb muscles such as abductor hallicus brevis and tibialis anterior (50, 56, 57, 66). The most commonly reported longitudinal neurophysiological indices include compound muscle action potential (CMAP) (51, 52), single motor unit action potential (SMUAP) (60), MUNE (55, 59), MUNIX (49, 56), neurophysiology index (NI) (54, 55), TMS measures (57, 58), and axonal excitability (52). Progressive neurophysiological changes have been detected by MUNIX (49, 51, 56), MUNE (51, 58, 60), CMAP (52, 61), NI (54), and TMS measures (57) and allowing for study-design limitations, the consensus is that degenerative changes are not linear.

Clinical Biomarkers and Instruments

Robust clinical longitudinal studies in ALS have up to 6 follow-up time points (88, 89, 91), the interval between the assessments can be as short as 3 months (95) and the sample size can be as big as several thousands (70, 93) (**Table 1**). Few multi-timepoint studies include disease controls such as motor neuropathies (91), alternative neuromuscular diseases (78), or neurodegenerative conditions (83). Large, multi-timepoint longitudinal studies invariably suffer from considerable attrition rates, but these are rarely explicitly reported in the manuscript abstracts (10). Detailed genotyping is only available in a minority of longitudinal studies (15, 77, 79, 94). The most widely utilized rating scale in longitudinal studies is the ALSFRS-r (70, 71, 128) which provides a composite score of bulbar, limb and respiratory dysfunction, and is invariably evaluated in clinical trials (72, 105). Quality of life (QoL) in ALS is increasingly evaluated by disease-specific instruments such as the 40-item ALS assessment questionnaire (ALSAQ-40) or the revised ALS-specific Quality of Life questionnaire (ALSSQoL-R) (129–131). A number of symptom-specific instruments are also commonly used such as the Center for Neurologic Study-Bulbar Function Scale (CNS-BFS), a 21-item self-report scale of bulbar function, and the Center for Neurologic Study-Lability Scale (CNS-LS), a 7-item self-report scale of pseudobulbar affect (PBA) (132). Tapping rates, composite reflex scores, The Penn UMN Score (133), the Modified Ashworth scale (MAS) are often used as proxies of UMN degeneration (132).

In clinical trials, muscle strength is often estimated by handheld dynamometry (HHD) (134), manual muscle testing (MMT) (105), scoring systems such as the Medical Research Council (MRC) Scale for muscle strength (135) and some studies also report limb circumference (136). Respiratory function in ALS is typically monitored by sniff nasal inspiratory pressure (SNIP), SVC, or FVC in addition to measures such as early morning arterial blood gas (ABG) and overnight pulse-oximetry (137, 138). Measures of typing ability (91), tongue movements (90), vital capacity (VC) (96), FVC (99), SNIP (97), and diaphragm amplitude (97) all show progressive longitudinal changes. Nutritional markers such as body mass index (BMI) and lipid profile are now established prognostic indicators (139, 140). Cognitive and behavioral domains are routinely assessed thanks to the availability of validated screening instruments such as the Edinburgh Cognitive and Behavioral ALS Screen (ECAS) (141), the Beaumont Behavioral Inventory (BBI) (142) and the ALS Cognitive Behavioral Screen (ALS-CBS) (143). In contrast to the relentlessly progressive motor deficits of ALS, the trajectory of cognitive and behavioral deficits is less clear due to considerable individual variations, genotype-associated profiles (144, 145), differences in assessment strategies and practice-effects (146). Several longitudinal neuropsychology studies do not detect progression (77, 147, 148), progressive behavioral impairment has been noted in the absence of cognitive change (149), and some studies report improved performance as a result of practice effects (77).

Wet Biomarkers

The findings, study design characteristics, and follow-up intervals of longitudinal biofluid studies are summarized in **Table 2**. Phosphorylated neurofilament heavy chain (pNFH), neurofilament light chain (NF-L), progranulin (PGRN), cytokines, TAR DNA-binding protein 43 (TDP-43), cystatin C, creatinine, micro-RNAs (miRNAs), chitotriosidase-1 (CHIT1), chitinase-3-like protein 1 (CHI3L1), chitinase-3-like protein 2 (CHI3L2) have been evaluated in both research studies (152, 153, 157, 158, 162, 164, 168, 171) and clinical trials (150, 156, 157, 160, 161). Markers of iron metabolism and ferroptosis are relatively recent domains of ALS biomarker research (172, 173). Most biofluid studies are either serum (150, 157) or CSF studies (152, 167), but urine (155) and skeletal

TABLE 2 | Longitudinal "wet biomarker" studies in ALS.

Author(s) and year of publication	Follow-up interval (months)	Number of patients / number of controls	Candidate biomarker evaluated	Biofluid	Assessment method used	Summary of conclusion
*Okada et al. (150)	12	57/0	creatinine	serum	NA	- progression detected (creatinine)
Raheja et al. (151)	NA	NA	microRNAs	serum	NA	- progression detected (miR-136-3p, miR-30b-5p, miR-331-3p, miR-496, miR-2110)
Thompson et al. (152)	30	49/52	chitotriosidase (CHIT1), chitinase-3-like protein 1 (CHI3L1), and chitinase-3-like protein 2 (CHI3L2), (phosphorylated neurofilament heavy chain) Pnfh	CSF	nano ultra-high performance liquid chromatography tandem mass spectrometry (nUHPLC LC-MS/MS), ELISA	- progression detected (CHI3L1)
Di Pietro et al. (153)	NA	14/24	micro-RNAs- MIR206, MIR208B, MIR499	skeletal muscle	quantitative real time PCR, Western blot analysis	- progression detected (MIR208B, MIR499, MIR206, HDAC4)
Murdock et al. (154)	Every 6–12 months	119/35	leukocytes	blood	flow cytometry	- progression detected (immune cells), associated with ALSFRS-R
Shepheard et al. (155)	NA	54/45	urinary p75ECD	urine	sandwich ELISA	- progression detected (urinary p75ECD), correlated with ALSFRS-R
van Ejik et al. (156)	NA	1241/0	creatinine	plasma	NA	- progression detected (plasma creatinine), correlated to ALSFRS-R, muscle strength, mortality
Waller et al. (157)	3	22/0	microRNAs, miR-17-5p, miR-223-3p, miR-24	serum	Qiagen miScript-based Qpcr	- progression detected (mir-206, mir-143-3p, mir-374b-5p)
McCombe et al. (158)	27	98/61	pNFH	serum	NA	- progression detected (pNFH)
Lu et al. (159)	36	136/104	neurofilament heavy chain-phosphoform	plasma	ELISA	- progression detected (NfH)
*Levine et al. (160)	6	28/0	tau, pNFH	CSF	ELISA	- progression detected (tau)
*Levine et al. (161)	12	20/0	tau, pNFH	CSF	ELISA	- progression detected (tau)
Wilson et al. (162)	24	44/60	cystatin C	CSF, plasma	quantitative enzyme linked immunosorbent assay (ELISA)	- progression detected (cystatin C)
Gaiani et al. (163)	36	94/82	ALSFRS-R, NFL	CSF	enzyme-linked immunosorbent assay (UmanDiagnostics AB)	- NFL may have role as a biomarker
Lu et al. (164)	48	95/88	CK, ferritin, tumor necrosis factor (TNF)–a, and interleukin (IL)−1b, IL-2, IL-8, IL-12p70, IL-4, IL-5, IL-10, and IL-13, IL-6, IFN-Y	plasma	multiplex electrochemiluminescence immunoassay	- no defined progression
Steinacker et al. (165)	24	125/28	neurofilament light chain (NF-L), progranulin (PGRN), S100	serum, CSF (baseline only)	ELISA, electrochemiluminescence (ECL) immunoassay, ECLIA Elecsys (Roche, Penzberg, Germany)	- no progression reported
Gibson et al. (166)	12	80/0	CK	NA	NA	- no progression detected
Gray et al. (167)	24	41/14	CSF- glucose, lactate, citric acid, ethanol	CSF	H-NMR	- no progression reported
Lu et al. (168)	36	167/78	neurofilament light chain (NFL)	serum, blood, CSF	electrochemiluminescence immunoassay	- no progression detected
Verstraete et al. (169)	NA	219/100	TDP-43	plasma	sandwich ELISA	- no defined progression
Nardo et al. (170)	6	94/64	PRDX2, GSTO1, CLIC1, HSC70, CypA, PDI, ERp57, CALR, PA28a, IRAK4, FUBP1, ROA2, actinNT, TDP-43	blood PBMC	2D-DIGE, mass spectometry	- no progression reported

**indicates clinical trial.*

muscle-based (153) studies have now also been published. Quantitative enzyme-linked immunosorbent assay (ELISA) is the most commonly used antibody-based technique (13, 174) which can be performed with one antibody (indirect ELISA), or with two antibodies (sandwich ELISA). Increased CSF (13) and serum (175) pNFH detected by ELISA is thought to be a sensitive marker of axonal degeneration in ALS (152, 171, 176, 177). The specificity of this marker however may be inadequate to reliably differentiate ALS from other neurodegenerative conditions (13, 176). Other antibody-based techniques such as Western blot (171) and electrochemiluminescence (ECL) (153, 168) may improve detection sensitivity and reliability (13). Panels of multiple proteins can be evaluated by multiplex immunoassays such as planar or microbead assays (13). Mass spectrometry based methods using chromatin-immunoprecipitation-based surfaces, two-dimensional gel electrophoresis or high-resolution mass spectrometry have identified cystatin-C and transthyretin as candidate biomarkers (178–180). The longest wet biomarker study followed patients for 4 years (164). The majority of studies have at least 2 follow-up timepoints (155, 162, 170) and one study included 13 follow-up timepoints (156, 159). Large multi-center trials include as much as 1,000 participants (156). One of the most striking shortcomings of existing longitudinal studies is that very few included disease controls such as Parkinson's disease cohorts, patients with multifocal motor neuropathy with conduction block, Kennedy's disease, chronic inflammatory demyelinating polyneuropathy (CIDP), cervical or lumbar radiculopathy, Charcot-Marie-Tooth disease (CMT), benign fasciculation, and cramp syndrome etc. (152, 159, 162). Another limitation of many longitudinal studies is the lack of comprehensive genotyping (12) as very few studies report comprehensive screening for ALS-associated mutations (153, 159, 169, 171). Exhaustive clinical profiling, such as medications (152, 164), neuropsychological assessments (171), quality of life indices are rarely reported in longitudinal studies. The majority of studies limit their clinical descriptions to ALSFRS-r, FVC, MRC, and Ashworth scores (153, 161, 162). Serum and plasma biomarkers such as creatinine (150, 156), pNfH (158, 159), and micro-RNAs (157), CSF biomarkers such as CHI3L1 (152), tau (160, 161), and cystatin-C (162), and urinary (155) and skeletal muscle (153) biomarkers are some of the promising tools for detecting disease progression. While no progressive changes have been detected in NFL levels, it is likely to be a useful as a diagnostic biomarker (168, 171).

Studies of Asymptomatic Mutation Carriers

Current clinical trials only recruit symptomatic cases despite accruing evidence that ALS has a long presymptomatic phase (5). Imaging studies of asymptomatic mutation carriers have consistently confirmed disease-specific cerebral and spinal cord changes prior to symptom onset (181–184) indicating that this disease-phase may represent a crucial window for therapeutic or neuroprotective intervention. The majority of presymptomatic studies assess a single time-point, as opposed to the longitudinal tracking of asymptomatic carriers of ALS-causing mutations (15). While the overwhelming majority of presymptomatic studies focus on *C9orf72* hexanucleotide carriers (183, 185–187), no prognostic markers have been validated to predict whether single patients will develop ALS or FTD. Compared to imaging studies, strikingly few presymptomatic neurophysiology studies have been undertaken (66). Studies of asymptomatic ALS-causing mutation carriers have enormous potential for academic research and may pave the way for asymptomatic pharmaceutical trials (5, 181).

DISCUSSION

Clinical trials currently evaluate the efficacy of candidate drugs using the revised ALS functional rating scale (ALSFRS-r), muscle strength assessment tools such as manual muscle testing (MMT), respiratory function indices such as forced vital capacity (FVC), slow vital capacity (SVC) and sniff nasal inspiratory pressure (SNIP), neurophysiological measures and survival (102, 116, 120, 188, 189). These measures however primarily reflect late-stage functional impairment and are not indicative of early stage pathology. Brain and spinal cord imaging has been evaluated as early-stage biomarkers with both diagnostic and monitoring potential (116, 120, 190). The core neuroimaging signature of ALS, irrespective of the disease-stage, includes corticospinal tract (191, 192), corpus callosum (193) and motor cortex degeneration (194). Atrophy in frontotemporal regions has been primarily associated with neuropsychological deficits (195–197) and linked to hexanucleotide repeats in C9orf72 (145, 198). Longitudinal imaging studies are superior to cross-sectional studies as they readily detect dynamic structural and functional changes and may elucidate compensatory processes (10, 14, 23, 28, 40, 120, 199). The emergence of multi-timepoint study designs (14, 20) enable the characterization of anatomical propagation patterns (200) and provide invaluable temporal insights into the disease trajectory of late-stage ALS. Inter-scan intervals as short as 3 months can detect longitudinal changes (14, 18, 120). Many longitudinal studies make use of multiple magnetic resonance (MR) metrics which is particularly useful in establishing an optimal panel of monitoring markers (120). Several longitudinal studies have indicated that white matter degeneration can be detected relatively early in the course of ALS with restricted further progression over time, whereas gray matter pathology shows relentless progression in the symptomatic phase of the disease (4, 14, 120). In addition to structural imaging studies, connectivity-based, metabolic, peripheral nerve, and, whole body muscle imaging have contributed to our understanding of longitudinal changes (20, 201–203).

Needle electromyography and nerve conduction studies play an important clinical role in ruling out alternative conditions and confirming a suspected diagnosis of ALS. Despite variations in local protocols, neurophysiological tests are recognized as objective, reliable and cost-effective tests of neuromuscular dysfunction, and have also been repeatedly proposed as longitudinal markers (55, 204). CMAP is generated by depolarization of muscle fibers through the stimulation of a single nerve, where amplitude reductions are interpreted as loss of motor axons (205, 206). While CMAP measurements capture longitudinal decline, it is confounded by variations in temperature, limb positioning and electrode placement (56, 207). CMAP-derived measures such as MUNE and MUNIX are now extensively utilized to characterize progressive changes in ALS. MUNE estimates motor neuron numbers, and may detect the rate of motor neuron loss, making it a more reliable method of appraising disease progression than CMAP (208, 209). However, its early-phase sensitivity has been questioned, as its use is limited to distal muscles, and the technique requires considerable training, especially for inter-rater and multi-site comparisons (205, 210). TMS allows the characterization of upper motor neuron dysfunction, and may be particularly useful in detecting progressive changes (57, 205).

Functional rating-scales are often the monitoring instruments of choice in clinical trials (55), as they are easy to administer, cost-effective to utilize and have acceptable inter- and intra-rater reliability profiles (7). The most widely used rating scale in clinical longitudinal studies is the ALSFRS-r. Despite its ease of administration, it has considerable limitations, as it may be disproportionately influenced by LMN dysfunction, does not account for laterality or asymmetry of symptoms, omits cognitive impairment, and may be affected by medications (14, 128, 188, 211).

Proteomics, metabolomics and lipidomics have seen significant advances in ALS research and CSF and serum markers are now used in longitudinal academic and pharmacological studies (172). Potential biomarkers for the detection of disease progression include serum and plasma biomarkers such as creatinine (150, 156), pNfH (158, 159), and micro-RNAs (157), CSF biomarkers such as CHI3L1 (152), tau (160, 161), and cystatin-C (162), and urinary (155) and skeletal muscle (153) biomarkers.

Prediction Analyses

Age at symptom onset (212), BMI (139), bulbar involvement (213), cognitive impairment (214), *C9orf72* genotype status (144), respiratory insufficiency (215), "definite ALS" by the El Escorial criteria (216), and functional disability (217) are the most commonly cited determinants of poor prognosis in ALS. SNIP (218) and less commonly used measures such as twitch trans-diaphragmatic pressure (Tw Pdi) (219) and maximal static expiratory mouth pressure (MEP) were shown to be good predictors of ventilator-free survival (219). A combined panel of several clinical, wet, and dry biomarkers is likely to offer the most accurate prognostic information (115, 120, 216, 217, 220). While cerebral (217, 221, 222) and spinal (115) imaging measures have been repeatedly linked to survival outcomes, these have not been utilized in a clinical setting. Neurophysiological variables, such as phrenic nerve stimulation outcomes (223) and biofluid markers, such as pNFH and NFL (165, 168, 224–226) are also thought to be accurate predictors.

Patient Stratification

Attempts to enroll patients in the early stages of the disease are hampered by the universally long diagnostic delay in ALS (227). Patient stratification in trials is typically based on site of onset (228), instead of other variables which have an established prognostic impact (138, 229). Admixed patient cohorts within a trial may hamper the ability to detect how different phenotypes and genotypes may exhibit a different response to a candidate drug (230–232). The stratification of heterogeneous cohorts is now aided by the development of validated staging systems, such as the King's (233), Milano-Torino (MITOS) (234) or the Fine'til 9 (FT9) (235) staging systems. The King's Staging system is based on the number of body regions affected, and the presence of nutritional or respiratory failure (233). The MITOS staging system is based on the ALSFRS-r, and is particularly sensitive to changes in later stages of the disease (236, 237). However, none of these staging systems account for cognitive or behavioral changes (236). Pathological staging systems suggest a four-stage model of ALS based on anatomical patterns of pTDP-43 load (238, 239). This system has now been validated by *in vivo* neuroimaging studies (240) and signals that accurate pathological staging and patient stratification may be possible based on neuroimaging (199, 240).

International Consortia

Only few ALS centers maintain dedicated biobanking facilities to store and process molecular markers in human biofluid locally. Similarly, relatively few centers are in a position to generate sufficient number of MRI and neurophysiology data sets of rare phenotypes to make meaningful inferences in a single center setting. Brain and tissue banks are also challenging to establish, maintain and fund, despite their invaluable contribution to ALS research (241–243).

Biospecimen samples are also often collected during clinical trials, and discarded after negative outcomes, despite their enormous potential for biomarker discovery (172). One of the most important achievements of biomarker development efforts is the establishment of national and international research consortia such as Association pour la recherche sur la SLA (ARSLA), Neuroimaging Society in ALS (NISALS), Research Motor Neuron (RMN), Canadian ALS Neuroimaging Consortium (CALSNIC), EU Joint Programme for Neurodegenerative Disease Research (JPND), European multidisciplinary ALS network identification to cure motor neurone degeneration (EUROMOTOR) which maintain vital biobanking facilities, registries, data repositories for multicenter data interpretation (121, 244). Clinical trial networks are also increasingly recognized as valuable platforms for multisite data collection and interpretation as they operate with carefully standardized protocols. Consortia such as the European Registry of ALS (EURALS) Consortium, the Western ALS (WALS) Consortium and the Northeast ALS (NEALS) Consortium are other examples (245). NEALS is one of the largest consortia with over 100 member sites from the US, Canada, Mexico, Italy, Lebanon and Australia (246). EURALS coordinates research studies and clinical trials relying on population-based European registries and include centers from Scotland, England, Netherlands, Spain, Ireland, Serbia, Italy, France, and Germany (241, 247, 248). ALS research consortia promote patient-oriented research, maintain biofluid, imaging and DNA banks, and have the potential to translate scientific advances into pragmatic clinical interventions.

Telehealth

Novel trends in longitudinal data collection include telemedicine-based technologies, wearable sensors and mobile phone applications (230). The continuous collection of data via telephone or telemedicine applications such as the Telehealth in Motor Neuron disease (TiM) system circumvent the inconvenience of patients and caregivers traveling long distances for research appointments (249). Once local data-protection and governance guidelines are complied with, information uploaded from these systems can be made available to healthcare professionals of multidisciplinary teams in real time (249). The feasibility of telehealth for ALS patients via live video-conferencing has also been evaluated (250) and is considered a particularly promising clinical and research platform (249, 250). A number of cognitive-behavioral screening tools have also been adapted for phone administration (251) including modified versions of the ALS Cognitive Behavior Screen (ALS-CBS), the Controlled Oral Word Association Test (COWAT), the Center for Neurologic Study-Lability Scale (CNS-LS) and found to be statistically equivalent to face-to-face assessments (251). Performance on other tests however, such as the telephone versions of the ALS-Frontal Behavioral Inventory (ALS-FBI) caregiver interview and the Written Verbal Fluency Index (WVFI) was not equivalent to clinic-based assessments (251). The continued development of telephone and internet-enabled devices are likely to provide further insights to longitudinal physical, cognitive and behavioral changes (251).

CONCLUSIONS

While clinical indicators of disease progression remain indispensable, neuroimaging, neurophysiology, and biofluid measures are particularly promising, objective, quantitative biomarker candidates. The validation of combined "wet" and "dry" biomarker panels will not only enable the detection of subtle progressive changes in ALS, but allow precision stratification of heterogeneous patient cohorts in clinical trials and improve existing prediction algorithms.

AUTHOR CONTRIBUTIONS

The manuscript was drafted by RC. EF, SL, OH and PB contributed to the conceptualization, editing, and revision of this paper.

FUNDING

This work was supported by the Andrew Lydon Scholarship, the Health Research Board (HRB–Ireland; HRB EIA-2017-019), the Irish Institute of Clinical Neuroscience (IICN)–Novartis Ireland Research Grant, the Iris O'Brien Foundation, the Perrigo Clinician-Scientist Research Fellowship, and the Research Motor Neuron (RMN–Ireland) Foundation.

REFERENCES

1. Katyal N, Govindarajan R. Shortcomings in the current amyotrophic lateral sclerosis trials and potential solutions for improvement. *Front Neurol.* (2017) 8:521. doi: 10.3389/fneur.2017.00521
2. Miller. Riluzole for amyotrophic lateral sclerosis (ALS)/motor neuron disease (MND). *Cochrane Database Syst Rev.* (2002) 14:CD001447. doi: 10.1002/14651858.CD001447
3. Al-Chalabi A, Jones A, Troakes C, King A, Al-Sarraj S, van den Berg LH. The genetics and neuropathology of amyotrophic lateral sclerosis. *Acta Neuropathol.* (2012) 124:339–52. doi: 10.1007/s00401-012-1022-4
4. Menke RA, Korner S, Filippini N, Douaud G, Knight S, Talbot K, et al. Widespread grey matter pathology dominates the longitudinal cerebral MRI and clinical landscape of amyotrophic lateral sclerosis. *Brain.* (2014) 137(Pt 9):2546–55. doi: 10.1093/brain/awu162
5. Eisen A, Kiernan M, Mitsumoto H, Swash M. Amyotrophic lateral sclerosis: a long preclinical period? *J Neurol Neurosurg Psychiatry.* (2014) 85:1232–8. doi: 10.1136/jnnp-2013-307135
6. Benatar M, Wuu J. Presymptomatic studies in ALS: rationale, challenges, and approach. *Neurology.* (2012) 79:1732–9. doi: 10.1212/WNL.0b013e31826e9b1d
7. Mitsumoto H, Brooks BR, Silani V. Clinical trials in amyotrophic lateral sclerosis: why so many negative trials and how can trials be improved? *Lancet Neurol.* (2014) 13:1127–38. doi: 10.1016/S1474-4422(14)70129-2
8. Beghi E, Chio A, Couratier P, Esteban J, Hardiman O, Logroscino G, et al. The epidemiology and treatment of ALS: focus on the heterogeneity of the disease and critical appraisal of therapeutic trials. *Amyotroph Lateral Scler.* (2011) 12:1–10. doi: 10.3109/17482968.2010.502940
9. de Carvalho M, Swash M. Can selection of rapidly progressing patients shorten clinical trials in amyotrophic lateral sclerosis? *Arch Neurol.* (2006) 63:557–60. doi: 10.1001/archneur.63.4.557
10. Schuster C, Elamin M, Hardiman O, Bede P. Presymptomatic and longitudinal neuroimaging in neurodegeneration–from snapshots to motion picture: a systematic review. *J Neurol Neurosurg Psychiatry.* (2015) 86:1089–96. doi: 10.1136/jnnp-2014-309888
11. Turner MR, Agosta F, Bede P, Govind V, Lule D, Verstraete E. Neuroimaging in amyotrophic lateral sclerosis. *Biomark Med.* (2012) 6:319–37. doi: 10.2217/bmm.12.26
12. Bede P, Hardiman O. Lessons of ALS imaging: pitfalls and future directions - a critical review. *NeuroImage Clin.* (2014) 4:436–43. doi: 10.1016/j.nicl.2014.02.011
13. Bowser R, Turner MR, Shefner J. Biomarkers in amyotrophic lateral sclerosis: opportunities and limitations. *Nat Rev Neurol.* (2011) 7:631–8. doi: 10.1038/nrneurol.2011.151
14. Bede P, Hardiman O. Longitudinal structural changes in ALS: a three time-point imaging study of white and gray matter degeneration. *Amyotroph Lateral Scler Frontotemporal Degener.* (2018) 19:232–41. doi: 10.1080/21678421.2017.1407795
15. Floeter MK, Danielian LE, Braun LE, Wu T. Longitudinal diffusion imaging across the C9orf72 clinical spectrum. *J Neurol Neurosurg Psychiatry.* (2018) 89:53–60. doi: 10.1136/jnnp-2017-316799
16. Kassubek J, Muller HP, Del Tredici K, Lule D, Gorges M, Braak H, et al. Imaging the pathoanatomy of amyotrophic lateral sclerosis *in vivo*: targeting a propagation-based biological marker. *J Neurol Neurosurg Psychiatry.* (2018) 89:374–81. doi: 10.1136/jnnp-2017-316365
17. Stampfli P, Sommer S, Czell D, Kozerke S, Neuwirth C, Weber M, et al. Investigation of neurodegenerative processes in amyotrophic lateral sclerosis using white matter fiber density. *Clin Neuroradiol.* (2018). doi: 10.1007/s00062-018-0670-8. [Epub ahead of print].
18. Baldaranov D, Khomenko A, Kobor I, Bogdahn U, Gorges M, Kassubek J, et al. Longitudinal diffusion tensor imaging-based assessment of tract alterations: an application to amyotrophic lateral

sclerosis. *Front Hum Neurosci.* (2017) 11:567. doi: 10.3389/fnhum.2017.00567

19. de Albuquerque M, Branco LM, Rezende TJ, de Andrade HM, Nucci A, Franca MC Jr. Longitudinal evaluation of cerebral and spinal cord damage in Amyotrophic Lateral Sclerosis. *NeuroImage Clin.* (2017) 14:269–76. doi: 10.1016/j.nicl.2017.01.024
20. Menke RAL, Proudfoot M, Talbot K, Turner MR. The two-year progression of structural and functional cerebral MRI in amyotrophic lateral sclerosis. *Neuroimage Clin.* (2018) 17:953–61. doi: 10.1016/j.nicl.2017.12.025
21. Simon NG, Lagopoulos J, Paling S, Pfluger C, Park SB, Howells J, et al. Peripheral nerve diffusion tensor imaging as a measure of disease progression in ALS. *J Neurol.* (2017) 264:882–90. doi: 10.1007/s00415-017-8443-x
22. Floeter MK, Bageac D, Danielian LE, Braun LE, Traynor BJ, Kwan JY. Longitudinal imaging in C9orf72 mutation carriers: relationship to phenotype. *NeuroImage Clin.* (2016) 12:1035–43. doi: 10.1016/j.nicl.2016.10.014
23. Schulthess I, Gorges M, Muller HP, Lule D, Del Tredici K, Ludolph AC, et al. Functional connectivity changes resemble patterns of pTDP-43 pathology in amyotrophic lateral sclerosis. *Sci Rep.* (2016) 6:38391. doi: 10.1038/srep38391
24. McMillan CT, Russ J, Wood EM, Irwin DJ, Grossman M, McCluskey L, et al. C9orf72 promoter hypermethylation is neuroprotective: neuroimaging and neuropathologic evidence. *Neurology.* (2015) 84:1622–30. doi: 10.1212/WNL.0000000000001495
25. Steinbach R, Loewe K, Kaufmann J, Machts J, Kollewe K, Petri S, et al. Structural hallmarks of amyotrophic lateral sclerosis progression revealed by probabilistic fiber tractography. *J Neurol.* (2015) 262:2257–70. doi: 10.1007/s00415-015-7841-1
26. Westeneng H-J, Verstraete E, Walhout R, Schmidt R, Hendrikse J, Veldink JH, et al. Subcortical structures in amyotrophic lateral sclerosis. *Neurobiol Aging.* (2015) 36:1075–82. doi: 10.1016/j.neurobiolaging.2014.09.002
27. Schuster C, Kasper E, Machts J, Bittner D, Kaufmann J, Benecke R, et al. Longitudinal course of cortical thickness decline in amyotrophic lateral sclerosis. *J Neurol.* (2014) 261:1871–80. doi: 10.1007/s00415-014-7426-4
28. Stoppel CM, Vielhaber S, Eckart C, Machts J, Kaufmann J, Heinze HJ, et al. Structural and functional hallmarks of amyotrophic lateral sclerosis progression in motor- and memory-related brain regions. *NeuroImage Clin.* (2014) 5:277–90. doi: 10.1016/j.nicl.2014.07.007
29. Verstraete E, Veldink JH, van den Berg LH, van den Heuvel MP. Structural brain network imaging shows expanding disconnection of the motor system in amyotrophic lateral sclerosis. *Hum Brain Mapp.* (2014) 35:1351–61. doi: 10.1002/hbm.22258
30. Ignjatovic A, Stevic Z, Lavrnic S, Dakovic M, Bacic G. Brain iron MRI: a biomarker for amyotrophic lateral sclerosis. *J Magn Reson Imaging.* (2013) 38:1472–9. doi: 10.1002/jmri.24121
31. Kwan JY, Meoded A, Danielian LE, Wu T, Floeter MK. Structural imaging differences and longitudinal changes in primary lateral sclerosis and amyotrophic lateral sclerosis. *Neuroimage Clin.* (2012) 2:151–60. doi: 10.1016/j.nicl.2012.12.003
32. Keil C, Prell T, Peschel T, Hartung V, Dengler R, Grosskreutz J. Longitudinal diffusion tensor imaging in amyotrophic lateral sclerosis. *BMC Neurosci.* (2012) 13:141. doi: 10.1186/1471-2202-13-141
33. Menke RA, Abraham I, Thiel CS, Filippini N, Knight S, Talbot K, et al. Fractional anisotropy in the posterior limb of the internal capsule and prognosis in amyotrophic lateral sclerosis. *Arch Neurol.* (2012) 69:1493–9. doi: 10.1001/archneurol.2012.1122
34. Ichikawa H, Ohno H, Murakami H, Ohnaka Y, Kawamura M. Writing error may be a predictive sign for impending brain atrophy progression in amyotrophic lateral sclerosis: a preliminary study using X-ray computed tomography. *Eur Neurol.* (2011) 65:346–51. doi: 10.1159/000328216
35. van der Graaff MM, Sage CA, Caan MW, Akkerman EM, Lavini C, Majoie CB, et al. Upper and extra-motoneuron involvement in early motoneuron disease: a diffusion tensor imaging study. *Brain.* (2011) 134(Pt 4):1211–28. doi: 10.1093/brain/awr016
36. Zhang Y, Schuff N, Woolley SC, Chiang GC, Boreta L, Laxamana J, et al. Progression of white matter degeneration in amyotrophic lateral sclerosis: a diffusion tensor imaging study. *Amyotroph Lateral Scler.* (2011) 12:421–9. doi: 10.3109/17482968.2011.593036
37. Agosta F, Gorno-Tempini ML, Pagani E, Sala S, Caputo D, Perini M, et al. Longitudinal assessment of grey matter contraction in amyotrophic lateral sclerosis: a tensor based morphometry study. *Amyotroph Lateral Scler.* (2009) 10:168–74. doi: 10.1080/17482960802603841
38. Agosta F, Rocca MA, Valsasina P, Sala S, Caputo D, Perini M, et al. A longitudinal diffusion tensor MRI study of the cervical cord and brain in amyotrophic lateral sclerosis patients. *J Neurol Neurosurg Psychiatry.* (2009) 80:53–5. doi: 10.1136/jnnp.2008.154252
39. Avants B, Khan A, McCluskey L, Elman L, Grossman M. Longitudinal cortical atrophy in amyotrophic lateral sclerosis with frontotemporal dementia. *Arch Neurol.* (2009) 66:138–9. doi: 10.1001/archneurol.2008.542
40. Lule D, Diekmann V, Kassubek J, Kurt A, Birbaumer N, Ludolph AC, et al. Cortical plasticity in amyotrophic lateral sclerosis: motor imagery and function. *Neurorehabil Neural Repair.* (2007) 21:518–26. doi: 10.1177/1545968307300698
41. Unrath A, Ludolph AC, Kassubek J. Brain metabolites in definite amyotrophic lateral sclerosis. A longitudinal proton magnetic resonance spectroscopy study. *J Neurol.* (2007) 254:1099–106. doi: 10.1007/s00415-006-0495-2
42. Suhy J, Miller RG, Rule R Schuff N, Licht J, Dronsky V, et al. Early detection and longitudinal changes in amyotrophic lateral sclerosis by 1H MRSI. *Neurology.* (2002) 58:773–9. doi: 10.1212/WNL.58.5.773
43. Block W, Karitzky J, Träber F, Pohl C, Keller E, Mundegar RR, et al. Proton magnetic resonance spectroscopy of the primary motor cortex in patients with motor neuron disease: subgroup analysis and follow-up measurements. *Arch Neurol.* (1998) 55:931–6. doi: 10.1001/archneur.55.7.931
44. Irwin DJ, McMillan CT, Brettschneider J, Libon DJ, Powers J, Rascovsky K, et al. Cognitive decline and reduced survival in C9orf72 expansion frontotemporal degeneration and amyotrophic lateral sclerosis. *J Neurol Neurosurg Psychiatry.* (2013) 84:163–9. doi: 10.1136/jnnp-2012-303507
45. Kolind S, Sharma R, Knight S, Johansen-Berg H, Talbot K, Turner MR. Myelin imaging in amyotrophic and primary lateral sclerosis. *Amyotroph Lateral Scler Frontotemporal Degener.* (2013) 14:562–73. doi: 10.3109/21678421.2013.794843
46. Verstraete E, Veldink JH, Hendrikse J, Schelhaas HJ, van den Heuvel MP, van den Berg LH. Structural MRI reveals cortical thinning in amyotrophic lateral sclerosis. *J Neurol Neurosurg Psychiatry.* (2012) 83:383–8. doi: 10.1136/jnnp-2011-300909
47. Blain CR, Williams VC, Johnston C, Stanton BR, Ganesalingam J, Jarosz JM, et al. A longitudinal study of diffusion tensor MRI in ALS. *Amyotroph Lateral Scler.* (2007) 8:348–55. doi: 10.1080/17482960701548139
48. Rule RR, Suhy J, Schuff N, Gelinas DF, Miller RG, Weiner MW. Reduced NAA in motor and non-motor brain regions in amyotrophic lateral sclerosis: a cross-sectional and longitudinal study. *Amyotroph Lateral Scler Other Motor Neuron Disord.* (2004) 5:141–9. doi: 10.1080/14660820410017109
49. Escorcio-Bezerra ML, Abrahao A, Santos-Neto D, de Oliveira Braga NI, Oliveira ASB, Manzano GM. Why averaging multiple MUNIX measures in the longitudinal assessment of patients with ALS? *Clin Neurophysiol.* (2017) 128:2392–6. doi: 10.1016/j.clinph.2017.09.104
50. de Carvalho M, Swash M. Fasciculation potentials and earliest changes in motor unit physiology in ALS. *J Neurol Neurosurg Psychiatry.* (2013) 84:963–8. doi: 10.1136/jnnp-2012-304545
51. Boekestein WA, Schelhaas HJ, van Putten MJ, Stegeman DF, Zwarts MJ, van Dijk JP. Motor unit number index (MUNIX) versus motor unit number estimation (MUNE): a direct comparison in a longitudinal study of ALS patients. *Clin Neurophysiol.* (2012) 123:1644–9. doi: 10.1016/j.clinph.2012.01.004
52. Cheah BC, Lin CS, Park SB, Vucic S, Krishnan AV, Kiernan MC. Progressive axonal dysfunction and clinical impairment in amyotrophic lateral sclerosis. *Clin Neurophysiol.* (2012) 123:2460–7. doi: 10.1016/j.clinph.2012.06.020
53. Ahn S-W, Kim J-E, Sung J-J, Lee K-W, Hong Y-H. Asymmetry of motor unit number estimate and its rate of decline in patients with amyotrophic lateral sclerosis. *J Clin Neurophysiol.* (2011) 28:528–32. doi: 10.1097/WNP.0b013e318231c9e0
54. Cheah BC, Vucic S, Krishnan AV, Boland RA, Kiernan MC. Neurophysiological index as a biomarker for ALS progression: validity of mixed effects models. *Amyotroph Lateral Scler.* (2011) 12:33–8. doi: 10.3109/17482968.2010.531742

55. de Carvalho M, Swash M. Sensitivity of electrophysiological tests for upper and lower motor neuron dysfunction in ALS: a six-month longitudinal study. *Muscle Nerve.* (2010) 41:208–11. doi: 10.1002/mus.21495
56. Neuwirth C, Nandedkar S, Stalberg E, Weber M. Motor unit number index (MUNIX): a novel neurophysiological technique to follow disease progression in amyotrophic lateral sclerosis. *Muscle Nerve.* (2010) 42:379–84. doi: 10.1002/mus.21707
57. Floyd AG, Yu QP, Piboolnurak P, Tang MX, Fang Y, Smith WA, et al. Transcranial magnetic stimulation in ALS: utility of central motor conduction tests. *Neurology.* (2009) 72:498–504. doi: 10.1212/01.wnl.0000341933.97883.a4
58. Gooch CL, Pullman SL, Shungu DC, Ulug AM, Chan S, Gordon PH, et al. Motor unit number estimation (MUNE) in diseases of the motor neuron: utility and comparative analysis in a multimodal biomarker study. *Suppl Clin Neurophysiol.* (2009) 60:153–62. doi: 10.1016/S1567-424X(08)00015-9
59. Liu XX, Zhang J, Zheng JY, Zhang S, Xu YS, Kang DX, et al. Stratifying disease stages with different progression rates determined by electrophysiological tests in patients with amyotrophic lateral sclerosis. *Muscle Nerve.* (2009) 39:304–9. doi: 10.1002/mus.21144
60. Albrecht E, Kuntzer T. Number of Edb motor units estimated using an adapted multiple point stimulation method: normal values and longitudinal studies in ALS and peripheral neuropathies. *Clin Neurophysiol.* (2004) 115:557–63. doi: 10.1016/j.clinph.2003.11.001
61. Wang FC, Bouquiaux O, De Pasqua V, Delwaide PJ. Changes in motor unit numbers in patients with ALS: a longitudinal study using the adapted multiple point stimulation method. *Amyotroph Lateral Scler Other Motor Neuron Disord.* (2002) 3:31–8. doi: 10.1080/146608202317576516
62. Chan KM, Stashuk DW, Brown WF. A longitudinal study of the pathophysiological changes in single human thenar motor units in amyotrophic lateral sclerosis. *Muscle Nerve.* (1998) 21:1714–23.
63. Felice KJ. A longitudinal study comparing thenar motor unit number estimates to other quantitative tests in patients with amyotrophic lateral sclerosis. *Muscle Nerve.* (1997) 20:179–85.
64. Yuen EC, Olney RK. Longitudinal study of fiber density and motor unit number estimate in patients with amyotrophic lateral sclerosis. *Neurology.* (1997) 49:573–8. doi: 10.1212/WNL.49.2.573
65. Vucic S, Lin CS, Cheah BC, Murray J, Menon P, Krishnan AV, et al. Riluzole exerts central and peripheral modulating effects in amyotrophic lateral sclerosis. *Brain.* (2013) 136(Pt 5):1361–70. doi: 10.1093/brain/awt085
66. Aggarwal A, Nicholson G. Detection of preclinical motor neurone loss in SOD1 mutation carriers using motor unit number estimation. *J Neurol Neurosurg Psychiatry.* (2002) 73:199–201. doi: 10.1136/jnnp.73.2.199
67. Arasaki K, Kato Y, Hyodo A, Ushijima R, Tamaki M. Longitudinal study of functional spinal alpha motor neuron loss in amyotrophic lateral sclerosis. *Muscle Nerve.* (2002) 25:520–6. doi: 10.1002/mus.10067
68. de Carvalho M, Miranda PC, Luis ML, Ducla-Soares E. Cortical muscle representation in amyotrophic lateral sclerosis patients: changes with disease evolution. *Muscle Nerve.* (1999) 22:1684–92.
69. Swash M, Schwartz MS. A longitudinal study of changes in motor units in motor neuron disease. *J Neurol Sci.* (1982) 56:185–97. doi: 10.1016/0022-510X(82)90141-1
70. Thakore NJ, Lapin BR, Pioro EP. Trajectories of impairment in amyotrophic lateral sclerosis: insights from the pooled resource open-access ALS clinical trials cohort. *Muscle Nerve.* (2018) 57:937–45. doi: 10.1002/mus.26042
71. Rooney J, Burke T, Vajda A, Heverin M, Hardiman O. What does the ALSFRS-R really measure? A longitudinal and survival analysis of functional dimension subscores in amyotrophic lateral sclerosis. *J Neurol Neurosurg Psychiatry.* (2016) 88:381–5. doi: 10.1136/jnnp-2016-314661
72. The amyotrophic lateral sclerosis functional rating scale. Assessment of activities of daily living in patients with amyotrophic lateral sclerosis. The ALS CNTF treatment study (ACTS) phase I-II Study Group. *Arch Neurol.* (1996) 53:141–7. doi: 10.1001/archneur.1996.00550020045014
73. Floeter MK, Traynor BJ, Farren J, Braun LE, Tierney M, Wiggs EA, et al. Disease progression in C9orf72 mutation carriers. *Neurology.* (2017) 89:234–41. doi: 10.1212/WNL.0000000000004115
74. Elamin M, Bede P, Byrne S, Jordan N, Gallagher L, Wynne B, et al. Cognitive changes predict functional decline in ALS: a population-based longitudinal study. *Neurology.* (2013) 80:1590–7. doi: 10.1212/WNL.0b013e31828f18ac
75. Roberts-South A, Findlater K, Strong MJ, Orange JB. Longitudinal changes in discourse production in amyotrophic lateral sclerosis. *Semin Speech Lang.* (2012) 33:79–94. doi: 10.1055/s-0031-1301165
76. Duning T, Schiffbauer H, Warnecke T, Mohammadi S, Floel A, Kolpatzik K, et al. G-CSF prevents the progression of structural disintegration of white matter tracts in amyotrophic lateral sclerosis: a pilot trial. *PLoS ONE.* (2011) 6:e17770. doi: 10.1371/journal.pone.0017770
77. Poletti B, Solca F, Carelli L, Faini A, Madotto F, Lafronza A, et al. Cognitive-behavioral longitudinal assessment in ALS: the Italian Edinburgh Cognitive and Behavioral ALS screen (ECAS). *Amyotroph Lateral Scler Frontotemporal Degener.* (2018) 19:387–95. doi: 10.1080/21678421.2018.1473443
78. Xu Z, Alruwaili ARS, Henderson RD, McCombe PA. Screening for cognitive and behavioural impairment in amyotrophic lateral sclerosis: frequency of abnormality and effect on survival. *J Neurol Sci.* (2017) 376:16–23. doi: 10.1016/j.jns.2017.02.061
79. Gillingham SM, Yunusova Y, Ganda A, Rogaeva E, Black SE, Stuss DT, et al. Assessing cognitive functioning in ALS: a focus on frontal lobe processes. *Amyotroph Lateral Scler Frontotemporal Degener.* (2017) 18:182–92. doi: 10.1080/21678421.2016.1248977
80. Mioshi E, Hsieh S, Caga J, Ramsey E, Chen K, Lillo P, et al. A novel tool to detect behavioural symptoms in ALS. *Amyotroph Lateral Scler Frontotemporal Degener.* (2014) 15:298–304. doi: 10.3109/21678421.2014.896927
81. Jakobsson Larsson B, Ozanne AG, Nordin K, Nygren I. A prospective study of quality of life in amyotrophic lateral sclerosis patients. *Acta Neurol Scand.* (2017) 136:631–8. doi: 10.1111/ane.12774
82. Beck M, Giess R, Magnus T, Puls I, Reiners K, Toyka KV, et al. Progressive sudomotor dysfunction in amyotrophic lateral sclerosis. *J Neurol Neurosurg Psychiatry.* (2002) 73:68–70. doi: 10.1136/jnnp.73.1.68
83. Garruto RM, Plato CC, Yanagihara R, Fox K, Dutt J, Gajdusek DC, et al. Bone mass in Guamanian patients with amyotrophic lateral sclerosis and parkinsonism-dementia. *Am J Phys Anthropol.* (1989) 80:107–13. doi: 10.1002/ajpa.1330800112
84. Ioannides ZA, Steyn FJ, Henderson RD, McCombe PA, Ngo ST. Anthropometric measures are not accurate predictors of fat mass in ALS. *Amyotroph Lateral Scler Frontotemporal Degener.* (2017) 18:486–91. doi: 10.1080/21678421.2017.1317811
85. Peter RS, Rosenbohm A, Dupuis L, Brehme T, Kassubek J, Rothenbacher D, et al. Life course body mass index and risk and prognosis of amyotrophic lateral sclerosis: results from the ALS registry Swabia. *Eur J Epidemiol.* (2017) 32:901–8. doi: 10.1007/s10654-017-0318-z
86. Nunes G, Santos CA, Grunho M, Fonseca J. Enteral feeding through endoscopic gastrostomy in amyotrophic lateral sclerosis patients. *Nutr Hosp.* (2016) 33:561. doi: 10.20960/nh.561
87. Jablecki CK, Berry C, Leach J. Survival prediction in amyotrophic lateral sclerosis. *Muscle Nerve.* (1989) 12:833–41. doi: 10.1002/mus.880121008
88. Andres PL, Allred MP, Stephens HE, Proffitt Bunnell M, Siener C, Macklin EA, et al. Fixed dynamometry is more sensitive than vital capacity or ALS rating scale. *Muscle Nerve.* (2017) 56:710–5. doi: 10.1002/mus.25586
89. de Bie E, Oskarsson B, Joyce NC, Nicorici A, Kurillo G, Han JJ. Longitudinal evaluation of upper extremity reachable workspace in ALS by Kinect sensor. *Amyotroph Lateral Scler Frontotemporal Degener.* (2017) 18:17–23. doi: 10.1080/21678421.2016.1241278
90. Shellikeri S, Green JR, Kulkarni M, Rong P, Martino R, Zinman L, et al. Speech movement measures as markers of bulbar disease in amyotrophic lateral sclerosis. *J Speech Lang Hear Res.* (2016) 59:887–99. doi: 10.1044/2016_JSLHR-S-15-0238
91. Londral A, Pinto S, de Carvalho M. Markers for upper limb dysfunction in Amyotrophic Lateral Sclerosis using analysis of typing activity. *Clin Neurophysiol.* (2016) 127:925–31. doi: 10.1016/j.clinph.2015.06.017
92. Panitz S, Kornhuber M, Hanisch F. The checklist individual strength (CIS20-R) in patients with amyotrophic lateral sclerosis - a longitudinal study. *Acta Neurol Scand.* (2015) 131:372–80. doi: 10.1111/ane.12349
93. Atassi N, Berry J, Shui A, Zach N, Sherman A, Sinani E, et al. The PRO-ACT database: design, initial analyses, and predictive features. *Neurology.* (2014) 83:1719–25. doi: 10.1212/WNL.0000000000000951

94. Watanabe H, Atsuta N, Nakamura R, Hirakawa A, Watanabe H, Ito M, et al. Factors affecting longitudinal functional decline and survival in amyotrophic lateral sclerosis patients. *Amyotroph Lateral Scler Frontotemporal Degener.* (2015) 16:230–6. doi: 10.3109/21678421.2014.990036
95. Leonardis L, Dolenc Groselj L, Vidmar G. Factors related to respiration influencing survival and respiratory function in patients with amyotrophic lateral sclerosis: a retrospective study. *Eur J Neurol.* (2012) 19:1518–24. doi: 10.1111/j.1468-1331.2012.03754.x
96. Mahajan KR, Bach JR, Saporito L, Perez N. Diaphragm pacing and noninvasive respiratory management of amyotrophic lateral sclerosis/motor neuron disease. *Muscle Nerve.* (2012) 46:851–5. doi: 10.1002/mus.23663
97. Pinto S, Geraldes R, Vaz N, Pinto A, de Carvalho M. Changes of the phrenic nerve motor response in amyotrophic lateral sclerosis: longitudinal study. *Clin Neurophysiol.* (2009) 120:2082–5. doi: 10.1016/j.clinph.2009.08.025
98. Montes J, Cheng B, Diamond B, Doorish C, Mitsumoto H, Gordon PH. The Timed Up and Go test: predicting falls in ALS. *Amyotroph Lateral Scler.* (2007) 8:292–5. doi: 10.1080/17482960701435931
99. Vender RL, Mauger D, Walsh S, Alam S, Simmons Z. Respiratory systems abnormalities and clinical milestones for patients with amyotrophic lateral sclerosis with emphasis upon survival. *Amyotroph Lateral Scler.* (2007) 8:36–41. doi: 10.1080/17482960600863951
100. Wilson SR, Quantz MA, Strong MJ, Ahmad D. Increasing peak expiratory flow time in amyotrophic lateral sclerosis. *Chest.* (2005) 127:156–60. doi: 10.1378/chest.127.1.156
101. Poloni M, Mento SA, Mascherpa C, Ceroni M. Value of spirometric investigations in amyotrophic lateral sclerosis. *Ital J Neurol Sci.* (1983) 4:39–46. doi: 10.1007/BF02043436
102. Andersen TM, Sandnes A, Fondenes O, Nilsen RM, Tysnes OB, Heimdal JH, et al. Laryngeal responses to mechanically assisted cough in progressing amyotrophic lateral sclerosis. *Respir Care.* (2018) 63:538–49. doi: 10.4187/respcare.05924
103. Quaranta VN, Carratu P, Damiani MF, Dragonieri S, Capozzolo A, Cassano A, et al. The prognostic role of obstructive sleep apnea at the onset of amyotrophic lateral sclerosis. *Neurodegener Dis.* (2017) 17:14–21. doi: 10.1159/000447560
104. Proudfoot M, Menke RA, Sharma R, Berna CM, Hicks SL, Kennard C, et al. Eye-tracking in amyotrophic lateral sclerosis: a longitudinal study of saccadic and cognitive tasks. *Amyotroph Lateral Scler Frontotemporal Degener.* (2015) 17:101–11. doi: 10.3109/21678421.2015.1054292
105. Lenglet T, Lacomblez L, Abitbol JL, Ludolph A, Mora JS, Robberecht W, et al. A phase II-III trial of olesoxime in subjects with amyotrophic lateral sclerosis. *Eur J Neurol.* (2014) 21:529–36. doi: 10.1111/ene.12344
106. Yamauchi R, Imai T, Tsuda E, Hozuki T, Yamamoto D, Shimohama S. Respiratory insufficiency with preserved diaphragmatic function in amyotrophic lateral sclerosis. *Intern Med.* (2014) 53:1325–31. doi: 10.2169/internalmedicine.53.2326
107. Mendoza M, Gelinas DF, Moore DH, Miller RG. A comparison of maximal inspiratory pressure and forced vital capacity as potential criteria for initiating non-invasive ventilation in amyotrophic lateral sclerosis. *Amyotroph Lateral Scler.* (2007) 8:106–11. doi: 10.1080/17482960601030188
108. Marti-Fabregas J, Dourado M, Sanchis J, Miralda R, Pradas J, Illa I. Respiratory function deterioration is not time-linked with upper-limb onset in amyotrophic lateral sclerosis. *Acta Neurol Scand.* (1995) 92:261–4. doi: 10.1111/j.1600-0404.1995.tb01699.x
109. Palmowski A, Jost WH, Prudlo J, Osterhage J, Kasmann B, Schimrigk K, et al. Eye movement in amyotrophic lateral sclerosis: a longitudinal study. *Ger J Ophthalmol.* (1995) 4:355–62.
110. El Mendili MM, Chen R, Tiret B, Villard N, Trunet S, Pelegrini-Issac M, et al. Fast and accurate semi-automated segmentation method of spinal cord MR images at 3T applied to the construction of a cervical spinal cord template. *PLoS ONE.* (2015) 10:e0122224. doi: 10.1371/journal.pone.0122224
111. Cohen-Adad J, El Mendili MM, Morizot-Koutlidis R, Lehericy S, Meininger V, Blancho S, et al. Involvement of spinal sensory pathway in ALS and specificity of cord atrophy to lower motor neuron degeneration. *Amyotroph Lateral Scler Frontotemporal Degener.* (2013) 14:30–8. doi: 10.3109/17482968.2012.701308
112. Bede P, Bokde AL, Byrne S, Elamin M, Fagan AJ, Hardiman O. Spinal cord markers in ALS: diagnostic and biomarker considerations. *Amyotroph Lateral Scler.* (2012) 13:407–15. doi: 10.3109/17482968.2011.649760
113. El Mendili MM, Cohen-Adad J, Pelegrini-Issac M, Rossignol S, Morizot-Koutlidis R, Marchand-Pauvert V, et al. Multi-parametric spinal cord MRI as potential progression marker in amyotrophic lateral sclerosis. *PLoS ONE.* (2014) 9:e95516. doi: 10.1371/journal.pone.0095516
114. Querin G, El Mendili MM, Bede P, Delphine S, Lenglet T, Marchand-Pauvert V, et al. Multimodal spinal cord MRI offers accurate diagnostic classification in ALS. *J Neurol Neurosurg Psychiatry.* (2018) 89:1220–1. doi: 10.1136/jnnp-2017-317214
115. Querin G, El Mendili MM, Lenglet T, Delphine S, Marchand-Pauvert V, Benali H, et al. Spinal cord multi-parametric magnetic resonance imaging for survival prediction in amyotrophic lateral sclerosis. *Eur J Neurol.* (2017) 24:1040–6. doi: 10.1111/ene.13329
116. Grolez G, Moreau C, Danel-Brunaud V, Delmaire C, Lopes R, Pradat PF, et al. The value of magnetic resonance imaging as a biomarker for amyotrophic lateral sclerosis: a systematic review. *BMC Neurol.* (2016) 16:155. doi: 10.1186/s12883-016-0672-6
117. Stroman PW, Wheeler-Kingshott C, Bacon M, Schwab JM, Bosma R, Brooks J, et al. The current state-of-the-art of spinal cord imaging: methods. *NeuroImage.* (2014) 84:1070–81. doi: 10.1016/j.neuroimage.2013.04.124
118. Verma T, Cohen-Adad J. Effect of respiration on the B0 field in the human spinal cord at 3T. *Magn Reson Med.* (2014) 72:1629–36. doi: 10.1002/mrm.25075
119. Finegan E, Chipika RH, Shing SLH, Hardiman O, Bede P. Primary lateral sclerosis: a distinct entity or part of the ALS spectrum? *Amyotroph Lateral Scler Frontotemporal Degener.* 2019:1–13. doi: 10.1080/21678421.2018.1550518
120. Bede P, Querin G, Pradat PF. The changing landscape of motor neuron disease imaging: the transition from descriptive studies to precision clinical tools. *Curr Opin Neurol.* (2018) 31:431–8. doi: 10.1097/WCO.0000000000000569
121. Muller HP, Turner MR, Grosskreutz J, Abrahams S, Bede P, Govind V, et al. A large-scale multicentre cerebral diffusion tensor imaging study in amyotrophic lateral sclerosis. *J Neurol Neurosurg Psychiatry.* (2016) 87:570–9. doi: 10.1136/jnnp-2015-311952
122. Atassi N, Xu M, Triantafyllou C, Keil B, Lawson R, Cernasov P, et al. Ultra high-field (7tesla) magnetic resonance spectroscopy in Amyotrophic Lateral Sclerosis. *PLoS ONE.* (2017) 12:e0177680. doi: 10.1371/journal.pone.0177680
123. Verstraete E, Biessels GJ, van Den Heuvel MP, Visser F, Luijten PR, van Den Berg LH. No evidence of microbleeds in ALS patients at 7 Tesla MRI. *Amyotroph Lateral Scler.* (2010) 11:555–7. doi: 10.3109/17482968.2010.513053
124. Dimond D, Ishaque A, Chenji S, Mah D, Chen Z, Seres P, et al. White matter structural network abnormalities underlie executive dysfunction in amyotrophic lateral sclerosis. *Hum Brain Mapp.* (2017) 38:1249–68. doi: 10.1002/hbm.23452
125. Cardenas AM, Sarlls JE, Kwan JY, Bageac D, Gala ZS, Danielian LE, et al. Pathology of callosal damage in ALS: an *ex-vivo*, 7 T diffusion tensor MRI study. *NeuroImage Clin.* (2017) 15:200–8. doi: 10.1016/j.nicl.2017.04.024
126. De Reuck J, Devos D, Moreau C, Auger F, Durieux N, Deramecourt V, et al. Topographic distribution of brain iron deposition and small cerebrovascular lesions in amyotrophic lateral sclerosis and in frontotemporal lobar degeneration: a post-mortem 7.0-tesla magnetic resonance imaging study with neuropathological correlates. *Acta Neurol Belg.* (2017) 117:873–8. doi: 10.1007/s13760-017-0832-5
127. Pugdahl K, Fuglsang-Frederiksen A, Johnsen B, Tankisi H, de Carvalho M, Fawcett PRW, et al. Variation in the neurophysiological examination of amyotrophic lateral sclerosis in Europe. *Amyotroph Lateral Scler.* (2010) 11:443–8. doi: 10.3109/17482960903552496
128. Cedarbaum JM, Stambler N, Malta E, Fuller C, Hilt D, Thurmond B, et al. The ALSFRS-R: a revised ALS functional rating scale that incorporates assessments of respiratory function. BDNF ALS Study Group (Phase III). *J Neurol Sci.* (1999) 169:13–21.
129. Petrov D, Mansfield C, Moussy A, Hermine O. ALS clinical trials review: 20 Years of failure. Are we any closer to registering a new treatment? *Front Aging Neurosci.* (2017) 9:68. doi: 10.3389/fnagi.2017.00068

130. Jenkinson C, Harris R, Fitzpatrick R. The Amyotrophic Lateral Sclerosis Assessment Questionnaire (ALSAQ-40): evidence for a method of imputing missing data. *Amyotroph Lateral Scler.* (2007) 8:90–5. doi: 10.1080/17482960600989343
131. Aggarwal SP, Zinman L, Simpson E, McKinley J, Jackson KE, Pinto H, et al. Safety and efficacy of lithium in combination with riluzole for treatment of amyotrophic lateral sclerosis: a randomised, double-blind, placebo-controlled trial. *Lancet Neurology.* (2010) 9:481–8. doi: 10.1016/S1474-4422(10)70068-5
132. Smith R, Pioro E, Myers K, Sirdofsky M, Goslin K, Meekins G, et al. Enhanced bulbar function in amyotrophic lateral sclerosis: the nuedexta treatment trial. *Neurotherapeutics.* (2017) 14:762–72. doi: 10.1007/s13311-016-0508-5
133. Woo JH, Wang S, Melhem ER, Gee JC, Cucchiara A, McCluskey L, et al. Linear associations between clinically assessed upper motor neuron disease and diffusion tensor imaging metrics in amyotrophic lateral sclerosis. *PLoS ONE.* (2014) 9:e105753. doi: 10.1371/journal.pone.0105753
134. Cudkowicz ME, Titus S, Kearney M, Yu H, Sherman A, Schoenfeld D, et al. Efficacy and safety of ceftriaxone for amyotrophic lateral sclerosis: results of a multi-stage, randomised, double-blind, placebo-controlled, phase 3 study. *Lancet Neurology.* (2014) 13:1083–91. doi: 10.1016/S1474-4422(14)70222-4
135. Bensimon G, Lacomblez L, Meininger V. A controlled trial of riluzole in amyotrophic lateral sclerosis. ALS/Riluzole Study Group. *N Engl J Med.* (1994) 330:585–91. doi: 10.1056/NEJM199403033300901
136. Kim S, Kim JK, Son MJ, Kim D, Song B, Son I, et al. Mecasin treatment in patients with amyotrophic lateral sclerosis: study protocol for a randomized controlled trial. *Trials.* (2018) 19:225. doi: 10.1186/s13063-018-2557-z
137. Shefner JM, Liu D, Leitner ML, Schoenfeld D, Johns DR, Ferguson T, et al. Quantitative strength testing in ALS clinical trials. *Neurology.* (2016) 87:617–24. doi: 10.1212/WNL.0000000000002941
138. Berry JD, Paganoni S, Atassi N, Macklin EA, Goyal N, Rivner M, et al. Phase IIa trial of fingolimod for amyotrophic lateral sclerosis demonstrates acceptable acute safety and tolerability. *Muscle Nerve.* (2017) 56:1077–84. doi: 10.1002/mus.25733
139. Jawaid A, Murthy SB, Wilson AM, Qureshi SU, Amro MJ, Wheaton M, et al. A decrease in body mass index is associated with faster progression of motor symptoms and shorter survival in ALS. *Amyotroph Lateral Scler.* (2010) 11:542–8. doi: 10.3109/17482968.2010.482592
140. Calvo A, Moglia C, Lunetta C, Marinou K, Ticozzi N, Ferrante GD, et al. Factors predicting survival in ALS: a multicenter Italian study. *J Neurol.* (2017) 264:54–63. doi: 10.1007/s00415-016-8313-y
141. Abrahams S, Newton J, Niven E, Foley J, Bak TH. Screening for cognition and behaviour changes in ALS. *Amyotroph Lateral Scler Frontotemporal Degener.* (2014) 15:9–14. doi: 10.3109/21678421.2013.805784
142. Elamin M, Pinto-Grau M, Burke T, Bede P, Rooney J, O'Sullivan M, et al. Identifying behavioural changes in ALS: validation of the Beaumont Behavioural Inventory (BBI). *Amyotroph Lateral Scler Frontotemporal Degener.* (2016) 8:68–73. doi: 10.1080/21678421.2016.1248976
143. Woolley SC, York MK, Moore DH, Strutt AM, Murphy J, Schulz PE, et al. Detecting frontotemporal dysfunction in ALS: utility of the ALS Cognitive Behavioral Screen (ALS-CBS). *Amyotroph Lateral Scler.* (2010) 11:303–11. doi: 10.3109/17482961003727954
144. Byrne S, Elamin M, Bede P, Shatunov A, Walsh C, Corr B, et al. Cognitive and clinical characteristics of patients with amyotrophic lateral sclerosis carrying a C9orf72 repeat expansion: a population-based cohort study. *Lancet Neurol.* (2012) 11:232–40. doi: 10.1016/S1474-4422(12)70014-5
145. Bede P, Bokde ALW, Byrne S, Elamin M, McLaughlin RL, Kenna K, et al. Multiparametric MRI study of ALS stratified for the C9orf72 genotype. *Neurology.* (2013) 81:361–9. doi: 10.1212/WNL.0b013e31829c5eee
146. Christidi F, Karavasilis E, Rentzos M, Kelekis N, Evdokimidis I, Bede P. Clinical and radiological markers of extra-motor deficits in amyotrophic lateral sclerosis. *Front Neurol.* (2018) 9:1005. doi: 10.3389/fneur.2018.01005
147. Burkhardt C, Neuwirth C, Weber M. Longitudinal assessment of the Edinburgh Cognitive and Behavioural Amyotrophic Lateral Sclerosis Screen (ECAS): lack of practice effect in ALS patients? *Amyotroph Lateral Scler Frontotemporal Degener.* (2017) 18:202–9. doi: 10.1080/21678421.2017.1283418
148. Kasper E, Zydatiss K, Schuster C, Machts J, Bittner D, Kaufmann J, et al. No change in executive performance in ALS patients: a longitudinal neuropsychological study. *Neurodegener Dis.* (2016) 16:184–91. doi: 10.1159/000440957
149. Woolley S, Goetz R, Factor-Litvak P, Murphy J, Hupf J, Lomen-Hoerth C, et al. Longitudinal screening detects cognitive stability and behavioral deterioration in ALS patients. *Behav Neurol.* (2018) 2018:5969137. doi: 10.1155/2018/5969137
150. Okada M, Yamashita S, Ueyama H, Ishizaki M, Maeda Y, Ando Y. Long-term effects of edaravone on survival of patients with amyotrophic lateral sclerosis. *eNeurologicalSci.* (2018) 11:11–4. doi: 10.1016/j.ensci.2018.05.001
151. Raheja R, Regev K, Healy BC, Mazzola MA, Beynon V, Von Glehn F, et al. Correlating serum micrornas and clinical parameters in amyotrophic lateral sclerosis. *Muscle Nerve.* (2018) 58:261–9. doi: 10.1002/mus.26106
152. Thompson AG, Gray E, Thezenas ML, Charles PD, Evetts S, Hu MT, et al. Cerebrospinal fluid macrophage biomarkers in amyotrophic lateral sclerosis. *Ann Neurol.* (2018) 83:258–68. doi: 10.1002/ana.25143
153. Di Pietro L, Baranzini M, Berardinelli MG, Lattanzi W, Monforte M, Tasca G, et al. Potential therapeutic targets for ALS: MIR206, MIR208b and MIR499 are modulated during disease progression in the skeletal muscle of patients. *Sci Rep.* (2017) 7:9538. doi: 10.1038/s41598-017-10161-z
154. Murdock BJ, Zhou T, Kashlan SR, Little RJ, Goutman SA, Feldman EL. Correlation of peripheral immunity with rapid amyotrophic lateral sclerosis progression. *JAMA Neurol.* (2017) 74:1446–54. doi: 10.1001/jamaneurol.2017.2255
155. Shepheard SR, Wuu J, Cardoso M, Wiklendt L, Dinning PG, Chataway T, et al. Urinary p75(ECD): a prognostic, disease progression, and pharmacodynamic biomarker in ALS. *Neurology.* (2017) 88:1137–43. doi: 10.1212/WNL.0000000000003741
156. van Eijk RPA, Eijkemans MJC, Ferguson TA, Nikolakopoulos S, Veldink JH, van den Berg LH. Monitoring disease progression with plasma creatinine in amyotrophic lateral sclerosis clinical trials. *J Neurol Neurosurg Psychiatry.* (2018) 89:156–61. doi: 10.1136/jnnp-2017-317077
157. Waller R, Goodall EF, Milo M, Cooper-Knock J, Da Costa M, Hobson E, et al. Serum miRNAs miR-206, 143-3p and 374b-5p as potential biomarkers for amyotrophic lateral sclerosis (ALS). *Neurobiol Aging.* (2017) 55:123–31. doi: 10.1016/j.neurobiolaging.2017.03.027
158. McCombe PA, Pfluger C, Singh P, Lim CY, Airey C, Henderson RD. Serial measurements of phosphorylated neurofilament-heavy in the serum of subjects with amyotrophic lateral sclerosis. *J Neurol Sci.* (2015) 353:122–9. doi: 10.1016/j.jns.2015.04.032
159. Lu CH, Petzold A, Topping J, Allen K, Macdonald-Wallis C, Clarke J, et al. Plasma neurofilament heavy chain levels and disease progression in amyotrophic lateral sclerosis: insights from a longitudinal study. *J Neurol Neurosurg Psychiatry.* (2015) 86:565–73. doi: 10.1136/jnnp-2014-307672
160. Levine TD, Bowser R, Hank NC, Gately S, Stephan D, Saperstein DS, et al. A pilot trial of pioglitazone HCl and tretinoin in ALS: cerebrospinal fluid biomarkers to monitor drug efficacy and predict rate of disease progression. *Neurol Res Int.* (2012) 2012:582075. doi: 10.1155/2012/582075
161. Levine TD, Bowser R, Hank N, Saperstein D. A pilot trial of memantine and riluzole in ALS: correlation to CSF biomarkers. *Amyotroph Lateral Scler.* (2010) 11:514–9. doi: 10.3109/17482968.2010.513052
162. Wilson ME, Boumaza I, Lacomis D, Bowser R. Cystatin C: a candidate biomarker for amyotrophic lateral sclerosis. *PLoS ONE.* (2010) 5:e15133. doi: 10.1371/journal.pone.0015133
163. Gaiani A, Martinelli I, Bello L, Querin G, Puthenparampil M, Ruggero S, et al. Diagnostic and prognostic biomarkers in amyotrophic lateral sclerosis: neurofilament light chain levels in definite subtypes of disease. *JAMA Neurol.* (2017) 74:525–32. doi: 10.1001/jamaneurol.2016.5398
164. Lu CH, Allen K, Oei F, Leoni E, Kuhle J, Tree T, et al. Systemic inflammatory response and neuromuscular involvement in amyotrophic lateral sclerosis. *Neurol Neuroimmunol Neuroinflamm.* (2016) 3:e244. doi: 10.1212/NXI.0000000000000244
165. Steinacker P, Feneberg E, Weishaupt J, Brettschneider J, Tumani H, Andersen PM, et al. Neurofilaments in the diagnosis of motoneuron diseases: a prospective study on 455 patients. *J Neurol Neurosurg Psychiatry.* (2016) 87:12–20. doi: 10.1136/jnnp-2015-311387

166. Gibson SB, Kasarskis EJ, Hu N, Pulst SM, Mendiondo MS, Matthews DE, et al. Relationship of creatine kinase to body composition, disease state, and longevity in ALS. *Amyotroph Lateral Scler Frontotemporal Degener.* (2015) 16:473–7. doi: 10.3109/21678421.2015.1062516

167. Gray E, Larkin JR, Claridge TD, Talbot K, Sibson NR, Turner MR. The longitudinal cerebrospinal fluid metabolomic profile of amyotrophic lateral sclerosis. *Amyotroph Lateral Scler Frontotemporal Degener.* (2015) 16:456–63. doi: 10.3109/21678421.2015.1053490

168. Lu CH, Macdonald-Wallis C, Gray E, Pearce N, Petzold A, Norgren N, et al. Neurofilament light chain: a prognostic biomarker in amyotrophic lateral sclerosis. *Neurology.* (2015) 84:2247–57. doi: 10.1212/WNL.0000000000001642

169. Verstraete E, Kuiperij HB, van Blitterswijk MM, Veldink JH, Schelhaas HJ, van den Berg LH, et al. TDP-43 plasma levels are higher in amyotrophic lateral sclerosis. *Amyotroph Lateral Scler.* (2012) 13:446–51. doi: 10.3109/17482968.2012.703208

170. Nardo G, Pozzi S, Pignataro M, Lauranzano E, Spano G, Garbelli S, et al. Amyotrophic lateral sclerosis multiprotein biomarkers in peripheral blood mononuclear cells. *PLoS ONE.* (2011) 6:e25545. doi: 10.1371/journal.pone.0025545

171. Steinacker P, Huss A, Mayer B, Grehl T, Grosskreutz J, Borck G, et al. Diagnostic and prognostic significance of neurofilament light chain NF-L, but not progranulin and S100B, in the course of amyotrophic lateral sclerosis: data from the German MND-net. *Amyotroph Lateral Scler Frontotemporal Degener.* (2017) 18:112–9. doi: 10.1080/21678421.2016.1241279

172. Blasco H, Patin F, Descat A, Garcon G, Corcia P, Gele P, et al. A pharmaco-metabolomics approach in a clinical trial of ALS: identification of predictive markers of progression. *PLoS ONE.* (2018) 13:e0198116. doi: 10.1371/journal.pone.0198116

173. Masaldan S, Bush AI, Devos D, Rolland AS, Moreau C. Striking while the iron is hot: iron metabolism and ferroptosis in neurodegeneration. *Free Radic Biol Med.* (2018) 133:221–33. doi: 10.1016/j.freeradbiomed.2018.09.033

174. Van Weemen BK, Schuurs AH. Immunoassay using antigen-enzyme conjugates. *FEBS Lett.* (1971) 15:232–6. doi: 10.1016/0014-5793(71)80319-8

175. Boylan K, Yang C, Crook J, Overstreet K, Heckman M, Wang Y, et al. Immunoreactivity of the phosphorylated axonal neurofilament H subunit (pNF-H) in blood of ALS model rodents and ALS patients: evaluation of blood pNF-H as a potential ALS biomarker. *J Neurochem.* (2009) 111:1182–91. doi: 10.1111/j.1471-4159.2009.06386.x

176. Reijn TS, Abdo WF, Schelhaas HJ, Verbeek MM. CSF neurofilament protein analysis in the differential diagnosis of ALS. *J Neurol.* (2009) 256:615–9. doi: 10.1007/s00415-009-0131-z

177. Strong MJ, Kesavapany S, Pant HC. The pathobiology of amyotrophic lateral sclerosis: a proteinopathy? *J Neuropathol Exp Neurol.* (2005) 64:649–64. doi: 10.1097/01.jnen.0000173889.71434.ea

178. Ranganathan S, Williams E, Ganchev P, Gopalakrishnan V, Lacomis D, Urbinelli L, et al. Proteomic profiling of cerebrospinal fluid identifies biomarkers for amyotrophic lateral sclerosis. *J Neurochem.* (2005) 95:1461–71. doi: 10.1111/j.1471-4159.2005.03478.x

179. Ryberg H, An J, Darko S, Lustgarten JL, Jaffa M, Gopalakrishnan V, et al. Discovery and verification of amyotrophic lateral sclerosis biomarkers by proteomics. *Muscle Nerve.* (2010) 42:104–11. doi: 10.1002/mus.21683

180. Pasinetti GM, Ungar LH, Lange DJ, Yemul S, Deng H, Yuan X, et al. Identification of potential CSF biomarkers in ALS. *Neurology.* (2006) 66:1218. doi: 10.1212/01.wnl.0000203129.82104.07

181. Menke RA, Proudfoot M, Wuu J, Andersen PM, Talbot K, Benatar M, et al. Increased functional connectivity common to symptomatic amyotrophic lateral sclerosis and those at genetic risk. *J Neurol Neurosurg Psychiatry.* (2016) 87:580–8. doi: 10.1136/jnnp-2015-311945

182. Carew JD, Nair G, Andersen PM, Wuu J, Gronka S, Hu X, et al. Presymptomatic spinal cord neurometabolic findings in SOD1-positive people at risk for familial ALS. *Neurology.* (2011) 77:1370–5. doi: 10.1212/WNL.0b013e318231526a

183. Lee SE, Sias AC, Mandelli ML, Brown JA, Brown AB, Khazenzon AM, et al. Network degeneration and dysfunction in presymptomatic C9ORF72 expansion carriers. *NeuroImage Clin.* (2017) 14:286–97. doi: 10.1016/j.nicl.2016.12.006

184. Ng MC, Ho JT, Ho SL, Lee R, Li G, Cheng TS, et al. Abnormal diffusion tensor in nonsymptomatic familial amyotrophic lateral sclerosis with a causative superoxide dismutase 1 mutation. *J Magn Reson Imaging.* (2008) 27:8–13. doi: 10.1002/jmri.21217

185. Wen J, Zhang H, Alexander DC, Durrleman S, Routier A, Rinaldi D, et al. Neurite density is reduced in the presymptomatic phase of C9orf72 disease. *J Neurol Neurosurg Psychiatry.* (2018). doi: 10.1136/jnnp-2018-318994. [Epub ahead of print].

186. Bertrand A, Wen J, Rinaldi D, Houot M, Sayah S, Camuzat A, et al. Early cognitive, structural, and microstructural changes in presymptomatic C9orf72 carriers younger than 40 Years. *JAMA Neurol.* (2018) 75:236–45. doi: 10.1001/jamaneurol.2017.4266

187. Papma JM, Jiskoot LC, Panman JL, Dopper EG, den Heijer T, Donker Kaat L, et al. Cognition and gray and white matter characteristics of presymptomatic C9orf72 repeat expansion. *Neurology.* (2017) 89:1256–64. doi: 10.1212/WNL.0000000000004393

188. Kollewe K, Mauss U, Krampfl K, Petri S, Dengler R, Mohammadi B. ALSFRS-R score and its ratio: a useful predictor for ALS-progression. *J Neurol Sci.* (2008) 275:69–73. doi: 10.1016/j.jns.2008.07.016

189. Rudnicki SA, Berry JD, Ingersoll E, Archibald D, Cudkowicz ME, Kerr DA, et al. Dexpramipexole effects on functional decline and survival in subjects with amyotrophic lateral sclerosis in a Phase II study: subgroup analysis of demographic and clinical characteristics. *Amyotroph Lateral Scler Frontotemporal Degener.* (2013) 14:44–51. doi: 10.3109/17482968.2012.723723

190. Bede P, Iyer PM, Finegan E, Omer T, Hardiman O. Virtual brain biopsies in amyotrophic lateral sclerosis: diagnostic classification based on *in vivo* pathological patterns. *NeuroImage Clin.* (2017) 15:653–8. doi: 10.1016/j.nicl.2017.06.010

191. Bede P, Elamin M, Byrne S, McLaughlin RL, Kenna K, Vajda A, et al. Patterns of cerebral and cerebellar white matter degeneration in ALS. *J Neurol Neurosurg Psychiatry.* (2015) 86:468–70. doi: 10.1136/jnnp-2014-308172

192. Schuster C, Elamin M, Hardiman O, Bede P. The segmental diffusivity profile of amyotrophic lateral sclerosis associated white matter degeneration. *Eur J Neurol.* (2016) 23:1361–71. doi: 10.1111/ene.13038

193. Filippini N, Douaud G, Mackay CE, Knight S, Talbot K, Turner MR. Corpus callosum involvement is a consistent feature of amyotrophic lateral sclerosis. *Neurology.* (2010) 75:1645–52. doi: 10.1212/WNL.0b013e3181fb84d1

194. Bede P, Bokde A, Elamin M, Byrne S, McLaughlin RL, Jordan N, et al. Grey matter correlates of clinical variables in amyotrophic lateral sclerosis (ALS): a neuroimaging study of ALS motor phenotype heterogeneity and cortical focality. *J Neurol Neurosurg Psychiatry.* (2013) 84:766–73. doi: 10.1136/jnnp-2012-302674

195. Christidi F, Karavasilis E, Zalonis I, Ferentinos P, Giavri Z, Wilde EA, et al. Memory-related white matter tract integrity in amyotrophic lateral sclerosis: an advanced neuroimaging and neuropsychological study. *Neurobiol Aging.* (2017) 49:69–78. doi: 10.1016/j.neurobiolaging.2016.09.014

196. Bede P, Elamin M, Byrne S, McLaughlin RL, Kenna K, Vajda A, et al. Basal ganglia involvement in amyotrophic lateral sclerosis. *Neurology.* (2013) 81:2107–15. doi: 10.1212/01.wnl.0000437313.80913.2c

197. Bede P, Omer T, Finegan E, Chipika RH, Iyer PM, Doherty MA, et al. Connectivity-based characterisation of subcortical grey matter pathology in frontotemporal dementia and ALS: a multimodal neuroimaging study. *Brain Imaging Behav.* (2018) 12:1696–707. doi: 10.1007/s11682-018-9837-9

198. Agosta F, Ferraro PM, Riva N, Spinelli EG, Domi T, Carrera P, et al. Structural and functional brain signatures of C9orf72 in motor neuron disease. *Neurobiol Aging.* (2017) 57:206–19. doi: 10.1016/j.neurobiolaging.2017.05.024

199. Bede P, Iyer PM, Schuster C, Elamin M, McLaughlin RL, Kenna K, et al. The selective anatomical vulnerability of ALS: 'disease-defining' and 'disease-defying' brain regions. *Amyotroph Lateral Scler Frontotemporal Degener.* (2016) 17:561–70. doi: 10.3109/21678421.2016.1173702

200. Ravits JM, La Spada AR. ALS motor phenotype heterogeneity, focality, and spread: deconstructing motor neuron degeneration. *Neurology.* (2009) 73:805–11. doi: 10.1212/WNL.0b013e3181b6bbbd

201. Loewe K, Machts J, Kaufmann J, Petri S, Heinze HJ, Borgelt C, et al. Widespread temporo-occipital lobe dysfunction in amyotrophic lateral sclerosis. *Sci Rep.* (2017) 7:40252. doi: 10.1038/srep40252
202. Jenkins TM, Alix JJP, David C, Pearson E, Rao DG, Hoggard N, et al. Imaging muscle as a potential biomarker of denervation in motor neuron disease. *J Neurol Neurosurg Psychiatry.* (2018) 89:248–55. doi: 10.1136/jnnp-2017-316744
203. Jongbloed BA, Haakma W, Goedee HS, Bos JW, Bos C, Hendrikse J, et al. Comparative study of peripheral nerve Mri and ultrasound in multifocal motor neuropathy and amyotrophic lateral sclerosis. *Muscle Nerve.* (2016) 54:1133–5. doi: 10.1002/mus.25391
204. de Carvalho M, Chio A, Dengler R, Hecht M, Weber M, Swash M. Neurophysiological measures in amyotrophic lateral sclerosis: markers of progression in clinical trials. *Amyotroph Lateral Scler.* (2005) 6:17–28. doi: 10.1080/14660820410020600
205. Rutkove SB. Clinical measures of disease progression in amyotrophic lateral sclerosis. *Neurotherapeutics.* (2015) 12:384–93. doi: 10.1007/s13311-014-0331-9
206. Kimura J. *Electrodiagnosis in Diseases of Nerve and Muscle: Principles and Practice.* Oxford: Oxford University Press (2001).
207. Lewelt A, Krosschell KJ, Scott C, Sakonju A, Kissel JT, Crawford TO, et al. Compound muscle action potential and motor function in children with spinal muscular atrophy. *Muscle Nerve.* (2010) 42:703–8. doi: 10.1002/mus.21838
208. Nandedkar SD, Nandedkar DS, Barkhaus PE, Stalberg EV. Motor unit number index (MUNIX). *IEEE Trans Biomed Eng.* (2004) 51:2209–11. doi: 10.1109/TBME.2004.834281
209. McComas AJ, Fawcett PR, Campbell MJ, Sica RE. Electrophysiological estimation of the number of motor units within a human muscle. *J Neurol Neurosurg Psychiatry.* (1971) 34:121–31. doi: 10.1136/jnnp.34.2.121
210. Neuwirth C, Braun N, Claeys KG, Bucelli R, Fournier C, Bromberg M, et al. Implementing Motor Unit Number Index (MUNIX) in a large clinical trial: real world experience from 27 centres. *Clin Neurophysiol.* (2018) 129:1756–62. doi: 10.1016/j.clinph.2018.04.614
211. Fastenau PS, Denburg NL, Mauer BA. Parallel short forms for the Boston Naming Test: psychometric properties and norms for older adults. *J Clin Exp Neuropsychol.* (1998) 20:828–34. doi: 10.1076/jcen.20.6.828.1105
212. Zoccolella S, Beghi E, Palagano G, Fraddosio A, Guerra V, Samarelli V, et al. Analysis of survival and prognostic factors in amyotrophic lateral sclerosis: a population based study. *J Neurol Neurosurg Psychiatry.* (2008) 79:33–7. doi: 10.1136/jnnp.2007.118018
213. Chio A, Logroscino G, Hardiman O, Swingler R, Mitchell D, Beghi E, et al. Prognostic factors in ALS: a critical review. *Amyotroph Lateral Scler.* (2009) 10:310–23. doi: 10.3109/17482960802566824
214. Elamin M, Phukan J, Bede P, Jordan N, Byrne S, Pender N, et al. Executive dysfunction is a negative prognostic indicator in patients with ALS without dementia. *Neurology.* (2011) 76:1263–9. doi: 10.1212/WNL.0b013e318214359f
215. Magnus T, Beck M, Giess R, Puls I, Naumann M, Toyka KV. Disease progression in amyotrophic lateral sclerosis: predictors of survival. *Muscle Nerve.* (2002) 25:709–14. doi: 10.1002/mus.10090
216. Westeneng HJ, Debray TPA, Visser AE, van Eijk RPA, Rooney JPK, Calvo A, et al. Prognosis for patients with amyotrophic lateral sclerosis: development and validation of a personalised prediction model. *Lancet Neurol.* (2018) 7:423–33. doi: 10.1016/S1474-4422(18)30089-9
217. Schuster C, Hardiman O, Bede P. Survival prediction in Amyotrophic lateral sclerosis based on MRI measures and clinical characteristics. *BMC Neurol.* (2017) 17:73. doi: 10.1186/s12883-017-0854-x
218. Capozzo R, Quaranta VN, Pellegrini F, Fontana A, Copetti M, Carratu P, et al. Sniff nasal inspiratory pressure as a prognostic factor of tracheostomy or death in amyotrophic lateral sclerosis. *J Neurol.* (2015) 262:593–603. doi: 10.1007/s00415-014-7613-3
219. Polkey MI, Lyall RA, Yang K, Johnson E, Leigh PN, Moxham J. Respiratory muscle strength as a predictive biomarker for survival in amyotrophic lateral sclerosis. *Am J Respir Crit Care Med.* (2017) 195:86–95. doi: 10.1164/rccm.201604-0848OC
220. Gordon PH, Salachas F, Lacomblez L, Le Forestier N, Pradat PF, Bruneteau G, et al. Predicting survival of patients with amyotrophic lateral sclerosis at presentation: a 15-year experience. *Neurodegener Dis.* (2013) 12:81–90. doi: 10.1159/000341316
221. Kalra S, Vitale A, Cashman NR, Genge A, Arnold DL. Cerebral degeneration predicts survival in amyotrophic lateral sclerosis. *J Neurol Neurosurg Psychiatry.* (2006) 77:1253–5. doi: 10.1136/jnnp.2006.090696
222. Agosta F, Pagani E, Petrolini M, Sormani MP, Caputo D, Perini M, et al. MRI predictors of long-term evolution in amyotrophic lateral sclerosis. *Eur J Neurosci.* (2010) 32:1490–6. doi: 10.1111/j.1460-9568.2010.07445.x
223. Pinto S, Pinto A, de Carvalho M. Phrenic nerve studies predict survival in amyotrophic lateral sclerosis. *Clin Neurophysiol.* (2012) 123:2454–9. doi: 10.1016/j.clinph.2012.05.012
224. Pijnenburg YA, Verwey NA, van der Flier WM, Scheltens P, Teunissen CE. Discriminative and prognostic potential of cerebrospinal fluid phosphoTau/tau ratio and neurofilaments for frontotemporal dementia subtypes. *Alzheimers Dement.* (2015) 1:505–12. doi: 10.1016/j.dadm.2015.11.001
225. Oberstadt M, Classen J, Arendt T, Holzer M. TDP-43 and cytoskeletal proteins in ALS. *Mol Neurobiol.* (2018) 55:3143–51. doi: 10.1007/s12035-017-0543-1
226. Ganesalingam J, An J, Shaw CE, Shaw G, Lacomis D, Bowser R. Combination of neurofilament heavy chain and complement C3 as CSF biomarkers for ALS. *J Neurochem.* (2011) 117:528–37. doi: 10.1111/j.1471-4159.2011.07224.x
227. Paganoni S, Macklin EA, Lee A, Murphy A, Chang J, Zipf A, et al. Diagnostic timelines and delays in diagnosing amyotrophic lateral sclerosis (ALS). *Amyotroph Lateral Scler Frontotemporal Degener.* (2014) 15:453–6. doi: 10.3109/21678421.2014.903974
228. Cudkowicz ME, van den Berg LH, Shefner JM, Mitsumoto H, Mora JS, Ludolph A, et al. Dexpramipexole versus placebo for patients with amyotrophic lateral sclerosis (EMPOWER): a randomised, double-blind, phase 3 trial. *Lancet Neurology.* (2013) 12:1059–67. doi: 10.1016/S1474-4422(13)70221-7
229. Kernan WN, Viscoli CM, Makuch RW, Brass LM, Horwitz RI. Stratified randomization for clinical trials. *J Clin Epidemiol.* (1999) 52:19–26. doi: 10.1016/S0895-4356(98)00138-3
230. Nicholson KA, Cudkowicz ME, Berry JD. Clinical trial designs in amyotrophic lateral sclerosis: does one design fit all? *Neurotherapeutics.* (2015) 12:376–83. doi: 10.1007/s13311-015-0341-2
231. Miller TM, Smith RA, Kordasiewicz H, Kaspar BK. Gene-targeted therapies for the central nervous system. *Arch Neurol.* (2008) 65:447–51. doi: 10.1001/archneur.65.4.nnr70007
232. Lagier-Tourenne C, Baughn M, Rigo F, Sun S, Liu P, Li HR, et al. Targeted degradation of sense and antisense C9orf72 RNA foci as therapy for ALS and frontotemporal degeneration. *Proc Natl Acad Sci USA.* (2013) 110:E4530–9. doi: 10.1073/pnas.1318835110
233. Roche JC, Rojas-Garcia R, Scott KM, Scotton W, Ellis CE, Burman R, et al. A proposed staging system for amyotrophic lateral sclerosis. *Brain.* (2012) 135(Pt 3):847–52. doi: 10.1093/brain/awr351
234. Chio A, Hammond ER, Mora G, Bonito V, Filippini G. Development and evaluation of a clinical staging system for amyotrophic lateral sclerosis. *J Neurol Neurosurg Psychiatry.* (2015) 86:38–44. doi: 10.1136/jnnp-2013-306589
235. Thakore NJ, Lapin BR, Kinzy TG, Pioro EP. Deconstructing progression of amyotrophic lateral sclerosis in stages: a Markov modeling approach. *Amyotroph Lateral Scler Frontotemporal Degener.* (2018) 19:483–494. doi: 10.1080/21678421.2018.1484925
236. Fang T, Al Khleifat A, Stahl DR, Lazo La Torre C, Murphy C, Uk-Mnd Lical S, et al. Comparison of the King's and MiToS staging systems for ALS. *Amyotroph Lateral Scler Frontotemporal Degener.* (2017) 18:227–32. doi: 10.1080/21678421.2016.1265565
237. Tramacere I, Dalla Bella E, Chio A, Mora G, Filippini G, Lauria G. The MITOS system predicts long-term survival in amyotrophic lateral sclerosis. *J Neurol Neurosurg Psychiatry.* (2015) 86:1180–5. doi: 10.1136/jnnp-2014-310176

238. Braak H, Brettschneider J, Ludolph AC, Lee VM, Trojanowski JQ, Del Tredici K. Amyotrophic lateral sclerosis–a model of corticofugal axonal spread. *Nat Rev Neurol.* (2013) 9:708–14. doi: 10.1038/nrneurol.2013.221
239. Brettschneider J, Del Tredici K, Toledo JB, Robinson JL, Irwin DJ, Grossman M, et al. Stages of pTDP-43 pathology in amyotrophic lateral sclerosis. *Ann Neurol.* (2013) 74:20–38. doi: 10.1002/ana.23937
240. Kassubek J, Muller HP, Del Tredici K, Brettschneider J, Pinkhardt EH, Lule D, et al. Diffusion tensor imaging analysis of sequential spreading of disease in amyotrophic lateral sclerosis confirms patterns of TDP-43 pathology. *Brain.* (2014) 137(Pt 6):1733–40. doi: 10.1093/brain/awu090
241. Sherman AV, Gubitz AK, Al-Chalabi A, Bedlack R, Berry J, Conwit R, et al. Infrastructure resources for clinical research in amyotrophic lateral sclerosis. *Amyotroph Lateral Scler Frontotemporal Degener.* (2013) 14(Suppl. 1):53–61. doi: 10.3109/21678421.2013.779058
242. Sherman A, Bowser R, Grasso D, Power B, Milligan C, Jaffa M, et al. Proposed BioRepository platform solution for the ALS research community. *Amyotroph Lateral Scler.* (2011) 12:11–6. doi: 10.3109/17482968.2010.539233
243. Otto M, Bowser R, Turner M, Berry J, Brettschneider J, Connor J, et al. Roadmap and standard operating procedures for biobanking and discovery of neurochemical markers in ALS. *Amyotroph Lateral Scler.* (2012) 13:1–10. doi: 10.3109/17482968.2011.627589
244. Turner MR, Grosskreutz J, Kassubek J, Abrahams S, Agosta F, Benatar M, et al. Towards a neuroimaging biomarker for amyotrophic lateral sclerosis. *Lancet Neurol.* (2011) 10:400–3. doi: 10.1016/S1474-4422(11)70049-7
245. Johnston MV, Adams HP, Fatemi A. *Neurobiology of Disease.* Oxford: Oxford University Press (2016).
246. *Northeast ALS Consortium. NEALS Member Sites.* Available online at: https://www.neals.org/about-us/neals-member-sites/
247. Beghi E. 127th ENMC International Workshop: implementation of a European registry of ALS. Naarden, The Netherlands, 8-10 October 2004. *Neuromuscul Disord.* (2006) 16:46–53. doi: 10.1016/j.nmd.2005.10.004
248. Beghi E, Logroscino G, Chio A, Hardiman O, Mitchell D, Swingler R, et al. The epidemiology of ALS and the role of population-based registries. *Biochim Biophys Acta.* (2006) 1762:1150–7. doi: 10.1016/j.bbadis.2006.09.008
249. Hobson EV, Baird WO, Partridge R, Cooper CL, Mawson S, Quinn A, et al. The TiM system: developing a novel telehealth service to improve access to specialist care in motor neurone disease using user-centered design. *Amyotroph Lateral Scler Frontotemporal Degener.* (2018) 19:351–61. doi: 10.1080/21678421.2018.1440408
250. Geronimo A, Wright C, Morris A, Walsh S, Snyder B, Simmons Z. Incorporation of telehealth into a multidisciplinary ALS Clinic: feasibility and acceptability. *Amyotroph Lateral Scler Frontotemporal Degener.* (2017) 18:555–61. doi: 10.1080/21678421.2017.1338298
251. Christodoulou G, Gennings C, Hupf J, Factor-Litvak P, Murphy J, Goetz RR, et al. Telephone based cognitive-behavioral screening for frontotemporal changes in patients with amyotrophic lateral sclerosis (ALS). *Amyotroph Lateral Scler Frontotemporal Degener.* (2016) 17:482–8. doi: 10.3109/21678421.2016.1173703

14

Ethical Principles in Patient-Centered Medical Care to Support Quality of Life in Amyotrophic Lateral Sclerosis

Dorothée Lulé [1], Andrea Kübler [2] and Albert C. Ludolph [1]*

[1] *Department of Neurology, University of Ulm, Ulm, Germany,*

[2] *Interventional Psychology, Psychology III, University of Würzburg, Würzburg, Germany*

Correspondence:
Dorothée Lulé
dorothee.lule@uni-ulm.de

It is one of the primary goals of medical care to secure good quality of life (QoL) while prolonging survival. This is a major challenge in severe medical conditions with a prognosis such as amyotrophic lateral sclerosis (ALS). Further, the definition of QoL and the question whether survival in this severe condition is compatible with a good QoL is a matter of subjective and culture-specific debate. Some people without neurodegenerative conditions believe that physical decline is incompatible with satisfactory QoL. Current data provide extensive evidence that psychosocial adaptation in ALS is possible, indicated by a satisfactory QoL. Thus, there is no fatalistic link of loss of QoL when physical health declines. There are intrinsic and extrinsic factors that have been shown to successfully facilitate and secure QoL in ALS which will be reviewed in the following article following the four ethical principles (1) Beneficence, (2) Non-maleficence, (3) Autonomy and (4) Justice, which are regarded as key elements of patient centered medical care according to Beauchamp and Childress. This is a JPND-funded work to summarize findings of the project NEEDSinALS (www.NEEDSinALS.com) which highlights subjective perspectives and preferences in medical decision making in ALS.

Keywords: ethics, quality of life (QoL), care, amyotrophic lateral sclerosis (ALS), well-being, depression, coping, psychosocial adaptation

QUALITY OF LIFE IN ALS

Amyotrophic lateral sclerosis (ALS) is among the most devastating neurological conditions: patients lose the ability to speak, to walk and eventually to breathe. On average, patients die within 3 years after symptom onset. If life-sustaining measures such as invasive ventilation are taken, patients may terminate in a locked-in state with a clear mind in a paralyzed body. There is no cure for ALS and care focuses on maintaining functional ability and providing palliative and symptomatic interventions to relieve the burden of symptoms (1). The communication of the diagnosis is a major stressful event for patients, families and caretakers and thus most challenging with regard to medical counseling (2).

There are different ways of how patients cope with these major changes. Quality of life (QoL) is one possible measure of good psychosocial adaptation to disability such as ALS, similarly to depression (3). There have been contradictory reports whether QoL is lost in the course of physical decline (4–6). This discrepancy is partly attributed to selection of patient subgroups (e.g., shortly after diagnosis vs. long-term survivors) and the use of different QoL definitions. QoL is the general well-being of a person and includes physical (individuals' perception of their physical state), psychological (individuals' perception of their cognitive and affective state) and social dimensions (individuals' perception of the interpersonal relationships and social roles in their life). It is therefore not simply a state of physical integrity (7). QoL is increasingly used to supplement objective clinical or biological measures to evaluate health care provision and interventions in research and clinical trials (8).

There is a debate which QoL measure is truly patient centered. Measures are either based on hedonic concepts focusing on subjective factors and emotional evaluation or eudaimonic concepts with more objective factors of QoL such as physical health or economic status (9). As physical health declines in ALS and mobility becomes heavily restricted, these QoL measures provide evidence for low QoL in ALS simply by the nature of the underlying concept. These clinimetric endpoints are increasingly considered overly reductionistic (10) as they include aspects, which are no longer relevant or are out of range of an immobile patient, e.g., physical activity (11); thus, patients often prefer more subjective scales of QoL as these better capture their emotional state of well-being (**Table 1**). They might as well be regarded as possible outcome measures in clinical trials to determine the subjective benefit of a treatment for a patient. Observations concerning hedonic QoL are often counter-intuitive: simultaneous deterioration of physical integrity and well-being does not necessarily occur (19). Accordingly, ALS patients may experience a surprisingly high subjective QoL and an only moderately increased affective state as compared to healthy subjects (6, 20–27) which can be maintained throughout the course of ALS (27–29). This may even be true in the final state of complete immobility, the locked-in state [LIS; (30, 31)].

The lack of association of severity of illness and subjective QoL has been shown for several diseases and is referred to as the "*well-being-paradox*" (32). Prerequisite for this paradox is a process of psychosocial adaptation to the altered circumstances of severe physical function loss. According to the theory of homeostasis in quality of life, everybody has his/her individual level of well-being which he/she aims to reach which is usually in the range of 70–80% of the maximum QoL (33). Provided that sufficient time (29) and intrinsic (e.g., successful coping) and extrinsic resources (e.g., strong family support) are given, patients may show a process of ongoing change and adaptation of their expectations to the actual circumstances [TOTE model; (34)]. The capability of adaptation is not simply a matter of disease state or general personality traits (21). It can be successfully supported by medical teams through patient centered medical care. The different intrinsic and extrinsic factors in medical care to facilitate QoL in ALS and the individualistic perspective in medical decision making have been evaluated within the JPND-funded project NEEDSinALS (www.NEEDSinALS.com). These factors may be subsumed under the four ethical principles of good medical care according to Beauchamp and Childress (35), namely beneficence, non-maleficence, autonomy and justice (**Figure 1**).

Beneficence

This principle requires that everything should be done in the best interest of the patient. Therapeutic interventions are usually introduced by the physician and their interdisciplinary teams to facilitate QoL in ALS. No cure is available yet, but different therapeutic interventions e.g., non-invasive ventilation (NIV) may be means also to prolong survival (36). Previous studies have provided extensive evidence that ALS patients with NIV have an increased QoL (20, 37, 38). Permanent respiratory insufficiency may lead to disturbed sleep, fatigue and reduced physical fitness, all these symptoms may be relieved by ventilation (39). Thus, ventilation may positively impact QoL and patients with ventilation may show even higher QoL than those without (20). Further, nutritional support is a major element of beneficence in ALS as a loss in BMI is a negative prognostic factor (40). Unfortunately, fear of choking during meals is widely prevalent in patients with bulbar symptoms (41), so many patients fear to eat at all. Thus, introduction of a PEG may be a highly useful approach to improve QoL as it allows for weight control while relieving the patient from the pressure to eat. As patients may nevertheless be able to have oral food intake, the pleasure and sensuality of eating can be maintained which additionally supports QoL. However, in some patients the positive effect of PEG insertion might be outbalanced by "particularly strong feelings of loss of control" (41), highlighting the subjective perspective on patient centered care (8). Other therapeutic interventions may as well-facilitate QoL such as application of botox to stop the debilitating syndrome of "drooling" (sialorrhoea). Also, therapies such as physiotherapy, occupational therapy (ergotherapy) and speech therapy (logopedics) may relieve physical symptoms of pain, muscle tension and stiffness which all finally may help to improve QoL (42).

Apart from therapeutics, there is one major extrinsic factor which may substantially improve QoL which is social support (23). Family is the most frequently named aspect of individual QoL in ALS (26, 29, 43). And, as satisfaction with family was often good among patients, the patient's QoL is also often good (44). For healthy subjects, there are other factors which are important for well-being (finances, career) whereas most ALS show a response shift toward social support in the course (20). Thus, inclusion of family members in clinical counseling and supporting the patient in refocusing on social resources may facilitate QoL.

Apart from these extrinsic factors, QoL in serious illness is highly depending on intrinsic factors, such as resilience which is a general characteristics addressing the capacity to recover quickly from difficulties (45). In this context, there has been evidence in ALS that appraisal of coping potential and mental attitudes may be crucial to adapt (23). A re-set of preferences referred to as response shift (46) may support these inner processes with the ability to see what is still there and what is untouched by the disease [e.g., spiritual well-being; (20)]. Further, reframing, the ability to see the same situation from a different perspective [e.g., instead of looking at what you lose, you pay attention to what is spared such as your emotions, feelings and desires; (20)] can be highly supportive for psychosocial adaptation. Finally, many years of research about adapting to and living with chronic diseases suggest that mindfulness in the sense of accepting the circumstances which cannot be changed without judgement and focus on the present (47) may reduce the negative psychological impact of the illness (48, 49).

TABLE 1 | Examples of most widely used measures of subjective, patient-centered QoL.

Abbreviation	Measure	Procedure	Outcome
MEASURES OF GLOBALE SUBJECTIVE QoL			
ACSA (12)	Anamnestic comparative self-assessment	Culturally independent and well-tolerated measure of general QoL; patient is asked to rate his or her current QoL on a scale from −5 to +5. Minus 5 indicates the worst, plus 5 the best ever experienced QoL. It is thus, a rating within each individual's own framework of QoL	ACSA score between −5 to +5
SEIQoL(-DW) (13)	Schedule for the Evaluation of Quality of Life direct weighting	Overall subjective QoL as judged by the patient through a semi-structured interview. The patients have to (1) name the life areas which are important to their QoL, (2) rate the current level of importance of each area and (3) rate the satisfaction with each of the areas	SEIQoL-Index-Score between 0 and 100%
Ganzini QoL (14)	QoL-single-item question	Single-item question to assess patients self-perceived overall QoL with end-points labeled 1 = "my quality of life is as good as it can be" and 6 = "my quality of life is very bad, horrible."	Score between 1 and 6
Krampe QoL (15)	QoL-single-item question	Single-item question to assess patients self-perceived overall QoL with end-points labeled: "Over the past 7 days, the quality of my life has been": very poor (0)–excellent (10).	Score between 0 and 10
ALSSQoL (16)	ALS-Specific Quality of Life Questionnaire	Fifty item disease-specific questionnaire on 6 domains adressing (1) Negative Emotion; (2) Interaction with People and the Environment; (3) Intimacy; (4) Religiosity; (5) Physical Symptoms; (6) Bulbar Function	Average total QOL score, and 6 domain scores
MEASURES OF GLOBALE SUBJECTIVE QoL COMBINED WITH PHYSICAL QoL			
WHOQOL-BREF (17)	Short version of the World Health Organization Quality of Life (WHOQOL)-Group questionnaire	Twenty-six item non-disease specific questionnaire on Physical, Psychological, Social Relations, Environment within cultural context	Domain scores between 0 and 100
MQoL (18)	The McGill Quality of Life Questionnaire	Subjective QoL according to five subscales: physical function, physical well-being, psychological symptoms, existential well-being and social support	MQoL score as mean of 5 subscales between 0 and 10
	Including MQOL single-item scale (SIS)	Single-item Score (SIS) of the MQoL for overall QoL on a visual analog scale	MQoL SIS score between 0 and 10

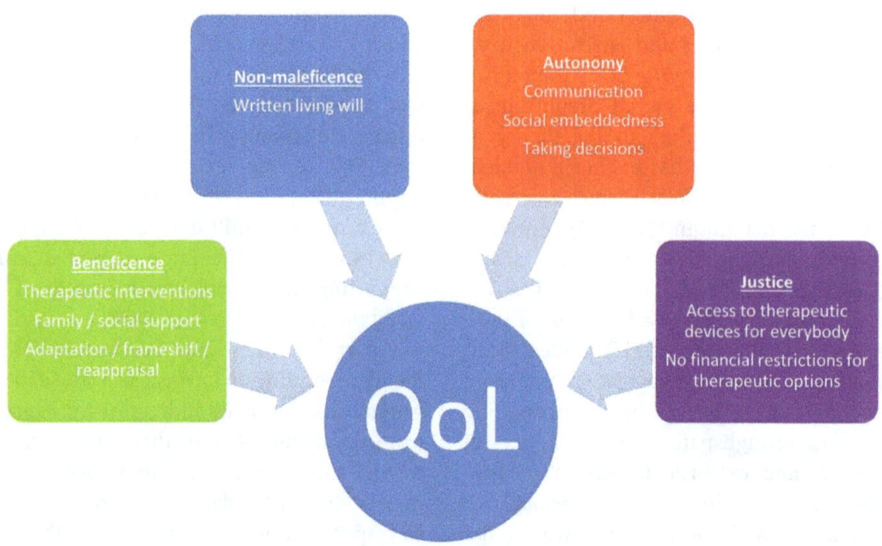

FIGURE 1 | Factors according to medical ethics which facilitate QoL in ALS.

Patients can be encouraged to use these inner resources mentioned above. Psychotherapeutic interventions may help to improve the QoL of patients and may even prolong survival as the psychoemotional state of the patient has impact on QoL (50) and survival time (49). The beneficence of the above mentioned intrinsic factors may as well be addressed in clinical routine by physicians and medical staff to encourage patients to give more room in life for any beneficial intrinsic process.

Beneficence requires the knowledge of the patient's wishes as peer evaluations might not meet the patient's actual needs.

There is evidence for discrepancy between patient's well-being and the perspective on patient's well-being of people without neurodegenerative conditions (27, 29). Peers judgement of patient's well-being is primarily based on personal opinion when they anticipate a low QoL in severely disabled patients. This is true for people without experience in ALS and is even true for caregivers and physicians if they lack experience with ALS (51). Healthy subjects may be blind toward the patient's process of ongoing change and adaptation and instead they may conclude from their personal perspective. The more experienced healthcare professionals are, the more they know about the capacity to adjust and are thus abled to correctly anticipate patient's quality of life, affective state, and wish for hastened death (51).

Thus, the knowledge of and believe in beneficence in ALS is a matter of the physician's experience. As many patients gradually adjust to their situation and also possibly change their therapeutic preferences in the course of the disease (52), beneficence from the patient's perspective is a dynamic construct which needs to be recognized and may be supported by caretakers and medical care teams.

Non-maleficence

Primum non-nocere, refrain from harm is the other side of the coin of beneficence and thus, similar aspects concern maleficence than beneficence. Non-maleficence needs to be considered the moment the diagnosis is communicated. "Breaking the news" is a highly delicate balance between patient's need to be informed which requires veracity and fidelity on the one hand and the right for denial on the other hand which can be a helpful strategy at least shortly after diagnosis (23). Maleficence in the sense of the emotional burden of diagnosis can be reduced by using a thorough approach for breaking the news as it may attenuate negative impact on QoL (53). But also providing sufficient information can prevent maleficence: patients with sudden respiratory insufficiency in an emergency situation who have been informed on all aspects of respiratory support may feel more competent to take the right decision (41).

Advance directives and living wills are crucial to prevent maleficence, e.g., insertion of a tracheostomy in an emergency if the patient does not want to [possibly because he/she is afraid of the burden for others; (52)]. Many therapeutic options secure QoL (e.g., ventilation) but most patients are unable to anticipate this shortly after diagnosis. During the course of ALS, some might dismiss the idea of maleficence of invasive ventilation and might realize the beneficial effect of this therapeutic treatment (29). Therefore, dynamic adjustment to living wills is a key aspect to prevent maleficence.

Preferences regarding therapeutic measures are highly determined by patient's personal values, religious beliefs and cultural background (54).

Cultural differences exist: in Japan, invasive ventilation is more regarded as routine therapeutic treatment than in other countries [33% in Japan; (55)]. In some countries, life prolongation might be regarded as maleficence and more life-shortening treatments are suggested (56). Thus, social context may define what is beneficence and maleficence in the context of cultural norms (54, 57).

Patient's Autonomy

Patient's sense of autonomy is a key issue of quality of life and goes beyond being physically autonomous to perform an action. Autonomy also encompasses the sense of capability to take decisions and the feeling of being an author of one's own action which is a key feature of self-efficacy and thus for QoL (58). Taking decisions also sustains the feeling of social embeddedness disregarding physical disability, e.g., the patient can be included in family decisions and may participate in daily routine if possible (59). This allows the patient to be an active part of daily routine: to participate in decision making, to be asked questions, to express concerns, address fears and anxieties, express wishes, values, desires, and hopes. It is noteworthy that possible minor cognitive deficits in some patients do not interfere with the competency to decide and participate (60).

It is especially challenging to secure patient's autonomy in LIS as there is lack of direct means to communicate in this state. Assisted communication (20, 29) becomes important for individual QoL in the course of ALS, but is not mentioned by patients in early stages of the disease (20). Many patients use letter board for communication which requires considerable effort from a second person to record which item the patient selected from the board. Technical devices may allow for communication but these are time consuming and strenuous to use and also additional assistance is required (59). Thus, knowledge on patient's wishes, desires and thoughts in advanced stages is sparse and there is substantial lack of understanding which factors may impact the dynamics of QoL and affective state in the course of ALS (30). Communication via eye-gaze control is possible, including standardized interviews (61, 62) but the latter are rarely performed. Brain Computer Interfaces (BCI) are promising technologies for communication and interaction (63, 64) but in a subgroup of patients only (65). Other means of BCI-use such as unrestricted access to web browsers of which some are adaptable to home based BCI systems (66) secure new degrees of freedom in severe paralysis (67–70). Some patients already use these techniques in their home environment for communication and painting (71–76) and first evidence support the notion that these techniques positively impact QoL (71, 77). In the future, with major advances in communication technology well-being in ALS might possibly be facilitated. BCIs might also be indirectly used in evaluation and recognition of well-being and emotional state in highly advanced patients (78) such as the amplitude of the N400, a negative deflection of the EEG curve following a meaningful event (79), which was higher in patients with high QoL compared to those with a poor. Thus, the N400 may serve as an objective physiological indicator of individual QoL in non-responsive ALS patients (80). Overall, there is still a long way to go until BCI will be a standard tool for home care for a majority of ALS patients (63, 81). But for patient-centered care, compensation for progressive loss of

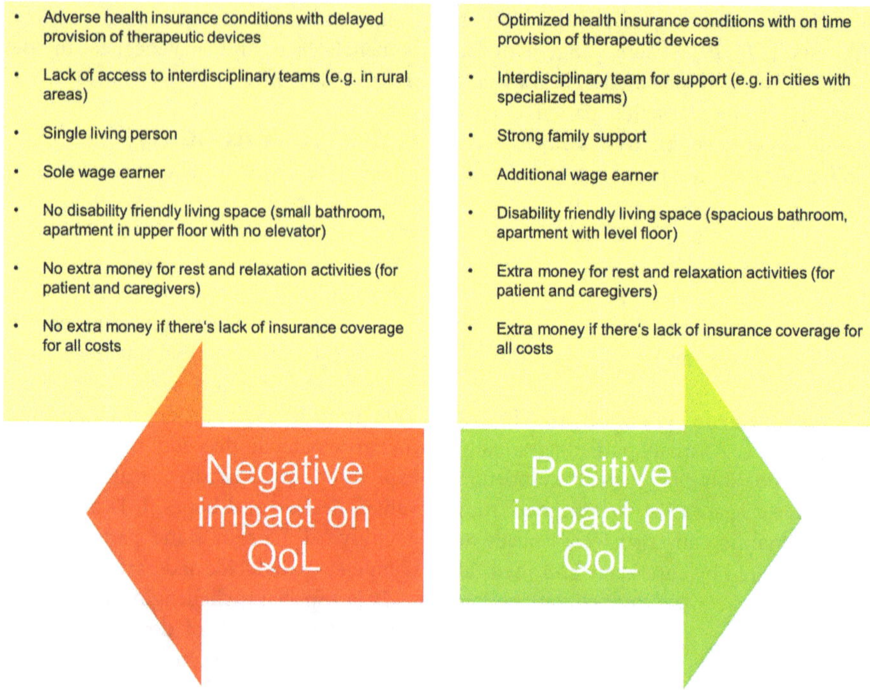

FIGURE 2 | Examples of setting differences which may interfere with justice in medical care despite optimized care provision by the medical team.

verbal speech is mandatory to secure patient's autonomy and QoL (52).

Justice

This ethical principle of care requires that all patients are treated in an equal way without prejudice or social discrimination.. In the sense of justice, patients in similar situations should have access to the same care options. Palliative care intervention improves quality of life in patients and caregivers (82) and medical care may facilitate this positive dynamics by offering this care to every patient. ALS patients expect dignified care (82) but instead, patients are often dissatisfied with health care services (83). Every patient needs to be treated differently according to the actual preferences and needs (54). There is no justice in defining every person by the diagnosis with a nihilistic view of the disease which has to be prevented under all circumstances (48). Instead, to grant justice every patient has to be regarded as an individual with specific needs and the right to be treated the same according to his/her preferences, disregarding mental, societal or financial status.

Further, providing sufficient information according to the patient's needs as outlined above is also a matter of justice. Thus, granting the patient the right for information is similarly a matter of justice as granting the right for not-knowing. In this sense, it is a matter of justice to grant patient's will even if it interferes with the physician's personal and professional opinion.

Finally, justice in medical care is secured in many countries as most healthcare systems secure this kind of justice by providing coverage of (most) costs. Despite that most medical systems are based on a solidary idea allowing for justice, the impact of the disease may vary between patients thus justice in clinical care is not easy to accomplish. There are basic settings which significantly hamper justice in care provision which cannot be changed by the medical team, e.g., there is variance of the paid costs by the insurance companies. Further, in some instances, only basic technical equipment is provided which possibly don't meet the patient's actual needs. Thus, patients have to cover the extra charges for the devices which fully meet their needs. And finally, there are personal settings (e.g., living and working conditions) which may heavily impact patient's life with ALS and which interfere with the principle of justice (**Figure 2**).

CONSEQUENCES AND FUTURE DIRECTIONS

There is evidence that considerate medical care within multidisciplinary teams (84) helps patients to find their own way of coping with the disease to gain or maintain a satisfactory QoL (48). Living with a fatal disease creates a crisis loaded environment and adapting to the disease is a psychological process rendering mandatory a strong support from these specialists' teams (41). Following the ethical principles of medical care as outlined in this text allows for a holistic support of the patient to secure QoL.

AUTHOR CONTRIBUTIONS

DL, AK, and AL have collected data underlying this review and discussion of data. Text writing was done by DL, thorough revision of the manuscript was performed by all authors.

ACKNOWLEDGMENTS

We thank all the patients and families for supporting our research. This is an EU Joint Programme–Neurodegenerative Disease Research (JPND) project. The project is supported through the following organizations under the aegis of JPND—www.jpnd.eu, e.g., Germany, Bundesministerium für Bildung und Forschung (BMBF, FKZ), Sweden, Vetenskapr å det Sverige, and Poland, Narodowe Centrum Badań i Rozwoju (NCBR). This work was supported by the Deutsche Forschungsgemeinschaft and the Bundesministerium für Bildung und Forschung (BMBF #01GM1103A, MND-Net).

REFERENCES

1. Andersen PM, Abrahams S, Borasio GD, de Carvalho M, Chio A, Van Damme P, et al. EFNS Task force on diagnosis and management of amyotrophic lateral sclerosis: EFNS guidelines on the clinical management of amyotrophic lateral sclerosis (MALS)–revised report of an EFNS task force. *Eur J Neurol.* (2012) 19:360–75. doi: 10.1111/j.1468-1331.2011.03501.x
2. McLeod JE, Clarke DM. A review of psychosocial aspects of motor neurone disease. *J Neurol Sci.* (2007) 258:4–10. doi: 10.1016/j.jns.2007.03.001
3. Livneh H. Psychosocial adaptation to chronic illness and disability: A conceptual framework. *Rehabil Counsel Bull.* (2001) 44:151. doi: 10.1177/003435520104400305
4. Kübler A, Winter S, Ludolph AC, Hautzinger M, Birbaumer N. Severity of depressive symptoms and quality of life in patients with amyotrophic lateral sclerosis. *Neurorehabil Neural Repair.* (2005) 19:182–93. doi: 10.1177/1545968305276583
5. Körner S, Kollewe K, Abdulla S, Zapf A, Dengler R, Petri S. Interaction of physical function, quality of life and depression in Amyotrophic lateral sclerosis: characterization of a large patient cohort. *BMC Neurol.* (2015) 15:84. doi: 10.1186/s12883-015-0340-2
6. Simmons Z, Bremer BA, Robbins RA, Walsh SM, Fischer S. Quality of life in ALS depends on factors other than strength and physical function. *Neurology.* (2000) 55:388–92. doi: 10.1212/WNL.55.3.388
7. World Health Organization. The World Health Organization Quality of Life assessment (WHOQOL): position paper from the World Health Organization. *Soc Sci Med.* (1995). 41:1403–9.
8. Carr AJ, Higginson IJ. Are quality of life measures patient centred? *BMJ.* (2001) 322:1357–60. doi: 10.1136/bmj.322.7298.1357
9. Simmons Z. Patient-perceived outcomes and quality of life in ALS. *Neurotherapeutics.* (2015) 12:394–402. doi: 10.1007/s13311-014-0322-x
10. Bernheim J. How to get serious answers to the serious question: "How have you been?": subjective quality of life (QOL) as an individual experiential emergent construct. *Bioethics.* (1999) 13:272–87. doi: 10.1111/1467-8519.00156
11. Neudert C, Wasner M, Borasio GD. Patients' assessment of quality of life instruments: a randomised study of SIP, SF-36 and SEIQoL-DW in patients with amyotrophic lateral sclerosis. *J Neurol Sci.* (2001) 191:103–9. doi: 10.1016/S0022-510X(01)00612-8
12. Bernheim JL, Buyse M. The anamnestic comparative self assessment for measuring the subjective quality of life of cancer patients. *J Psychosoc Oncol.* (1984) 1:25–38. doi: 10.1300/J077v01n04_03
13. O'Boyle C, McGee HM, Hickey A, Joyce C, Browne J, O'Malley K, et al. *The Schedule for the Evaluation of Individual Quality of Life (SEIQoL): Administration Manual.* Dublin: Department of Psychology Royal College of Surgeons in Ireland (1993).
14. Ganzini L, Johnston WS, Hoffman WF. Correlates of suffering in amyotrophic lateral sclerosis. *Neurology.* (1999) 52:1434–40. doi: 10.1212/WNL.52.7.1434
15. Krampe H, Bartels C, Victorson D, Enders CK, Beaumont J, Cella D, et al. The influence of personality factors on disease progression and healthrelated quality of life in people with ALS. *Amyotroph Lateral Scler.* (2008) 9:99–107. doi: 10.1080/17482960701875805
16. Simmons Z, Felgoise SH, Bremer BA, Walsh SM, Hufford DJ, Bromberg MB, et al. The ALSSQOL: balancing physical and nonphysical factors in assessing quality of life in ALS. *Neurology.* (2006) 67:1659–64. doi: 10.1212/01.wnl.0000242887.79115.19
17. WHOQOL Group. The World Health Organization quality of life assessment (WHOQOL): development and general psychometric properties. *Soc Sci Med.* (1998) 46:1569–85. doi: 10.1016/S0277-9536(98)00009-4
18. Cohen SR, Mount BM, Strobel MG, Bui F. The McGill quality of life questionnaire: a measure of quality of life appropriate for people with advanced disease. A preliminary study of validity and acceptability. *Palliat Med.* (1995) 9:207–19. doi: 10.1177/026921639500900306
19. Joyce CR, Hickey A, McGee HM, O'Boyle CA. A theory-based method for the evaluation of individual quality of life: the SEIQoL. *Qual Life Res.* (2003) 12:275–80. doi: 10.1023/A:1023273117040
20. Lulé D, Häcker S, Ludolph A, Birbaumer N, Kübler A. Depression and quality of life in patients with amyotrophic lateral sclerosis. *Dtsch Arztebl Int.* (2008) 105:397–403. doi: 10.3238/arztebl.2008.0397
21. Lulé D, Pauli S, Altintas E, Singer U, Merk T, Uttner I, et al. Emotional adjustment in amyotrophic lateral sclerosis (ALS). *J Neurol.* (2012). 259:334–41. doi: 10.1007/s00415-011-6191-x
22. Chiò A, Gauthier A, Montuschi A, Calvo A, Di Vito N, Ghiglione P, et al. A cross sectional study on determinants of quality of life in ALS. *J Neurol Neurosurg Psychiatry.* (2004) 75:1597–601. doi: 10.1136/jnnp.2003.033100
23. Matuz T, Birbaumer N, Hautzinger M, Kübler A. Coping with amyotrophic lateral sclerosis: an integrative view. *J Neurol Neurosurg Psychiatry.* (2010) 81:893–8. doi: 10.1136/jnnp.2009.201285
24. Cupp J, Simmons Z, Berg A, Felgoise SH, Walsh SM, Stephens HE. Psychological health in patients with ALS is maintained as physical function declines. *Amyotroph Lateral Scler.* (2011) 12:290–6. doi: 10.3109/17482968.2011.554555
25. Hardiman O, Hickey A, O'Donerty LJ. Physical decline and quality of life in amyotrophic lateral sclerosis. *Amyotroph Lateral Scler Other Motor Neuron Disord.* (2004) 5:230–4. doi: 10.1080/226-14660820410021294
26. Neudert C, Wasner M, Borasio GD. Individual quality of life is not correlated with health-related quality of life or physical function in patients with amyotrophic lateral sclerosis. *J Palliat Med.* (2004) 7:551–7 doi: 10.1089/jpm.2004.7.551
27. Grehl T, Rupp M, Budde P, Tegenthoff M, Fangerau H. Depression and QOL in patients with ALS: how do self-ratings and ratings by relatives differ? *Qual Life Res.* (2011) 20:569–74. doi: 10.1007/s11136-010-9781-7
28. Matuz T, Birbaumer N, Hautzinger M, Kübler A. Psychosocial adjustment to ALS: a longitudinal study. *Front Psychol.* (2015) 6:1197. doi: 10.3389/fpsyg.2015.01197
29. Lulé D, Ehlich B, Lang D, Sorg S, Heimrath J, Kübler A, et al. Quality of life in fatal disease: the flawed judgement of the social environment. *J Neurol.* (2013) 260:2836–43. doi: 10.1007/s00415-013-7068-y
30. Linse K, Rüger W, Joos M, Schmitz-Peiffer H, Storch A, Hermann A. Eye-tracking-based assessment suggests preserved well-being in locked-in patients. *Ann Neurol.* (2017) 81:310–5. doi: 10.1002/ana.24871
31. Lulé D, Zickler C, Häcker S, Bruno MA, Demertzi A, Pellas F, et al. Life can be worth living in locked-in syndrome. *Prog Brain Res.* (2009) 177:339–51. doi: 10.1016/S0079-6123(09)17723-3

32. Herschbach P. The well-being paradox in quality-of-life research - on what does our sense of well-being depend? *Psychother Psych Med.* (2002) 52:141–50. doi: 10.1055/s-2002-24953
33. Cummins RA. Subjective Wellbeing, Homeostatically protected mood and depression: a synthesis. *Journal of Happiness Studies.* (2010) 11:1–17. doi: 10.1007/s10902-009-9167-0
34. Miller GA, Galanter E, Pribram KA. *Plans and the Structure of Behavior.* New York, NY: Holt, Rhinehart, & Winston (1960).
35. Beauchamp TL, Childress JF. *Principles of Biomedical Ethics.* 6th ed. Oxford: Oxford University Press (2008).
36. Bourke SC, Bullock RE, Williams TL, Shaw PJ, Gibson GJ. Noninvasive ventilation in ALS: indications and effect on quality of life. *Neurology.* (2003) 61:171–7. doi: 10.1212/01.WNL.0000076182.13137.38
37. Kaub-Wittemer D, Steinbüchel NV, Wasner M, Laier-Groeneveld G, Borasio GD. Quality of life and psychosocial issues in ventilated patients with amyotrophic lateral sclerosis and their caregivers. *J Pain Symptom Manage.* (2003) 26:890–6. doi: 10.1016/S0885-3924(03)00323-3
38. Piepers S, van den Berg JP, Kalmijn S, van der Pol WL, Wokke JH, Lindeman E, et al. Effect of non-invasive ventilation on survival, quality of life, respiratory function and cognition: a review of the literature. *Amyotroph Lateral Scler.* (2006) 7:195–200. doi: 10.1080/14660820500514974
39. Bourke SC, Tomlinson M, Williams TL, Bullock RE, Shaw PJ, Gibson GJ. Effects of non-invasive ventilation on survival and quality of life in patients with amyotrophic lateral sclerosis: a randomised controlled trial. *Lancet Neurol.* 2006 5:140–7. doi: 10.1016/S1474-4422(05)70326-4
40. Peter RS, Rosenbohm A, Dupuis L, Brehme T, Kassubek J, Rothenbacher D, et al. Life course body mass index and risk and prognosis of amyotrophic lateral sclerosis: results from the ALS registry Swabia. *Eur J Epidemiol.* (2017) 32:901–8. doi: 10.1007/s10654-017-0318-z
41. Oliver DJ, Turner MR. Some difficult decisions in ALS/MND. *Amyotroph Lateral Scler.* (2010) 11:339–43. doi: 10.3109/17482968.2010.487532
42. van Groenestijn AC, van de Port IG, Schröder CD, Post MW, Grupstra HF, Kruitwagen ET, et al. Effects of aerobic exercise therapy and cognitive behavioural therapy on functioning and quality of life in amyotrophic lateral sclerosis: protocol of the FACTS-2-ALS trial. *BMC Neurol.* (2011) 11:70. doi: 10.1186/1471-2377-11-70
43. Felgoise SH, Stewart JL, Bremer BA, Walsh SM, Bromberg MB, Simmons Z. The SEIQoL-DW for assessing quality of life in ALS: strengths and limitations. *Amyotroph Lateral Scler.* (2009) 10:456–62. doi: 10.3109/17482960802444840
44. Olsson AG, Markhede I, Strang S, Persson LI. Differences in quality of life modalities give rise to needs of individual support in patients with ALS and their next of kin. *Palliat Support Care.* (2010) 8:75–82. doi: 10.1017/S1478951509990733
45. Rabkin JG, Wagner GJ, Del Bene M. Resilience and distress among amyotrophic lateral sclerosis patients and caregivers. *Psychosom Med.* (2000) 62:271–9. doi: 10.1097/00006842-200003000-00020
46. Schwartz CE. Applications of response shift theory and methods to participation measurement: a brief history of a young field. *Arch Phys Med Rehabil.* (2010) 91:38–43. doi: 10.1016/j.apmr.2009.11.029
47. Langer E. *Mindfulness.* Reading, MA:Addison-Wesley (1989).
48. Pagnini F, Phillips D, Langer E. A mindful approach with end-of-life thoughts. *Front Psychol.* 5:138. doi: 10.3389/fpsyg.2014.00138
49. Pagnini F, Phillips D, Bosma CM, Reece A, Langer E. Mindfulness, physical impairment and psychological well-being in people with amyotrophic lateral sclerosis. *Psychol Health.* (2015) 30:503–17. doi: 10.1080/08870446.2014.982652
50. van Groenestijn AC, Schröder CD, Visser-Meily JM, Reenen ET, Veldink JH, van den Berg LH. Cognitive behavioural therapy and quality of life in psychologically distressed patients with amyotrophic lateral sclerosis and their caregivers: results of a prematurely stopped randomized controlled trial. *Amyotroph Lateral Scler Frontotemporal Degener.* (2015) 16:309–15. doi: 10.3109/21678421.2015.1038276
51. Aho-Özhan HE, Böhm S, Keller J, Dorst J, Uttner I, Ludolph AC, et al. Experience matters: neurologists' perspectives on ALS patients' well-being. *J Neurol.* (2017) 264:639–46. doi: 10.1007/s00415-016-8382-y
52. Lulé D, Nonnenmacher S, Sorg S, Heimrath J, Hautzinger M, Meyer T, et al. Live and let die: existential decision processes in a fatal disease. *J Neurol.* (2014) 261:518–25. doi: 10.1007/s00415-013-7229-z
53. Creemers H, de Morée S, Veldink JH, Nollet F, van den Berg LH, Beelen A. Factors related to caregiver strain in ALS: a longitudinal study. *J Neurol Neurosurg Psychiatry.* (2016). 87:775–81. doi: 10.1136/jnnp-2015-311651
54. Andersen PM, Kuzma-Kozakiewicz M, Keller J, Aho-Oezhan HEA, Ciecwierska K, Szejko N, et al. Therapeutic decisions in ALS patients: cross-cultural differences and clinical implications. *J Neurol.* (2018) 265:1600–06. doi: 10.1007/s00415-018-8861-4
55. Tagami M, Kimura F, Nakajima H, Ishida S, Fujiwara S, Doi Y, et al. Tracheostomy and invasive ventilation in Japanese ALS patients: decision-making and survival analysis: 1990-2010. *J Neurol Sci.* (2014) 344:158–64. doi: 10.1016/j.jns.2014.06.047
56. Veldink JH, Wokke JH, van der Wal G, Vianney de Jong JM, van den Berg LH. Euthanasia and physician-assisted suicide among patients with amyotrophic lateral sclerosis in the Netherlands. *N Engl J Med.* (2002) 346:1638–44. doi: 10.1056/NEJMsa012739
57. Christodoulou G, Goetz R, Ogino M, Mitsumoto H, Rabkin J. Opinions of Japanese and American ALS caregivers regarding tracheostomy with invasive ventilation (TIV). *Amyotroph Lateral Scler Frontotemporal Degener.* (2015) 17:47–54. doi: 10.3109/21678421.2015.1069850
58. Galin S, Heruti I, Barak N, Gotkine M. Hope and self-efficacy are associated with better satisfaction with life in people with ALS. *Amyotroph Lateral Scler Frontotemporal Degener.* (2018) 2018:1–8. doi: 10.1080/21678421.2018.1476546
59. Linse K, Rüger W, Joos M, Schmitz-Peiffer H, Storch A, Hermann A. Usability of eyetracking computer systems and impact on psychological wellbeing in patients with advanced amyotrophic lateral sclerosis. *Amyotroph Lateral Scler Frontotemporal Degener.* (2018) 19:212–9. doi: 10.1080/21678421.2017.1392576
60. Böhm S, Aho-Özhan HE, Keller J, Dorst J, Uttner I, Ludolph AC, et al. Medical decisions are independent of cognitive impairment in amyotrophic lateral sclerosis. *Neurology.* (2016) 87:1737–8. doi: 10.1212/WNL.0000000000003232
61. Keller J, Gorges M, Horn HT, Aho-Özhan HE, Pinkhardt EH, Uttner I, et al. Eye-tracking controlled cognitive function tests in patients with amyotrophic lateral sclerosis: a controlled proof-of-principle study. *J Neurol.* (2015) 262:1918–26. doi: 10.1007/s00415-015-7795-3
62. Lakerveld J, Kotchoubey B, Kübler A. Cognitive function in patients with late stage amyotrophic lateral sclerosis. *J Neurol Neurosurg Psychiatry.* (2008) 79:25–9. doi: 10.1136/jnnp.2007.116178
63. Kübler A, Holz EM, Riccio A, Zickler C, Kaufmann T, Kleih SC, et al. The user-centered design as novel perspective for evaluating the usability of BCI-controlled applications. *PLoS ONE.* (2014) 9:e112392. doi: 10.1371/journal.pone.0112392
64. Lulé D, Hörner K, Vazquez C, Aho-Özhan H, Keller J, Gorges M, et al. Screening for cognitive function in complete immobility using brain-machine interfaces: a proof of principle study. *Front Neurosci.* (2018) 12:517. doi: 10.3389/fnins.2018.00517
65. Mochizuki Y, Hayashi K, Nakayama Y, Shimizu T, Kamide M, Ogino M, et al. ALS patients with ability to communicate after long-term mechanical ventilation have confined degeneration to the motor neuron system. *J Neurol Sci.* (2016) 363:245–8. doi: 10.1016/j.jns.2016.02.068
66. Miralles F, Vargiu E, Dauwalder S, Solà M, Müller-Putz G, Wriessnegger SC, et al. Brain computer interface on track to home. *Scientif World J.* (2015) 2015:623896. doi: 10.1155/2015/623896
67. Mugler EM, Ruf CA, Halder S, Bensch M, Kubler A. Design and implementation of a P300-based brain-computer interface for controlling an internet browser. *IEEE Trans Neural Syst Rehabil Eng.* (2010) 18:599–609. doi: 10.1109/TNSRE.2010.2068059
68. Pinegger A, Deckert L, Halder S, Barry N, Faller J, Käthner I, et al. Write, read and answer emails with a dry 'n' wireless brain-computer interface system. *Conf Proc IEEE Eng Med Biol Soc.* (2014) 2014:1286–9. doi: 10.1109/EMBC.2014.6943833
69. Millán JD, Rupp R, Müller-Putz GR, Murray-Smith R, Giugliemma C, Tangermann M, et al. Combining brain-computer interfaces and assistive technologies: state-of-the-art and challenges. *Front Neurosci.* (2010) 4:161. doi: 10.3389/fnins.2010.00161
70. Blankertz B, Tangermann M, Vidaurre C, Fazli S, Sannelli C, Haufe S, et al. The Berlin brain-computer interface: non-medical uses of BCI technology. *Front Neurosci.* (2010) 4:198. doi: 10.3389/fnins.2010.00198

71. Holz EM, Botrel L, Kaufmann T, Kübler A. Long-term independent brain-computer interface home use improves quality of life of a patient in the locked-in state: a case study. *Arch Phys Med Rehabil.* (2015) 96:16–26. doi: 10.1016/j.apmr.2014.03.035
72. Holz EM, Botrel L, Kübler A. Independent home use of Brain Painting improves quality of life of two artists in the locked-in state diagnosed with amyotrophic lateral sclerosis. *Brain Comput Interfaces.* (2015) 2:117–34. doi: 10.1080/2326263X.2015.1100048
73. Botrel L, Holz EM, Kübler A. Brain Painting V2: evaluation of P300-based brain-computer interface for creative expression by an end-user following the user-centered design. *Brain Comput Interfaces.* (2015) 2:135–49. doi: 10.1080/2326263X.2015.1100038
74. Sellers EW, Vaughan TM, Wolpaw JR. A brain-computer interface for long-term independent home use. *Amyotroph Lateral Scler.* (2010) 11:449–55. doi: 10.3109/17482961003777470
75. Münßinger JI, Halder S, Kleih SC, Furdea A, Raco V, Hösle A, et al. Brain painting: first evaluation of a new brain-computer interface application with ALS-patients and healthy volunteers. *Front Neurosci.* (2010). 4:182. doi: 10.3389/fnins.2010.00182
76. Kübler A, Mattia D, Rupp R, Tangermann M. Facing the challenge: bringing brain-computer interfaces to end-users. *Artif Intell Med.* (2013) 59:55–60. doi: 10.1016/j.artmed.2013.08.002
77. Mora JS, Salas T, Fajardo ML, Iváñez L, Rodríguez-Santos F. Self perceived emotional functioning of spanish patients with amyotrophic lateral sclerosis: a longitudinal study. *Front Psychol.* (2013) 3:609. doi: 10.3389/fpsyg.2012.00609
78. Kashihara K. A brain-computer interface for potential non-verbal facial communication based on EEG signals related to specific emotions. *Front Neurosci.* (2014) 8:244. doi: 10.3389/fnins.2014.00244
79. Kutas M, Hillyard SA. Reading senseless sentences: Brain potentials reflect semantic incongruity. *Science.* (1980) 207:203–8. doi: 10.1126/science.7350657
80. Real RG, Herbert C, Kotchoubey B, Wessig C, Volkmann J, Kübler A. Psychophysiological correlates of coping and quality of life in patients with ALS. *Clin Neurophysiol.* (2014) 125:955–61. doi: 10.1016/j.clinph.2013.09.040
81. Kübler A, Holz EM, Sellers EW, Vaughan TM. Toward independent home use of brain-computer interfaces: a decision algorithm for selection of potential end-users. *Arch Phys Med Rehabil.* (2015) 96:27–32. doi: 10.1016/j.apmr.2014.03.036
82. Bede P, Oliver D, Stodart J, van den Berg L, Simmons ZO, Hardiman O. Palliative care in amyotrophic lateral sclerosis: a review of current international guidelines and initiatives. *J Neurol Neurosurg Psychiatry.* (2011) 82:413–18. doi: 10.1136/jnnp.2010.232637
83. Foley G, Timonen V, Hardiman O. Patients' perceptions of services and preferences for care in amyotrophic lateral sclerosis: a review. *Amyotroph Lateral Scler.* (2012) 13:11–24. doi: 10.3109/17482968.2011.607500
84. Seeber AA, Pols AJ, Hijdra A, Grupstra HF, Willems DL, de Visser M. Experiences and reflections of patients with motor neuron disease on breaking the news in a two-tiered appointment: a qualitative study. *BMJ Support Palliat Care.* (2016) 9:e8. doi: 10.1136/bmjspcare-2015-000977

15

Imaging Cerebral Activity in Amyotrophic Lateral Sclerosis

Malcolm Proudfoot [1], *Peter Bede* [2] *and Martin R. Turner* [1,3]*

[1] Nuffield Department of Clinical Neurosciences, University of Oxford, Oxford, United Kingdom, [2] Computational Neuroimaging Group, Academic Unit of Neurology, Trinity College Dublin, Dublin, Ireland, [3] Wellcome Centre for Integrative Neuroimaging, University of Oxford, Oxford, United Kingdom

***Correspondence:**
Martin R. Turner
martin.turner@ndcn.ox.ac.uk

Advances in neuroimaging, complementing histopathological insights, have established a multi-system involvement of cerebral networks beyond the traditional neuromuscular pathological view of amyotrophic lateral sclerosis (ALS). The development of effective disease-modifying therapy remains a priority and this will be facilitated by improved biomarkers of motor system integrity against which to assess the efficacy of candidate drugs. Functional MRI (FMRI) is an established measure of both cerebral activity and connectivity, but there is an increasing recognition of neuronal oscillations in facilitating long-distance communication across the cortical surface. Such dynamic synchronization vastly expands the connectivity foundations defined by traditional neuronal architecture. This review considers the unique pathogenic insights afforded by the capture of cerebral disease activity in ALS using FMRI and encephalography.

Keywords: amyotrophic lateral sclerosis, motor neurone disease, biomarker, neuroimaging, neurophysiology, cortex

INTRODUCTION

Neurodegenerative disorders are increasingly understood as a disintegration of complex cerebral functional networks (1). Amyotrophic lateral sclerosis (ALS) is characterized by loss of upper and lower motor neurones of the corticospinal tract, brainstem, and spinal anterior horns, resulting in progressive weakness of downstream muscles. In addition to protean upstream causes (2, 3), there is firmly established clinical, pathological, and genetic overlap of ALS with frontotemporal dementia (FTD). The diagnosis remains a clinical one, with a lack of biomarkers being a significant barrier to the development of highly-effective disease-modifying therapy. Advanced neuroimaging, in combination with histopathological insights, has brought the brain to the forefront of biomarker development (4).

The earliest studies of cerebral blood flow in ALS employed positron emission tomography, and demonstrated a widened region of cortical activation in response to a simple motor task (5). Among the hypotheses for this "boundary shift effect" was loss of local inhibitory GABA-ergic interneuronal circuits [reviewed in (6)]. A consistent pathological feature of ALS has been the observation of increased cortical excitability, possibly reflecting reduced local inhibitory influences, measured using short-interval paired transcranial magnetic stimulation (TMS) (7, 8). Through the characterization of monogenetic associations, ALS research has expanded to include the study of what is now thought to be a long presymptomatic phase (9), in which cortical functional abnormalities may be the among the earliest detectable manifestations (10).

Blood oxygenation level-dependent (BOLD)-based functional (FMRI), with the major advantages of avoiding ionizing radiation and the greater availability of MRI technology, confirmed a profound alteration in cortical activity inherent to the pathogenesis of ALS. Tools to study cortical neurophysiology in real-time have also undergone significant development in both sensitivity and analysis. This review will consider the unique insights that FMRI and encephalography bring to the understanding of the pathogenesis of ALS at the systems level, which is increasingly of greatest relevance to the long-term goal of neuroprotective therapy.

FUNCTIONAL MRI

FMRI has been extensively used to characterize network dysfunction in ALS in cross-sectional, longitudinal, and presymptomatic study designs. The practical advantages of FMRI in ALS include the widespread availability of MRI platforms, the large number of freely available analysis suites and the ability to provide crucial biological insights in relatively simple, cost-effective, and non-invasive study designs (11). Despite some inconsistencies in the literature (12), two main themes have consistently emerged from the application of FMRI to ALS: (i) the characterization of compensatory changes, such as the recruitment of additional cortical (13–16), subcortical (14, 17, 18), and cerebellar (17, 19) regions to execute motor and cognitive tasks, and ii) the concept of inhibitory dysfunction as a key facet of ALS-associated pathophysiology (6, 20).

Methodological Considerations

Functional MRI has been extensively used to characterize network dysfunction in ALS in cross-sectional, longitudinal, and presymptomatic study designs (21) (**Table 1**), but method-associated limitations are rarely articulated. The protracted hemodynamic response to neural activity hampers the temporal resolution of fMRI. Blood oxygen-level dependent (BOLD) signal typically peaks only 5–6s after focal activation therefore careful study designs are indispensable for meaningful temporal inferences (22, 23). Spatial distortions and signal dropout due to susceptibility gradients near air-tissue interfaces lead to decreased BOLD signal in lateral parietal, orbitofrontal and dorsolateral prefrontal regions necessitating meticulous sequence optimization before data acquisition (24–26). Scanner noise may also impact on the interpretation of BOLD signal, particularly in the default-mode network (27), and careful experimental designs are required to minimize the influence of background noise (28). While fMRI findings are often presented by overlaying activation maps upon high-resolution structural images, the inherent spatial resolution of fMRI is limited by the signal-to-noise ratio profile of consecutive, rapid whole-brain imaging. In the majority ALS studies, the voxel size of fMRI protocols is two to four times larger than what is used for structural acquisitions (21).

Motor Paradigms

Pioneering FMRI studies in ALS relied initially on hand movement paradigms (15, 16), which were gradually complemented by innovative bulbar studies (13, 29, 30). In motor-task FMRI studies, different strategies have been utilized to control for limb weakness, motor effort and lower motor neuron involvement for the interpretation of cerebral activation. Motor imagery (31) has attracted considerable attention, not only for emerging brain-machine interface applications (32) but also as an FMRI paradigm for a condition like ALS in which patients typically develop severe motor disability (33). The execution and imagination of specific movements manifest in similar activation patterns in ALS and controls (15) suggesting that this approach may be particularly pertinent to patient cohorts with mixed disability profiles. Some ALS studies however report divergent activation maps in motor imagery and execution (34). Similarly to motor imagery, action observation is also thought to result in comparable cortical activity to action execution which has been used to study the mirror-neuron system in ALS (35, 36). Another approach to control for motor disability and establish ALS-specific activation patterns is the inclusion of disease-controls, i.e., non-ALS patients with motor disability (16, 37). Very few FMRI studies to date have specifically evaluated functional changes in other rarer motor neurone disorders such as the upper motor neurone-only primary lateral sclerosis (PLS) (38, 39) and lower motor neurone-dominated Kennedy's disease (30) using motor paradigms. Patient stratification into separate study groups based on motor disability is another strategy to interpret functional alterations in the context of disability (14). In light of the fundamentally divergent study designs, the inclusion of patients in different stages of their disease and small sample sizes, the inconsistent findings of motor activation studies are not surprising. Whilst, hypo- (29, 30, 40) and hyper-activation (13, 14, 16, 35, 36) of the somatosensory cortex have both been reported in response to motor tasks, the recruitment of premotor areas is a relatively consistent finding. An integrative explanation of the seemingly divergent findings is that the initial hyper-activation represents an early-stage adaptive process to execute movement (14), which gradually gives place to hypo-activation as progressive structural changes ensue (41, 42). Robust multi-timepoint longitudinal studies are required to clarify the timeline of functional changes in ALS as very few task-based longitudinal FMRI studies have been published to date (33, 43). One longitudinal study identified reduced motor activation on 3-month follow-up which was interpreted as compensatory failure due to progressive neural loss (43), while another study reported increased precentral gyrus activity 6-month after initial scanning as evidence of ongoing adaptation (33). In addition to compensatory processes in motor, premotor and supplementary motor areas (44), evidence also exist that the basal ganglia (17, 18, 45, 46), the ipsilateral motor cortex (14, 47), and the cerebellum (17, 19, 47, 48) also contribute to adaptive network reorganization.

Extra-Motor Studies

With the increasing recognition of cognitive impairment in ALS (49, 50), a series of elegant language (51), executive (52), theory-of-mind (36), and memory (43, 53, 54) task-based activation studies have also been published. In addition to the cognitive activation paradigms, visual, auditory and somatosensory stimulation studies have further characterized the spectrum of extra-motor involvement in ALS (55, 56). Other innovative non-motor activation studies in ALS include an anti-saccade study with concurrent eye tracking to investigate dorsolateral prefrontal cortex (DLPFC) function (57). Similar to the divergent findings of motor-task studies, increased activation

TABLE 1 | Selected motor task-based and resting-state fMRI studies in ALS.

Authors	Year	Study design	ALS (n)	Controls (n)	Main study findings/interpretation
Li et al. (29)	2009	Motor task: swallowing, Cross-sectional study	10	10 HC	Reduced somatosensory cortex activation in patients with dysphagia
Mohammadi et al. (30)	2009	Motor: tongue movement, Cross-sectional study	22	22 HC 5 DC (SBMA)	ALS patients with bulbar symptoms showed decreased cortical and thalamic activation
Palmieri et al. (53)	2010	Emotional attribution and recognition task, Cross-sectional study	9	10 HC	Altered emotional processing similar to patents observed in FTD.
Lule et al. (55)	2010	visual, auditory and somatosensory stimulation, Cross-sectional study	14	18 HC	Decreased response in secondary visual areas in ALS, delayed response in secondary auditory areas, reduced response to somatosensory stimulation
Goldstein et al. (52)	2011	Cognitive task, Cross-sectional study	14	8 HC	Increased left temporal and decreased precentral and left medial frontal activation: altered inhibitory processing in ALS
Kollewe et al. (13)	2011	Motor task: hand and tongue movement, Cross-sectional study	20	20 HC	Decreased cortical activation during tongue movements in patients with bulbar symptoms. Increased activation during hand movements. Different functional reorganization in limb and bulbar impairment.
Mohammadi et al. (14)	2011	Motor task, Cross-sectional study	22	22 HC	Patients stratified into three groups based on disability, Increased activation in early-stage, decreased activation in later stage disease.
Poujois et al. (15)	2013	Hand motor task Motor imagery, Cross-sectional study	19	13 HC	Motor execution and imagery yields to similar activation patterns. Increased contra- and ipsilateral somatosensory cortex activation.
Passamonti (59)	2013	Emotional processing task, Cross-sectional study	11	12 HC	Increased activation in prefrontal areas and altered amygdala-prefrontal cortex connectivity in ALS, suggestive of limbic system dysfunction
Witiuk et al. (57)	2014	Antisaccade task with eye tracking, Cross-sectional study	12	12 HC	ALS patients make more antisaccade direction errors and exhibit reduced DLPFC activation compared to controls i.e. deficits in automatic response inhibition are associated with impaired DLPFC activation
Stoppel et al. (43)	2014	Go/No-Go paradigm, Longitudinal design	14	14 HC	Increased motor activation compared to controls with subsequent decline on follow-up scanning suggestive of failing adaptive compensation
Mohammadi et al. (61)	2015	Movement inhibition task (go/no-go), Cross-sectional study	17	17 HC	Increased motor inhibition and execution related activation in patients with ALS compared to controls.
Jelsone-Swain et al. (36)	2015	Action Observation and Execution task, Cross-sectional study	19	18 HC	Increased activation during action-execution and observation in ALS patients in opercular, premotor and primary motor regions. Mirror neuron system mediated compensation.
Li et al. (35)	2015	Action observation paradigm, Cross-sectional study	30	30 HC	Action observation activates similar networks to action execution. Increased activation observed in the DLPFC and supplementary motor regions of ALS patients.
Aho-Ozhan (60)	2016	Cognitive task Cross-sectional study	15	14 HC	Impaired processing of negative emotions such as fear and disgust in ALS
Vellage et al. (54)	2016	Cognitive task: working memory Cross-sectional study	14	14 HC	Reduced hemodynamic responses in the left occipital cortex and right prefrontal cortex in ALS patients compared to healthy controls
Keller et al. (58)	2018	Cognitive task: ToM and executive task, Cross-sectional study	65	33	Increased activation in all ALS patients compared to HC. High performing patients exhibit more activation than those with neuropsychological deficits suggestive of compensation.
Mohammadi et al. (66)	2009	Resting-state fMRI, Cross-sectional study	20	20 HC	ICA analyses: decreased DMN activation in the anterior and posterior cingulate and parietal regions
Jelsone-Swain et al. (84)	2010	Resting-state fMRI, Cross-sectional study	20	20 HC	ROI analyses: decreased functional connectivity between the right and left motor cortices
Douaud et al. (20)	2011	Resting-state fMRI, Cross-sectional study	25	15 HC	Increased SMN, premotor, prefrontal and thalamic functional connectivity, interpreted as compensation and inhibitory dysfunction

(Continued)

TABLE 1 | Continued

Authors	Year	Study design	ALS (n)	Controls (n)	Main study findings/interpretation
Agosta et al. (42)	2011	Resting-state fMRI, Cross-sectional study	26	15 HC	Increased SMN, cingulate, cerebellar connectivity interpreted as compensation.
Fekete et al. (76)	2013	Resting state fMRI, Cross-sectional study	40	30 HC	Widespread motor, cerebellar and basal ganglia functional connectivity alterations in the ALS cohort. Accurate subject classification using multiple kernel learning.
Zhou et al. (82)	2013	Resting-state fMRI, Cross-sectional study	12	12 HC	Positive correlation between disability and functional connectivity
Agosta et al. (65)	2013	Resting-state fMRI, Cross-sectional study	20	15 HC	ICA analyses: Increased parietal connectivity is associated with cognitive deficits which may represent compensation
Welsh et al. (67)	2013	Resting state fMRI, Cross-sectional study	32	31 HC	Machine learning (support-vector machine) based on fMRI metrics achieves over 71% accuracy for disease state classification
Zhou et al. (73)	2014	Resting state fMRI, Cross-sectional study	12	12 HC	Decreased regional brain synchrony in the superior medial SMN detected by regional coherence measures
Meoded et al. (38)	2015	Resting state fMRI, Cross-sectional study		14 HC 16 PLS	Increased functional connectivity between the cerebellum and cortical motor areas and between the cerebellum and frontal and temporal cortex in primary lateral sclerosis
Schmidt et al. (77)	2014	Resting state fMRI, Cross-sectional study	64	27 HC	A strong positive correlation exist between changes in SC and FC averaged per brain region; suggesting that structural and functional network degeneration in ALS is coupled
Chenji et al. (75)	2016	Resting state fMRI, Cross-sectional study	21	40 HC	Increased DMN and reduced SMN connectivity associated with greater disability interpreted as inhibitory dysfunction
Zhou et al. (69)	2016	Resting state fMRI, Cross-sectional study	44	44 HC	Increased cerebellar, occipital and prefrontal degree centrality (DC) and decreased DC in the primary motor cortex and sensory motor regions of ALS patients
Menke et al. (79)	2016	Resting state fMRI, Presymptomatic study design	12	12 psALS 12 HC	Increased FC between the cerebellum and precuneus-cingulate-frontal lobe network in asymptomatic mutation carriers compared to controls
Trojsi et al. (72)	2017	Resting state fMRI, Cross-sectional study	21	15	Decreased FC in DMN, salience and fronto-parietal network. More significant SLN connectivity changes observed in bulbar onset patients compared to those with spinal onset.
Zhang et al. (74)	2017	Resting state fMRI, Cross-sectional study	38	35 HC	Impaired interhemispheric functional connectivity eidenceed by voxel mirrored homotopic connectivity (VMHC) reductions, correlations with CC diffusivity metrics
Zhang et al. (166)	2017	Resting state fMRI, Cross-sectional study	25	25 HC	Reduced occipital surface-based local gyrification index (LGI) is associated with decreased functional connectivity in the bilateral precuneus.
Lee et al. (80)	2017	Resting state fMRI, Presymptomatic study design		13 psALS 46 HC	Connectivity deficits detected in salience, sensorimotor, default mode and thalamic networks in presymptomatic *C9orf72* carriers
Li et al. (68)	2018	Resting state fMRI, Cross-sectional study	38	35 HC	Graph theory method (functional connectivity density FCD) Decreased FCD in the primary motor cortex, increased long-range FCD in the premotor cortex in ALS patients.
Bueno et al. (167)	2018	Resting state fMRI, Cross-sectional study	20	15 HC	Focus on Papez circuit integrity. Decreased functional connectivity in ALS patients between hippocampal, parahippocampal and cingulate regions.
Menke et al. (39)	2018	Resting state fMRI, Longitudinal study	13	3 PLS	Multi-timepoint structural-functional study, ICA and DRA, decreased FC between SMN and frontal pole, increased FC between primary motor cortex and fronto-parietal network

HC healthy control, DC Disease Control, DLPFC DorsoLateral PreFrontal Cortex, FC functional connectivity, SC Structural Connectivity, SBMA Kennedy's disease, FTD FrontoTemporal Dementia, PLS Primary Lateral Sclerosis, DMN Default Mode Network, SMN SensoriMotor Network, ToM Theory of Mind.

(36, 52, 58, 59) and impaired activation (51, 60) have both been noted on cognitive tasks, which is likely to represent stages of successful and failing adaptation. More often however a pattern of coexisting hypo- and hyper- activation is reported (37, 54, 61).

Resting-State Studies

The analysis of task-free BOLD signal in the so-called resting-state (rsFMRI) benefits from fast acquisition times with a data-driven, more consistent experimental design, making them an attractive add-on to high-resolution structural protocols. With the establishment of the internationally collaborative Neuroimaging Society in ALS (NiSALS) (62) and successful multi-site initiatives (63), there is interest in FMRI sequence harmonization and potential for multicentre data pooling (12, 64). rsFMRI studies differ considerably in their analysis approaches and their methods span from independent component analysis (65–67), to graph theory (68, 69) and amplitude of low frequency fluctuation (ALFF) (70, 71). rsFMRI studies in ALS identified decreased frontotemporal (72), sensorimotor (70, 73–75), and cortical-subcortical (76) network integrity and increased default mode network (75), and cerebellar (38, 69) connectivity. Large combined structural-FMRI studies suggest that patterns of structural degeneration overlap with functionally impaired regions and that a strong positive correlation exists between functional and structural connectivity alterations (77). Longitudinal rsFMRI studies indicate declining functional connectivity in sensorimotor, thalamic, and visual networks and increasing connectivity in fronto-parietal and temporal circuits (39). Multimodal, structural-functional, multi-timepoint longitudinal studies (39) are best suited to characterize the natural history of progressive neurodegenerative changes (78). Data from presymptomatic carriers of ALS-causing gene mutations revealed increased cerebello-cerebral functional connectivity (79) and decreased salience, sensorimotor, default-mode, and thalamic networks connectivity (80). Despite the controversy around direct clinico-radiological correlations (81), some studies in ALS have reported significant associations, most often with functional measures (73, 82–84), disease duration (59, 73), and progression rates (20, 40, 85).

Practical Limitations

For a condition in which accumulation of physical disability is accompanied by ventilatory compromise with orthopnoea, supine MRI limits longitudinal assessment to those with slower rates of progression (39). The application of such a biomarker as an outcome measure in a small-scale clinical trial would then entail costly statistical compromises, since no ideal solution exists for the imputation of data points selectively lost from those patients with more aggressive disease (86).

ENCEPHALOGRAPHY

Cortical processes, and the diseases that impact on them, are inadequately described without reference to dynamic neural communication (87, 88), but this necessitates temporal precision, without the dispersive effects of the haemodynamic response function that smears neural signals across several seconds (89). Surface electroencephalography (EEG) as a biomarker in ALS is appealingly practical, well tolerated and non-invasive.

Methodological Limitations

Even a high-density array of surface EEG electrodes still sacrifices spatial resolution owing to the attenuation and mutation of neural signals as they pass through several tissue layers with varying electrical conductivity (89). Magnetoencephalography (MEG) permits recording of tiny (femtoTesla) fluctuations in the magnetic field external to (and undispersed by) the scalp (90). Yet reconstruction of cortical sources remains a mathematically "ill-posed" problem—any given recorded signal could in theory be generated by multiple neural sources and the analytical choice to address this (for example "beamforming") necessitates certain assumptions (91). MEG's improvement in spatial precision is also offset by expenses and susceptibility to artifact from ferromagnetic interference, albeit mitigated by acquisition and analysis standardization (92, 93). The resulting data is feature-rich, subsequent analysis may necessarily be restricted to a frequency-band of interest or a selected connectivity metric, these choices may in turn influence study conclusions (94) (**Table 2**).

Evoked Potentials

Small-scale EEG studies have addressed the utility of somatosensory, visual and brainstem evoked potentials in ALS (95–100). Reflecting the inconsistency of reported results, these well-established and standardized assessments have failed to find any routine clinical application in ALS, although they may yet find a role in multimodal assessment (101, 102).

To better reflect the pathological burden in ALS studies have therefore moved toward either motor or cognitive activation paradigms, initially appraising cortical processes via evoked response potentials [ERPs, previously reviewed in (103)]. The "Bereitschaftspotential," a classical lateralized change in cortical electrical potential, easily recordable during movement preparation, appeared robustly decreased in ALS (104, 105). More recent studies have considered the implications of abnormal movement-related cortical potentials (MRCPs) in ALS in terms of clinical and structural correlates. While a study of 21 ALS patients demonstrated higher MRCPs overall, the effect was shown to be driven by patients with a low burden of clinically detectable UMN morbidity (106). The inference that increased MRCPs reflect cortical compensatory mechanisms was born out by longitudinal study of a sub-set in whom MRCPs declined over 10 months. A comparable study of finger movement in 32 ALS patients revealed reduced MRCPs only in patients with a high UMN burden, alongside evidence of ipsilateral premotor activation to suggest a compensatory "boundary shift" (107). MRCPs are also elicited during imagined movements, but only a limited study in ALS has thus far been performed (108), mandating replication before application of these measures in control and communication devices is to be seriously considered.

Motor Paradigms

Motor events (including self-generated movement) are reflected in frequency-specific changes to continuous "background" neuronal oscillations (109). As might be expected, the neurodegeneration associated with ALS results in distinct alteration to pre-central sensorimotor rhythms. While studies are yet to be widely replicated, they show promise both in terms of relevance to daily motor tasks, and sensitivity to detect early cortical dysfunction in patients still capable of performing the task in question. The results may also contribute to the ongoing efforts to characterize a presymptomatic phase to ALS and have implications for the development of brain-computer interfaces

TABLE 2 | Selected motor task-based and resting-state encephalographic studies in ALS.

Authors	Year	*n*	EEG/MEG (channels)	Protocol	Main measure	Phenotype correlations
Westphal et al. (104)	1998	16 ALS 16 HC	EEG (11c)	Self-paced R fist closure	Reduced BP	Spasticity correlation
Thorns et al. (105)	2010	13 ALS 13 HC	EEG (19c)	Cued R or L index finger button press	Reduced BP	N/A
Inuggi et al. (107)	2011	32 ALS 12 HC	EEG (29c)	Self-paced R thumb extension	Reduced MRCPs (only in UMN+ ALS)	Ipsilateral MRCP correlation with movement speed
Riva et al. (119)	2012	16 ALS 15 HC	EEG (29c)	Self-paced R thumb extension	Reduced beta ERS; Unaltered beta ERD	ERS correlation with CST damage via MRI and TMS
Gu et al. (108)	2013	4 ALS 7 HC	EEG (15c)	Imaginary R wrist extension	Slower MRCP rebound	N/A
Bizovičar et al. (120)	2014	21 ALS 19 HC	EEG (30c)	Self-paced R index finger flexion	Reduced beta ERD; Lateralised ERS	None
Proudfoot et al. (122)	2017	11 ALS 9 PLS 12 Presymp 10 HC	MEG (306c)	Cued R or L index finger extension	Excess beta ERD; Delayed ERS	Altered ERS lateralisation in PLS
Proudfoot et al. (126)	2018	17 ALS 11 HC 5 Presymp	MEG (306c)	Cued R and L hand grips	Reduced beta CMC; Reduced inter-hemispheric beta FC	CMC unaltered in Presymp
Mai et al. (143)	1998	18 ALS 14 HC	EEG (18c)	Resting	Reduced central alpha power	Alpha correlation with MRC and Norris scales
Santhosh et al. (144)	2005	12 ALS 12 ALS	EEG (8c)	Resting	Reduced alpha power	N/A
Jayaram et al. (145)	2015	6 ALS 32 HC	EEG (124c)	Resting	Reduced central theta power; Widespread increased high gamma power	Gamma reduced only in patient with ALSFRS=0
Iyer et al. (147)	2015	18 ALS 17 HC	EEG (128c)	Resting	Increased FC especially within salience and default-mode networks	N/A
Nasseroleslami et al. (148)	2017	100 ALS 34 HC	EEG (128c)	Resting	Increased FC especially interhemispheric theta and fronto-parietal gamma	FC correlation with structural MRI degeneration
Fraschini et al. (150)	2018	21 ALS 16 HC	EEG (61c)	Resting	Widespread reduced alpha FC	N/A
Proudfoot et al. (151)	2018	24 ALS 24 HC 15 Presymp 9 PLS	MEG (306c)	Resting	Widespread increased broadband FC	Similar changes in PLS. More subtle changes in Presymp.
Sorrentino et al. (154)	2018	50 ALS 25 HC	MEG (163c)	Resting	Broadband increased FC with disorganized topology	Advanced ALS associated with a more centralized, "vulnerable" network

HC healthy control, FC functional connectivity, Presymp asymptomatic ALS-causing gene carriers, BP Bereitschaftspotential, MRCP movement related cortical potential, ERD event related desynchronization, ERS event related synchronization PLS primary lateral sclerosis, CMC cortico-muscular coherence UMN+ above average quantity of upper motor neuron signs, CST cortico-spinal tract, ALSFRS ALS functional rating scale (disability metric).

aiming to facilitate environmental control by patients with advanced ALS (110).

Movement is accompanied by reliable and well-characterized fluctuations in neural signal power, particularly within the beta (15–30 Hz) band, with recognizable anatomical localization to motor cortex. Beta-band power is reduced (event related desynchronization, ERD) prior to and during movement execution; movement termination is followed by an equally reliable increase in power well above baseline levels (synchronization, ERS or post-movement beta-rebound) (111). Temporally corresponding to fluctuations in cortical excitability (112), ERD and ERS are adjusted to meet task requirements [including force (113), speed (114), and complexity (115)], are sensitive to pharmacological manipulation [particularly synaptic GABA levels via benzodiazepines (116) or tiagabine (117)] and may be disrupted by other disease states including Parkinson's (118).

Motor Studies (EEG)

Two independent EEG studies have demonstrated attenuation of ERS in ALS. The first involved 16 patients efficiently performing self-paced thumb extensions (119). The degree of

ERS attenuation was shown to correlate with corticospinal pathological burden as measured by both mean diffusivity on structural MRI and diminished motor evoked potentials in APB in response to TMS stimulation. The second study included 21 patients performing both sniffing and right index finger flexion (120). Although the patients had detectable weakness in terms of both maximal grip strength and sniff nasal-inspiratory pressure, there were no group differences in the precise pressure produced during the task performance. Neural data from the sniff task were heavily contaminated by facial muscle artifact, but the finger flexion task resulted in reliable ERD/S. The ALS patients were observed to have diminished beta ERD, interpreted as a consequence of pyramidal cell degeneration. Both motor preparation and execution timepoints were affected, while the lateralization of beta ERS was also altered. The study failed to establish clinical correlations with these measures, nor was there any successful correlation with F-wave elicitability (an imperfect measure of corticospinal tract integrity in any case).

Motor Studies (MEG)

The neural signal acquired by MEG is far less susceptible to distortion as it passes through skull and scalp, source modeling is therefore likely to be more accurate than EEG, and an expanding range of MEG studies have specifically appraised sensorimotor rhythms (121). A MEG study involving 11 ALS patients, 9 with PLS, and 12 asymptomatic genetic mutation carriers, investigated sensorimotor rhythms during a laterally-cued motor preparation task requiring speeded index finger extension of either hand (122). Whole-brain source-space data were analyzed pre, during, and post movement, specifically focusing on beta-band frequencies. Although the task was behaviorally performed comparably by ALS patients, the neural data revealed larger beta ERD, 500 ms after cue presentation, during the period of maximal motor preparation, particularly within contra and ipsilateral gyri. Beta ERS, after movement termination, was delayed in both patient groups. The asymptomatic carriers produced excessive beta ERD during motor execution. Conceptually the results are concordant with cross-modality support for cortical hyperexcitability in ALS (123, 124).

The integrity of upper motor neurone pathways can also be non-invasively appraised using MEG. Cortico-muscular coherence (CMC), by which neural oscillations and surface electromyography correlate temporally (particularly during sustained contraction), principally reflects direct corticospinal drive to the peripheral musculature (125). A MEG study of 17 ALS patients was designed to measure CMC during a bilateral forearm grip task (126). As expected, source-space beta CMC was distinctly strongest from the contra-lateral precentral gyrus, but this frequency specific peak was markedly attenuated in the ALS group, despite adequate grip production and without any correlation to force production. The analysis also took advantage of MEG spatial precision to consider motoric cortico-cortical communication during the same task performance. Interhemispheric functional connectivity, in terms of beta band amplitude envelope correlation, was reduced in ALS patients. The inference of reduced CMC, a measure that in health indexes the quality of motor performance (127), is that beta coherence may serve as a novel UMN specific biomarker at the disposal of future therapeutic efforts (128).

Extra-Motor Studies

Taking advantage of the high temporal resolution of encephalographic data, component steps in the complex cognitive dysfunction associated with the ALS-FTD syndrome may be examined. The mismatch negativity (MMN) paradigm considers the attentional modulation of auditory perception. An early EEG study failed to show any abnormalities within ALS patients (129). However, using MEG, plus subtle experimental design adjustments in 12 participants all with bulbar symptoms, MMN response amplitudes were shown to increase relative to healthy controls (130). Given the previously demonstrated sensitivity of MMN responses to ketamine administration, the authors tentatively linked their findings to the glutamatergic excitotoxicity ALS pathogenesis theory. This rare example of "gain of function" was not consistently replicated in two later EEG studies, which interpreted delayed MMN responses as evidence of sub-clinical extra-motor dysfunction (131, 132).

Less well-replicated methodologies have also been applied to ALS patients to consider neural processes underlying working memory (133, 134), selective attention (135, 136), and executive control (137, 138). Broadly, these studies have provided further evidence in favor of sub-clinical disruption to "frontal" cognitive processes in keeping with the extended non-motor ALS phenotype (139). Parietal cortex dysfunction was also implicated in an EEG study involving the Wisconsin Card Sorting Test. While 26 ALS patients did not differ in performance of a "set-shifting" task, even patients without mild cognitive impairment failed to produce the expected enhancement of parietal ERPs during a task-switch (140). Although the attenuation of the "switch potential" failed to correlate with neuropsychological indices, the authors speculated whether such sub-clinical deficits could predict future behavioral disorder.

A study requiring cognitive task performance during data acquisition took a very different analytical approach, using 200 s of data to measure "transfer entropy" between scalp electrodes rather than the millisecond granularity of evoked potentials. The directionality of functional connectivity was appraised via EEG in 18 ALS patients, revealing only feedforward (parietal to frontal) connectivity to increase across a broad frequency band (141). As the patients engaged in a spelling task with a view to brain-computer interfacing, sensory (visual) stimuli were hypothesized to be more readily processed in compensation for the diminished proprioceptive input resulting from physical disability, but an alternative explanation in terms of failing cortical inhibition was also acknowledged (20).

Resting-State Studies (EEG)

The earliest EEG investigations of ALS reflected the emerging concept of cognitive dysfunction within the ALS clinical spectrum, with slowed cortical rhythms noted in non-demented patients (142). A more systematic study of 18 ALS patients conversely revealed sparse differences to healthy controls (143). Only at central electrodes, and only within the alpha band (8–13 Hz), was the power of neural oscillations reduced in ALS. The reduction was interpreted to reflect selective neuronal loss within the sensorimotor cortices. A comparable result was described in a subsequent smaller study (144), and increases in the gamma band (30–90 Hz) power beyond central regions was also reported (145).

Further ALS electrophysiology studies have reflected a growing interest in the so-called "dynome" (146), the extent to which the organization of cortical function is reflected in particular patterns of active connectivity. High-density (128 channel) surface EEG was used to calculate connectivity between both scalp points and projected source nodes in an initial study of 18 patients (147). Fronto-central areas were shown to have increased connectivity, and this was explored across a broad range of measures. A subsequent study expanded this work to 100 patients, including some longitudinal analyses (148), and confirmed EEG-derived connectivity changes in ALS to be more striking than limited group differences in the scalp-recorded power spectrum. This more parsimonious analysis appraised only sensor-space, deriving coherence estimates within 8 consecutive frequency bands. Widespread increases in connectivity were again demonstrated relative to healthy controls, particularly theta band interhemispheric sensorimotor connectivity and gamma band fronto-parietal connectivity. As 59 of the ALS patients had undergone contemporaneous structural MRI, mathematically derived structural "degeneration modes" (accounting for the large-scale gray and white matter changes typical in ALS) were shown to correlate with EEG change, conceptually aligned with the concept of progressive network decline overlying structural disintegration.

Network structures can also be summarized using graph theory metrics, this was explored in sensor-space in 21 patients, demonstrating a more "de-centralised" organization (149). The connectivity metric chosen in this study was phase-based, thus insensitive to any group differences in spectral power, and furthermore was significantly correlated with disability between individuals. This group later re-analyzed the same data reconstructed into source-space (150) and filtered into 3 classical frequency bands to show spatially distributed decreases in connectivity, albeit restricted to the alpha band spectrum.

Resting-State Studies (MEG)

A resting-state MEG study explored functional connectivity in 24 ALS patients using source-space data acquired after co-registration with structural MRI (151). Ten minutes of continuous data was parcellated into 39 regions of interest and the broad-band (3–40 Hz) signal used to calculate "edge" strength between these 39 "nodes," In keeping with many FMRI studies, functional connectivity was broadly increased in ALS patients relative to age-matched healthy controls, particularly affecting communication links to the posterior cingulate cortex. This finding was aligned with the hypothesis of loss of cortical inhibitory neuronal influences underlying cortical excitability in ALS (5). Comparable posterior non-motor connectivity changes were described using FMRI (152). Nevertheless, the diversity of reported results and interpretations serves to highlight a need for replication and standardization between centers and where possible across modalities (153). A further study of 50 patients, using a different (phase-based) connectivity measure, also described widespread connectivity increases in ALS (154). The increases were not restricted to specific frequency bands and the extracted graph theory metrics suggest global network hyper-centralization to accompany disease progression.

FUTURE DIRECTIONS

MEG is providing broader insight into cognitive mechanisms underpinning higher cortical function in health (155), and comparable results may eventually prove achievable using surface EEG (156). The next generation of wearable sensors may yet dramatically expand MEG's application (157). The spinal cord is a core but functionally understudied aspect of the motor system disintegration that characterizes ALS. Spinal FMRI is in its infancy (158), but a number of promising studies have already been published in animal models (159, 160), healthy populations (161, 162) and other clinical cohorts (163, 164). The goal of non-invasively studying the integrated activity of upper and lower motor neurone pools looks more feasible with the success in studies involving the dorsal pathways (165). Cerebral FMRI parameters are likely to take an increasing role in emerging machine-learning and classification studies both in diagnostic and prognostic applications (67, 76). Future studies need robust longitudinal design and to capitalize on the growing infrastructure for multicentre studies. This will permit the testing of pathogenic hypotheses within larger cohorts of clinically more homogeneous ALS patients, and define the earliest markers of pathology in presymptomatic individuals essential for the assessment of future neurotherapeutic interventions.

AUTHOR CONTRIBUTIONS

All authors listed have made a substantial, direct and intellectual contribution to the work, and approved it for publication.

FUNDING

PB is supported by the Health Research Board (HRB–Ireland; HRB EIA-2017-019), the Irish Institute of Clinical Neuroscience IICN–Novartis Ireland Research Grant, the Iris O'Brien Foundation, and the Research Motor Neuron (RMN-Ireland) Foundation.

REFERENCES

1. Seeley WW, Crawford RK, Zhou J, Miller BL, Greicius MD. Neurodegenerative diseases target large-scale human brain networks. *Neuron* (2009) 62:42–52. doi: 10.1016/j.neuron.2009.03.024
2. Turner MR, Swash M. The expanding syndrome of amyotrophic lateral sclerosis: a clinical and molecular odyssey. *J Neurol Neurosurg Psychiatry* (2015) 86:667–73. doi: 10.1136/jnnp-2014-308946
3. Talbot K, Feneberg E, Scaber J, Thompson AG, Turner MR. Amyotrophic lateral sclerosis: the complex path to precision medicine. *J Neurol.* (2018) 265:2454–62. doi: 10.1007/s00415-018-8983-8

4. Turner MR, Verstraete E. What does imaging reveal about the pathology of amyotrophic lateral sclerosis? *Curr Neurol Neurosci Rep.* (2015) 15:45. doi: 10.1007/s11910-015-0569-6
5. Kew JJM, Leigh PN, Playford ED, Passingham RE, Goldstein LH, Frackowiak RSJ, et al. Cortical function in amyotrophic lateral sclerosis: a positron emission tomography study. *Brain* (1993) 116:655–80. doi: 10.1093/brain/116.3.655
6. Turner MR, Kiernan MC. Does interneuronal dysfunction contribute to neurodegeneration in amyotrophic lateral sclerosis? *Amyotroph Lateral Scler.* (2012) 13:245–50. doi: 10.3109/17482968.2011.636050
7. Yokota T, Yoshino A, Inaba A, Saito Y. Double cortical stimulation in amyotrophic lateral sclerosis. *J Neurol Neurosurg Psychiatry* (1996) 61:596–600. doi: 10.1136/jnnp.61.6.596
8. Menon P, Geevasinga N, Yiannikas C, Howells J, Kiernan MC, Vucic S. Sensitivity and specificity of threshold tracking transcranial magnetic stimulation for diagnosis of amyotrophic lateral sclerosis: a prospective study. *Lancet Neurol.* (2015) 14:478–84. doi: 10.1016/S1474-4422(15)00 014-9
9. Benatar M, Wuu J, Ravits J. Opportunity and innovation in studying pre-symptomatic amyotrophic lateral sclerosis. *Muscle Nerve* (2013) 47:629–31. doi: 10.1002/mus.23782
10. Vucic S, Nicholson G A, Kiernan MC. Cortical hyperexcitability may precede the onset of familial amyotrophic lateral sclerosis. *Brain* (2008) 131:1540–50. doi: 10.1093/brain/awn071
11. Bede P. Deciphering neurodegeneration. *Neurology* (2017) 89:1758–9. doi: 10.1212/WNL.0000000000 004582
12. Bede P, Querin G, Pradat P-F. The changing landscape of motor neuron disease imaging: the transition from descriptive studies to precision clinical tools. *Curr Opin Neurol.* (2018) 31:431–8. doi: 10.1097/WCO.0000000000000569
13. Kollewe K, Münte TF, Samii A, Dengler R, Petri S, Mohammadi B. Patterns of cortical activity differ in ALS patients with limb and/or bulbar involvement depending on motor tasks. *J Neurol.* (2011) 258:804–10. doi: 10.1007/s00415-010-5842-7
14. Mohammadi B, Kollewe K, Samii A, Dengler R, Münte TF. Functional neuroimaging at different disease stages reveals distinct phases of neuroplastic changes in amyotrophic lateral sclerosis. *Hum Brain Mapp.* (2011) 32:750–8. doi: 10.1002/hbm.21064
15. Poujois A, Schneider FC, Faillenot I, Camdessanché J-P, Vandenberghe N, Thomas-Antérion C, et al. Brain plasticity in the motor network is correlated with disease progression in amyotrophic lateral sclerosis. *Hum Brain Mapp.* (2013) 34:2391–401. doi: 10.1002/hbm.22070
16. Stanton BR, Williams VC, Leigh PN, Williams SCR, Blain CRV, Jarosz JM, et al. Altered cortical activation during a motor task in ALS. Evidence for involvement of central pathways. *J Neurol.* (2007) 254:1260–7. doi: 10.1007/s00415-006-0513-4
17. Konrad C, Jansen A, Henningsen H, Sommer J, Turski PA, Brooks BR, et al. Subcortical reorganization in amyotrophic lateral sclerosis. *Exp Brain Res.* (2006) 172:361–9. doi: 10.1007/s00221-006-0352-7
18. Tessitore A, Esposito F, Monsurrò MR, Graziano S, Panza D, Russo A, et al. Subcortical motor plasticity in patients with sporadic ALS: An fMRI study. *Brain Res Bull.* (2006) 69:489–94. doi: 10.1016/j.brainresbull.2006.01.013
19. Prell T, Grosskreutz J. The involvement of the cerebellum in amyotrophic lateral sclerosis. *Amyotroph Lateral Scler Frontotemporal Degener.* (2013) 14:507–15. doi: 10.3109/21678421.2013.812661
20. Douaud G, Filippini N, Knight S, Talbot K, Turner MR. Integration of structural and functional magnetic resonance imaging in amyotrophic lateral sclerosis. *Brain* (2011) 134:3470–9. doi: 10.1093/brain/awr279
21. Bede P, Hardiman O. Lessons of ALS imaging: pitfalls and future directions - A critical review. *NeuroImage Clin.* (2014) 4:436–43. doi: 10.1016/j.nicl.2014.02.011
22. Buckner RL, Bandettini PA, O'Craven KM, Savoy RL, Petersen SE, Raichle ME, et al. Detection of cortical activation during averaged single trials of a cognitive task using functional magnetic resonance imaging. *Proc Natl Acad Sci USA.* (1996) 93:14878–83. doi: 10.1073/pnas.93.25.14878
23. Ogawa S, Lee T-M, Stepnoski R, Chen W, Zhu X-H, Ugurbil K. An approach to probe some neural systems interaction by functional MRI at neural time scale down to milliseconds. *Proc Natl Acad Sci USA.* (2000) 97:11026–31. doi: 10.1073/pnas.97.20.11026
24. Yang QX, Dardzinski BJ, Li S, Eslinger PJ, Smith MB. Multi-gradient echo with susceptibility inhomogeneity compensation (MGESIC): demonstration of fMRI in the olfactory cortex at 3.0 T. *Magn Reson Med.* (1997) 37:331–5. doi: 10.1002/mrm.1910370304
25. Weiger M, Pruessmann KP, Österbauer R, Börnert P, Boesiger P, Jezzard P. Sensitivity-encoded single-shot spiral imaging for reduced susceptibility artifacts in BOLD fMRI. *Magn Reson Med.* (2002) 48:860–6. doi: 10.1002/mrm.10286
26. Stenger VA, Boada FE, Noll DC. Three-dimensional tailored RF pulses for the reduction of susceptibility artifacts in T2/(*)-weighted functional MRI. *Magn Reson Med.* (2000) 44:525–31. doi: 10.1002/1522-2594(200010)44:4<525::AID-MRM5>3.0.CO;2-L
27. Gaab N, Gabrieli JDE, Glover GH. Resting in peace or noise: Scanner background noise suppresses default-mode network. *Hum Brain Mapp.* (2008) 29:858–67. doi: 10.1002/hbm.20578
28. Gaab N, Gabrieli JDE, Glover GH. Assessing the influence of scanner background noise on auditory processing. I. An fMRI study comparing three experimental designs with varying degrees of scanner noise. *Hum Brain Mapp.* (2007) 28:703–20. doi: 10.1002/hbm.20298
29. Li S, Chen Q, Yu B, Xue K, Luo C, Xu Y, et al. Structural and functional changes mapped in the brains of amyotrophic lateral sclerosis patients with/without dysphagia: A pilot study. *Amyotroph Lateral Scler.* (2009) 10:280–7. doi: 10.3109/17482960902893342
30. Mohammadi B, Kollewe K, Samii A, Krampfl K, Dengler R, Münte TF. Decreased brain activation to tongue movements in amyotrophic lateral sclerosis with bulbar involvement but not Kennedy syndrome. *J Neurol.* (2009) 256:1263–9. doi: 10.1007/s00415-009-5112-8
31. Szameitat AJ, Shen S, Sterr A. Motor imagery of complex everyday movements. An fMRI study. *Neuroimage* (2007) 34:702–13. doi: 10.1016/j.neuroimage.2006.09.033
32. Marchesotti S, Bassolino M, Serino A, Bleuler H, Blanke O. Quantifying the role of motor imagery in brain-machine interfaces. *Sci Rep.* (2016) 6:24076. doi: 10.1038/srep24076
33. Lulé D, Diekmann V, Kassubek J, Kurt A, Birbaumer N, Ludolph AC, et al. Cortical plasticity in amyotrophic lateral sclerosis: motor imagery and function. *Neurorehabil Neural Repair.* (2007) 21:518–26. doi: 10.1177/1545968307300698
34. Stanton BR, Williams VC, Leigh PN, Williams SCR, Blain CRV, Giampietro VP, et al. Cortical activation during motor imagery is reduced in Amyotrophic Lateral Sclerosis. *Brain Res.* (2007) 1172:145–51. doi: 10.1016/j.brainres.2007.07.044
35. Li H, Chen Y, Li Y, Yin B, Tang W, Yu X, et al. Altered cortical activation during action observation in amyotrophic lateral sclerosis patients: a parametric functional MRI study. *Eur Radiol.* (2015) 25:2584–92. doi: 10.1007/s00330-015-3671-x
36. Jelsone-Swain L, Persad C, Burkard D, Welsh RC. Action processing and mirror neuron function in patients with amyotrophic lateral sclerosis: an fMRI study. *PLoS ONE* (2015) 10:e0119862. doi: 10.1371/journal.pone.0119862
37. Lulé D, Diekmann V, Anders S, Kassubek J, Kübler A, Ludolph AC, et al. Brain responses to emotional stimuli in patients with amyotrophic lateral sclerosis (ALS). *J Neurol.* (2007) 254:519–27. doi: 10.1007/s00415-006-0409-3
38. Meoded A, Morrissette AE, Katipally R, Schanz O, Gotts SJ, Floeter MK. Cerebro-cerebellar connectivity is increased in primary lateral sclerosis. *NeuroImage Clin.* (2015) 7:288–96. doi: 10.1016/j.nicl.2014.12.009
39. Menke RAL, Proudfoot M, Talbot K, Turner MR. The two-year progression of structural and functional cerebral MRI in amyotrophic lateral sclerosis. *NeuroImage Clin.* (2018) 17:953–61. doi: 10.1016/j.nicl.2017.12.025
40. Cosottini M, Pesaresi I, Piazza S, Diciotti S, Cecchi P, Fabbri S, et al. Structural and functional evaluation of cortical motor areas in Amyotrophic Lateral Sclerosis. *Exp Neurol.* (2012) 234:169–80. doi: 10.1016/j.expneurol.2011.12.024
41. Bede P, Hardiman O. Longitudinal structural changes in ALS: a three time-point imaging study of white and gray matter

degeneration. *Amyotroph Lateral Scler Front Degener.* (2018) 19:232–41. doi: 10.1080/21678421.2017.1407795
42. Agosta F, Valsasina P, Absinta M, Riva N, Sala S, Prelle A, et al. Sensorimotor functional connectivity changes in amyotrophic lateral sclerosis. *Cereb Cortex* (2011) 21:2291–8. doi: 10.1093/cercor/bhr002
43. Stoppel CM, Vielhaber S, Eckart C, Machts J, Kaufmann J, Heinze H-J, et al. Structural and functional hallmarks of amyotrophic lateral sclerosis progression in motor- and memory-related brain regions. *NeuroImage Clin.* (2014) 5:277–90. doi: 10.1016/j.nicl.2014.07.007
44. Konrad C, Henningsen H, Bremer J, Mock B, Deppe M, Buchinger C, et al. Pattern of cortical reorganization in amyotrophic lateral sclerosis: a functional magnetic resonance imaging study. *Exp brain Res.* (2002) 143:51–6. doi: 10.1007/s00221-001-0981-9
45. Bede P, Omer T, Finegan E, Chipika RH, Iyer PM, Doherty MA, et al. Connectivity-based characterisation of subcortical grey matter pathology in frontotemporal dementia and ALS: a multimodal neuroimaging study. *Brain Imaging Behav.* (2018) 12:1696–1707. doi: 10.1007/s11682-018-9837-9
46. Feron M, Couillandre A, Mseddi E, Termoz N, Abidi M, Bardinet E, et al. Extrapyramidal deficits in ALS: a combined biomechanical and neuroimaging study. *J Neurol.* (2018) 265:1–12. doi: 10.1007/s00415-018-8964-y
47. Schoenfeld MA, Tempelmann C, Gaul C, Kühnel GR, Düzel E, Hopf J-M, et al. Functional motor compensation in amyotrophic lateral sclerosis. *J Neurol.* (2005) 252:944–52. doi: 10.1007/s00415-005-0787-y
48. Han J, Ma L. Functional magnetic resonance imaging study of the brain in patients with amyotrophic lateral sclerosis. *Chinese Med Sci J.* (2006) 21:228–33.
49. Elamin M, Bede P, Byrne S, Jordan N, Gallagher L, Wynne B, et al. Cognitive changes predict functional decline in ALS: a population-based longitudinal study. *Neurology* (2013) 80:1590–7. doi: 10.1212/WNL.0b013e31828f18ac
50. Elamin M, Phukan J, Bede P, Jordan N, Byrne S, Pender N, et al. Executive dysfunction is a negative prognostic indicator in patients with ALS without dementia. *Neurology* (2011) 76:1263–9. doi: 10.1212/WNL.0b013e318214359f
51. Abrahams S, Goldstein LH, Simmons A, Brammer M, Williams SCR, Giampietro V, et al. Word retrieval in amyotrophic lateral sclerosis: a functional magnetic resonance imaging study. *Brain* (2004) 127:1507–17. doi: 10.1093/brain/awh170
52. Goldstein LH, Newsom-Davis IC, Bryant V, Brammer M, Leigh PN, Simmons A. Altered patterns of cortical activation in ALS patients during attention and cognitive response inhibition tasks. *J Neurol.* (2011) 258:2186–98. doi: 10.1007/s00415-011-6088-8
53. Palmieri A, Naccarato M, Abrahams S, Bonato M, D'Ascenzo C, Balestreri S, et al. Right hemisphere dysfunction and emotional processing in ALS: An fMRI study. *J Neurol.* (2010) 257:1970–8. doi: 10.1007/s00415-010-5640-2
54. Vellage AK, Veit M, Kobeleva X, Petri S, Vielhaber S, Müller NG. Working memory network changes in ALS: An fMRI study. *Front Neurosci.* (2016) 10:158. doi: 10.3389/fnins.2016.00158
55. Lulé D, Diekmann V, Müller HP, Kassubek J, Ludolph AC, Birbaumer N. Neuroimaging of multimodal sensory stimulation in amyotrophic lateral sclerosis. *J Neurol Neurosurg Psychiatry* (2010) 81:899–906. doi: 10.1136/jnnp.2009.192260
56. Bede P, Iyer PM, Schuster C, Elamin M, Mclaughlin RL, Kenna K, et al. The selective anatomical vulnerability of ALS: 'disease-defining' and 'disease-defying' brain regions. *Amyotroph Lateral Scler Front Degener.* (2016) 8421:1–10. doi: 10.3109/21678421.2016.1173702
57. Witiuk K, Fernandez-Ruiz J, McKee R, Alahyane N, Coe BC, Melanson M, et al. Cognitive deterioration and functional compensation in ALS measured with fMRI using an inhibitory task. *J Neurosci.* (2014) 34:14260–71. doi: 10.1523/JNEUROSCI.1111-14.2014
58. Keller J, Böhm S, Aho-Özhan HEA, Loose M, Gorges M, Kassubek J, et al. Functional reorganization during cognitive function tasks in patients with amyotrophic lateral sclerosis. *Brain Imaging Behav.* (2018) 12:771–84. doi: 10.1007/s11682-017-9738-3
59. Passamonti L, Fera F, Tessitore A, Russo A, Cerasa A, Gioia CM, et al. Dysfunctions within limbic-motor networks in amyotrophic lateral sclerosis. *Neurobiol Aging* (2013) 34:2499–509. doi: 10.1016/j.neurobiolaging.2013.05.016
60. Aho-Özhan HEA, Keller J, Heimrath J, Uttner I, Kassubek J, Birbaumer N, et al. Perception of emotional facial expressions in amyotrophic lateral sclerosis (ALS) at behavioural and brain metabolic level. *PLoS ONE* (2016) 11:e0164655. doi: 10.1371/journal.pone.0164655
61. Mohammadi B, Kollewe K, Cole DM, Fellbrich A, Heldmann M, Samii A, et al. Amyotrophic lateral sclerosis affects cortical and subcortical activity underlying motor inhibition and action monitoring. *Hum Brain Mapp.* (2015) 36:2878–89. doi: 10.1002/hbm.22814
62. Turner MR, Grosskreutz J, Kassubek J, Abrahams S, Agosta F, Benatar M, et al. Towards a neuroimaging biomarker for amyotrophic lateral sclerosis. *Lancet Neurol.* (2011) 10:400–3. doi: 10.1016/S1474-4422(11)70049-7
63. Müller H-P, Turner MR, Grosskreutz J, Abrahams S, Bede P, Govind V, et al. A large-scale multicentre cerebral diffusion tensor imaging study in amyotrophic lateral sclerosis. *J Neurol Neurosurg Psychiatry* (2016) 87:570–9. doi: 10.1136/jnnp-2015-311952
64. Dansereau C, Benhajali Y, Risterucci C, Pich EM, Orban P, Arnold D, et al. Statistical power and prediction accuracy in multisite resting-state fMRI connectivity. *Neuroimage* (2017) 149:220–32. doi: 10.1016/J.NEUROIMAGE.2017.01.072
65. Agosta F, Canu E, Valsasina P, Riva N, Prelle A, Comi G, et al. Divergent brain network connectivity in amyotrophic lateral sclerosis. *Neurobiol Aging* (2013) 34:419–27. doi: 10.1016/j.neurobiolaging.2012.04.015
66. Mohammadi B, Kollewe K, Samii A, Krampfl K, Dengler R, Münte TF. Changes of resting state brain networks in amyotrophic lateral sclerosis. *Exp Neurol.* (2009) 217:147–53. doi: 10.1016/j.expneurol.2009.01.025
67. Welsh RC, Jelsone-Swain LM, Foerster BR. The utility of independent component analysis and machine learning in the identification of the amyotrophic lateral sclerosis diseased brain. *Front Hum Neurosci.* (2013) 7:251. doi: 10.3389/fnhum.2013.00251
68. Li W, Zhang J, Zhou C, Hou W, Hu J, Feng H, et al. Abnormal functional connectivity density in amyotrophic lateral sclerosis. *Front Aging Neurosci.* (2018) 10:215. doi: 10.3389/fnagi.2018.00215
69. Zhou C, Hu X, Hu J, Liang M, Yin X, Chen L, et al. Altered brain network in amyotrophic lateral sclerosis: a resting graph theory-based network study at voxel-wise level. *Front Neurosci.* (2016) 10:204. doi: 10.3389/fnins.2016.00204
70. Sako W, Abe T, Izumi Y, Yamazaki H, Matsui N, Harada M, et al. Spontaneous brain activity in the sensorimotor cortex in amyotrophic lateral sclerosis can be negatively regulated by corticospinal fiber integrity. *Neurol Sci.* (2017) 38:755–60. doi: 10.1007/s10072-017-2831-y
71. Luo C, Chen Q, Huang R, Chen X, Chen K, Huang X, et al. Patterns of spontaneous brain activity in amyotrophic lateral sclerosis: a resting-state fMRI study. *PLoS ONE* (2012) 7:e45470. doi: 10.1371/journal.pone.0045470
72. Trojsi F, Di Nardo F, Santangelo G, Siciliano M, Femiano C, Passaniti C, et al. Resting state fMRI correlates of theory of mind impairment in amyotrophic lateral sclerosis. *Cortex* (2017) 97:1–16. doi: 10.1016/j.cortex.2017.09.016
73. Zhou F, Xu R, Dowd E, Zang Y, Gong H, Wang Z. Alterations in regional functional coherence within the sensory-motor network in amyotrophic lateral sclerosis. *Neurosci Lett.* (2014) 558:192–6. doi: 10.1016/j.neulet.2013.11.022
74. Zhang J, Ji B, Hu J, Zhou C, Li L, Li Z, et al. Aberrant interhemispheric homotopic functional and structural connectivity in amyotrophic lateral sclerosis. *J Neurol Neurosurg Psychiatry* (2017) 88:369.1–70. doi: 10.1136/jnnp-2016-314567
75. Chenji S, Jha S, Lee D, Brown M, Seres P, Mah D, et al. Investigating default mode and sensorimotor network connectivity in amyotrophic lateral sclerosis. *PLoS ONE* (2016) 11:e0157443. doi: 10.1371/journal.pone.0157443
76. Fekete T, Zach N, Mujica-Parodi LR, Turner MR. Multiple kernel learning captures a systems-level functional connectivity biomarker signature in amyotrophic lateral sclerosis. *PLoS ONE* (2013) 8:e85190. doi: 10.1371/journal.pone.0085190
77. Schmidt R, Verstraete E, de Reus MA, Veldink JH, van den Berg LH, van den Heuvel MP. Correlation between structural and functional connectivity impairment in amyotrophic lateral sclerosis. *Hum Brain Mapp.* (2014) 35:4386–95. doi: 10.1002/hbm.22481
78. Schuster C, Elamin M, Hardiman O, Bede P. Presymptomatic and longitudinal neuroimaging in neurodegeneration–from snapshots to motion

picture: a systematic review. *J Neurol Neurosurg Psychiatry* (2015) 86:1089–96. doi: 10.1136/jnnp-2014-309888

79. Menke RAL, Proudfoot M, Wuu J, Andersen PM, Talbot K, Benatar M, et al. Increased functional connectivity common to symptomatic amyotrophic lateral sclerosis and those at genetic risk. *J Neurol Neurosurg Psychiatry* (2016) 87:580–8. doi: 10.1136/jnnp-2015-311945
80. Lee SE, Sias AC, Mandelli ML, Brown JA, Brown AB, Khazenzon AM, et al. Network degeneration and dysfunction in presymptomatic C9ORF72 expansion carriers. *NeuroImage Clin.* (2017) 14:286–97. doi: 10.1016/j.nicl.2016.12.006
81. Verstraete E, Turner MR, Grosskreutz J, Filippi M, Benatar M. Mind the gap: The mismatch between clinical and imaging metrics in ALS. *Amyotroph Lateral Scler Front Degener.* (2015) 16:524–9. doi: 10.3109/21678421.2015.1051989
82. Zhou F, Gong H, Li F, Zhuang Y, Zang Y, Xu R, et al. Altered motor network functional connectivity in amyotrophic lateral sclerosis: a resting-state functional magnetic resonance imaging study. *Neuroreport* (2013) 24:657–62. doi: 10.1097/WNR.0b013e328363148c
83. Geevasinga N, Korgaonkar MS, Menon P, Van den Bos M, Gomes L, Foster S, et al. Brain functional connectome abnormalities in amyotrophic lateral sclerosis are associated with disability and cortical hyperexcitability. *Eur J Neurol.* (2017) 24:1507–17. doi: 10.1111/ene.13461
84. Jelsone-Swain LM, Fling BW, Seidler RD, Hovatter R, Gruis K, Welsh RC. Reduced interhemispheric functional connectivity in the motor cortex during rest in limb-onset amyotrophic lateral sclerosis. *Front Syst Neurosci.* (2010) 4:158. doi: 10.3389/fnsys.2010.00158
85. Verstraete E, van den Heuvel MP, Veldink JH, Blanken N, Mandl RC, Hulshoff Pol HE, et al. Motor network degeneration in amyotrophic lateral sclerosis: a structural and functional connectivity study. *PLoS ONE* (2010) 5:e13664. doi: 10.1371/journal.pone.0013664
86. Proudfoot M, Jones A, Talbot K, Al-Chalabi A, Turner MR. The ALSFRS as an outcome measure in therapeutic trials and its relationship to symptom onset. *Amyotroph Lateral Scler Frontotemporal Degener.* (2016) 17:414–25. doi: 10.3109/21678421.2016.1140786
87. Fries P. Rhythms for cognition: communication through coherence. *Neuron* (2015) 88:220–35. doi: 10.1016/j.neuron.2015.09.034
88. Voytek B, Knight RT. Dynamic network communication as a unifying neural basis for cognition, development, aging, and disease. *Biol Psychiatry* (2015) 77:1089–97. doi: 10.1016/j.biopsych.2015.04.016
89. Lopes da Silva F. EEG and MEG: relevance to neuroscience. *Neuron* (2013) 80:1112–28. doi: 10.1016/j.neuron.2013.10.017
90. Proudfoot M, Woolrich MW, Nobre AC, Turner MR. Magnetoencephalography. *Pract Neurol.* (2014) 14:336–43. doi: 10.1136/practneurol-2013-000768
91. Hall EL, Robson SE, Morris PG, Brookes MJ. The relationship between MEG and fMRI. *Neuroimage* (2014) 102:80–91. doi: 10.1016/j.neuroimage.2013.11.005
92. Gross J, Baillet S, Barnes GR, Henson RN, Hillebrand A, Jensen O, et al. Good practice for conducting and reporting MEG research. *Neuroimage* (2013) 65:349–63. doi: 10.1016/j.neuroimage.2012.10.001
93. Hari R, Baillet S, Barnes G, Burgess R, Forss N, Gross J, et al. IFCN-endorsed practical guidelines for clinical magnetoencephalography (MEG). *Clin Neurophysiol.* (2018) 129:1720–47. doi: 10.1016/j.clinph.2018.03.042
94. van Diessen E, Numan T, van Dellen E, van der Kooi AW, Boersma M, Hofman D, et al. Opportunities and methodological challenges in EEG and MEG resting state functional brain network research. *Clin Neurophysiol.* (2015) 126:1468–81. doi: 10.1016/j.clinph.2014.11.018
95. Bosch EP, Yamada T, Kimura J. Somatosensory evoked potentials in motor neuron disease. *Muscle Nerve* (1985) 8:556–62. doi: 10.1002/mus.880080703
96. Ghezzi A, Mazzalovo E, Locatelli C, Zibetti A, Zaffaroni M, Montanini R. Multimodality evoked potentials in amyotrophic lateral sclerosis. *Acta Neurol Scand.* (1989) 79:353–6. doi: 10.1111/j.1600-0404.1989.tb03799.x
97. Radtke RA, Erwin A, Erwin CW. Abnormal sensory evoked potentials in amyotrophic lateral sclerosis. *Neurology* (1986) 36:796–801. doi: 10.1212/WNL.36.6.796
98. Cosi V, Poloni M, Mazzini L, Callieco R. Somatosensory evoked potentials in amyotrophic lateral sclerosis. *J Neurol Neurosurg Psychiatry* (1984) 47:857–61. doi: 10.1136/jnnp.47.8.857
99. Subramaniam JS, Yiannikas C. Multimodality evoked potentials in motor neuron disease. *Arch Neurol.* (1990) 47:989–94. doi: 10.1001/archneur.1990.00530090063014
100. Soares JJF, Lawoko S, Nolan P. The nature, extent and determinants of violence against psychiatric personnel. *Work Stress* (2000) 14:105–20. doi: 10.1080/026783700750051630
101. Iglesias C, Sangari S, El Mendili M-M, Benali H, Marchand-Pauvert V, Pradat P-F. Electrophysiological and spinal imaging evidences for sensory dysfunction in amyotrophic lateral sclerosis. *BMJ Open* (2015) 5:e007659. doi: 10.1136/bmjopen-2015-007659
102. Sangari S, Iglesias C, El Mendili MM, Benali H, Pradat PF, Marchand-Pauvert V. Impairment of sensory-motor integration at spinal level in amyotrophic lateral sclerosis. *Clin Neurophysiol.* (2016) 127:1968–77. doi: 10.1016/j.clinph.2016.01.014
103. Raggi A, Iannaccone S, Cappa SF. Event-related brain potentials in amyotrophic lateral sclerosis: a review of the international literature. *Amyotroph Lateral Scler.* (2010) 11:16–26. doi: 10.3109/174829609029 12399
104. Westphal KP, Heinemann HA, Grözinger B, Kotchoubey BJ, Diekmann V, Becker W, et al. Bereitschaftspotential in amyotrophic lateral sclerosis (ALS): lower amplitudes in patients with hyperreflexia (spasticity). *Acta Neurol Scand.* (1998) 98:15–21. doi: 10.1111/j.1600-0404.1998.tb07372.x
105. Thorns J, Wieringa BM, Mohammadi B, Hammer A, Dengler R, Münte TF. Movement initiation and inhibition are impaired in amyotrophic lateral sclerosis. *Exp Neurol.* (2010) 224:389–94. doi: 10.1016/j.expneurol.2010.04.014
106. Bizovičar N, Koritnik B, Zidar I, Dreo J, Zidar J. Movement-related cortical potentials in ALS increase at lower and decrease at higher upper motor neuron burden scores. *Amyotroph Lateral Scler Frontotemporal Degener.* (2013) 14:380–9. doi: 10.3109/21678421.2012.760604
107. Inuggi A, Riva N, González-Rosa JJ, Amadio S, Amato N, Fazio R, et al. Compensatory movement-related recruitment in amyotrophic lateral sclerosis patients with dominant upper motor neuron signs: an EEG source analysis study. *Brain Res.* (2011) 1425:37–46. doi: 10.1016/j.brainres.2011.09.007
108. Gu Y, Farina D, Murguialday AR, Dremstrup K, Birbaumer N. Comparison of movement related cortical potential in healthy people and amyotrophic lateral sclerosis patients. *Front Neurosci.* (2013) 7:65. doi: 10.3389/fnins.2013.00065
109. Pfurtscheller G, Lopes Da Silva FH. Event-related EEG/MEG synchronization and desynchronization: basic principles. *Clin Neurophysiol.* (1999) 110:1842–57. doi: 10.1016/S1388-2457(99)00141-8
110. Vansteensel MJ, Pels EGM, Bleichner MG, Branco MP, Denison T, Freudenburg Z V, et al. Fully implanted brain–computer interface in a locked-in patient with ALS. *N Engl J Med.* (2016) 375:2060–6. doi: 10.1056/NEJMoa1608085
111. Kilavik BE, Zaepffel M, Brovelli A, MacKay WA, Riehle A. The ups and downs of β oscillations in sensorimotor cortex. *Exp Neurol.* (2013) 245:15–26. doi: 10.1016/j.expneurol.2012.09.014
112. Chen R, Yaseen Z, Cohen LG, Hallett M. Time course of corticospinal excitability in reaction time and self-paced movements. *Ann Neurol.* (1998) 44:317–25. doi: 10.1002/ana.410440306
113. Stančák A, Riml A, Pfurtscheller G. The effects of external load on movement-related changes of the sensorimotor EEG rhythms. *Electroencephalogr Clin Neurophysiol.* (1997) 102:495–504. doi: 10.1016/S0013-4694(96)96623-0
114. Toma K, Mima T, Matsuoka T, Gerloff C, Ohnishi T, Koshy B, et al. Movement rate effect on activation and functional coupling of motor cortical areas. *J Neurophysiol.* (2002) 88:3377–85. doi: 10.1152/jn.0028 1.2002
115. Hummel F, Kirsammer R, Gerloff C. Ipsilateral cortical activation during finger sequences of increasing complexity: representation of movement difficulty or memory load? *Clin Neurophysiol.* (2003) 114:605–13. doi: 10.1016/S1388-2457(02)00417-0
116. Hall SD, Stanford IM, Yamawaki N, McAllister CJ, Rönnqvist KC, Woodhall GL, et al. The role of GABAergic modulation in motor function related neuronal network activity. *Neuroimage* (2011) 56:1506–10. doi: 10.1016/j.neuroimage.2011.02.025

117. Muthukumaraswamy SD, Myers JFM, Wilson SJ, Nutt DJ, Lingford-Hughes A, Singh KD, et al. The effects of elevated endogenous GABA levels on movement-related network oscillations. *Neuroimage* (2012) 66C:36–41. doi: 10.1016/j.neuroimage.2012.10.054
118. Little S, Pogosyan A, Kuhn AA, Brown P. Beta band stability over time correlates with Parkinsonian rigidity and bradykinesia. *Exp Neurol.* (2012) 236:383–8. doi: 10.1016/j.expneurol.2012.04.024
119. Riva N, Falini A, Inuggi A, Gonzalez-Rosa JJ, Amadio S, Cerri F, et al. Cortical activation to voluntary movement in amyotrophic lateral sclerosis is related to corticospinal damage: electrophysiological evidence. *Clin Neurophysiol.* (2012) 123:1586–92. doi: 10.1016/j.clinph.2011.12.013
120. Bizovičar N, Dreo J, Koritnik B, Zidar J. Decreased movement-related beta desynchronization and impaired post-movement beta rebound in amyotrophic lateral sclerosis. *Clin Neurophysiol.* (2014) 125:1689–99. doi: 10.1016/j.clinph.2013.12.108
121. Cheyne DO. MEG studies of sensorimotor rhythms: a review. *Exp Neurol.* (2013) 245:27–39. doi: 10.1016/j.expneurol.2012.08.030
122. Proudfoot M, Rohenkohl G, Quinn A, Colclough GL, Wuu J, Talbot K, et al. Altered cortical beta-band oscillations reflect motor system degeneration in amyotrophic lateral sclerosis. *Hum Brain Mapp.* (2017) 38:237–54. doi: 10.1002/hbm.23357
123. Vucic S, Ziemann U, Eisen A, Hallett M, Kiernan MC. Transcranial magnetic stimulation and amyotrophic lateral sclerosis: pathophysiological insights. *J Neurol Neurosurg Psychiatry* (2013) 84:1161–70. doi: 10.1136/jnnp-2012-304019
124. Turner MR, Hammers A, Al-Chalabi A, Shaw CE, Andersen PM, Brooks DJ, et al. Distinct cerebral lesions in sporadic and "D90A" SOD1 ALS: studies with [11C]flumazenil PET. *Brain* (2005) 128:1323–9. doi: 10.1093/brain/awh509
125. Baker SN, Kilner JM, Pinches EM, Lemon RN. The role of synchrony and oscillations in the motor output. *Exp. Brain Res.* 128, 109–17. doi: 10.1007/s002210050825
126. Proudfoot M, van Ede F, Quinn A, Colclough GL, Wuu J, Talbot K, et al. Impaired corticomuscular and interhemispheric cortical beta oscillation coupling in amyotrophic lateral sclerosis. *Clin Neurophysiol.* (2018) 129:1479–89. doi: 10.1016/j.clinph.2018.03.019
127. Kristeva R, Patino L, Omlor W. Beta-range cortical motor spectral power and corticomuscular coherence as a mechanism for effective corticospinal interaction during steady-state motor output. *Neuroimage* (2007) 36:785–92. doi: 10.1016/j.neuroimage.2007.03.025
128. Fisher KM, Zaaimi B, Williams TL, Baker SN, Baker MR. Beta-band intermuscular coherence: a novel biomarker of upper motor neuron dysfunction in motor neuron disease. *Brain* (2012) 135:2849–64. doi: 10.1093/brain/aws150
129. Hanagasi HA, Gurvit IH, Ermutlu N, Kaptanoglu G, Karamursel S, Idrisoglu HA, et al. Cognitive impairment in amyotrophic lateral sclerosis: evidence from neuropsychological investigation and event-related potentials. *Cogn Brain Res.* (2002) 14:234–44. doi: 10.1016/S0926-6410(02)00 110-6
130. Pekkonen E, Osipova D, Laaksovirta H. Magnetoencephalographic evidence of abnormal auditory processing in amyotrophic lateral sclerosis with bulbar signs. *Clin Neurophysiol.* (2004) 115:309–15. doi: 10.1016/S1388-2457(03)00360-2
131. Raggi A, Consonni M, Iannaccone S, Perani D, Zamboni M, Sferrazza B, et al. Auditory event-related potentials in non-demented patients with sporadic amyotrophic lateral sclerosis. *Clin Neurophysiol.* (2008) 119:342–50. doi: 10.1016/j.clinph.2007.10.010
132. Mannarelli D, Pauletti C, Locuratolo N, Vanacore N, Frasca V, Trebbastoni A, et al. Attentional processing in bulbar- and spinal-onset amyotrophic lateral sclerosis: insights from event-related potentials. *Amyotroph Lateral Scler Frontotemporal Degener.* (2014) 15:30–8. doi: 10.3109/21678421.2013.787628
133. Volpato C, Piccione F, Silvoni S, Cavinato M, Palmieri A, Meneghello F, et al. Working memory in amyotrophic lateral sclerosis: auditory event-related potentials and neuropsychological evidence. *J Clin Neurophysiol.* (2010) 27:198–206. doi: 10.1097/WNP.0b013e3181e0aa14
134. Zaehle T, Becke A, Naue N, Machts J, Abdulla S, Petri S, et al. Working memory in ALS patients: preserved performance but marked changes in underlying neuronal networks. *PLoS ONE* (2013) 8:e71973. doi: 10.1371/journal.pone.0071973
135. Pinkhardt EH, Jürgens R, Becker W, Mölle M, Born J, Ludolph AC, et al. Signs of impaired selective attention in patients with amyotrophic lateral sclerosis. *J Neurol.* (2008) 255:532–8. doi: 10.1007/s00415-008-0734-9
136. Volpato C, Prats Sedano MA, Silvoni S, Segato N, Cavinato M, Merico A, et al. Selective attention impairment in amyotrophic lateral sclerosis. *Amyotroph Lateral Scler Front Degener.* (2016) 17:236–44. doi: 10.3109/21678421.2016.1143514
137. Seer C, Fürkötter S, Vogts M-B, Lange F, Abdulla S, Dengler R, et al. Executive dysfunctions and event-related brain potentials in patients with amyotrophic lateral sclerosis. *Front Aging Neurosci.* (2015) 7:225. doi: 10.3389/fnagi.2015.00225
138. Seer C, Joop M, Lange F, Lange C, Dengler R, Petri S, et al. Attenuated error-related potentials in amyotrophic lateral sclerosis with executive dysfunctions. *Clin Neurophysiol.* (2017) 128:1496–503. doi: 10.1016/j.clinph.2017.05.007
139. Goldstein LH, Abrahams S. Changes in cognition and behaviour in amyotrophic lateral sclerosis: nature of impairment and implications for assessment. *Lancet Neurol.* (2013) 12:368–80. doi: 10.1016/S1474-4422(13)70026-7
140. Lange F, Lange C, Joop M, Seer C, Dengler R, Kopp B, et al. Neural correlates of cognitive set shifting in amyotrophic lateral sclerosis. *Clin Neurophysiol.* (2016) 127:3537–45. doi: 10.1016/j.clinph.2016.09.019
141. Blain-Moraes S, Mashour GA, Lee H, Huggins JE, Lee U. Altered cortical communication in amyotrophic lateral sclerosis. *Neurosci Lett.* (2013) 543:172–6. doi: 10.1016/j.neulet.2013.03.028
142. Gallassi R, Montagna P, Morreale A, Lorusso S, Tinuper P, Daidone R, et al. Neuropsychological, electroencephalogram and brain computed tomography findings in motor neuron disease. *Eur Neurol.* (1989) 29:115–20. doi: 10.1159/000116391
143. Mai R, Facchetti D, Micheli A, Poloni M. Quantitative electroencephalography in amyotrophic lateral sclerosis. *Electroencephalogr Clin Neurophysiol.* (1998) 106:383–6. doi: 10.1016/S0013-4694(97)00159-4
144. Santhosh J, Bhatia M, Sahu S, Anand S. Decreased electroencephalogram alpha band [8-13 Hz] power in amyotrophic lateral sclerosis patients: a study of alpha activity in an awake relaxed state. *Neurol India* (2005) 53:99–101. doi: 10.4103/0028-3886.15071
145. Jayaram V, Widmann N, Förster C, Fomina T, Hohmann M, Müller Vom Hagen J, et al. Brain-computer interfacing in amyotrophic lateral sclerosis: Implications of a resting-state EEG analysis. *Conf Proc.* (2015) 2015:6979–82. doi: 10.1109/EMBC.2015.7319998
146. Kopell NJ, Gritton HJ, Whittington MA, Kramer MA. Beyond the connectome: the dynome. *Neuron* (2014) 83:1319–28. doi: 10.1016/j.neuron.2014.08.016
147. Iyer PM, Egan C, Pinto-Grau M, Burke T, Elamin M, Nasseroleslami B, et al. Functional connectivity changes in resting-state EEG as potential biomarker for amyotrophic lateral sclerosis. *PLoS ONE* (2015) 10:e0128682. doi: 10.1371/journal.pone.0128682
148. Nasseroleslami B, Dukic S, Broderick M, Mohr K, Schuster C, Gavin B, et al. Characteristic increases in EEG connectivity correlate with changes of structural MRI in amyotrophic lateral sclerosis. *Cereb Cortex* (2017) 29:27–41. doi: 10.1093/cercor/bhx301
149. Fraschini M, Demuru M, Hillebrand A, Cuccu L, Porcu S, Di Stefano F, et al. EEG functional network topology is associated with disability in patients with amyotrophic lateral sclerosis. *Sci Rep.* (2016) 6:38653. doi: 10.1038/srep38653
150. Fraschini M, Lai M, Demuru M, Puligheddu M, Floris G, Borghero G, et al. Functional brain connectivity analysis in amyotrophic lateral sclerosis: an EEG source-space study. *Biomed Phys Eng Express* (2018) 4:037004. doi: 10.1088/2057-1976/aa9c64
151. Proudfoot M, Colclough GL, Quinn A, Wuu J, Talbot K, Benatar M, et al. Increased cerebral functional connectivity in ALS: a resting-state magnetoencephalography study. *Neurology* (2018) 90:e1418–24. doi: 10.1212/WNL.0000000000005333
152. Loewe K, Machts J, Kaufmann J, Petri S, Heinze H-J, Borgelt C, et al. Widespread temporo-occipital lobe dysfunction in amyotrophic lateral sclerosis. *Sci Rep.* (2017) 7:40252. doi: 10.1038/srep40252

153. Höller Y, Uhl A, Bathke A, Thomschewski A, Butz K, Nardone R, et al. Reliability of EEG measures of interaction: a paradigm shift is needed to fight the reproducibility crisis. *Front Hum Neurosci.* (2017) 11:1–15. doi: 10.3389/fnhum.2017.00441
154. Sorrentino P, Rucco R, Jacini F, Trojsi F, Lardone A, Baselice F, et al. Brain functional networks become more connected as amyotrophic lateral sclerosis progresses: a source level magnetoencephalographic study. *NeuroImage Clin.* (2018) 20:564–71. doi: 10.1016/j.nicl.2018.08.001
155. Cope TE, Sohoglu E, Sedley W, Patterson K, Jones PS, Wiggins J, et al. Evidence for causal top-down frontal contributions to predictive processes in speech perception. *Nat Commun.* (2017) 8:2154. doi: 10.1038/s41467-017-01958-7
156. Baillet S. Magnetoencephalography for brain electrophysiology and imaging. *Nat Neurosci.* (2017) 20:327–39. doi: 10.1038/nn.4504
157. Boto E, Holmes N, Leggett J, Roberts G, Shah V, Meyer SS, et al. Moving magnetoencephalography towards real-world applications with a wearable system. *Nature* (2018) 555:657–61. doi: 10.1038/nature26147
158. Bede P, Bokde ALW, Byrne S, Elamin M, Fagan AJ, Hardiman O. Spinal cord markers in ALS: diagnostic and biomarker considerations. *Amyotroph Lateral Scler.* (2012) 13:407–15. doi: 10.3109/17482968.2011.649760
159. Lawrence J, Stroman PW, Malisza KL. Functional MRI of the cervical spinal cord during noxious and innocuous thermal stimulation in the alpha-chloralose- and halothane-anesthetized rat. *Magn Reson Imaging* (2008) 26:1–10. doi: 10.1016/j.mri.2007.05.001
160. Malisza KL, Stroman PW. Functional imaging of the rat cervical spinal cord. *J Magn Reson Imaging* (2002) 16:553–8. doi: 10.1002/jmri.10185
161. Stroman PW, Krause V, Malisza KL, Frankenstein UN, Tomanek B. Functional magnetic resonance imaging of the human cervical spinal cord with stimulation of different sensory dermatomes. *Magn Reson Imaging* (2002) 20:1–6. doi: 10.1016/S0730-725X(02)00468-X
162. Kornelsen J, Stroman PW. fMRI of the lumbar spinal cord during a lower limb motor task. *Magn Reson Med.* (2004) 52:411–4. doi: 10.1002/mrm.20157
163. Agosta F, Valsasina P, Caputo D, Stroman PW, Filippi M. Tactile-associated recruitment of the cervical cord is altered in patients with multiple sclerosis. *Neuroimage* (2008) 39:1542–8. doi: 10.1016/J.NEUROIMAGE.2007.10.048
164. Stroman PW, Kornelsen J, Bergman A, Krause V, Ethans K, Malisza KL, et al. Noninvasive assessment of the injured human spinal cord by means of functional magnetic resonance imaging. *Spinal Cord.* (2004) 42:59–66. doi: 10.1038/sj.sc.3101559
165. Eippert F, Kong Y, Winkler AM, Andersson JL, Finsterbusch J, Büchel C, et al. Investigating resting-state functional connectivity in the cervical spinal cord at 3T. *Neuroimage* (2017) 147:589–601. doi: 10.1016/j.neuroimage.2016.12.072
166. Zhang Y, Fang T, Wang Y, Guo X, Alarefi A, Wang J, et al. Occipital cortical gyrification reductions associate with decreased functional connectivity in amyotrophic lateral sclerosis. *Brain Imaging Behav.* (2017) 11:1–7. doi: 10.1007/s11682-015-9499-9
167. Bueno APA, Pinaya WHL, Moura LM, Bertoux M, Radakovic R, Kiernan MC, et al. Structural and functional papez circuits integrity in amyotrophic lateral sclerosis. *Brain Imaging Behav.* (2018) 12:1622–30. doi: 10.1007/s11682-018-9825-0

16

A Systematic Review of Suggested Molecular Strata, Biomarkers and their Tissue Sources in ALS

*Udaya Geetha Vijayakumar†, Vanessa Milla†, Mei Yu Cynthia Stafford, Anthony J. Bjourson, William Duddy and Stephanie Marie-Rose Duguez**

Northern Ireland Center for Stratified Medicine, Biomedical Sciences Research Institute, Londonderry, United Kingdom

***Correspondence:**
Stephanie Duguez
s.duguez@ulster.ac.uk

† These authors have contributed equally to this work

Amyotrophic lateral sclerosis (ALS), also known as motor neuron disease, is an incurable neurodegenerative condition, characterized by the loss of upper and lower motor neurons. It affects 1–1.8/100,000 individuals worldwide, and the number of cases is projected to increase as the population ages. Thus, there is an urgent need to identify both therapeutic targets and disease-specific biomarkers–biomarkers that would be useful to diagnose and stratify patients into different sub-groups for therapeutic strategies, as well as biomarkers to follow the efficacy of any treatment tested during clinical trials. There is a lack of knowledge about pathogenesis and many hypotheses. Numerous "omics" studies have been conducted on ALS in the past decade to identify a disease-signature in tissues and circulating biomarkers. The first goal of the present review was to group the molecular pathways that have been implicated in monogenic forms of ALS, to enable the description of patient strata corresponding to each pathway grouping. This strategy allowed us to suggest 14 strata, each potentially targetable by different pharmacological strategies. The second goal of this review was to identify diagnostic/prognostic biomarker candidates consistently observed across the literature. For this purpose, we explore previous biomarker-relevant "omics" studies of ALS and summarize their findings, focusing on potential circulating biomarker candidates. We systematically review 118 papers on biomarkers published during the last decade. Several candidate markers were consistently shared across the results of different studies in either cerebrospinal fluid (CSF) or blood (leukocyte or serum/plasma). Although these candidates still need to be validated in a systematic manner, we suggest the use of combinations of biomarkers that would likely reflect the "health status" of different tissues, including motor neuron health (e.g., pNFH and NF-L, cystatin C, Transthyretin), inflammation status (e.g., MCP-1, miR451), muscle health (miR-338-3p, miR-206) and metabolism (homocysteine, glutamate, cholesterol). In light of these studies and because ALS is increasingly perceived as a multi-system disease, the identification of a panel of biomarkers that accurately reflect features of pathology is a priority, not only for diagnostic purposes but also for prognostic or predictive applications.

Keywords: circulating biomarkers, ALS, patients stratification, multi-system biomarkers, motor neuron disease

INTRODUCTION

Amyotrophic lateral sclerosis (ALS) is a fatal neurological disorder with an adult onset around 54-67 years old (1). Its clinical hallmark is the degeneration of both upper and lower motor neurons (2, 3), leading to progressive muscle atrophy and weakness, and ultimately to paralysis. Death, often resulting from swallowing problems and respiratory failure (4, 5), generally occurs within 2–4 years from disease onset (6–8), although 5–10% of ALS patients survive over 10 years (7). ALS has a median incidence of about 2.8 cases per 100,000 persons per year and a median prevalence about 5.4 cases per 100,000 persons for a median age at 61.8 ± 3.8 years (1). The incidence and prevalence thus increases with age and reaches a cumulative lifetime risk of 1 in 400 after 80 years old (9, 10). Due to the projected aging of the global population, ALS cases are expected to increase by 69% in the next 25 years (11), underlining the urgent need to identify causes, biomarkers and therapeutic targets for ALS.

The causes of ALS are largely unknown, with ~90% of cases being sporadic (sALS) while only ~10% are familial ALS (fALS) (12). Intensive research since the 1990's has aimed to unravel the mechanisms involved in motor neuron degeneration. These studies suggest that ALS is a complex disease driven by a combination of several systemic parameters. To date, up to 30 genes (**Figure 1**) are described as monogenic causes of ALS, with the most frequent being C9orf72, SOD1, FUS, and TARDBP/TDP43 (13–15). In motor neurons, these identified mutations are functionally associated with an alteration of electrophysiological properties (16), accumulation of stress marks (17) and sensitivity to stress (18) (**Figure 2**). However, these monogenic forms

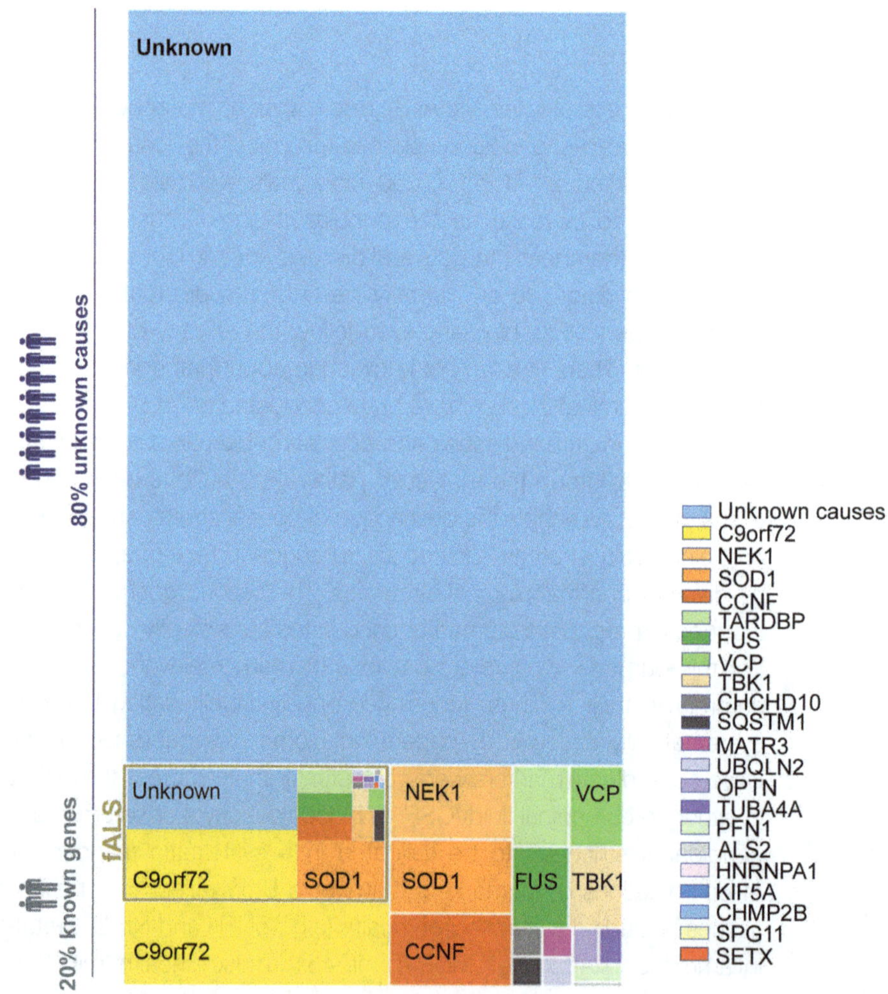

FIGURE 1 | Distribution of genetic basis among the ALS population. A treemap representation of the proportion of ALS patients carrying known causative mutation. The full rectangle represents 100% of all ALS cases. The fALS are highlighted in gold with a frequency adjusted to represent 7.5% of the total (as fALS is estimated at 5–10% of all ALS cases). The two light blue blocks represent those with no known ALS-associated gene mutation among sporadic and familial cases. Cases with known mutations are represented in the other blocks, broken down by affected gene. The color code for each gene is preserved between familial and sporadic cases. The size of each block is proportional to the percentage of ALS associated to the considered genes–proportions given in Volk et al. (13). Overall, some 80% of ALS cases (sALS and fALS combined) are not explained by a known mutation.

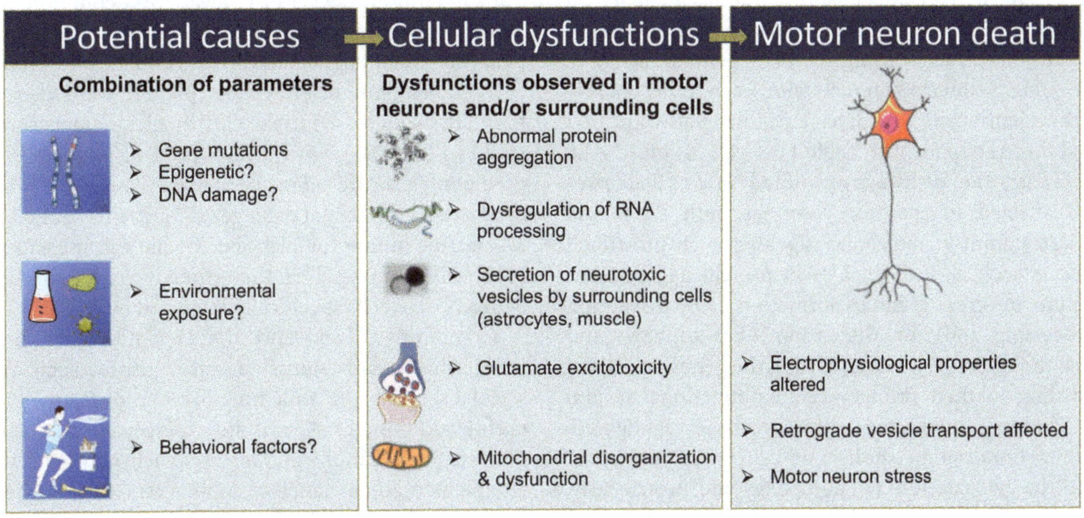

FIGURE 2 | Sequential events that could be involved in motor neuron death in ALS. Gene mutations, epigenetic changes, or DNA damage that occur either spontaneously or due to environmental risk factors such as exposure to toxins or infectious agents, or behavioral factors, have all been proposed as potentially leading to cellular dysfunction (9, 13, 14, 20–23). Cellular dysfunction could include abnormal protein aggregations, alteration of RNA processing, secretion of neurotoxic vesicles by surrounding cells such as astrocyte, muscle cells, glutamate excitotoxicity, and mitochondrial disorganization and dysfunction leading to oxidative stress (24–30). These cellular dysfunctions may take place in motor neurons and/or surrounding cells and, combined or alone, could lead to an alteration of the electrophysiological properties of the motor neuron, and/or to an induction of secretion of neurotoxic elements by surrounding cells, in either case ultimately leading to motor neuron death (16–18).

explain only 15% of sporadic cases and 66% of familial cases (12) (**Figure 1**).

Furthermore, the penetrance of these disease-associated mutations is quite variable and can increase with age (12, 19). The variability in penetrance as well as the lack of identification of a single associated gene mutations in 85% of sALS suggests that some ALS cases have a multigenic component, and/or involve epigenetic modification, and/or result from DNA damage, environmental risk factors, or viral infections (9, 14, 20–23) (**Figure 2**). In these cases, it is likely a combination of these factors that leads to cellular dysfunction such as glutamate-mediated excitotoxicity (24), abnormal protein aggregation (25), mitochondrial disorganization and dysfunction (26, 27) contributing to the oxidative stress (28–30) (**Figure 2**). Adding to the complexity of ALS, several studies suggest that not only the motor neurons are affected but also the surrounding cells, and that these cells participate in the propagation and burden of the disease. For instance, activated microglia cells release superoxide and nitric oxide metabolites, elements that are toxic to neuronal cells (31). Astrocytes can also participate in the propagation of neurotoxic elements (32, 33) such as SOD1 aggregates (34–36), and a failure of astrocytes to remove extracellular glutamate may mediate excitotoxicity (37–39). Ultimately, the intracellular dysfunction of the motor neuron combined with aberrant secretion of neurotoxic elements of surrounding cells leads to motor neuron stress, aberrant electrophysiological properties, and consequently to motor neuron death (**Figure 2**).

In the absence of a reliable diagnostic test for ALS, diagnosis is based on clinical and electrophysiological criteria such as evidence for progressive involvement of both upper and lower motor neurons and exclusion of diseases mimicking ALS as set out in the Revised El Escorial Criteria (REEC), Airlie House criteria (AHC) and Awaji criteria (2, 40). The process of diagnosis can be lengthy and there is a typical diagnostic delay of 9-15 months from onset to diagnostic confirmation (41). Considering that the average survival from onset is 2–4 years (6–8) and that efficacy of Riluzole is improved by early treatment (42), there is an urgent need to improve diagnostic speed and accuracy for ALS. One way of achieving this is the identification of biomarkers specific to ALS pathology, to enable the development a reliable fast diagnostic test. As well as diagnostics, it is also important to identify prognostic biomarkers that can be used to monitor the status of the pathology-various candidates may serve both these purposes. The identification of ALS biomarkers will contribute to a better understanding of the disease pathogenesis, and permit targeted drug development and patient stratification for more efficient clinical trials, assuming that different sub-cohorts of ALS patients respond differently to treatments. Biomarker discovery can be achieved by examining the "omics" contents of ALS patient tissues.

The present review has two aims: (1) to identify pathways commonly affected in genetic forms of ALS, and stratify the patients accordingly, and (2) to explore previous genomic, transcriptomic, proteomic, metabolomic and miRNomic studies of ALS published during the last decade, and summarize the findings, highlighting potential biomarker candidates for ALS disease management and treatment.

Genetic Markers for ALS Patient Stratification

The first gene identified to be associated with ALS was SOD1 in 1993 (43). Since then 29 new genes have been identified (13–15), representing the most frequent genetic mutations included in current diagnostic processes (13, 44) (**Figure 1**). These 30 genes offer crucial clues in understanding the pathogenesis of ALS—some of the gene products interact with each other (14)—and enable the identification of diverse cellular pathways that are disrupted in ALS patients (**Table 1**). Even if most ALS cases are sporadic, the pathways disrupted in familial cases may also be affected in sporadic cases, as both sALS and fALS can share common molecular signatures or functional biological effects such as FUS or TDP43 protein aggregations or accumulation of stress granules formation (45), disruption in RNA processing (46), or disruption of autophagy and mitochondrial functions (47). When sorting the genes associated to ALS according to their primary cellular functions, several categories of dominantly affected pathway can be highlighted, such as (1) mitochondrial metabolism and turnover, (2) axonal transport and the cytoskeleton, (3) autophagy and proteostasis, (4) endosomal and vesicular trafficking, (5) DNA repair, and (6) ribostasis/RNA alteration/Nucleocytoplasmic transport—with most of the genes being involved in multiple pathways. It may be possible to group patients into strata depending on which combination of pathways is dysregulated, and to recruit patients accordingly for translational research and clinical trials. We have cautiously assigned each causal gene to one of 14 strata, depending on the profile of its affected pathways (**Table 1**). These groupings represent our effort to summarize current understanding and are not intended to be definitive—indeed, it will be important to modify and update them on an ongoing basis with improvements in the knowledge of protein function and the impact of mutations. Although these 14 strata are directly applicable to only 20% of total ALS cases (**Figure 1**), future work may determine whether (and which of) these molecular signatures are implicated in the remaining cases.

The Search for Circulating Biomarkers

The identification of circulating markers associated with ALS pathology would be important tools to provide early disease diagnosis and to track progression or treatment. There has been a concerted focus aimed at identifying such biomarkers in different body fluids over the past 20 years. In **Table S1**, we summarized 76 studies that investigated proteins, miRs, mRNAs, and metabolites as potential biomarkers in cerebrospinal fluid (CSF) or blood (blood cells, serum or plasma). To date, little has been done investigating urine-based biomarkers, and thus urine biomarker analyses are not reported in the current review. CSF is the most frequently used sample source, and several studies (**Table S1**) report a consistent decrease in protein levels of transthyretin—involved in neurogenesis, nerve repair and axonal growth (171)—and cystatin c—an endogenous cysteine protease inhibitor that can protect motor neurons against neurotoxicity by stimulating autophagy and inhibition of cathepsin B (172). In addition, CSF cystatin C protein levels positively correlated with the survival of ALS patients and could be thus potentially used as a prognostic biomarker (173). However, both transthyretin and cystatin C decreases are not specific to ALS patients and a similar pattern is observed in other neurodegenerative diseases (173) such as Alzheimer's (171), suggesting that the protein levels of both transthyretin and cystatin C level are a common signature for neuron vulnerabilities and neurodegeneration. The protein levels of neurofilament light chain (NF-L) and the phosphorylated form of neurofilament heavy chain (pNFH) were also consistently found to be increased in the CSF of ALS patients across multiple studies (**Table S1**), with a high level of either NF-L or pNFH predicting a shorter life expectancy (174–178). NF-L and pNFH are markers for axonal damage (179). In this context, similarly to M-creatine kinase for myofiber fragility in muscular dystrophy (180), NF-L and pNFH thus directly reflect the health of the neurons -the cells specifically impacted by ALS.

Combining NF-L and pNFH with other markers that reflect the "health status" of other tissues such as glial cells, skeletal muscle, or inflammatory response, may represent a useful addition, as ALS is now perceived as a multisystemic disease. Such a multi-marker approach may represent a useful complement to a panel of biomarkers to test the efficacy of drugs in clinical trials. In this respect, miR-451—an inhibitor of microglial cell activation (181)—was consistently decreased in leukocytes of ALS patients (**Table S1**), while the pro-inflammatory MCP-1, secreted by the glial cells and neurons (182), was found to be increased in both serum and plasma (**Table S1**). Both miR-451 and MCP-1 could thus potentially inform the status of inflammatory cell recruitment and activation (181, 182). In addition, miR-206, which is essential for skeletal muscle growth and regeneration (183), as well as miR-338-3p, a regulator of neuromuscular junctions (184), are consistently upregulated in leukocytes—with miR-206 also consistently reported to be upregulated in serum and plasma samples across multiple studies (**Table S1**). In this context, miR-206 and miR-338-3p could be clinically useful candidate biomarkers of the health status of skeletal muscle (185).

Regarding circulating mRNAs, no obvious consistent candidates have been identified yet across previous studies (**Table S1**). With regard to analyses of circulating metabolite candidates, huge variation is observed between studies, though there was a general tendency for upregulation of specific metabolites in serum and plasma (**Table S1**), which is consistent with the hypermetabolism observed in some ALS patients (186). For instance, creatine, which is linked to cell energy metabolism, was consistently increased in CSF and plasma across studies (**Table S1**). Pyruvate and glucose were also found to be increased in CSF and plasma of ALS patients (**Table S1**), potentially reflecting a dysregulation of glycolytic metabolism as observed in SOD1-G93A motor neurons (187), and in some ALS cases (188, 189). This upregulation of glycolysis correlates with a shorter survival time and thus could be used as a prognostic biomarker (188, 189). Similarly, the upregulation of cholesterol and LDL observed in CSF and plasma across studies (**Table S1**) could also reflect a global dysregulation of lipid metabolism in ALS patients (190, 191). Other neurotoxic metabolites, such as homocysteine, were consistently increased in all body fluids (**Table S1**). Altogether, these data suggest a global dysregulation of the energy metabolism in ALS patients.

Other types of molecules could be investigated as biomarkers in ALS, such as long non-coding RNA (lncRNA), which can act in cis to either silence or enhance the expression of proximal genes

TABLE 1 | Summary of the 30 genes presently known to have monogenic association with ALS, and their primary functions.

Gene name, full name	References	Pathways affected: Mitochondria	Axonal transport	Cytoskeleton	Autophagy	Proteostasis	Endosomal trafficking	Vesicular traficking	DNA repair	Ribostasis	Global RNA alteration	Nucleocytoplasmic transport	Suggestion of possible Strata
SOD1, Cu,Zn-xuperoxide dismutase-1	(48–52)	x			x	x							
OPTN, Optineurin	(53–58)	x			x								1
CHCHD10, Coiled-coil-helix-coiled-coil-helix domain containing 10	(59–63)	x				x							
NEK1, NIMA related kinase 1	(64–71)	x		x					x				2
KIF5A, kinesin family member 5A	(15,72,73)			x									
NEFH, Neurofilament heavy subunit	(74–80)		x	x									3
TUBA4A, Tubulin alpha 4a	(81–86)		x	x									
DCTN1, Dynactin subunit 1	(87–90)		x					x					4
PFN1 , Profilin 1	(55,91–94)		x	x		x							5
ELP3, Elongator protein 3	(95–98)			x						x	x		6
C9orf72, Chromosome 9 open reading frame 72	(18,99–106)				x	x	x				x	x	7
CHMP2B, Charged multivesicular body protein 2B	(50,107–114)				x	x	x						
VCP, Valosin-containing protein	(50,55,115–121)				x	x	x						
FIG4, Phosphoinositide 5-phosphatase	(18,50,122–124)				x		x	x					8
VAPB, Vesicle-associated membrane protein B	(55,125–129)					x		x					
UBQLN2, Ubiquilin 2	(55,130–134)				x	x							
TBK1 , TANK binding kinase 1	(55,58,64,135)				x	x							
SQSTM1, Sequestosome 1	(50,55,136,137)				x								9
CCNF, Cyclin F	(55,138–140)					x							
TARDBP, TAR DNA binding protein	(45,50,138,141,142)					x				x	x		10
hnRNPA1, Heterogeneous nuclear ribonucleoprotein A1	(138,143,144)					x				x	x		
hnRNPA2B1, Heterogeneous nuclear ribonucleoprotein A2/B1	(144–148)					x				x	x		
ALS2, Alsin	(65,149–151)						x						11
SPG11, Spatacsin vesicle trafficking associated	(152,153)							x					
C21orf2, Cilia and flagella associated protein 410	(154)								x				12
SETX, Senataxin	(155–158)								x	x	x		13
FUS, Fused in sarcoma	(55,138,159–162)								x	x	x		
ATXN2, Ataxin 2	(45,138,163,164)									x	x		
ANG, Angiogenin	(165–168)									x			14
MATR3, Matrin 3	(138,169,170)										x		

The list of genes is taken from Volk et al. (13) and Chia et al (14). The references given in the second column indicate papers providing experimental evidence of the primary pathways (or molecular functions) affected in cell and animal models harboring the respective mutation. These pathways are given in columns 3-13–it should be noted that our understanding of the implicated pathways may change in future as more is known regarding the effects of mutations. We grouped together pathways commonly affected across genetic forms of ALS, and we suggest 14 potential strata based on the profiles of affected pathways. These groupings represent our effort to summarize current understanding and are not intended to be definitive–indeed, it will be important to modify and update them on an ongoing basis as the knowledge of protein loss and gain of function improves.

TABLE 2 | Circulating biomarker candidates consistently observed and confirmed across studies.

Biomarker categories	Biomarker name	CSF	Serum	Plasma	BMC/ Leukocytes	References
Proteins	Transthyretin	↓↓				*(203,204)*
	Cystatin C	↓↓↓↓↓				*(173,175,203–205*
	A peptic fragment of the neurosecretory protein VGF	↓		↓		*(205,206)*
	C-reactive protein (CRP)	↑	↑			*(204,207)*
	Neurofilament heavy chain phosphorylated pNFH	↑↑↑↑	↑	↑		*(174–178)*
	Neurofilament light chain (NF-L)	↑↑				*(174,208)*
	Chitotriosidase	↑↑				*(175,179)*
	MCP1- alpha		↑	↑		*(209,210)*
	TDP43				↑↑	*(211,212)*
miRs	miR-451				↓↓	*(184,213)*
	miR-338-3p				↑↑	*(184,214)*
	miR-206		↑↑↑	↑	↑	*(169,202,215–217*
	miR-133b		↑↑			*(217,218)*
Metabolites	Pyruvate	↑		↑		*(219,220)*
	Ascorbate	↑↑				*(219,221)*
	Glutamine	↓	↓	↓		*(222–224)*
	Aspartate	↑		↑		*(225,226)*
	Serine	↑		↑		*(224,225)*
	Glucose	↑↑				*(227,228)*
	Creatine	↑		↑↑		*(220,224,228)*
	Creatinine	↓		↓↓		*(220,224,228)*
	α-hydroxybutyrate	↑		↑↑		*(220,224,228)*
	Cholesterol	↑		↑↑		*(190,224,229)*
	Homocysteine	↑	↑	↑↑		*(230–232)*
	Glutamate		↑	↑↑		*(223,226,233)*

This table is a summary of the detailed ***Table S1****. Data are organized per category of molecule investigated. In each category, the source material is indicated as follows: Gold = CSF, Light blue = Serum, Dark Blue = Plasma, Gray = Blood cells. ↑ = Concentration increased in ALS patients compared to controls, ↓ = Concentration decreased in ALS patients compared to controls. The number of arrows indicates the number of papers describing the increase or decrease of the biomarker considered, in a given tissue. The papers describing these changes are referenced in the last column.*

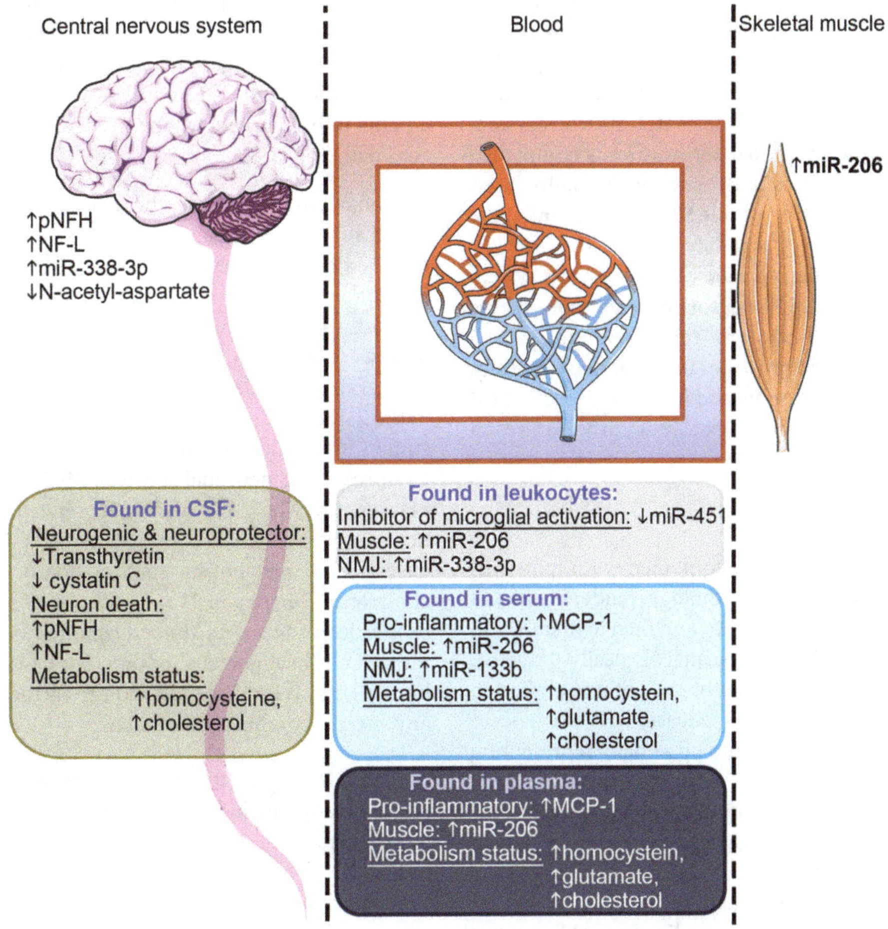

FIGURE 3 | Summary of candidate biomarkers consistently found across studies. Candidates observed in CSF are highlighted in brown, in leukocytes in gray, in serum light blue and in plasma dark blue. These candidate biomarkers reflect the motor neuron health, the inflammatory status, skeletal muscle health, and metabolism status–as indicated in each text block. Some of these candidates were found in postmortem central nervous tissue or on muscle biopsies. NMJ, neuromuscular junction.

(192) and which are known to have a key role in normal neuronal development, as well as in development and progression of neurodegenerative diseases [see (193) for review]. The lncRNA have also been detected in body fluids and have been suggested as potential diagnostic and/or prognostic biomarkers in, but not only, lung cancer (194), triple negative breast cancer (195) and cardiovascular diseases (196). In this context, lncRNA could be investigated as new biomarker candidates for neurodegenerative diseases (193), including ALS.

EXPLORING POTENTIAL ALS SIGNATURES IN TISSUE

Studying changes at the molecular level of specific tissues affected in ALS should improve our understanding of the disease mechanisms and multi-systemic impact.

Postmortem brain or spinal cord have been widely investigated. Accumulation of pNF-H and NF-L in brain tissue (**Table S2**) positively correlate with the accumulation of these markers in CSF (**Table S1**), and may be reflective of motor neuron breakdown (179). Similarly, miR-146a and miR-338-3p, both increased in spinal cord (**Table S2**), are also detected at a greater level in circulating blood cells of ALS patients (**Table S1**). These two miRNAs are involved in the regulation of the inflammatory response (197) and the neuromuscular junction (184, 198). In addition, miR-206, a skeletal muscle growth regulator (183), is increased in ALS muscles across studies [**Table S1**, 2 studies show significant increases (199, 200), the third study only shows a tendency toward an increase in levels (201)]. Together these data reinforce the suggestion that these candidate biomarkers may have utility in determining the status of motor neurons, inflammatory cells and muscle in ALS at different stages of the disease.

When looking at the proteomic and transcriptomic signature of ALS tissues, most observations have not been reproduced across studies. This lack of repeatability could be attributed to numerous factors, such as: different study populations; different types of control subject; different sample sources; different stages of the disease; and the use of different methodological strategies (**Table S2**).

However, when looking at the different pathways affected in nervous or muscle tissues, we can identify dominant signatures. For instance, skeletal muscle exhibits a dysregulation of pathways involved in muscle atrophy/growth, cytoskeletal maintenance and metabolism, while the central nervous system exhibits inflammatory and excitotoxicity features accompanied by disruptions in axonal transport, cell death, autophagy, metabolism, and RNA processing (**Table S2**). Concordantly, the systematic decrease of N-acetyl-aspartate observed *in vivo* by magnetic resonance spectrometry in the central nervous system across studies reflects (**Table S2**) neuron degeneration. These markers likely capture most strongly the endpoints of ALS disease, including degeneration processes in motor neuron death, and muscle denervation and atrophy, and it will be important for future studies to identify biomarkers that track early features of the disease.

CONCLUSION

The number of monogenic forms, combined with potential multisystemic contributions to ALS pathology, render it difficult first to unravel physiopathological events, and then to understand which of these events could be pharmacologically targeted. However, by taking a wide-angle view of the pathways affected in different monogenic forms of the disease, it is possible to discern patient strata, with each stratum potentially representing a separate target for therapeutic intervention. Such a strategy is directly applicable to monogenic forms of ALS—known in ~20% of current ALS cases—and future work may discover the extent to which each of these potential targets are transferrable to the 80% of cases in which causal links (genetic or otherwise) have not been identified. Identifying biomarkers to diagnose ALS patients and predict their progression (prognostic biomarkers) may also lead to the identification of patient strata in these non-causally linked forms of ALS.

Identifying such biomarkers in ALS is a significant challenge as it involves the assessment, not only of motor neuron health status, but also that of other cell types affected in ALS such as astrocytes, microglia, skeletal muscle and inflammatory cells. In this review, we collated across a large number of recently published studies on ALS biomarkers covering several different cell and tissue types (76 studies on body fluids and 42 studies on tissues), and identified only a relatively few candidates that are consistently identified as potential biomarkers across multiple independent studies. These candidate biomarkers are predominantly reflective of motor neuron health, the inflammatory status, and skeletal muscle health (**Figure 3**). As ALS is increasingly recognized as a multi-systemic disease, it is thus important to track the progression or the recovery of these multiple tissues during clinical trials. In addition, some of these candidates have been confirmed in murine models, e.g., miR-206 in SOD1-G93A mice reflects disease progression in the murine model (202), making them interesting candidates for assessment in pre-clinical studies. As a multi-systemic disease, it is likely that a panel of biomarkers will be needed to fully capture features of ALS pathology.

Considering the different source tissues and the potential implication of each of these in the pathology, our capacity to detect them in accessible fluids, and also the desire to have biomarkers that are confirmed in multiple studies, we would suggest that a useful approach to obtain an overall picture of disease progress in any given patient, may be to combine biomarker candidate molecules from across those listed in **Table 2**. For example, of biomarkers confirmed in multiple studies, we could suggest a panel of Cystatin C, pNFH and NF-L, all reflecting neuronal survival, MCP1 as a pro-inflammatory marker, the MiRs 206 and 133b reflecting muscle origin and neuromuscular junction, respectively, and some indicators of dysregulated metabolism such as homocysteine, glutamate, or cholesterol. Such a panel (or a variation of it with similarly diverse properties in terms of tissue origin), would be useful to assess the overall "health status" of different tissues. However, all of the biomarkers so far proposed require further validation, as would any specific combination of them.

The development of a heterogeneous multi-biomarker panel—likely including robust new biomarkers and the biomarkers cited in this report—could be seen as a priority, not only for diagnostic purposes but also for prognostic or predictive applications.

AUTHOR CONTRIBUTIONS

UV, VM, and MS collated the data from the literature, and wrote the paper. WD and SD organized the data, wrote the paper. AB, WD, and SD edited the paper.

ACKNOWLEDGMENTS

This work was financed by TARGET-ALS (ViTAL consortium, PI: SD), ARsLA (TEAM consortium, PI: SD), European Union Regional Development Fund (ERDF) EU Sustainable Competitiveness Programme for N. Ireland, Northern Ireland Public Health Agency (HSC R&D) & Ulster University (PI: AB). UV's post-doctoral position is financed by Target-ALS.

REFERENCES

1. Chiò A, Logroscino G, Traynor BJ, Collins J, Simeone JC, Goldstein LA, et al. Global epidemiology of amyotrophic lateral sclerosis: a systematic review of the published literature. *Neuroepidemiology.* (2013) 41:118–30. doi: 10.1159/000351153
2. Al-Chalabi A, Hardiman O, Kiernan MC, Chiò A, Rix-Brooks B, van den Berg LH. Amyotrophic lateral sclerosis: moving towards

a new classification system. *Lancet Neurol.* (2016) 15:1182–94. doi: 10.1016/S1474-4422(16)30199-5
3. Talbot K, Feneberg E, Scaber J, Thompson AG, Turner MR. Amyotrophic lateral sclerosis: the complex path to precision medicine. *J Neurol.* (2018) 265:2454–62. doi: 10.1007/s00415-018-8983-8
4. Niedermeyer S, Murn M, Choi PJ. Respiratory failure in amyotrophic lateral sclerosis. *Chest.* (2018) 155:401–8. doi: 10.1016/j.chest.2018.06.035
5. Luchesi KF, Kitamua S, Mourão LF. Amyotrophic Lateral Sclerosis survival analysis: swallowing and non-oral feeding. *NeuroRehabilitation.* (2014) 35:535–42. doi: 10.3233/NRE-141149
6. Talbott EO, Malek AM, Lacomis D. The epidemiology of amyotrophic lateral sclerosis. *Handb Clin Neurol.* 138:225–38. doi: 10.1016/B978-0-12-802973-2.00013-6
7. Chiò A, Logroscino G, Hardiman O, Swingler R, Mitchell D, Beghi E, et al. Prognostic factors in ALS: a critical review. *Amyotroph Lateral Scler.* (2009) 10:310–23. doi: 10.3109/17482960802566824
8. del Aguila MA, Longstreth WT, McGuire V, Koepsell TD, van Belle G. Prognosis in amyotrophic lateral sclerosis: a population-based study. *Neurology.* (2003) 60:813–9. doi: 10.1212/01.WNL.0000049472.47709.3B
9. Brown RH, Al-Chalabi A. Amyotrophic lateral sclerosis. *N Engl J Med.* (2017) 377:1602. doi: 10.1056/NEJMc1710379
10. Broussalis E, Grinzinger S, Kunz AB, Killer-Oberpfalzer M, Haschke-Becher E, Hartung H-P, et al. Late age onset of amyotrophic lateral sclerosis is often not considered in elderly people. *Acta Neurol Scand.* (2018) 137:329–34. doi: 10.1111/ane.12869
11. Arthur KC, Calvo A, Price TR, Geiger JT, Chiò A, Traynor BJ. Projected increase in amyotrophic lateral sclerosis from 2015 to 2040. *Nat Commun.* (2016) 7:12408. doi: 10.1038/ncomms12408
12. Turner MR, Al-Chalabi A, Chio A, Hardiman O, Kiernan MC, Rohrer JD, et al. Genetic screening in sporadic ALS and FTD. *J Neurol Neurosurg Psychiatry.* (2017) 88:1042–4. doi: 10.1136/jnnp-2017-315995
13. Volk AE, Weishaupt JH, Andersen PM, Ludolph AC, Kubisch C. Current knowledge and recent insights into the genetic basis of amyotrophic lateral sclerosis. *Med Genet.* (2018) 30:252–8. doi: 10.1007/s11825-018-0185-3
14. Chia R, Chiò A, Traynor BJ. Novel genes associated with amyotrophic lateral sclerosis: diagnostic and clinical implications. *Lancet Neurol.* (2018) 17:94–102. doi: 10.1016/S1474-4422(17)30401-5
15. Nicolas A, Kenna KP, Renton AE, Ticozzi N, Faghri F, Chia R, et al. Genome-wide analyses identify KIF5A as a novel ALS gene. *Neuron.* (2018) 97:1268–83.e6. doi: 10.1016/j.neuron.2018.02.027
16. Wainger BJ, Kiskinis E, Mellin C, Wiskow O, Han SSW, Sandoe J, et al. Intrinsic membrane hyperexcitability of amyotrophic lateral sclerosis patient-derived motor neurons. *Cell Rep.* (2014) 7:1–11. doi: 10.1016/j.celrep.2014.03.019
17. Seminary ER, Sison SL, Ebert AD. Modeling protein aggregation and the heat shock response in ALS iPSC-derived motor neurons. *Front Neurosci.* (2018) 12:86. doi: 10.3389/fnins.2018.00086
18. Shi Y, Lin S, Staats KA, Li Y, Chang W-H, Hung S-T, et al. Haploinsufficiency leads to neurodegeneration in C9ORF72 ALS/FTD human induced motor neurons. *Nat Med.* (2018) 24:313–25. doi: 10.1038/nm.4490
19. Majounie E, Renton AE, Mok K, Dopper EGP, Waite A, Rollinson S, et al. Frequency of the C9orf72 hexanucleotide repeat expansion in patients with amyotrophic lateral sclerosis and frontotemporal dementia: a cross-sectional study. *Lancet Neurol.* (2012) 11:323–30. doi: 10.1016/S1474-4422(12)70043-1
20. Armon C. From snow to hill to ALS: an epidemiological odyssey in search of ALS causation. *J Neurol Sci.* (2018) 391:134–40. doi: 10.1016/j.jns.2018.05.016
21. Xue YC, Feuer R, Cashman N, Luo H. Enteroviral infection: the forgotten link to amyotrophic lateral sclerosis? *Front Mol Neurosci.* (2018) 11:63. doi: 10.3389/fnmol.2018.00063
22. Mackenzie IR, Nicholson AM, Sarkar M, Messing J, Purice MD, Pottier C, et al. TIA1 mutations in amyotrophic lateral sclerosis and frontotemporal dementia promote phase separation and alter stress granule dynamics. *Neuron.* (2017) 95:808–16.e9. doi: 10.1016/j.neuron.2017.07.025
23. Al-Chalabi A, Van Den Berg LH, Veldink J. Gene discovery in amyotrophic lateral sclerosis: implications for clinical management. *Nat Rev Neurol.* (2017) 13:96–104. doi: 10.1038/nrneurol.2016.182
24. Blasco H, Mavel S, Corcia P, Gordon PH. The glutamate hypothesis in ALS: pathophysiology and drug development. *Curr Med Chem.* (2014) 21:3551–75. doi: 10.2174/0929867321666140916120118
25. Ross CA, Poirier MA. Protein aggregation and neurodegenerative disease. *Nat Med.* (2004) 10:S10–S17. doi: 10.1038/nm1066
26. Cappello V, Francolini M. Neuromuscular junction dismantling in amyotrophic lateral sclerosis. *Int J Mol Sci.* (2017) 18:2092. doi: 10.3390/ijms18102092
27. Delic V, Kurien C, Cruz J, Zivkovic S, Barretta J, Thomson A, Hennessey D, Joseph J, Ehrhart J, Willing AE, et al. Discrete mitochondrial aberrations in the spinal cord of sporadic ALS patients. *J Neurosci Res.* (2018) 96:1353–66. doi: 10.1002/jnr.24249
28. Anand A, Thakur K, Gupta PK. ALS and oxidative stress: the neurovascular scenario. *Oxid Med Cell Longev.* (2013) 2013:1–14. doi: 10.1155/2013/635831
29. Sharma A, Varghese AM, Vijaylakshmi K, Sumitha R, Prasanna VK, Shruthi S, et al. Cerebrospinal fluid from sporadic amyotrophic lateral sclerosis patients induces mitochondrial and lysosomal dysfunction. *Neurochem Res.* (2016) 41:965–84. doi: 10.1007/s11064-015-1779-7
30. Onesto E, Colombrita C, Gumina V, Borghi MO, Dusi S, Doretti A, et al. Gene-specific mitochondria dysfunctions in human TARDBP and C9ORF72 fibroblasts. *Acta Neuropathol Commun.* (2016) 4:47. doi: 10.1186/s40478-016-0316-5
31. Beers DR, Henkel JS, Xiao Q, Zhao W, Wang J, Yen AA, et al. Wild-type microglia extend survival in PU.1 knockout mice with familial amyotrophic lateral sclerosis. *Proc Natl Acad Sci USA.* (2006) 103:16021–6. doi: 10.1073/pnas.0607423103
32. Nagai M, Re DB, Nagata T, Chalazonitis A, Jessell TM, Wichterle H, et al. Astrocytes expressing ALS-linked mutated SOD1 release factors selectively toxic to motor neurons. *Nat Neurosci.* (2007) 10:615–22. doi: 10.1038/nn1876
33. Haidet-Phillips AM, Hester ME, Miranda CJ, Meyer K, Braun L, Frakes A, et al. Astrocytes from familial and sporadic ALS patients are toxic to motor neurons. *Nat Biotechnol.* (2011) 29:824–8. doi: 10.1038/nbt.1957
34. Basso M, Pozzi S, Tortarolo M, Fiordaliso F, Bisighini C, Pasetto L, et al. Mutant copper-zinc superoxide dismutase (SOD1) induces protein secretion pathway alterations and exosome release in astrocytes: implications for disease spreading and motor neuron pathology in amyotrophic lateral sclerosis. *J Biol Chem.* (2013) 288:15699–711. doi: 10.1074/jbc.M112.425066
35. Di Giorgio FP, Boulting GL, Bobrowicz S, Eggan KC. Human embryonic stem cell-derived motor neurons are sensitive to the toxic effect of glial cells carrying an ALS-causing mutation. *Cell Stem Cell.* (2008) 3:637–48. doi: 10.1016/j.stem.2008.09.017
36. Marchetto MCN, Muotri AR, Mu Y, Smith AM, Cezar GG, Gage FH. Non-cell-autonomous effect of human SOD1G37R astrocytes on motor neurons derived from human embryonic stem cells. *Cell Stem Cell.* (2008) 3:649–57. doi: 10.1016/j.stem.2008.10.001
37. Rothstein JD, Martin LJ, Kuncl RW. Decreased glutamate transport by the brain and spinal cord in amyotrophic lateral sclerosis. *N Engl J Med.* (1992) 326:1464–8. doi: 10.1056/NEJM199205283262204
38. Rothstein JD, Dykes-Hoberg M, Pardo CA, Bristol LA, Jin L, Kuncl RW, et al. Knockout of glutamate transporters reveals a major role for astroglial transport in excitotoxicity and clearance of glutamate. *Neuron.* (1996) 16:675–86.
39. Medina L, Figueredo-Cardenas G, Rothstein JD, Reiner A. Differential abundance of glutamate transporter subtypes in amyotrophic lateral sclerosis (ALS)-vulnerable versus ALS-resistant brain stem motor cell groups. *Exp Neurol.* (1996) 142:287–95. doi: 10.1006/exnr.1996.0198
40. Okita T, Nodera H, Shibuta Y, Nodera A, Asanuma K, Shimatani Y, et al. Can Awaji ALS criteria provide earlier diagnosis than the revised El Escorial criteria? *J Neurol Sci.* (2011) 302:29–32. doi: 10.1016/j.jns.2010.12.007
41. Hardiman O, van den Berg LH, Kiernan MC. Clinical diagnosis and management of amyotrophic lateral sclerosis. *Nat Rev Neurol.* (2011) 7:639–49. doi: 10.1038/nrneurol.2011.153
42. Miller RG, Mitchell JD, Moore DH. Riluzole for amyotrophic lateral sclerosis (ALS)/motor neuron disease (MND). *Cochrane database Syst Rev.* (2012) 2012:CD001447. doi: 10.1002/14651858.CD001447.pub3
43. Rosen DR, Siddique T, Patterson D, Figlewicz DA, Sapp P, Hentati A, et al. Mutations in Cu/Zn superoxide dismutase gene are associated

with familial amyotrophic lateral sclerosis. *Nature.* (1993) 362:59–62. doi: 10.1038/362059a0
44. Bocker MT, Hellwig I, Breiling A, Eckstein V, Ho AD, Lyko F. Genome-wide promoter DNA methylation dynamics of human hematopoietic progenitor cells during differentiation and aging. *Blood.* (2011) 117:e182-9. doi: 10.1182/blood-2011-01-331926
45. Monahan Z, Shewmaker F, Pandey UB. Stress granules at the intersection of autophagy and ALS. *Brain Res.* (2016) 1649:189–200. doi: 10.1016/j.brainres.2016.05.022
46. Ajroud-Driss S, Siddique T. Sporadic and hereditary amyotrophic lateral sclerosis (ALS). *Biochim Biophys Acta.* (2015) 1852:679–84. doi: 10.1016/j.bbadis.2014.08.010
47. Edens BM, Miller N, Ma Y-C. Impaired autophagy and defective mitochondrial function: converging paths on the road to motor neuron degeneration. *Front Cell Neurosci.* (2016) 10:44. doi: 10.3389/fncel.2016.00044
48. Kitamura A, Inada N, Kubota H, Matsumoto G, Kinjo M, Morimoto RI, et al. Dysregulation of the proteasome increases the toxicity of ALS-linked mutant SOD1. *Genes to Cells.* (2014) 19:209–24. doi: 10.1111/gtc.12125
49. An T, Shi P, Duan W, Zhang S, Yuan P, Li Z, et al. Oxidative stress and autophagic alteration in brainstem of SOD1-G93A mouse model of ALS. *Mol Neurobiol.* (2014) 49:1435–48. doi: 10.1007/s12035-013-8623-3
50. Otomo A, Pan L, Hadano S. Dysregulation of the autophagy-endolysosomal system in amyotrophic lateral sclerosis and related motor neuron diseases. *Neurol Res Int.* (2012) 2012:498428. doi: 10.1155/2012/498428
51. Kaur SJ, McKeown SR, Rashid S. Mutant SOD1 mediated pathogenesis of amyotrophic lateral sclerosis. *Gene.* (2016) 577:109–18. doi: 10.1016/j.gene.2015.11.049
52. Lautenschläger J, Lautenschläger C, Tadic V, Süße H, Ortmann W, Denzler J, et al. Novel computer vision algorithm for the reliable analysis of organelle morphology in whole cell 3D images—A pilot study for the quantitative evaluation of mitochondrial fragmentation in amyotrophic lateral sclerosis. *Mitochondrion.* (2015) 25:49–59. doi: 10.1016/J.MITO.2015.10.003
53. Moore AS, Holzbaur ELF. Dynamic recruitment and activation of ALS-associated TBK1 with its target optineurin are required for efficient mitophagy. *Proc Natl Acad Sci USA.* (2016) 113:E3349-58. doi: 10.1073/pnas.1523810113
54. Richter B, Sliter DA, Herhaus L, Stolz A, Wang C, Beli P, et al. Phosphorylation of OPTN by TBK1 enhances its binding to Ub chains and promotes selective autophagy of damaged mitochondria. *Proc Natl Acad Sci USA.* (2016) 113:4039–44. doi: 10.1073/pnas.1523926113
55. Shahheydari H, Ragagnin A, Walker AK, Toth RP, Vidal M, Jagaraj CJ, et al. Protein quality control and the amyotrophic lateral sclerosis/frontotemporal dementia continuum. *Front Mol Neurosci.* (2017) 10:119: doi: 10.3389/FNMOL.2017.00119
56. Heo J-M, Ordureau A, Paulo JA, Rinehart J, Harper JW. The PINK1-PARKIN mitochondrial ubiquitylation pathway drives a program of OPTN/NDP52 recruitment and TBK1 activation to promote mitophagy. *Mol Cell.* (2015) 60:7–20. doi: 10.1016/j.molcel.2015.08.016
57. Ying H, Yue BYJT. Optineurin: the autophagy connection. *Exp Eye Res.* (2016) 144:73–80. doi: 10.1016/j.exer.2015.06.029
58. Oakes JA, Davies MC, Collins MO. TBK1: a new player in ALS linking autophagy and neuroinflammation. *Mol Brain.* (2017) 10:5. doi: 10.1186/s13041-017-0287-x
59. Lehmer C, Schludi MH, Ransom L, Greiling J, Junghänel M, Exner N, et al. A novel CHCHD10 mutation implicates a Mia40-dependent mitochondrial import deficit in ALS. *EMBO Mol Med.* (2018) 10:8558. doi: 10.15252/emmm.201708558
60. Genin EC, Plutino M, Bannwarth S, Villa E, Cisneros-Barroso E, Roy M, et al. CHCHD10 mutations promote loss of mitochondrial cristae junctions with impaired mitochondrial genome maintenance and inhibition of apoptosis. *EMBO Mol Med.* (2016) 8:58–72. doi: 10.15252/emmm.201505496
61. Woo J-AA, Liu T, Trotter C, Fang CC, De Narvaez E, LePochat P, et al. Loss of function CHCHD10 mutations in cytoplasmic TDP-43 accumulation and synaptic integrity. *Nat Commun.* (2017) 8:15558. doi: 10.1038/ncomms 15558
62. Anderson CJ, Bredvik K, Burstein SR, Davis C, Meadows SM, Dash J, et al. ALS/FTD mutant CHCHD10 mice reveal a tissue-specific toxic gain-of-function and mitochondrial stress response. *Acta Neuropathol.* (2019) doi: 10.1007/s00401-019-01989-y. [Epub ahead of print].
63. Burstein SR, Valsecchi F, Kawamata H, Bourens M, Zeng R, Zuberi A, et al. *In vitro* and *in vivo* studies of the ALS-FTLD protein CHCHD10 reveal novel mitochondrial topology and protein interactions. *Hum Mol Genet.* (2018) 27:160–77. doi: 10.1093/hmg/ddx397
64. Cirulli ET, Lasseigne BN, Petrovski S, Sapp PC, Dion PA, Leblond CS, et al. Exome sequencing in amyotrophic lateral sclerosis identifies risk genes and pathways. *Science.* (2015) 347:1436–41. doi: 10.1126/science.aaa3650
65. Walker C, El-Khamisy SF. Perturbed autophagy and DNA repair converge to promote neurodegeneration in amyotrophic lateral sclerosis and dementia. *Brain.* (2018) 141:1247–62. doi: 10.1093/brain/awy076
66. Melo-Hanchuk TD, Slepicka PF, Meirelles GV, Basei FL, Lovato DV, Granato DC, et al. NEK1 kinase domain structure and its dynamic protein interactome after exposure to Cisplatin. *Sci Rep.* (2017) 7:5445. doi: 10.1038/s41598-017-05325-w
67. Chen Y, Chen C-F, Riley DJ, Chen P-L. Nek1 kinase functions in DNA damage response and checkpoint control through a pathway independent of ATM and ATR. *Cell Cycle.* (2011) 10:655–63. doi: 10.4161/cc.10.4.14814
68. Singh V, Connelly ZM, Shen X, De Benedetti A. Identification of the proteome complement of humanTLK1 reveals it binds and phosphorylates NEK1 regulating its activity. *Cell Cycle.* (2017) 16:915–26. doi: 10.1080/15384101.2017.1314421
69. Liu S, Ho CK, Ouyang J, Zou L. Nek1 kinase associates with ATR-ATRIP and primes ATR for efficient DNA damage signaling. *Proc Natl Acad Sci USA.* (2013) 110:2175–80. doi: 10.1073/pnas.1217781110
70. Al-Jassar C, Andreeva A, Barnabas DD, McLaughlin SH, Johnson CM, Yu M, et al. The Ciliopathy-Associated Cep104 Protein Interacts with Tubulin and Nek1 Kinase. *Structure.* (2017) 25:146–56. doi: 10.1016/j.str.2016.11.014
71. Chen Y, Craigen WJ, Riley DJ. Nek1 regulates cell death and mitochondrial membrane permeability through phosphorylation of VDAC1. *Cell Cycle.* (2009) 8:257–67. doi: 10.4161/cc.8.2.7551
72. Füger P, Sreekumar V, Schüle R, Kern J V., Stanchev DT, Schneider CD, et al. Spastic Paraplegia Mutation N256S in the Neuronal Microtubule Motor KIF5A Disrupts Axonal Transport in a Drosophila HSP Model. *PLoS Genet.* (2012) 8:e1003066. doi: 10.1371/journal.pgen.1003066
73. Liu M, Nadar VC, Kozielski F, Kozlowska M, Yu W, Baas PW. Kinesin-12, a mitotic microtubule-associated motor protein, impacts axonal growth, navigation, and branching. *J Neurosci.* (2010) 30:14896–906. doi: 10.1523/JNEUROSCI.3739-10.2010
74. Jacquier A, Delorme C, Belotti E, Juntas-Morales R, Solé G, Dubourg O, et al. Cryptic amyloidogenic elements in mutant NEFH causing Charcot-Marie-Tooth 2 trigger aggresome formation and neuronal death. *Acta Neuropathol Commun.* (2017) 5:55. doi: 10.1186/s40478-017-0457-1
75. Xu Z, Henderson RD, David M, McCombe PA. Neurofilaments as biomarkers for amyotrophic lateral sclerosis: a systematic review and meta-analysis. *PLoS ONE.* (2016) 11:e0164625. doi: 10.1371/journal.pone.0164625
76. Figlewicz DA, Krizus A, Martinoli MG, Meininger V, Dib M, Rouleau GA, et al. Variants of the heavy neurofilament subunit are associated with the development of amyotrophic lateral sclerosis. *Hum Mol Genet.* (1994) 3:1757–61.
77. Rebelo AP, Abrams AJ, Cottenie E, Horga A, Gonzalez M, Bis DM, et al. Cryptic amyloidogenic elements in the 3′ UTRs of neurofilament genes trigger axonal neuropathy. *Am J Hum Genet.* (2016) 98:597–614. doi: 10.1016/j.ajhg.2016.02.022
78. Julien J-P. Neurofilament functions in health and disease. *Curr Opin Neurobiol.* (1999) 9:554–60. doi: 10.1016/S0959-4388(99)00004-5
79. Thyagarajan A, Strong MJ, Szaro BG. Post-transcriptional control of neurofilaments in development and disease. *Exp Cell Res.* (2007) 313:2088–97. doi: 10.1016/j.yexcr.2007.02.014
80. Lobsiger CS, Garcia ML, Ward CM, Cleveland DW. Altered axonal architecture by removal of the heavily phosphorylated neurofilament tail domains strongly slows superoxide dismutase 1 mutant-mediated ALS. *Proc Natl Acad Sci USA.* (2005) 102:10351–6. doi: 10.1073/pnas.0503862102

81. Howes SC, Alushin GM, Shida T, Nachury M V, Nogales E. Effects of tubulin acetylation and tubulin acetyltransferase binding on microtubule structure. *Mol Biol Cell.* (2014) 25:257–66. doi: 10.1091/mbc.E13-07-0387
82. Laird FM, Farah MH, Ackerley S, Hoke A, Maragakis N, Rothstein JD, et al. Motor neuron disease occurring in a mutant dynactin mouse model is characterized by defects in vesicular trafficking. *J Neurosci.* (2008) 28:1997–2005. doi: 10.1523/JNEUROSCI.4231-07.2008
83. Smith BN, Ticozzi N, Fallini C, Gkazi AS, Topp S, Kenna KP, et al. Exome-wide rare variant analysis identifies TUBA4A mutations associated with familial ALS. *Neuron.* (2014) 84:324–31. doi: 10.1016/j.neuron.2014.09.027
84. Helferich AM, Brockmann SJ, Reinders J, Deshpande D, Holzmann K, Brenner D, et al. Dysregulation of a novel miR-1825/TBCB/TUBA4A pathway in sporadic and familial ALS. *Cell Mol Life Sci.* (2018) 75:4301–19. doi: 10.1007/s00018-018-2873-1
85. Schäfer MK, Bellouze S, Jacquier A, Schaller S, Richard L, Mathis S, et al. Sensory neuropathy in progressive motor neuronopathy *(pmn)* mice is associated with defects in microtubule polymerization and axonal transport. *Brain Pathol.* (2017) 27:459–71. doi: 10.1111/bpa.12422
86. Clark JA, Yeaman EJ, Blizzard CA, Chuckowree JA, Dickson TC. A case for microtubule vulnerability in amyotrophic lateral sclerosis: altered dynamics during disease. *Front Cell Neurosci.* (2016) 10:204. doi: 10.3389/fncel.2016.00204
87. Liu X, Yang L, Tang L, Chen L, Liu X, Fan D. DCTN1 gene analysis in Chinese patients with sporadic amyotrophic lateral sclerosis. *PLoS ONE.* (2017) 12:e0182572. doi: 10.1371/journal.pone.0182572
88. Hafezparast M, Ahmad-Annuar A, Hummerich H, Shah P, Ford M, Baker C, et al. Paradigms for the identification of new genes in motor neuron degeneration. *Amyotroph Lateral Scler Other Motor Neuron Disord.* (2003) 4:249–57. doi: 10.1080/14660820310016084
89. Vohra BPS, Sasaki Y, Miller BR, Chang J, DiAntonio A, Milbrandt J. Amyloid precursor protein cleavage-dependent and -independent axonal degeneration programs share a common nicotinamide mononucleotide adenylyltransferase 1-sensitive pathway. *J Neurosci.* (2010) 30:13729–38. doi: 10.1523/JNEUROSCI.2939-10.2010
90. Ikenaka K, Katsuno M, Kawai K, Ishigaki S, Tanaka F, Sobue G. Disruption of axonal transport in motor neuron diseases. *Int J Mol Sci.* (2012) 13:1225–38. doi: 10.3390/ijms13011225
91. Henty-Ridilla JL, Juanes MA, Goode BL. Profilin directly promotes microtubule growth through residues mutated in amyotrophic lateral sclerosis. *Curr Biol.* (2017) 27:3535–43.e4. doi: 10.1016/j.cub.2017.10.002
92. Wu C-H, Fallini C, Ticozzi N, Keagle PJ, Sapp PC, Piotrowska K, et al. Mutations in the profilin 1 gene cause familial amyotrophic lateral sclerosis. *Nature.* (2012) 488:499–503. doi: 10.1038/nature11280
93. Nekouei M, Ghezellou P, Aliahmadi A, Arjmand S, Kiaei M, Ghassempour A. Changes in biophysical characteristics of PFN1 due to mutation causing amyotrophic lateral sclerosis. *Metab Brain Dis.* (2018) 33:1975–84. doi: 10.1007/s11011-018-0305-4
94. Kiaei M, Balasubramaniam M, Govind Kumar V, Shmookler Reis RJ, Moradi M, Varughese KI. ALS-causing mutations in profilin-1 alter its conformational dynamics: a computational approach to explain propensity for aggregation. *Sci Rep.* (2018) 8:13102. doi: 10.1038/s41598-018-31199-7
95. Simpson CL, Lemmens R, Miskiewicz K, Broom WJ, Hansen VK, van Vught PWJ, et al. Variants of the elongator protein 3 (ELP3) gene are associated with motor neuron degeneration. *Hum Mol Genet.* (2009) 18:472–481. doi: 10.1093/hmg/ddn375
96. Bento-Abreu A, Jager G, Swinnen B, Rué L, Hendrickx S, Jones A, et al. Elongator subunit 3 (ELP3) modifies ALS through tRNA modification. *Hum Mol Genet.* (2018) 27:1276–89. doi: 10.1093/hmg/ddy043
97. Nguyen L, Humbert S, Saudou F, Chariot A. Elongator–an emerging role in neurological disorders. *Trends Mol Med.* (2010) 16:1–6. doi: 10.1016/j.molmed.2009.11.002
98. Tielens S, Huysseune S, Godin JD, Chariot A, Malgrange B, Nguyen L. Elongator controls cortical interneuron migration by regulating actomyosin dynamics. *Cell Res.* (2016) 26:1131–48. doi: 10.1038/cr.2016.112
99. Zhang K, Donnelly CJ, Haeusler AR, Grima JC, Machamer JB, Steinwald P, et al. The C9orf72 repeat expansion disrupts nucleocytoplasmic transport. *Nature.* (2015) 525:56–61. doi: 10.1038/nature 14973
100. Farg MA, Sundaramoorthy V, Sultana JM, Yang S, Atkinson RAK, Levina V, et al. C9ORF72, implicated in amytrophic lateral sclerosis and frontotemporal dementia, regulates endosomal trafficking. *Hum Mol Genet.* (2014) 23:3579–95. doi: 10.1093/hmg/ddu068
101. Bäumer D, Talbot K, Turner MR. Advances in motor neurone disease. *J R Soc Med.* (2014) 107:14–21. doi: 10.1177/0141076813511451
102. DeJesus-Hernandez M, Mackenzie IRR, Boeve BFF, Boxer ALL, Baker M, Rutherford NJJ, et al. Expanded GGGGCC hexanucleotide repeat in noncoding region of C9ORF72 causes chromosome 9p-linked FTD and ALS. *Neuron.* (2011) 72:245–56. doi: 10.1016/j.neuron.2011.09.011
103. Babić Leko M, Županski V, Kirincich J, Smilović D, Hortobágyi T, Hof PR, et al. Molecular mechanisms of neurodegeneration related to *C9orf72* hexanucleotide repeat expansion. *Behav Neurol.* (2019) 2019:1–18. doi: 10.1155/2019/2909168
104. Burk K, Pasterkamp RJ. Disrupted neuronal trafficking in amyotrophic lateral sclerosis. *Acta Neuropathol.* (2019) doi: 10.1007/s00401-019-01964-7. [Epub ahead of print].
105. Guo Q, Lehmer C, Martínez-Sánchez A, Rudack T, Beck F, Hartmann H, et al. *In situ* structure of neuronal C9orf72 Poly-GA aggregates reveals proteasome recruitment. *Cell.* (2018) 172:696–705.e12. doi: 10.1016/j.cell.2017. 12.030
106. Ho WY, Tai YK, Chang J-C, Liang J, Tyan S-H, Chen S, et al. The ALS-FTD-linked gene product, C9orf72, regulates neuronal morphogenesis via autophagy. *Autophagy.* (2019) 15:827–42. doi: 10.1080/15548627.2019.1569441
107. Han J-H, Ryu H-H, Jun M-H, Jang D-J, Lee J-A. The functional analysis of the CHMP2B missense mutation associated with neurodegenerative diseases in the endo-lysosomal pathway. *Biochem Biophys Res Commun.* (2012) 421:544–9. doi: 10.1016/j.bbrc.2012.04.041
108. Zaglia T, Milan G, Ruhs A, Franzoso M, Bertaggia E, Pianca N, et al. Atrogin-1 deficiency promotes cardiomyopathy and premature death via impaired autophagy. *J Clin Invest.* (2014) 124:2410–24. doi: 10.1172/JCI66339
109. Parkinson N, Ince PG, Smith MO, Highley R, Skibinski G, Andersen PM, et al. ALS phenotypes with mutations in CHMP2B (charged multivesicular body protein 2B). *Neurology.* (2006) 67:1074–7. doi: 10.1212/01.wnl.0000231510.89311.8b
110. Filimonenko M, Stuffers S, Raiborg C, Yamamoto A, Malerød L, Fisher EMC, et al. Functional multivesicular bodies are required for autophagic clearance of protein aggregates associated with neurodegenerative disease. *J Cell Biol.* (2007) 179:485–500. doi: 10.1083/jcb.200702115
111. Vandal S, Zheng X, Ahmad S. Molecular genetics of frontotemporal dementia elucidated by drosophila models–defects in endosomal–lysosomal pathway. *Int J Mol Sci.* (2018) 19:1714. doi: 10.3390/ijms19061714
112. Krasniak CS, Ahmad ST. The role of CHMP2BIntron5 in autophagy and frontotemporal dementia. *Brain Res.* (2016) 1649:151–7. doi: 10.1016/j.brainres.2016.02.051
113. Clayton EL, Mizielinska S, Edgar JR, Nielsen TT, Marshall S, Norona FE, et al. Frontotemporal dementia caused by CHMP2B mutation is characterised by neuronal lysosomal storage pathology. *Acta Neuropathol.* (2015) 130:511–23. doi: 10.1007/s00401-015-1475-3
114. Tanikawa S, Mori F, Tanji K, Kakita A, Takahashi H, Wakabayashi K. Endosomal sorting related protein CHMP2B is localized in Lewy bodies and glial cytoplasmic inclusions in α-synucleinopathy. *Neurosci Lett.* (2012) 527:16–21. doi: 10.1016/j.neulet.2012.08.035
115. Franz A, Ackermann L, Hoppe T. Create and preserve: proteostasis in development and aging is governed by Cdc48/p97/VCP. *Biochim Biophys Acta.* (2014) 1843:205–15. doi: 10.1016/j.bbamcr.2013.03.031
116. Shaw CE. Capturing VCP: another molecular piece in the ALS jigsaw puzzle. *Neuron.* (2010) 68:812–14. doi: 10.1016/j.neuron.2010.11.040
117. Johnson JO, Mandrioli J, Benatar M, Abramzon Y, Van Deerlin VM, Trojanowski JQ, et al. Exome sequencing reveals VCP mutations as a cause of familial ALS. *Neuron.* (2010) 68:857–64. doi: 10.1016/j.neuron.2010.11.036
118. Yin HZ, Nalbandian A, Hsu C-I, Li S, Llewellyn KJ, Mozaffar T, et al. Slow development of ALS-like spinal cord pathology in mutant valosin-containing protein gene knock-in mice. *Cell Death Dis.* (2012) 3:e374. doi: 10.1038/cddis.2012.115
119. Wang T, Xu W, Qin M, Yang Y, Bao P, Shen F, et al. Pathogenic mutations in the valosin-containing Protein/p97(VCP) N-domain Inhibit

the SUMOylation of VCP and lead to impaired stress response. *J Biol Chem.* (2016) 291:14373–84. doi: 10.1074/jbc.M116.729343

120. Llewellyn KJ, Walker N, Nguyen C, Tan B, BenMohamed L, Kimonis VE, et al. A fine balance of dietary lipids improves pathology of a murine model of VCP-associated multisystem proteinopathy. *PLoS ONE.* (2015) 10:e0131995. doi: 10.1371/journal.pone.0131995
121. Papadopoulos C, Kirchner P, Bug M, Grum D, Koerver L, Schulze N, et al. VCP/p97 cooperates with YOD1, UBXD1 and PLAA to drive clearance of ruptured lysosomes by autophagy. *EMBO J.* (2017) 36:135–50. doi: 10.15252/embj.201695148
122. Kon T, Mori F, Tanji K, Miki Y, Toyoshima Y, Yoshida M, et al. ALS-associated protein FIG4 is localized in Pick and Lewy bodies, and also neuronal nuclear inclusions, in polyglutamine and intranuclear inclusion body diseases. *Neuropathology.* (2014) 34:19–26. doi: 10.1111/neup.12056
123. Chow CY, Landers JE, Bergren SK, Sapp PC, Grant AE, Jones JM, et al. Deleterious variants of FIG4, a phosphoinositide phosphatase, in patients with ALS. *Am J Hum Genet.* (2009) 84:85–8. doi: 10.1016/j.ajhg.2008.12.010
124. Lenk GM, Meisler MH. Mouse models of PI(3,5)P2 deficiency with impaired lysosome function. *Methods Enzymol.* (2014) 534:245–60. doi: 10.1016/B978-0-12-397926-1.00014-7
125. Nishimura AL, Mitne-Neto M, Silva HCAA, Richieri-Costa A, Middleton S, Cascio D, et al. A mutation in the vesicle-trafficking protein VAPB causes late-onset spinal muscular atrophy and amyotrophic lateral sclerosis. *Am J Hum Genet.* (2004) 75:822–31. doi: 10.1086/425287
126. Genevini P, Colombo MN, Venditti R, Marcuzzo S, Colombo SF, Bernasconi P, et al. VAPB depletion alters neuritogenesis and phosphoinositide balance in motoneuron-like cells: relevance to VAPB-linked ALS. *J Cell Sci.* (2019) 2019:jcs.220061. doi: 10.1242/jcs.220061
127. Vinay Kumar C, Kumar KM, Swetha R, Ramaiah S, Anbarasu A. Protein aggregation due to nsSNP resulting in P56S VABP protein is associated with amyotrophic lateral sclerosis. *J Theor Biol.* (2014) 354:72–80. doi: 10.1016/j.jtbi.2014.03.027
128. Kabashi E, El Oussini H, Bercier V, Gros-Louis F, Valdmanis PN, McDearmid J, et al. Investigating the contribution of VAPB/ALS8 loss of function in amyotrophic lateral sclerosis. *Hum Mol Genet.* (2013) 22:2350–60. doi: 10.1093/hmg/ddt080
129. Aliaga L, Lai C, Yu J, Chub N, Shim H, Sun L, et al. Amyotrophic lateral sclerosis-related VAPB P56S mutation differentially affects the function and survival of corticospinal and spinal motor neurons. *Hum Mol Genet.* (2013) 22:4293–305. doi: 10.1093/hmg/ddt279
130. Hjerpe R, Bett JS, Keuss MJ, Solovyova A, McWilliams TG, Johnson C, et al. UBQLN2 mediates autophagy-independent protein aggregate clearance by the proteasome. *Cell.* (2016) 166:935–49. doi: 10.1016/j.cell.2016.07.001
131. Blokhuis AM, Groen EJN, Koppers M, van den Berg LH, Pasterkamp RJ. Protein aggregation in amyotrophic lateral sclerosis. *Acta Neuropathol.* (2013) 125:777–94. doi: 10.1007/s00401-013-1125-6
132. Deng H-X, Chen W, Hong S-T, Boycott KM, Gorrie GH, Siddique N, et al. Mutations in UBQLN2 cause dominant X-linked juvenile and adult-onset ALS and ALS/dementia. *Nature.* (2011) 477:211–15. doi: 10.1038/nature10353
133. Chen T, Huang B, Shi X, Gao L, Huang C. Mutant UBQLN2P497H in motor neurons leads to ALS-like phenotypes and defective autophagy in rats. *Acta Neuropathol Commun.* (2018) 6:122. doi: 10.1186/s40478-018-0627-9
134. Jantrapirom S, Lo Piccolo L, Yoshida H, Yamaguchi M. Depletion of ubiquilin induces an augmentation in soluble ubiquitinated drosophila TDP-43 to drive neurotoxicity in the fly. *Biochim Biophys Acta.* (2018) 1864:3038–49. doi: 10.1016/j.bbadis.2018.06.017
135. Brenner D, Sieverding K, Bruno C, Lüningschrör P, Buck E, Mungwa S, et al. Heterozygous *Tbk1* loss has opposing effects in early and late stages of ALS in mice. *J Exp Med.* (2019) 216:jem.20180729. doi: 10.1084/jem.20180729
136. Williams KL, Topp S, Yang S, Smith B, Fifita JA, Warraich ST, et al. CCNF mutations in amyotrophic lateral sclerosis and frontotemporal dementia. *Nat Commun.* (2016) 7:11253. doi: 10.1038/ncomms11253
137. Goode A, Rea S, Sultana M, Shaw B, Searle MS, Layfield R. ALS-FTLD associated mutations of SQSTM1 impact on Keap1-Nrf2 signalling. *Mol Cell Neurosci.* (2016) 76:52–8. doi: 10.1016/j.mcn.2016.08.004
138. Zhao M, Kim JR, van Bruggen R, Park J. RNA-binding proteins in amyotrophic lateral sclerosis. *Mol Cells.* (2018) 41:818–29. doi: 10.14348/molcells.2018.0243
139. Kabashi E, Valdmanis PN, Dion P, Spiegelman D, McConkey BJ, Velde CV, et al. TARDBP mutations in individuals with sporadic and familial amyotrophic lateral sclerosis. *Nat Genet.* (2008) 40:572–4. doi: 10.1038/ng.132
140. Sreedharan J, Blair IP, Tripathi VB, Hu X, Vance C, Rogelj B, et al. TDP-43 mutations in familial and sporadic amyotrophic lateral sclerosis. *Science.* (2008) 319:1668–72. doi: 10.1126/science.1154584
141. Kim HJ, Kim NC, Wang Y-D, Scarborough EA, Moore J, Diaz Z, et al. Mutations in prion-like domains in hnRNPA2B1 and hnRNPA1 cause multisystem proteinopathy and ALS. *Nature.* (2013) 495:467–73. doi: 10.1038/nature11922
142. Higashi S, Kabuta T, Nagai Y, Tsuchiya Y, Akiyama H, Wada K. TDP-43 associates with stalled ribosomes and contributes to cell survival during cellular stress. *J Neurochem.* (2013) 126:288–300. doi: 10.1111/jnc.12194
143. Villarroya-Beltri C, Gutiérrez-Vázquez C, Sánchez-Cabo F, Pérez-Hernández D, Vázquez J, Martin-Cofreces N, et al. Sumoylated hnRNPA2B1 controls the sorting of miRNAs into exosomes through binding to specific motifs. *Nat Commun.* (2013) 4:2980. doi: 10.1038/ncomms3980
144. Guo L, Kim HJ, Wang H, Monaghan J, Freyermuth F, Sung JC, et al. Nuclear-import receptors reverse aberrant phase transitions of RNA-binding proteins with prion-like domains. *Cell.* (2018) 173:677–92.e20. doi: 10.1016/j.cell.2018.03.002
145. Lai C, Xie C, Shim H, Chandran J, Howell BW, Cai H. Regulation of endosomal motility and degradation by amyotrophic lateral sclerosis 2/alsin. *Mol Brain.* (2009) 2:23. doi: 10.1186/1756-6606-2-23
146. Hadano S, Yanagisawa Y, Skaug J, Fichter K, Nasir J, Martindale D, et al. Cloning and characterization of three novel genes, ALS2CR1, ALS2CR2, and ALS2CR3, in the juvenile amyotrophic lateral sclerosis (ALS2) critical region at chromosome 2q33–q34: candidate genes for ALS2. *Genomics.* (2001) 71:200–13. doi: 10.1006/geno.2000.6392
147. Uversky VN. The roles of intrinsic disorder-based liquid-liquid phase transitions in the "Dr. Jekyll-Mr. Hyde" behavior of proteins involved in amyotrophic lateral sclerosis and frontotemporal lobar degeneration. *Autophagy.* (2017) 13:2115–2162. doi: 10.1080/15548627.2017.1384889
148. Martinez FJ, Pratt GA, Van Nostrand EL, Batra R, Huelga SC, Kapeli K, et al. Protein-RNA networks regulated by normal and ALS-associated mutant HNRNPA2B1 in the nervous system. *Neuron.* (2016) 92:780–95. doi: 10.1016/j.neuron.2016.09.050
149. van Rheenen W, Shatunov A, Dekker AM, McLaughlin RL, Diekstra FP, Pulit SL, et al. Genome-wide association analyses identify new risk variants and the genetic architecture of amyotrophic lateral sclerosis. *Nat Genet.* (2016) 48:1043–8. doi: 10.1038/ng.3622
150. Sato K, Otomo A, Ueda MT, Hiratsuka Y, Suzuki-Utsunomiya K, Sugiyama J, et al. Altered oligomeric states in pathogenic ALS2 variants associated with juvenile motor neuron diseases cause loss of ALS2-mediated endosomal function. *J Biol Chem.* (2018) 293:17135–53. doi: 10.1074/jbc.RA118.003849
151. Hadano S, Otomo A, Kunita R, Suzuki-Utsunomiya K, Akatsuka A, Koike M, et al. Loss of ALS2/Alsin exacerbates motor dysfunction in a SOD1H46R-expressing mouse ALS model by disturbing endolysosomal trafficking. *PLoS ONE.* (2010) 5:e9805. doi: 10.1371/journal.pone.0009805
152. Branchu J, Boutry M, Sourd L, Depp M, Leone C, Corriger A, et al. Loss of spatacsin function alters lysosomal lipid clearance leading to upper and lower motor neuron degeneration. *Neurobiol Dis.* (2017) 102:21–37. doi: 10.1016/j.nbd.2017.02.007
153. Orlacchio A, Babalini C, Borreca A, Patrono C, Massa R, Basaran S, et al. SPATACSIN mutations cause autosomal recessive juvenile amyotrophic lateral sclerosis. *Brain.* (2010) 133:591–598. doi: 10.1093/brain/awp325
154. Fang X, Lin H, Wang X, Zuo Q, Qin J, Zhang P. The NEK1 interactor, C21ORF2, is required for efficient DNA damage repair. *Acta Biochim Biophys Sin.* (2015) 47:834–41. doi: 10.1093/abbs/gmv076
155. Hirano M, Quinzii CM, Mitsumoto H, Hays AP, Roberts JK, et al. Senataxin mutations and amyotrophic lateral sclerosis. *Amyotroph Lateral Scler.* (2011) 12:223–7. doi: 10.3109/17482968.2010.545952

156. Becherel OJ, Yeo AJ, Stellati A, Heng EYH, Luff J, Suraweera AM, et al. Senataxin plays an essential role with DNA damage response proteins in meiotic recombination and gene silencing. *PLoS Genet.* (2013) 9:e1003435. doi: 10.1371/journal.pgen.1003435
157. Bennett CL, La Spada AR. Senataxin, a novel helicase at the interface of RNA transcriptome regulation and neurobiology: from normal function to pathological roles in motor neuron disease and cerebellar degeneration. *Adv Neurobiol.* 20:265–81. doi: 10.1007/978-3-319-89689-2_10
158. Grunseich C, Wang IX, Watts JA, Burdick JT, Guber RD, Zhu Z, et al. Senataxin mutation reveals how R-loops promote transcription by blocking DNA methylation at gene promoters. *Mol Cell.* (2018) 69:426–37.e7. doi: 10.1016/j.molcel.2017.12.030
159. Kwiatkowski TJ, Bosco DA, LeClerc AL, Tamrazian E, Vanderburg CR, Russ C, et al. Mutations in the FUS/TLS gene on chromosome 16 cause familial amyotrophic lateral sclerosis. *Science.* (2009) 323:1205–8. doi: 10.1126/science.1166066
160. Wang H, Guo W, Mitra J, Hegde PM, Vandoorne T, Eckelmann BJ, Mitra S, Tomkinson AE, Van Den Bosch L, Hegde ML. Mutant FUS causes DNA ligation defects to inhibit oxidative damage repair in Amyotrophic Lateral Sclerosis. *Nat Commun.* (2018) 9:3683. doi: 10.1038/s41467-018-06111-6
161. Devoy A, Kalmar B, Stewart M, Park H, Burke B, Noy SJ, et al. Humanized mutant FUS drives progressive motor neuron degeneration without aggregation in "FUSDelta14" knockin mice. *Brain.* (2017) 140:2797–805. doi: 10.1093/brain/awx248
162. Butti Z, Patten SA. RNA Dysregulation in amyotrophic lateral sclerosis. *Front Genet.* (2019) 9:712. doi: 10.3389/fgene.2018.00712
163. Elden AC, Kim H-J, Hart MP, Chen-Plotkin AS, Johnson BS, Fang X, et al. Ataxin-2 intermediate-length polyglutamine expansions are associated with increased risk for ALS. *Nature.* (2010) 466:1069–75. doi: 10.1038/nature09320
164. Ostrowski L, Hall A, Mekhail K. Ataxin-2: from RNA control to human health and disease. *Genes (Basel).* (2017) 8:157. doi: 10.3390/genes8060157
165. Thiyagarajan N, Ferguson R, Subramanian V, Acharya KR. Structural and molecular insights into the mechanism of action of human angiogenin-ALS variants in neurons. *Nat Commun.* (2012) 3:1121. doi: 10.1038/ncomms2126
166. Greenway MJ, Andersen PM, Russ C, Ennis S, Cashman S, Donaghy C, et al. ANG mutations segregate with familial and "sporadic" amyotrophic lateral sclerosis. *Nat Genet.* (2006) 38:411–3. doi: 10.1038/ng1742
167. Cronin S, Greenway MJ, Ennis S, Kieran D, Green A, Prehn JHM, et al. Elevated serum angiogenin levels in ALS. *Neurology.* (2006) 67:1833–6. doi: 10.1212/01.wnl.0000244466.46020.47
168. Li S, Hu G-F. Angiogenin-mediated rRNA transcription in cancer and neurodegeneration. *Int J Biochem Mol Biol.* (2010) 1:26–35.
169. Johnson JO, Pioro EP, Boehringer A, Chia R, Feit H, Renton AE, et al. Mutations in the Matrin 3 gene cause familial amyotrophic lateral sclerosis. *Nat Neurosci.* (2014) 17:664–6. doi: 10.1038/nn.3688
170. Malik AM, Miguez RA, Li X, Ho Y-S, Feldman EL, Barmada SJ. Matrin 3-dependent neurotoxicity is modified by nucleic acid binding and nucleocytoplasmic localization. *Elife.* (2018) 7:eLife.35977. doi: 10.7554/eLife.35977
171. Vieira M, Saraiva MJ. Transthyretin: a multifaceted protein. *Biomol Concepts.* (2014) 5:45–54. doi: 10.1515/bmc-2013-0038
172. Watanabe S, Hayakawa T, Wakasugi K, Yamanaka K. Cystatin C protects neuronal cells against mutant copper-zinc superoxide dismutase-mediated toxicity. *Cell Death Dis.* (2014) 5:e1497. doi: 10.1038/cddis.2014.459
173. Wilson ME, Boumaza I, Lacomis D, Bowser R. Cystatin C: a candidate biomarker for amyotrophic lateral sclerosis. *PLoS ONE.* (2010) 5:e15133. doi: 10.1371/journal.pone.0015133
174. Rossi D, Volanti P, Brambilla L, Colletti T, Spataro R, La Bella V. CSF neurofilament proteins as diagnostic and prognostic biomarkers for amyotrophic lateral sclerosis. *J Neurol.* (2018) 265:510–21. doi: 10.1007/s00415-017-8730-6
175. Chen X, Chen Y, Wei Q, Ou R, Cao B, Zhao B, et al. Assessment of a multiple biomarker panel for diagnosis of amyotrophic lateral sclerosis. *BMC Neurol.* (2016) 16:173. doi: 10.1186/s12883-016-0689-x
176. Gonçalves M, De Carvalho M, Peixoto C, Alves P, Barreto C, Oliva A, et al. Phosphoneurofilament heavy chain and vascular endothelial growth factor as cerebrospinal fluid biomarkers for ALS. *Amyotroph Lateral Scler Front Degener.* (2017) 18:134–6. doi: 10.1080/21678421.2016.1212894
177. Gendron TF, C9ORF72 Neurofilament Study Group LM, Daughrity LM, Heckman MG, Diehl NN, Wuu J, et al. Phosphorylated neurofilament heavy chain: a biomarker of survival for C9ORF72-associated amyotrophic lateral sclerosis. *Ann Neurol.* (2017) 82:139–46. doi: 10.1002/ana.24980
178. Boylan KB, Glass JD, Crook JE, Yang C, Thomas CS, Desaro P, et al. Phosphorylated neurofilament heavy subunit (pNF-H) in peripheral blood and CSF as a potential prognostic biomarker in amyotrophic lateral sclerosis. *J Neurol Neurosurg Psychiatry.* (2013) 84:467–72. doi: 10.1136/jnnp-2012-303768
179. Thompson AG, Gray E, Thézénas M-L, Charles PD, Evetts S, Hu MT, et al. Cerebrospinal fluid macrophage biomarkers in amyotrophic lateral sclerosis. *Ann Neurol.* (2018) 83:258–68. doi: 10.1002/ana.25143
180. Hathout Y, Seol H, Han MHJ, Zhang A, Brown KJ, Hoffman EP. Clinical utility of serum biomarkers in Duchenne muscular dystrophy. *Clin Proteomics.* (2016) 13:9. doi: 10.1186/s12014-016-9109-x
181. Sun X, Zhang H. miR-451 elevation relieves inflammatory pain by suppressing microglial activation-evoked inflammatory response via targeting TLR4. *Cell Tissue Res.* (2018) doi: 10.1007/s00441-018-2898-7
182. Yao Y, Tsirka SE. Monocyte chemoattractant protein-1 and the blood-brain barrier. *Cell Mol Life Sci.* (2014) 71:683–97. doi: 10.1007/s00018-013-1459-1
183. Boettger T, Wüst S, Nolte H, Braun T. The miR-206/133b cluster is dispensable for development, survival and regeneration of skeletal muscle. *Skelet Muscle.* (2014) 4:23. doi: 10.1186/s13395-014-0023-5
184. De Felice B, Guida M, Guida M, Coppola C, De Mieri G, Cotrufo R. A miRNA signature in leukocytes from sporadic amyotrophic lateral sclerosis. *Gene.* (2012) 508:35–40. doi: 10.1016/j.gene.2012.07.058
185. Horak M, Novak J, Bienertova-Vasku J. Muscle-specific microRNAs in skeletal muscle development. *Dev Biol.* (2016) 410:1–13. doi: 10.1016/J.YDBIO.2015.12.013
186. Turner MR, Hardiman O, Benatar M, Brooks BR, Chio A, De Carvalho M, et al. Controversies and priorities in amyotrophic lateral sclerosis. *Lancet Neurol.* (2013) 12:310–22. doi: 10.1016/S1474-4422(13)70036-X
187. Valbuena GN, Rizzardini M, Cimini S, Siskos AP, Bendotti C, Cantoni L, et al. Metabolomic analysis reveals increased aerobic glycolysis and amino acid deficit in a cellular model of amyotrophic lateral sclerosis. *Mol Neurobiol.* (2016) 53:2222–40. doi: 10.1007/s12035-015-9165-7
188. Funalot B, Desport J-C, Sturtz F, Camu W, Couratier P. High metabolic level in patients with familial amyotrophic lateral sclerosis. *Amyotroph Lateral Scler.* (2009) 10:113–117. doi: 10.1080/17482960802295192
189. Steyn FJ, Ioannides ZA, van Eijk RPA, Heggie S, Thorpe KA, Ceslis A, et al. Hypermetabolism in ALS is associated with greater functional decline and shorter survival. *J Neurol Neurosurg Psychiatry.* (2018) 89:1016–23. doi: 10.1136/jnnp-2017-317887
190. Abdel-Khalik J, Yutuc E, Crick PJ, Gustafsson J-Å, Warner M, Roman G, et al. Defective cholesterol metabolism in amyotrophic lateral sclerosis. *J Lipid Res.* (2017) 58:267–78. doi: 10.1194/jlr.P071639
191. Blasco H, Patin F, Molinier S, Vourc'h P, Le Tilly O, Bakkouche S, et al. A decrease in blood cholesterol after gastrostomy could impact survival in ALS. *Eur J Clin Nutr.* (2017) 71:1133–5. doi: 10.1038/ejcn.2017.54
192. Vieira AS, Dogini DB, Lopes-Cendes I. Role of non-coding RNAs in non-aging-related neurological disorders. *Braz J Med Biol Res.* (2018) 51:e7566. doi: 10.1590/1414-431X20187566
193. Wan P, Su W, Zhuo Y. The Role of Long Noncoding RNAs in neurodegenerative diseases. *Mol Neurobiol.* (2017) 54:2012–21. doi: 10.1007/s12035-016-9793-6
194. Peng W, Wang J, Shan B, Peng Z, Dong Y, Shi W, et al. Diagnostic and prognostic potential of circulating long non-coding RNAs in non small cell lung cancer. *Cell Physiol Biochem.* (2018) 49:816–27. doi: 10.1159/000493043
195. Bermejo JL, Huang G, Manoochehri M, Mesa KG, Schick M, Silos RG, et al. Long intergenic noncoding RNA 299 methylation in peripheral blood is a biomarker for triple-negative breast cancer. *Epigenomics.* (2018) 2018:epi-2018-0121. doi: 10.2217/epi-2018-0121

196. Li M, Wang Y-F, Yang X-C, Xu L, Li W-M, Xia K, et al. Circulating long noncoding RNA LIPCAR acts as a novel biomarker in patients with ST-segment elevation myocardial infarction. *Med Sci Monit.* (2018) 24:5064–70. doi: 10.12659/MSM.909348
197. Nagaraj S, Zoltowska KM, Laskowska-Kaszub K, Wojda U. microRNA diagnostic panel for Alzheimer's disease and epigenetic trade-off between neurodegeneration and cancer. *Ageing Res Rev.* (2018) 49:125–43. doi: 10.1016/J.ARR.2018.10.008
198. Punga T, Bartoccioni E, Lewandowska M, Damato V, Evoli A, Punga AR. Disease specific enrichment of circulating let-7 family microRNA in MuSK+ myasthenia gravis. *J Neuroimmunol.* (2016) 292:21–6. doi: 10.1016/j.jneuroim.2016.01.003
199. de Andrade HMT, de Albuquerque M, Avansini SH, de S Rocha C, Dogini DB, Nucci A, et al. MicroRNAs-424 and 206 are potential prognostic markers in spinal onset amyotrophic lateral sclerosis. *J Neurol Sci.* (2016) 368:19–24. doi: 10.1016/j.jns.2016.06.046
200. Russell AP, Wada S, Vergani L, Hock MB, Lamon S, Léger B, et al. Disruption of skeletal muscle mitochondrial network genes and miRNAs in amyotrophic lateral sclerosis. *Neurobiol Dis.* (2013) 49:107–17. doi: 10.1016/j.nbd.2012.08.015
201. Si Y, Cui X, Crossman DK, Hao J, Kazamel M, Kwon Y, et al. Muscle microRNA signatures as biomarkers of disease progression in amyotrophic lateral sclerosis. *Neurobiol Dis.* (2018) 114:85–94. doi: 10.1016/J.NBD.2018.02.009
202. Toivonen JM, Manzano R, Oliván S, Zaragoza P, García-Redondo A, Osta R. MicroRNA-206: a potential circulating biomarker candidate for amyotrophic lateral sclerosis. *PLoS ONE.* (2014) 9:e89065. doi: 10.1371/journal.pone.0089065
203. Ranganathan S, Williams E, Ganchev P, Gopalakrishnan V, Lacomis D, Urbinelli L, et al. Proteomic profiling of cerebrospinal fluid identifies biomarkers for amyotrophic lateral sclerosis. *J Neurochem.* (2005) 95:1461–71. doi: 10.1111/j.1471-4159.2005.03478.x
204. Ryberg H, An J, Darko S, Lustgarten JL, Jaffa M, Gopalakrishnan V, et al. Discovery and verification of amyotrophic lateral sclerosis biomarkers by proteomics. *Muscle Nerve.* (2010) 42:104–11. doi: 10.1002/mus.21683
205. Pasinetti GM, Ungar LH, Lange DJ, Yemul S, Deng H, Yuan X, et al. Identification of potential CSF biomarkers in ALS. *Neurology.* (2006) 66:1218–22. doi: 10.1212/01.wnl.0000203129.82104.07
206. Brancia C, Noli B, Boido M, Pilleri R, Boi A, Puddu R, et al. TLQP Peptides in amyotrophic lateral sclerosis: possible blood biomarkers with a neuroprotective role. *Neuroscience.* (2018) 380:152–63. doi: 10.1016/j.neuroscience.2018.03.023
207. Lunetta C, Lizio A, Maestri E, Sansone VA, Mora G, Miller RG, et al. Serum C-reactive protein as a prognostic biomarker in amyotrophic lateral sclerosis. *JAMA Neurol.* (2017) 74:660–7. doi: 10.1001/jamaneurol.2016.6179
208. Gaiani A, Martinelli I, Bello L, Querin G, Puthenparampil M, Ruggero S, et al. Diagnostic and Prognostic Biomarkers in amyotrophic lateral sclerosis: neurofilament light chain levels in definite subtypes of disease. *JAMA Neurol.* (2017) 74:525–32. doi: 10.1001/jamaneurol.2016.5398
209. Mitchell RM, Simmons Z, Beard JL, Stephens HE, Connor JR. Plasma biomarkers associated with ALS and their relationship to iron homeostasis. *Muscle Nerve.* (2010) 42:95–103. doi: 10.1002/mus.21625
210. Simpson EP, Henry YK, Henkel JS, Smith RG, Appel SH. Increased lipid peroxidation in sera of ALS patients: a potential biomarker of disease burden. *Neurology.* (2004) 62:1758–65. doi: 10.1212/WNL.62.10.1758
211. Nardo G, Pozzi S, Pignataro M, Lauranzano E, Spano G, Garbelli S, et al. Amyotrophic lateral sclerosis multiprotein biomarkers in peripheral blood mononuclear cells. *PLoS ONE.* (2011) 6:e25545. doi: 10.1371/journal.pone.0025545
212. Filareti M, Luotti S, Pasetto L, Pignataro M, Paolella K, Messina P, et al. Decreased levels of foldase and chaperone proteins are associated with an early-onset amyotrophic lateral sclerosis. *Front Mol Neurosci.* (2017) 10:99. doi: 10.3389/fnmol.2017.00099
213. Chen Y, Wei Q, Chen X, Li C, Cao B, Ou R, et al. Aberration of miRNAs expression in leukocytes from sporadic amyotrophic lateral sclerosis. *Front Mol Neurosci.* (2016) 9:69. doi: 10.3389/fnmol.2016.00069
214. De Felice B, Annunziata A, Fiorentino G, Borra M, Biffali E, Coppola C, et al. miR-338-3p is over-expressed in blood, CFS, serum and spinal cord from sporadic amyotrophic lateral sclerosis patients. *Neurogenetics.* (2014) 15:243–53. doi: 10.1007/s10048-014-0420-2
215. Vrabec K, Boštjančič E, Koritnik B, Leonardis L, Dolenc Grošelj L, Zidar J, et al. Differential expression of several miRNAs and the host genes AATK and DNM2 in leukocytes of sporadic ALS patients. *Front Mol Neurosci.* (2018) 11:106. doi: 10.3389/fnmol.2018.00106
216. Waller R, Goodall EF, Milo M, Cooper-Knock J, Da Costa M, Hobson E, et al. Serum miRNAs miR-206, 143-3p and 374b-5p as potential biomarkers for amyotrophic lateral sclerosis (ALS). *Neurobiol Aging.* (2017) 55:123–31. doi: 10.1016/j.neurobiolaging.2017.03.027
217. Tasca E, Pegoraro V, Merico A, Angelini C. Circulating microRNAs as biomarkers of muscle differentiation and atrophy in ALS. *Clin Neuropathol.* (2016) 35:22–30. doi: 10.5414/NP300889
218. Raheja R, Regev K, Healy BC, Mazzola MA, Beynon V, Von Glehn F, et al. Correlating serum micrornas and clinical parameters in amyotrophic lateral sclerosis. *Muscle Nerve.* (2018) 58:261–9. doi: 10.1002/mus.26106
219. Blasco H, Corcia P, Moreau C, Veau S, Fournier C, Vourc'h P, et al. 1H-NMR-based metabolomic profiling of CSF in early amyotrophic lateral sclerosis. *PLoS ONE.* (2010) 5:e13223. doi: 10.1371/journal.pone.0013223
220. Lawton KA, Cudkowicz ME, Brown MV, Alexander D, Caffrey R, Wulff JE, et al. Biochemical alterations associated with ALS. *Amyotroph Lateral Scler.* (2012) 13:110–8. doi: 10.3109/17482968.2011.619197
221. Ihara Y, Nobukuni K, Takata H, Hayabara T. Oxidative stress and metal content in blood and cerebrospinal fluid of amyotrophic lateral sclerosis patients with and without a Cu, Zn-superoxide dismutase mutation. *Neurol Res.* (2005) 27:105–8. doi: 10.1179/016164105X18430
222. Wuolikainen A, Andersen PM, Moritz T, Marklund SL, Antti H. ALS patients with mutations in the SOD1 gene have an unique metabolomic profile in the cerebrospinal fluid compared with ALS patients without mutations. *Mol Genet Metab.* (2012) 105:472–8. doi: 10.1016/j.ymgme.2011.11.201
223. Kumar A, Bala L, Kalita J, Misra UK, Singh RL, Khetrapal CL, et al. Metabolomic analysis of serum by (1) H NMR spectroscopy in amyotrophic lateral sclerosis. *Clin Chim Acta.* (2010) 411:563–7. doi: 10.1016/j.cca.2010.01.016
224. Lawton KA, Brown MV, Alexander D, Li Z, Wulff JE, Lawson R, et al. Plasma metabolomic biomarker panel to distinguish patients with amyotrophic lateral sclerosis from disease mimics. *Amyotroph Lateral Scler Frontotemporal Degener.* (2014) 15:362–70. doi: 10.3109/21678421.2014.908311
225. Rothstein JD, Tsai G, Kuncl RW, Clawson L, Cornblath DR, Drachman DB, et al. Abnormal excitatory amino acid metabolism in amyotrophic lateral sclerosis. *Ann Neurol.* (1990) 28:18–25. doi: 10.1002/ana.410280106
226. Iwasaki Y, Ikeda K, Kinoshita M. Plasma amino acid levels in patients with amyotrophic lateral sclerosis. *J Neurol Sci.* (1992) 107:219–22.
227. Gray E, Larkin JR, Claridge TDW, Talbot K, Sibson NR, Turner MR. The longitudinal cerebrospinal fluid metabolomic profile of amyotrophic lateral sclerosis. *Amyotroph Lateral Scler Frontotemporal Degener.* (2015) 16:456–63. doi: 10.3109/21678421.2015.1053490
228. Wuolikainen A, Jonsson P, Ahnlund M, Antti H, Marklund SL, Moritz T, et al. Multi-platform mass spectrometry analysis of the CSF and plasma metabolomes of rigorously matched amyotrophic lateral sclerosis, Parkinson's disease and control subjects. *Mol Biosyst.* (2016) 12:1287–98. doi: 10.1039/c5mb00711a
229. Dupuis L, Corcia P, Fergani A, Gonzalez De Aguilar J-L, Bonnefont-Rousselot D, Bittar R, et al. Dyslipidemia is a protective factor in amyotrophic lateral sclerosis. *Neurology.* (2008) 70:1004–9. doi: 10.1212/01.wnl.0000285080.70324.27
230. Valentino F, Bivona G, Butera D, Paladino P, Fazzari M, Piccoli T, et al. Elevated cerebrospinal fluid and plasma homocysteine levels in ALS. *Eur J Neurol.* (2010) 17:84–9. doi: 10.1111/j.1468-1331.2009.02752.x
231. Levin J, Bötzel K, Giese A, Vogeser M, Lorenzl S. Elevated levels of methylmalonate and homocysteine in Parkinson's disease, progressive supranuclear palsy and amyotrophic lateral sclerosis. *Dement Geriatr Cogn Disord.* (2010) 29:553–9. doi: 10.1159/000314841
232. Zoccolella S, Simone IL, Lamberti P, Samarelli V, Tortelli R, Serlenga L, et al. Elevated plasma homocysteine levels in patients

with amyotrophic lateral sclerosis. *Neurology.* (2008) 70:222–5. doi: 10.1212/01.wnl.0000297193.53986.6f

233. Cieslarova Z, Lopes FS, do Lago CL, França MC, Colnaghi Simionato AV. Capillary electrophoresis tandem mass spectrometry determination of glutamic acid and homocysteine's metabolites: potential biomarkers of amyotrophic lateral sclerosis. *Talanta.* (2017) 170:63–8. doi: 10.1016/J.TALANTA.2017.03.103
234. Brettschneider J, Lehmensiek V, Mogel H, Pfeifle M, Dorst J, Hendrich C, et al. Proteome analysis reveals candidate markers of disease progression in amyotrophic lateral sclerosis (ALS). *Neurosci Lett.* (2010) 468:23–7. doi: 10.1016/j.neulet.2009.10.053
235. Zhou J-Y, Afjehi-Sadat L, Asress S, Duong DM, Cudkowicz M, Glass JD, et al. Galectin-3 is a candidate biomarker for amyotrophic lateral sclerosis: discovery by a proteomics approach. *J Proteome Res.* (2010) 9:5133–41. doi: 10.1021/pr100409r
236. Liu J, Gao L, Zang D. Elevated levels of IFN-γ in CSF and serum of patients with amyotrophic lateral sclerosis. *PLoS ONE.* (2015) 10:e0136937. doi: 10.1371/journal.pone.0136937
237. Gao L, Zhou S, Cai H, Gong Z, Zang D. VEGF levels in CSF and serum in mild ALS patients. *J Neurol Sci.* (2014) 346:216–20. doi: 10.1016/j.jns.2014.08.031
238. Lind A-L, Wu D, Freyhult E, Bodolea C, Ekegren T, Larsson A, et al. A multiplex protein panel applied to cerebrospinal fluid reveals three new biomarker candidates in ALS but none in neuropathic pain patients. *PLoS ONE.* (2016) 11:e0149821. doi: 10.1371/journal.pone.0149821
239. Kano O, Tanaka K, Kanno T, Iwasaki Y, Ikeda J-E. Neuronal apoptosis inhibitory protein is implicated in amyotrophic lateral sclerosis symptoms. *Sci Rep.* (2018) 8:6. doi: 10.1038/s41598-017-18627-w
240. Lima C, Pinto S, Napoleão P, Pronto-Laborinho AC, Barros MA, Freitas T, et al. Identification of erythrocyte biomarkers in amyotrophic lateral sclerosis. *Clin Hemorheol Microcirc.* (2016) 63:423–37. doi: 10.3233/CH-162066
241. Edri-Brami M, Rosental B, Hayoun D, Welt M, Rosen H, Wirguin I, et al. Glycans in sera of amyotrophic lateral sclerosis patients and their role in killing neuronal cells. *PLoS ONE.* (2012) 7:e35772. doi: 10.1371/journal.pone.0035772
242. Otto M, Bahn E, Wiltfang J, Boekhoff I, Beuche W. Decrease of S100 beta protein in serum of patients with amyotrophic lateral sclerosis. *Neurosci Lett.* (1998) 240:171–3.
243. Häggmark A, Mikus M, Mohsenchian A, Hong M-G, Forsström B, Gajewska B, et al. Plasma profiling reveals three proteins associated to amyotrophic lateral sclerosis. *Ann Clin Transl Neurol.* (2014) 1:544–53. doi: 10.1002/acn3.83
244. Williams SM, Khan G, Harris BT, Ravits J, Sierks MR. TDP-43 protein variants as biomarkers in amyotrophic lateral sclerosis. *BMC Neurosci.* (2017) 18:20. doi: 10.1186/s12868-017-0334-7
245. Freischmidt A, Müller K, Ludolph AC, Weishaupt JH. Systemic dysregulation of TDP-43 binding microRNAs in amyotrophic lateral sclerosis. *Acta Neuropathol Commun.* (2013) 1:42. doi: 10.1186/2051-5960-1-42
246. Benigni M, Ricci C, Jones AR, Giannini F, Al-Chalabi A, Battistini S. Identification of miRNAs as potential biomarkers in cerebrospinal fluid from amyotrophic lateral sclerosis patients. *Neuromolecular Med.* (2016) 18:551–60. doi: 10.1007/s12017-016-8396-8
247. Waller R, Wyles M, Heath PR, Kazoka M, Wollff H, Shaw PJ, et al. Small RNA sequencing of sporadic amyotrophic lateral sclerosis cerebrospinal fluid reveals differentially expressed miRNAs related to neural and glial activity. *Front Neurosci.* (2017) 11:731. doi: 10.3389/fnins.2017.00731
248. Butovsky O, Siddiqui S, Gabriely G, Lanser AJ, Dake B, Murugaiyan G, et al. Modulating inflammatory monocytes with a unique microRNA gene signature ameliorates murine ALS. *J Clin Invest.* (2012) 122:3063–87. doi: 10.1172/JCI62636
249. Freischmidt A, Müller K, Zondler L, Weydt P, Volk AE, BoŽič AL, et al. Serum microRNAs in patients with genetic amyotrophic lateral sclerosis and pre-manifest mutation carriers. *Brain.* (2014) 137:2938–50. doi: 10.1093/brain/awu249
250. Freischmidt A, Müller K, Zondler L, Weydt P, Mayer B, von Arnim CAF, et al. Serum microRNAs in sporadic amyotrophic lateral sclerosis. *Neurobiol Aging.* (2015) 36:2660.e15-2660.e20. doi: 10.1016/j.neurobiolaging.2015.06.003
251. Matamala JM, Arias-Carrasco R, Sanchez C, Uhrig M, Bargsted L, Matus S, et al. Genome-wide circulating microRNA expression profiling reveals potential biomarkers for amyotrophic lateral sclerosis. *Neurobiol Aging.* (2018) 64:123–38. doi: 10.1016/j.neurobiolaging.2017.12.020
252. Takahashi I, Hama Y, Matsushima M, Hirotani M, Kano T, Hohzen H, et al. Identification of plasma microRNAs as a biomarker of sporadic amyotrophic lateral sclerosis. *Mol Brain.* (2015) 8:67. doi: 10.1186/s13041-015-0161-7
253. Saris CG, Horvath S, van Vught PW, van Es MA, Blauw HM, Fuller TF, et al. Weighted gene co-expression network analysis of the peripheral blood from Amyotrophic Lateral Sclerosis patients. *BMC Genomics.* (2009) 10:405. doi: 10.1186/1471-2164-10-405
254. Mougeot J-LC, Li Z, Price AE, Wright FA, Brooks BR. Microarray analysis of peripheral blood lymphocytes from ALS patients and the SAFE detection of the KEGG ALS pathway. *BMC Med Genomics.* (2011) 4:74. doi: 10.1186/1755-8794-4-74
255. Zhao W, Beers DR, Hooten KG, Sieglaff DH, Zhang A, Kalyana-Sundaram S, et al. Characterization of gene expression phenotype in amyotrophic lateral sclerosis monocytes. *JAMA Neurol.* (2017) 74:677. doi: 10.1001/jamaneurol.2017.0357
256. Nachmany H, Wald S, Abekasis M, Bulvik S, Weil M. Two potential biomarkers identified in mesenchymal stem cells and leukocytes of patients with sporadic amyotrophic lateral sclerosis. *Dis Markers.* (2012) 32:211–20. doi: 10.3233/DMA-2011-0885
257. Lilo E, Wald-Altman S, Solmesky LJ, Ben Yaakov K, Gershoni-Emek N, Bulvik S, et al. Characterization of human sporadic ALS biomarkers in the familial ALS transgenic mSOD1(G93A) mouse model. *Hum Mol Genet.* (2013) 22:4720–5. doi: 10.1093/hmg/ddt325
258. Wuolikainen A, Moritz T, Marklund SL, Antti H, Andersen PM. Disease-related changes in the cerebrospinal fluid metabolome in amyotrophic lateral sclerosis detected by GC/TOFMS. *PLoS ONE.* (2011) 6:e17947. doi: 10.1371/journal.pone.0017947
259. Spreux-Varoquaux O, Bensimon G, Lacomblez L, Salachas F, Pradat PF, Le Forestier N, et al. Glutamate levels in cerebrospinal fluid in amyotrophic lateral sclerosis: a reappraisal using a new HPLC method with coulometric detection in a large cohort of patients. *J Neurol Sci.* (2002) 193:73–8. doi: 10.1016/S0022-510X(01)00661-X
260. Dupuis L, Spreux-Varoquaux O, Bensimon G, Jullien P, Lacomblez L, Salachas F, et al. Platelet serotonin level predicts survival in amyotrophic lateral sclerosis. *PLoS ONE.* (2010) 5:e13346. doi: 10.1371/journal.pone.0013346
261. Simone IL, Ruggieri M, Tortelli R, Ceci E, D'Errico E, Leo A, et al. Serum N-acetylaspartate level in amyotrophic lateral sclerosis. *Arch Neurol.* (2011) 68:1308. doi: 10.1001/archneurol.2011.217
262. Keizman D, Ish-Shalom M, Berliner S, Maimon N, Vered Y, Artamonov I, .et al. Low uric acid levels in serum of patients with ALS: further evidence for oxidative stress? *J Neurol Sci.* (2009) 285:95–9. doi: 10.1016/j.jns.2009.06.002
263. Dorst J, Kühnlein P, Hendrich C, Kassubek J, Sperfeld AD, Ludolph AC. Patients with elevated triglyceride and cholesterol serum levels have a prolonged survival in amyotrophic lateral sclerosis. *J Neurol.* (2011) 258:613–7. doi: 10.1007/s00415-010-5805-z
264. Dedic SIK, Stevic Z, Dedic V, Stojanovic VR, Milicev M, Lavrnic D. Is hyperlipidemia correlated with longer survival in patients with amyotrophic lateral sclerosis? *Neurol Res.* (2012) 34:576–80. doi: 10.1179/1743132812Y.0000000049
265. Rozen S, Cudkowicz ME, Bogdanov M, Matson WR, Kristal BS, Beecher C, et al. Metabolomic analysis and signatures in motor neuron disease. *Metabolomics.* (2005) 1:101–8. doi: 10.1007/s11306-005-4810-1

266. Patin F, Corcia P, Vourc'h P, Nadal-Desbarats L, Baranek T, Goossens J-F, et al. Omics to explore amyotrophic lateral sclerosis evolution: the central role of arginine and proline metabolism. *Mol Neurobiol.* (2017) 54:5361–74. doi: 10.1007/s12035-016-0078-x
267. Conti A, Riva N, Pesca M, Iannaccone S, Cannistraci CV, Corbo M, et al. Increased expression of Myosin binding protein H in the skeletal muscle of amyotrophic lateral sclerosis patients. *Biochim Biophys Acta.* (2014) 1842:99–106. doi: 10.1016/J.BBADIS.2013.10.013
268. Yin F, Ye F, Tan L, Liu K, Xuan Z, Zhang J, et al. Alterations of signaling pathways in muscle tissues of patients with amyotrophic lateral sclerosis. *Muscle Nerve.* (2012) 46:856–60. doi: 10.1002/mus.23411
269. Elf K, Shevchenko G, Nygren I, Larsson L, Bergquist J, Askmark H, et al. Alterations in muscle proteome of patients diagnosed with amyotrophic lateral sclerosis. *J Proteomics.* (2014) 108:55–64. doi: 10.1016/j.jprot.2014.05.004
270. Narayan M, Seeley KW, Jinwal UK. Identification of Apo B48 and other novel biomarkers in amyotrophic lateral sclerosis patient fibroblasts. *Biomark Med.* (2016) 10:453–462. doi: 10.2217/bmm-2016-0025
271. Paré B, Touzel-Deschênes L, Lamontagne R, Lamarre M-S, Scott F-D, Khuong HT, et al. Early detection of structural abnormalities and cytoplasmic accumulation of TDP-43 in tissue-engineered skins derived from ALS patients. *Acta Neuropathol Commun.* (2015) 3:5. doi: 10.1186/s40478-014-0181-z
272. Mendonça DMF, Chimelli L, Martinez AMB. Quantitative evidence for neurofilament heavy subunit aggregation in motor neurons of spinal cords of patients with amyotrophic lateral sclerosis. *Brazilian J Med Biol Res.* (2005) 38:925–33. doi: 10.1590/S0100-879X2005000600015
273. Kovanda A, Leonardis L, Zidar J, Koritnik B, Dolenc-Groselj L, Ristic Kovacic S, et al. Differential expression of microRNAs and other small RNAs in muscle tissue of patients with ALS and healthy age-matched controls. *Sci Rep.* (2018) 8:5609. doi: 10.1038/s41598-018-23139-2
274. Campos-Melo D, Droppelmann CA, He Z, Volkening K, Strong MJ. Altered microRNA expression profile in amyotrophic lateral sclerosis: a role in the regulation of NFL mRNA levels. *Mol Brain.* (2013) 6:26. doi: 10.1186/1756-6606-6-26
275. Koval ED, Shaner C, Zhang P, du Maine X, Fischer K, Tay J, et al. Method for widespread microRNA-155 inhibition prolongs survival in ALS-model mice. *Hum Mol Genet.* (2013) 22:4127–35. doi: 10.1093/hmg/ddt261
276. Ishtiaq M, Campos-Melo D, Volkening K, Strong MJ. Analysis of novel NEFL mRNA targeting microRNAs in amyotrophic lateral sclerosis. *PLoS ONE.* (2014) 9:e85653. doi: 10.1371/journal.pone.0085653
277. Emde A, Eitan C, Liou L-L, Libby RT, Rivkin N, Magen I, et al. Dysregulated miRNA biogenesis downstream of cellular stress and ALS-causing mutations: a new mechanism for ALS. *EMBO J.* (2015) 34:2633–2651. doi: 10.15252/embj.201490493
278. Si Y, Cui X, Kim S, Wians R, Sorge R, Oh SJ, et al. Smads as muscle biomarkers in amyotrophic lateral sclerosis. *Ann Clin Transl Neurol.* (2014) 1:778–87. doi: 10.1002/acn3.117
279. Shtilbans A, Choi S-G, Fowkes ME, Khitrov G, Shahbazi M, Ting J, et al. Differential gene expression in patients with amyotrophic lateral sclerosis. *Amyotroph Lateral Scler.* (2011) 12:250–6. doi: 10.3109/17482968.2011.560946
280. Bernardini C, Censi F, Lattanzi W, Barba M, Calcagnini G, Giuliani A, et al. Mitochondrial network genes in the skeletal muscle of amyotrophic lateral sclerosis patients. *PLoS ONE.* (2013) 8:e57739. doi: 10.1371/journal.pone.0057739
281. Si Y, Kim S, Cui X, Zheng L, Oh SJ, Anderson T, et al. Transforming growth factor beta (TGF-β) Is a muscle biomarker of disease progression in ALS and correlates with smad expression. *PLoS ONE.* (2015) 10:e0138425. doi: 10.1371/journal.pone.0138425
282. Dupuis L, Gonzalez de Aguilar J-L, di Scala F, Rene F, de Tapia M, Pradat P-F, et al. Nogo provides a molecular marker for diagnosis of amyotrophic lateral sclerosis. *Neurobiol Dis.* (2002) 10:358–365. doi: 10.1006/NBDI.2002.0522
283. Malaspina A, Kaushik N, De Belleroche J. Differential expression of 14 genes in amyotrophic lateral sclerosis spinal cord detected using gridded cDNA arrays. *J Neurochem.* (2008) 77:132–45. doi: 10.1046/j.1471-4159.2001.00231.x
284. Jiang Y-M, Yamamoto M, Kobayashi Y, Yoshihara T, Liang Y, Terao S, et al. Gene expression profile of spinal motor neurons in sporadic amyotrophic lateral sclerosis. *Ann Neurol.* (2005) 57:236–51. doi: 10.1002/ana.20379
285. Ishigaki S, Niwa J, Ando Y, Yoshihara T, Sawada K, Doyu M, et al. Differentially expressed genes in sporadic amyotrophic lateral sclerosis spinal cords-screening by molecular indexing and subsequent cDNA microarray analysis. *FEBS Lett.* (2002) 531:354–8. doi: 10.1016/S0014-5793(02)03546-9
286. Dangond F, Hwang D, Camelo S, Pasinelli P, Frosch MP, Stephanopoulos G, et al. Molecular signature of late-stage human ALS revealed by expression profiling of postmortem spinal cord gray matter. *Physiol Genomics.* (2004) 16:229–39. doi: 10.1152/physiolgenomics.00087.2001
287. Wang X-S, Simmons Z, Liu W, Boyer PJ, Connor JR. Differential expression of genes in amyotrophic lateral sclerosis revealed by profiling the post mortem cortex. *Amyotroph Lateral Scler.* (2006) 7:201–10. doi: 10.1080/17482960600947689
288. Lederer CW, Torrisi A, Pantelidou M, Santama N, Cavallaro S. Pathways and genes differentially expressed in the motor cortex of patients with sporadic amyotrophic lateral sclerosis. *BMC Genomics.* (2007) 8:26. doi: 10.1186/1471-2164-8-26
289. Offen D, Barhum Y, Melamed E, Embacher N, Schindler C, Ransmayr G. Spinal cord mRNA profile in patients with ALS: comparison with transgenic mice expressing the human SOD-1 mutant. *J Mol Neurosci.* (2009) 38:85–93. doi: 10.1007/s12031-007-9004-z
290. Cox LE, Ferraiuolo L, Goodall EF, Heath PR, Higginbottom A, Mortiboys H, et al. Mutations in CHMP2B in lower motor neuron predominant amyotrophic lateral sclerosis (ALS). *PLoS ONE.* (2010) 5:e9872. doi: 10.1371/journal.pone.0009872
291. Riva N, Clarelli F, Domi T, Cerri F, Gallia F, Trimarco A, et al. Unraveling gene expression profiles in peripheral motor nerve from amyotrophic lateral sclerosis patients: insights into pathogenesis. *Sci Rep.* (2016) 6:39297. doi: 10.1038/srep39297
292. Wiedemann FR, Manfredi G, Mawrin C, Beal MF, Schon EA. Mitochondrial DNA and respiratory chain function in spinal cords of ALS patients. *J Neurochem.* (2002) 80:616–25. doi: 10.1046/j.0022-3042.2001.00731.x
293. Jones AP, Gunawardena WJ, Coutinho CM, Gatt JA, Shaw IC, Mitchell JD. Preliminary results of proton magnetic resonance spectroscopy in motor neurone disease (amytrophic lateral sclerosis). *J Neurol Sci.* (1995) 129(Suppl.):85–9.
294. Gredal O, Rosenbaum S, Topp S, Karlsborg M, Strange P, Werdelin L. Quantification of brain metabolites in amyotrophic lateral sclerosis by localized proton magnetic resonance spectroscopy. *Neurology.* (1997) 48:878–81.
295. Cwik VA, Hanstock CC, Allen PS, Martin WR. Estimation of brainstem neuronal loss in amyotrophic lateral sclerosis with *in vivo* proton magnetic resonance spectroscopy. *Neurology.* (1998) 50:72–7.
296. Ikeda K, Iwasaki Y, Kinoshita M, Ichijo M, Fujii H, Matsuoka Y, et al. Quantification of brain metabolites in ALS by localized proton magnetic spectroscopy. *Neurology.* (1998) 50:576–7.
297. Carew JD, Nair G, Pineda-Alonso N, Usher S, Hu X, Benatar M. Magnetic resonance spectroscopy of the cervical cord in amyotrophic lateral sclerosis. *Amyotroph Lateral Scler.* (2011) 12:185–191. doi: 10.3109/17482968.2010.515223
298. Ikeda K, Murata K, Kawase Y, Kawabe K, Kano O, Yoshii Y, et al. Relationship between cervical cord ^{1}H-magnetic resonance spectroscopy and clinoco-electromyographic profile in amyotrophic lateral sclerosis. *Muscle Nerve.* (2013) 47:61–7. doi: 10.1002/mus.23467
299. Cistaro A, Pagani M, Montuschi A, Calvo A, Moglia C, Canosa A, et al. The metabolic signature of C9ORF72-related ALS: FDG PET comparison

with nonmutated patients. *Eur J Nucl Med Mol Imaging.* (2014) 41:844–52. doi: 10.1007/s00259-013-2667-5

300. Cheong I, Marjanska M, Deelchand DK, Eberly LE, Walk D, Öz G. Ultra-high field proton MR spectroscopy in early-stage amyotrophic lateral sclerosis. *Neurochem Res.* (2017) 42:1833–44. doi: 10.1007/s11064-017-2248-2
301. Foerster BR, Pomper MG, Callaghan BC, Petrou M, Edden RAE, Mohamed MA, et al. An imbalance between excitatory and inhibitory neurotransmitters in amyotrophic lateral sclerosis revealed by use of 3-T proton magnetic resonance spectroscopy. *JAMA Neurol.* (2013) 70:1009–16. doi: 10.1001/jamaneurol.2013.234
302. Unrath A, Ludolph AC, Kassubek J. Brain metabolites in definite amyotrophic lateral sclerosis. A longitudinal proton magnetic resonance spectroscopy study. *J Neurol.* (2007) 254:1099–106. doi: 10.1007/s00415-006-0495-2
303. Kalra S, Hanstock CC, Martin WRW, Allen PS, Johnston WS. Detection of cerebral degeneration in amyotrophic lateral sclerosis using high-field magnetic resonance spectroscopy. *Arch Neurol.* (2006) 63:1144–8. doi: 10.1001/archneur.63.8.1144

17

Suboptimal Baseline Serum Vitamin B12 is Associated with Cognitive Decline in People with Alzheimer's Disease Undergoing Cholinesterase Inhibitor Treatment

Hsiao Shan Cho[1†], Li Kai Huang[1,2†], Yao Tung Lee[3,4], Lung Chan[1,5] and Chien Tai Hong[1,5]*

[1] Department of Neurology, Shuang Ho Hospital, Taipei Medical University, New Taipei City, Taiwan, [2] Graduate Institute of Humanities in Medicine, Taipei Medical University, Taipei, Taiwan, [3] Department of Psychiatry, Shuang Ho Hospital, Taipei Medical University, New Taipei City, Taiwan, [4] Department of Psychiatry, School of Medicine, College of Medicine, Taipei Medical University, Taipei, Taiwan, [5] Department of Neurology, School of Medicine, College of Medicine, Taipei Medical University, Taipei, Taiwan

***Correspondence:**
Chien Tai Hong
ct.hong@tmu.edu.tw

†These authors have contributed equally to this work.

Objectives: Cholinesterase inhibitors (ChEIs) are the mainstream treatment for delaying cognitive decline in Alzheimer's disease (AD). Low vitamin B12 is associated with cognitive dysfunction, and its supplementation has been applied as the treatment for certain types of reversible dementia. The present study hypothesized that baseline serum vitamin B12 is associated with the deterioration of cognitive function in people with AD undergoing ChEI treatment.

Materials and methods: Between 2009 and 2016, medical records from 165 Taiwanese with mild to moderate AD who underwent ChEI treatment for at least 2 years were reviewed. Their baseline serum vitamin B12 levels were measured before treatment initiation. Their cognitive function was assessed using the Mini–Mental State Examination (MMSE) and Cognitive Abilities Screening Instrument (CASI). Student's *t* test and multivariable logistic regression were used to analyze the association between cognitive decline and vitamin B12 level. Statistical analyses were performed using SPSS 19.0.

Results: Overall, 122 participants were women. Their median age was 76 years (ranging from 54 to 91). For people with optimal baseline vitamin B12 (above the median level of 436 ng/L), the rates of MMSE and CASI decline were 0.78 ± 1.28 and 2.84 ± 4.21 per year, respectively, which were significantly slower than those with suboptimal vitamin B12 (1.42 ± 1.67 and 4.94 ± 5.88 per year; $p = 0.007$ and 0.009, respectively). After adjustment for age, sex, education level, hypertension, diabetes, history of stroke, and baseline cognitive function, the baseline serum vitamin B12 level was negatively associated with MMSE and CASI decline.

Conclusion: Suboptimal baseline serum vitamin B12 level is associated with cognitive decline in people with AD undergoing ChEI treatment.

Keywords: cholinesterase inhibitors, Alzheimer's disease, vitamin B12, cognition, Mini–Mental State Status Examination, Cognitive Abilities Screening Instrument

INTRODUCTION

Alzheimer's disease (AD) is the most common cause of dementia. Estimates have revealed that in 2050, the number of people with AD aged 65 years and older will be triple (1). Presently, no curative treatment is available for AD. The most effective symptomatic pharmacological treatment for AD is cholinesterase inhibitors (ChEIs), which delay the progress of cognitive dysfunction (2). However, the response to ChEI treatment is variable. Higher cognitive profile, a previous intellectual occupation, healthier lifestyles, being married and not living alone, a higher degree of autonomy, and lower degree of brain atrophy at baseline were associated with better response to ChEI (3). The genotype of apolipoprotein E (ApoE), a cholesterol-transporting enzyme is strongly associated with AD. However, whether ApoE genotype affects the response to ChEI in people with AD is controversial. It had been demonstrated that ApoE ε4 allele carriers were poor responders to tacrine (4); nevertheless, other studies revealed that this detrimental genotype carriers exhibited better response to donepezil (5, 6). Evidence from several prospective, randomized, placebo-controlled trials with large samples were consistent with that ApoE was not a good predictor of response to ChEIs (7–10).

Vitamin B12 has been identified to be associated with cognitive function. Vitamin B12 deficiency because of a vegetarian diet, gastric surgery, malnutrition, or alcoholism results in cognitive dysfunction, and vitamin B12 supplementation can be applied as a rescue treatment for "reversible dementia" (11). A low vitamin B12 level is associated with increasing risks of AD and behavioral and psychological symptoms of dementia in people with AD (12, 13). Although a previous study reported that vitamin B12 supplementation failed to demonstrate neuroprotection in AD (14), the significance of vitamin B12 in AD should not be underestimated.

According to the Taiwan National Health Insurance (NHI) guideline, the insurance-coverage of ChEI treatment is only available to people with AD after vitamin B12 deficiency has been ruled out. Therefore, baseline serum vitamin B12 level measurements were available for all people with approval for the ChEI prescription. The present study investigated whether the baseline vitamin B12 level was associated with the deterioration of cognitive function in Taiwanese people with AD undergoing ChEI treatment.

MATERIALS AND METHODS

Patient Selection

This retrospective study was approved by the Joint Institutional Review Board of Taipei Medical University (TMU-JIRB) (Approval No. N201707049) and waived of informed consent was agreed by TMU-JIRB due to (1) the risk of participants is minimal and (2) waiving of informed consent is no harmful for the right of participants. Medical records from Shuang Ho Hospital between August 2009 and December 2016 were reviewed. During this period, there were 165 people with mild to moderate AD [baseline Mini–Mental State Examination (MMSE) between 10 and 26] who (1) underwent NHI-approved ChEI treatment (2) regular follow-up through cognitive function tests for at least two years. To avail of the insurance-coverage of ChEI treatment, the Taiwan NHI requires that patients should fulfill the following criteria: 1. AD diagnosis (DSM-IV diagnostic criteria of AD) and without any comorbidity affecting cognitive function, such as obvious vascular insults, vitamin B12 (≥206 ng/L), or folate deficiency, or metabolic disorder; 2. a review process to assess all medical records of the patient. The review is conducted by an NHI committee consisting of either neurologists or psychiatrists. After receiving NHI approval for ChEI treatment, patients are required to receive at least annual follow-up through the MMSE, and ChEI treatment would be discontinued for patients with MMSE decline of more than 2 points year-by-year.

The present study collected baseline medical and personal records, including age; sex; education years; medical history of hypertension, diabetes, and cerebrovascular accident (CVA); and serum vitamin B12 and folate. Since vitamin B12 level is known to be affected by several drugs (colchicine, proton pump inhibitors, histamine H2-receptor antagonists, metformin, and antiepileptic agents) and medical conditions (alcohol consumption, peptic ulcer, or gastric operation), specific drug and medical history were also recorded. All patients received MMSE and Cognitive Abilities Screening Instrument (CASI) tests at least three times: at the baseline, first follow-up, and second follow-up, with a 1-year interval. The longest follow-up period was 8 years. For ChEI treatment, donepezil (5 and 10 mg) and rivastigmine (1.5 and 4.5-mg pill and 10-mg patch) were available in Shuang Ho Hospital. People with AD were allowed to switch medications if side effects were intolerable. The deterioration of MMSE and CASI was determined by calculating the ratio of the difference in scores between the baseline and last cognitive tests (unit: score) to the time interval between two tests (unit: year).

Statistical Analyses

All statistical analyses were performed using SPSS for Windows 10 (version 19; SPSS Inc., Chicago, IL, USA). Continuous variables are presented as mean ± SD, and categorical variables are presented as percentages with corresponding 95% confidence intervals. The differences were analyzed using Student's t test. The multivariate logistic regression model was adjusted for the following variables: age; sex; education level; initial cognitive function test (either the MMSE or CASI); history of hypertension, diabetes, and CVA; and baseline folate level. A p-value of <0.05 was considered statistically significant.

RESULTS

All 165 people with AD underwent ChEI treatment for at least 2 years and were followed through annual cognitive examination (the MMSE and CASI). Their median age was 76 years (ranging from 54 to 91) while initiating treatment; 112 of them were women; and their median education years was 6 years (ranging from 0 to 16). The median level of vitamin B12 was 436 ng/L (ranging from 206 to 5,454). The distribution of serum vitamin B12 was a two-tailed normal distribution pattern (Figure S1 in Supplementary Material).

Furthermore, people with AD were categorized into two groups based on their baseline vitamin B12 levels: the group with optimal baseline vitamin B12 level (above median, 436 ng/L, n = 82) and suboptimal baseline vitamin B12 level (n = 83) (**Table 1**). Comparison between these two groups revealed no significant difference in most of the background demographic characteristics, including age, education years, major medical history, and baseline MMSE and CASI scores. However, more women (65 versus 47, p = 0.003) were in the optimal vitamin B12 group. Moreover, patients in the optimal B12 group had a significantly higher folate level. In both groups, donepezil was the main choice of ChEI treatment and the dosage of donepezil among the majority of them were titrated up to 10 mg daily. Only few of participants in both groups were exposure to drugs which may affect vitamin B12, mainly metformin.

TABLE 1 | Demographic data of all patients categorized into optimal vitamin B12 (>436 ng/L) and suboptimal (≤436 ng/L) groups.

	Optimal vitamin B12 (n = 82)	Suboptimal vitamin B12 (n = 83)	p-Value
Women (%)	65 (79.3)	47 (56.6)	0.003
Age (years)	76.01 ± 6.93	75.41 ± 8.46	0.618
Education (years)	5.46 ± 4.81	7.10 ± 4.23	0.019
Hypertension (%)	30 (36.6)	38 (45.8)	0.269
Diabetes (%)	17 (20.7)	25 (30.1)	0.211
CVA (%)	9 (11.0)	9 (10.8)	1.000
Folate (ng/mL)	15.79 ± 10.52	11.14 ± 10.46	0.005
Baseline MMSE	18.33 ± 5.00	19.28 ± 4.38	0.197
Baseline CASI	60.30 ± 16.57	64.83 ± 13.67	0.057
ChEIs	Donepezil 5 mg, n = 12 Donepezil 10 mg, n = 50 Rivastigmine, n = 20	Donepezil 5 mg, n = 21 Donepezil 10 mg, n = 43 Rivastigmine, n = 19	0.253
Medications affecting Vitamin B12	Metformin, n = 7 PPI, n = 4 AED, n = 1 H2 blockers, n = 1	Metformin, n = 11 AED, n = 3 Colchicine, n = 1	
MMSE decline/year	0.78 ± 1.28	1.42 ± 1.67	0.007
CASI decline/year	2.84 ± 4.21	4.95 ± 5.88	0.009

CVA, cerebrovascular accident; MMSE, Mini-Mental State Examination; CASI, Cognitive Abilities Screening Instrument; ChEI, cholinesterase inhibitor; PPI, proton pump inhibitor; AED, antiepileptic drug; H2, histamine H2 receptors.

The present study aimed to investigate the effect of baseline vitamin B12 on the response to ChEI treatment for cognitive decline in people with AD. After the first 2-year treatment, participants in both groups demonstrated a decline in the MMSE and CASI with highly variable results of cognitive function test within the group (**Figure 1**). However, if extending the follow-up period to the end of ChEI treatment (maximum follow-up period: 8 years), for patients with optimal vitamin B12 level, the corresponding cognitive decline was significantly slower than suboptimal vitamin B12 group of patients (MMSE decline: 0.78 ± 1.28 versus 1.42 ± 1.67 point/year, p = 0.007; CASI decline: 2.84 ± 4.21 versus 4.95 ± 5.88 point/year, p = 0.009) (**Table 1**).

If further categorized all the patients into four groups by first, second, and third quartile, the results demonstrated a similar pattern that people with higher baseline vitamin B12 level demonstrated less cognitive decline (Table S1 in Supplementary Material).

Because several factors affect cognitive decline, including age, education years, comorbidities, and baseline cognitive function before treatment, we applied a multivariable regression model to investigate the association between the baseline serum vitamin B12 level and cognitive decline. After adjustment for the aforementioned factors, the baseline vitamin B12 level was significantly and negatively associated with cognitive decline (MMSE decline, p = 0.009; CASI decline, p = 0.014) (**Table 2**).

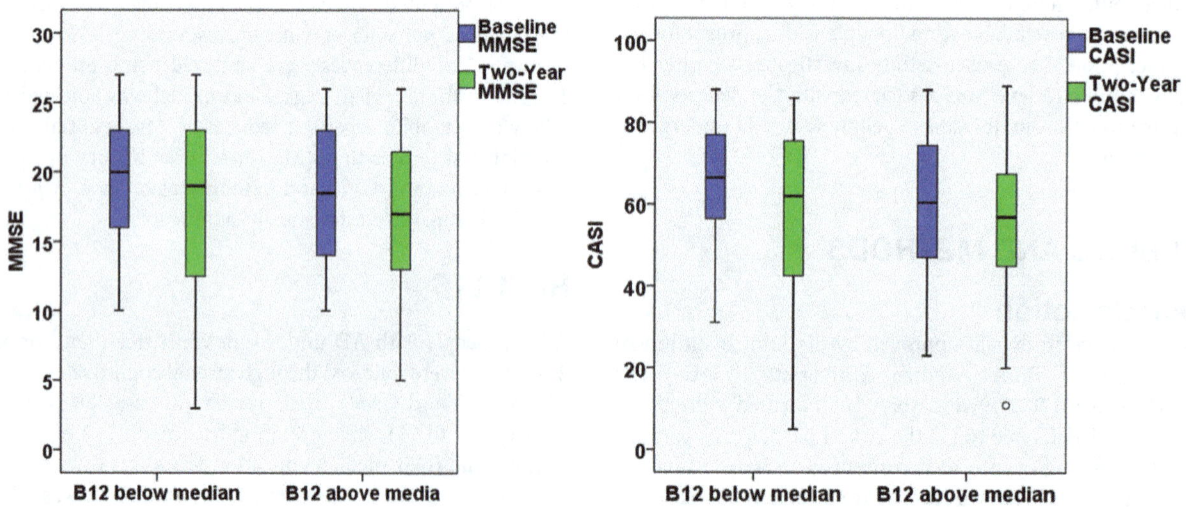

FIGURE 1 | The box plots demonstrated the results of Mini-Mental State Examination (MMSE) and Cognitive Abilities Screening Instrument (CASI) at baseline and 2-year follow-up for patients with optimal (>436 ng/L) or suboptimal baseline vitamin B12 level.

TABLE 2 | Multivariable regression model of the association between high vitamin B12 level and deterioration of cognitive function.

	Deterioration of Mini-Mental State Examination (MMSE)		Deterioration of Cognitive Abilities Screening Instrument (CASI)	
	Normalized beta coefficient	*p*-Value	Normalized beta coefficient	*p*-Value
Vitamin B12	−0.214	0.009	−0.195	0.014

The model was adjusted for age; sex; education level; initial cognitive function test (either MMSE or CASI); history of diabetes, and CVA; and baseline folate level.

DISCUSSION

The present study showed that the baseline vitamin B12 level was negatively associated with cognitive decline in people with AD undergoing ChEI treatment. The deterioration of cognitive function, as assessed by the MMSE and CASI, was significantly slower in patients with optimal baseline vitamin B12 level. Moreover, after adjustment of age, sex, education level, comorbidity, and baseline cognitive function, the baseline vitamin B12 level was negatively associated with cognitive decline. The results demonstrate that the suboptimal baseline vitamin B12 level was associated with poorer response to ChEI treatment in people with AD.

Vitamin B12 deficiency is associated with damage to the white matter in the spinal cord and in the brain, which adversely affects neuronal function. The exact mechanism underlying this association remains unknown. Damage to myelin as a result of defective methylation of myelin basic protein (MBP) has been postulated as an underlying mechanism. MBP accounts for approximately one-third of myelin protein, and demyelination in the setting of vitamin B12 deficiency may explain many of the neurologic findings, including the association with cognitive decline (15, 16). Another hypothesis is the alteration of the concentrations of cytokines, such as tumor necrosis factor-α or epidermal growth factor (17). A low vitamin B12 status leads to S-adenosylmethionine deficiency, which results in defective methylation reactions in the central nervous system (18). In a longitudinal study, the serum holotranscobalamin level was found to be related to cognitive performance 7 years later, even in elderly subjects without dementia, and a higher holotranscobalamin level tended to be related to higher performance in executive functions and psychomotor speed (19). Another study conducted in participants aged 45–69 years showed that participants whose vitamin B12 level was in the highest quartile had significantly higher verbal fluency scores (20). The Framingham Heart Study that included community-dwelling individuals aged 74.8 ± 4.6 years showed that plasma vitamin B12 levels ranging from 187 to 256.8 pmol/L predicted cognitive decline (21). Cohort studies have also demonstrated the association of low vitamin B12 status with cognitive dysfunction and cognitive decline (22, 23). A longitudinal cohort study that included 97 people with AD also revealed that baseline homocysteine levels showed a concentration–response relationship with the subsequent rate of decline in cognitive tests (24). However, in clinical practice, it was found that people with cognitive impairment, which is associated with vitamin B12 deficiency, did not always improve on treatment, whereas those with obvious dementia usually showed no improvement (25). Connelly suggested that the isolated use of B vitamins and folic acid is ineffective in improving cognition in people with AD, although homocysteine levels were normal or mildly increased (26). In a systematic review of four randomized controlled trials, vitamin B supplementation was found to be effective in reducing serum homocysteine levels but not in facilitating cognitive improvement (27). In a meta-analysis of 11 randomized trials involving 22,000 participants, Clarke et al. argued that 5-year dietary supplementation with B vitamins did not have any effect on cognitive domains, global cognitive function, or cognitive aging in older people (28).

The present study has some limitations. Although the medical chart review could identify numerous useful information, it was shortage of certain valuable factors for research. For instance, the present study failed to provide the ApoE genetic information, which is the strongest genetic determinant of AD. However, as aforementioned, whether ApoE genotype affects the response of ChEI was controversial. In addition, activities of daily living and instrumental activities of daily living assessments were not routinely performed in the clinical setting, so authors were not able to provide this information. On the other hand, according to the NHI guidelines about the insurance-coverage ChEI treatment, all people with AD with approved ChEI treatment are required to receive the cognitive function test annually. However, this treatment may be discontinued in patients with cognitive decline of more than 2 points in MMSE year-by-year; thus, the follow-up of cognitive function may stop. Our patients received ChEI treatment for at least 2 years, indicating that they were not the early non-responders to ChEI treatment in the first 12 months. Patients with a longer follow-up duration had a more benign course of AD. Therefore, this population was not exactly real-world people with AD but a group of partial or good responders to ChEI treatment. In addition, the vitamin B12 level of the study patients was not followed up annually. Without follow-up, no information was available to determine the correlation between the change in vitamin B12 and cognitive function and the effect of vitamin B12 supplementation on cognitive decline.

In conclusion, the present study demonstrated that suboptimal baseline serum vitamin B12 level was associated with rapid cognitive decline in people with AD undergoing ChEI treatment. Additional studies are required to delineate whether the alteration of the vitamin B12 level during the ChEI treatment period is correlated with cognitive change and to identify the specific people with AD who may be the responders to vitamin B12 supplementation.

AUTHOR CONTRIBUTIONS

Conception or design of the work: YL, LC, and CH. The acquisition, analysis: HC and LH. Interpretation of data for the work: HC, LH, and YL. Drafting the work or revising it critically for important intellectual content, final approval of the version to be published, agreement to be accountable for all aspects of the work in ensuring that questions related to the accuracy or integrity of any part of the work are appropriately investigated and resolved: HC, LH, YL, LC, and CH. HC and LH: both authors contributed equally to this study.

REFERENCES

1. Alzheimer's Association. 2016 Alzheimer's disease facts and figures. *Alzheimers Dement* (2016) 12:459–509. doi:10.1016/j.jalz.2016.03.001
2. Rabins PV, Blacker D, Rovner BW, Rummans T, Schneider LS, Tariot PN, et al. American Psychiatric Association practice guideline for the treatment of patients with Alzheimer's disease and other dementias. Second edition. *Am J Psychiatry* (2007) 164:5–56.
3. Gallucci M, Spagnolo P, Arico M, Grossi E. Predictors of response to cholinesterase inhibitors treatment of Alzheimer's disease: date mining from the TREDEM registry. *J Alzheimers Dis* (2016) 50:969–79. doi:10.3233/JAD-150747
4. Sjögren M, Hesse C, Basun H, Köl G, Thostrup H, Kilander L, et al. Tacrine and rate of progression in Alzheimer's disease – relation to ApoE allele genotype. *J Neural Transm (Vienna)* (2001) 108:451–8. doi:10.1007/s007020170066
5. Petersen RC, Smith GE, Waring SC, Ivnik RJ, Tangalos EG, Kokmen E. Mild cognitive impairment: clinical characterization and outcome. *Arch Neurol* (1999) 56:303–8. doi:10.1001/archneur.56.3.303
6. Bizzarro A, Marra C, Acciarri A, Valenza A, Tiziano FD, Brahe C, et al. Apolipoprotein E epsilon4 allele differentiates the clinical response to donepezil in Alzheimer's disease. *Dement Geriatr Cogn Disord* (2005) 20:254–61. doi:10.1159/000087371
7. Wilcock GK, Lilienfeld S, Gaens E. Efficacy and safety of galantamine in patients with mild to moderate Alzheimer's disease: multicentre randomised controlled trial. Galantamine International-1 Study Group. *BMJ* (2000) 321:1445–9. doi:10.1136/bmj.321.7274.1445
8. Aerssens J, Raeymaekers P, Lilienfeld S, Geerts H, Konings F, Parys W. APOE genotype: no influence on galantamine treatment efficacy nor on rate of decline in Alzheimer's disease. *Dement Geriatr Cogn Disord* (2001) 12:69–77. doi:10.1159/000051238
9. Winblad B, Engedal K, Soininen H, Verhey F, Waldemar G, Wimo A, et al. A 1-year, randomized, placebo-controlled study of donepezil in patients with mild to moderate AD. *Neurology* (2001) 57:489–95. doi:10.1212/WNL.57.3.489
10. Farlow MR, Cyrus PA, Nadel A, Lahiri DK, Brashear A, Gulanski B. Metrifonate treatment of AD: influence of APOE genotype. *Neurology* (1999) 53:2010–6. doi:10.1212/WNL.53.9.2010
11. Health Quality Ontario. Vitamin B12 and cognitive function: an evidence-based analysis. *Ont Health Technol Assess Ser* (2013) 13:1–45.
12. Chan A, Paskavitz J, Remington R, Rasmussen S, Shea TB. Efficacy of a vitamin/nutriceutical formulation for early-stage Alzheimer's disease: a 1-year, open-label pilot study with an 16-month caregiver extension. *Am J Alzheimers Dis Other Demen* (2008) 23:571–85. doi:10.1177/1533317508325093
13. Shen L, Ji HF. Associations between homocysteine, folic acid, vitamin B12 and Alzheimer's disease: insights from meta-analyses. *J Alzheimers Dis* (2015) 46:777–90. doi:10.3233/JAD-150140
14. Sun Y, Lu CJ, Chien KL, Chen ST, Chen RC. Efficacy of multivitamin supplementation containing vitamins B6 and B12 and folic acid as adjunctive treatment with a cholinesterase inhibitor in Alzheimer's disease: a 26-week, randomized, double-blind, placebo-controlled study in Taiwanese patients. *Clin Ther* (2007) 29:2204–14. doi:10.1016/j.clinthera.2007.10.012
15. Scott JM. Folate and vitamin B12. *Proc Nutr Soc* (1999) 58:441–8. doi:10.1017/S0029665199000580
16. Ikram MA, Vrooman HA, Vernooij MW, den Heijer T, Hofman A, Niessen WJ, et al. Brain tissue volumes in relation to cognitive function and risk of dementia. *Neurobiol Aging* (2010) 31:378–86. doi:10.1016/j.neurobiolaging.2008.04.008
17. Scalabrino G, Veber D, Mutti E. Experimental and clinical evidence of the role of cytokines and growth factors in the pathogenesis of acquired cobalamin-deficient leukoneuropathy. *Brain Res Rev* (2008) 59:42–54. doi:10.1016/j.brainresrev.2008.05.001
18. Weir DG, Scott JM. Brain function in the elderly: role of vitamin B12 and folate. *Br Med Bull* (1999) 55:669–82. doi:10.1258/0007142991902547
19. Hooshmand B, Solomon A, Kåreholt I, Rusanen M, Hänninen T, Leiviskä J, et al. Associations between serum homocysteine, holotranscobalamin, folate and cognition in the elderly: a longitudinal study. *J Intern Med* (2012) 271: 204–12. doi:10.1111/j.1365-2796.2011.02484.x
20. Horvat P, Gardiner J, Kubinova R, Pajak A, Tamosiunas A, Schöttker B, et al. Serum folate, vitamin B-12 and cognitive function in middle and older age: the HAPIEE study. *Exp Gerontol* (2016) 76:33–8. doi:10.1016/j.exger.2016.01.011
21. Morris MS, Selhub J, Jacques PF. Vitamin B-12 and folate status in relation to decline in scores on the mini-mental state examination in the Framingham heart study. *J Am Geriatr Soc* (2012) 60:1457–64. doi:10.1111/j.1532-5415.2012.04076.x
22. Nie T, Lu T, Xie L, Huang P, Lu Y, Jiang M. Hyperhomocysteinemia and risk of cognitive decline: a meta-analysis of prospective cohort studies. *Eur Neurol* (2014) 72:241–8. doi:10.1159/000363054
23. O'Leary F, Allman-Farinelli M, Samman S. Vitamin B 12 status, cognitive decline and dementia: a systematic review of prospective cohort studies. *Br J Nutr* (2012) 108:1948–61. doi:10.1017/S0007114512004175
24. Oulhaj A, Refsum H, Beaumont H, Williams J, King E, Jacoby R, et al. Homocysteine as a predictor of cognitive decline in Alzheimer's disease. *Int J Geriatr Psychiatry* (2010) 25:82–90. doi:10.1002/gps.2303
25. Malouf R, Areosa Sastre A. Vitamin B12 for cognition. *Cochrane Database Syst Rev* (2003):CD004326. doi:10.1002/14651858.CD004326
26. Connelly P. High dose vitamin B supplementation does not slow cognitive decline in mild to moderate Alzheimer's disease. *Evid Based Ment Health* (2009) 12:86. doi:10.1136/ebmh.12.3.86
27. Zhang D-M, Ye J-X, Mu J-S, Cui X-P. Efficacy of vitamin B supplementation on cognition in elderly patients with cognitive-related diseases: a systematic review and meta-analysis. *J Geriatr Psychiatry Neurol* (2017) 30:50–9. doi:10.1177/0891988716673466
28. Clarke R, Bennett D, Parish S, Lewington S, Skeaff M, Eussen SJ, et al. Effects of homocysteine lowering with B vitamins on cognitive aging: meta-analysis of 11 trials with cognitive data on 22,000 individuals. *Am J Clin Nutr* (2014) 100:657–66. doi:10.3945/ajcn.113.076349

18

The Impact of Cognitive and Behavioral Symptoms on ALS Patients and their Caregivers

Jashelle Caga[1,2], *Sharpley Hsieh*[3], *Patricia Lillo*[4], *Kaitlin Dudley*[5] *and Eneida Mioshi*[5*]

[1] *Sydney Medical School, University of Sydney, Camperdown, NSW, Australia,* [2] *Brain & Mind Centre, University of Sydney, Camperdown, NSW, Australia,* [3] *Faculty of Health and Behavioural Sciences, School of Psychology, University of Queensland, QLD, Australia,* [4] *Departamento de Neurología Sur/Neurociencia, Facultad de Medicina, Universidad de Chile & Geroscience Center for Brain Health and Metabolism, Santiago, Chile,* [5] *School of Health Sciences, University of East Anglia, Norwich, United Kingdom*

Correspondence:
Eneida Mioshi
e.mioshi@uea.ac.uk

Previously thought to be a pure motor disease, amyotrophic lateral sclerosis (ALS) is now established as multisystem neurodegenerative disorder that lies on a continuum with frontotemporal dementia (FTD). Cognitive and behavioral symptoms primarily extend to executive function, personality, social conduct, and emotion processing. The assessment and management of cognitive and behavioral symptoms is complicated as they must be differentiated from psychological responses to a terminal diagnosis and progressive physical impairment. This is made more difficult by the limited number of studies investigating how these symptoms specifically affect patients and caregivers well-being. The current review focuses on the impact of cognitive and behavioral symptoms on patient and caregiver well-being and their implications for future research and interventions in ALS. This is an important area of research that could form the basis for more tailored, and potentially more successful, non-pharmacological interventions to improve psychological well-being among patients with ALS and their caregivers.

Keywords: amyotrophic lateral sclerosis, dementia, depression, quality of life, caregiver, burden, adherence, non-pharmacological interventions

BACKGROUND

Amyotrophic lateral sclerosis (ALS) is a multisystem neurodegenerative disorder which includes a broad spectrum of non-motor symptoms that can dominate the clinical presentation (1, 2). Cognitive and behavioral symptoms include impaired executive function, deficits in social and emotional cognition, apathy, disinhibition, and perseveration similar to that seen in frontotemporal dementia (FTD). Frontotemporal dysfunction of varying severity can affect more than 50% of ALS patients (3), with ~8–14% meeting full diagnostic criteria for FTD (4–8). As such, early detection and timely management of cognitive and behavioral symptoms is widely acknowledged as an important aspect of contemporary ALS care (9). However, fully assessing cognitive and behavioral symptoms in ALS is made difficult by the fact that these symptoms must be distinguished from psychological reactions to a terminal diagnosis and the progressive physical loss that comes alongside it. Our narrative review focuses on evaluating the impact of cognitive and behavioral symptoms on patient and caregiver well-being and their implications for developing future non-pharmacological interventions in ALS. Gathering this research can help form more appropriate and effective non-pharmacological interventions to improve psychological well-being among patients with ALS and their caregivers.

SEARCH STRATEGY AND SELECTION CRITERIA

For this narrative review references were primarily searched through PubMed. The following terms were systematically searched: "amyotrophic lateral sclerosis"; "motor neuron(e) disease"; "cognitive"; "behavioral"; "depression"; "anxiety"; "quality of life"; "psychological health"; "caregiver"; "carer"; "burden"; "strain"; "stress"; "compliance"; "adherence"; "psychosocial intervention"; "non-pharmacological intervention"; "support"; "manage"; "intervention"; "care"; "caring"; "coping"; "cope"; "frontotemporal dementia." The section on non-pharmacological interventions for cognitive and behavioral symptoms in ALS also used the MEDLINE, EMBASE, PsycINFO, AMED, and CINAHL databases. Searches included papers published in English between May/2013 and July/2018. Research articles relevant to ALS and FTD were included in the review.

PSYCHOLOGICAL SYMPTOMS IN ALS

The psychological impact of ALS has been widely addressed in the literature. Anxiety and depression, particularly depression are often used as clinical markers of psychological morbidity in patients diagnosed with ALS. Self-report measures, particularly the Hospital Anxiety and Depression Scale and Beck's Depression Inventory remain the most widely used measures. Based on the Structured Clinical Interview for the Diagnostic and Statistical Manual of Mental Disorders, the "gold standard" for assessment of depression, the rate of clinical depression ranges between 9 and 12% in ALS (10, 11). Perhaps not surprisingly, self-report measures of depression tend to show more variable rates of depression ranging from 20 to 64% (12–20). Similarly, the prevalence rates of anxiety vary widely, with rates ranging as low as 8% to as high as 88% among patients with ALS (12, 14, 18, 19, 21). The severity of symptoms appear to be predominantly in the mild range. Despite the low rates of clinical depression and anxiety, patients with ALS have been shown to be at increased risk of being diagnosed with depression, anxiety and other neurotic or stress-related disorders following diagnosis (21–25), however this may be attributable to the clinicopathological overlap between ALS and FTD (24).

Management of psychological symptoms is crucial to maintaining quality of life. ALS patients provided with an assistive communication device in the early stages of the disease have been found to experience higher quality of life, particularly in the domains related to psychological and existential well-being (26). Quality of life and depression appear to be largely unrelated to patients' desire for hastened death (27) and end-of-life choices (28). This may be due to satisfactory levels of quality of life typically reported by ALS patients (29, 30). In fact, several studies have shown that caregivers and healthy controls tend to underestimate ALS patients quality of life and psychological well-being (31), possibly reflecting a "disability paradox" (32). However, it should be noted that many quality of life measurements used were not ALS specific.

THE IMPACT OF COGNITIVE AND BEHAVIORAL SYMPTOMS ON ALS PATIENT'S PSYCHOLOGICAL WELL-BEING

To date, there is a paucity of research specifically examining cognitive/behavioral symptoms and patients' psychological well-being. The majority of recent studies on patients' psychological well-being have either excluded patients with cognitive/behavioral symptoms or have not specifically discussed findings in relation to cognitive/behavioral symptoms. This is an important area for future research given emerging findings showing a relationship between depression and cognitive/behavioral changes. Higher levels of depression have been associated with lower cognitive performance on the Edinburgh Cognitive and Behavioral ALS Screen (17), specifically the subtests measuring social cognitive deficits and inhibitory control (12). Findings regarding anxiety and cognitive function are inconsistent, with one recent study finding no relationship (12) and another showing a weak association between anxiety and cognitive performance, perhaps reflecting underlying behavioral changes, namely disinhibition (17). Indeed, the findings available on behavioral and psychological symptoms appear to be more consistent. A large scale study of cognitive and behavioral impairment, and depression showed that patients with behavioral impairment exhibited higher levels of depression and hopelessness (10). This may partly reflect the overlap between depression and behavioral symptoms, namely apathy (33, 34).

THE IMPACT OF COGNITIVE AND BEHAVIORAL SYMPTOMS ON TREATMENT ADHERENCE IN ALS

Adherence to treatment recommendations in ALS can extend survival (e.g., non-invasive ventilation or Riluzole), improve patients' quality of life (35, 36), and likely to reduce caregiver burden. Review articles of cognition and behavioral symptoms in ALS discuss the likely impact of these symptoms on treatment adherence (37–40), however only one study to date has investigated the effect of non-motor symptoms on treatment adherence in ALS (41). Non-adherence to non-invasive positive-pressure ventilation and percutaneous endoscopic gastrostomy recommendations was 75 and 72% respectively for patients with ALS-FTD compared to 38 and 31% those with "motor only" symptoms. Therefore, the presence of a frontotemporal syndrome reduced adherence by half in ALS.

In general, ALS patients are compliant with recommendations made in multidisciplinary clinics (36). Out of a total of 287 recommendations made to 25 patients with ALS, patients complied fully with 59% of the recommendations made by the team. Not surprisingly, recommendations were greatest for physical needs (e.g., medications for symptoms such as spasm, saliva, sleep difficulties and interventions for nutrition and speech) and adherence was also highest for this category of recommendations. Interestingly, while patients with marked cognitive impairment were excluded in this study, patients with milder cognitive and behavioral symptoms (e.g., executive dysfunction) were included and may help explain why less than half of all recommendations were recalled (40%) and only a small proportion of patients (32%) had retained the written list of recommendations provided after the clinic visit. In total, <5% of the total recommendations were for mental health needs of patients (e.g., anti-depressants) and almost no recommendations (<2% of total recommendations) were made for caregivers (e.g., increase caregiver hours, ALS respite care program, and caregiver training to aid in patient transport).

In general, studies of treatment adherence in ALS have not typically characterized non-motor symptoms in patient cohorts [e.g., physiotherapy exercises (42); respiratory support (43); tolerability of oral vs. tablet Riluzole (44); tolerability of early non-invasive ventilation use (45)] and is an exclusionary criteria in some studies [e.g., aerobic exercise therapy vs. cognitive behavioral therapy (46)]. It is therefore not surprising that motor predictors of treatment adherence are often reported. For example, symptomatic orthopnoea and dyspnoea, nocturnal hypoventilation, and spinal onset of symptoms have been associated with adherence to non-invasive ventilation (47–50). Functional scores (forced volume vital capacity and the revised ALS Functional Rating Scale) have also been identified as independent predictors of adherence to clinical trials and fewer protocol deviations (51).

CAREGIVER BURDEN IN ALS

Several studies have shown that caregiving in ALS affects caregivers' level of distress and quality of life (52). The psychological symptoms experienced by caregivers have a significant impact on caregiver burden (53). Burke et al. (54) demonstrated that caregiver distress explained 39% of the variance in caregiver burden (54). In another study where caregivers were dichotomized into low and high burden groups, there were no differences across groups with respect to motor function (revised ALS Functional Rating Scale), bulbar/spinal onset, or survival time. Significant differences were only found when high and low-burden caregivers were compared on levels of anxiety, depression, distress and quality of life (55). A longitudinal study involving ALS patients with relatively preserved cognition demonstrated that anxiety and depression in caregivers were the best long-term predictors of burden (56).

An interesting study using a mixed methods approach (quantitative and qualitative) to assess burden in 81 informal ALS caregivers, showed that increased psychological distress, hours of care provided, and lower quality of life were the best predictors of caregiver burden, explaining 53% of variance. These caregivers identified difficulties related to four main themes: (a) the caregiving role and tasks associated with management of the condition, (b) psychosocial and emotional impact, (c) limitated time and restricted social life, and (d) significant impact in relationships with others and also identity (the process of "becoming" and "being" a caregiver) (57). Longitudinal studies have also demonstrated that disease severity causes strain and burden in caregivers over time (58, 59).

THE IMPACT OF COGNITIVE AND BEHAVIORAL SYMPTOMS ON CAREGIVER BURDEN

Recent evidence has demonstrated that both cognitive and behavioral symptoms contribute to caregiver burden in ALS (54, 60). A study involving 33 ALS patient-caregiver dyads showed that caregiver burden (Zarit Scale) was associated with executive dysfunction and behavioral changes, such as apathy and disinhibition (54). Similarly, findings from a Chinese study revealed that the degree of frontal dysfunction and behavioral changes (predominantly disinhibition) was significantly associated with caregiver burden (60).

More severe cognitive deficits have also been shown to predict caregiver burden in ALS (61). Conversely, a study involving 84 ALS patient-caregiver dyads found no correlation between caregiver burden (Caregiver Burden Inventory) and cognitive functioning (ALS-Cognitive Behavioral Screen). Only disease progression and behavioral symptoms were correlated with caregiver burden (62). Indeed, the level of burden for caregivers of ALS-FTD patients appears to increase with disease progression compared to a persistently high level of burden among caregivers of FTD patients (63).

Few studies have found specific motor symptoms associated with caregiver burden. One study linked poor motivation and difficulties with everyday skills to higher burden (64), while another study revealed that caregiver burden was predicted by behavioral problems and severity of limb involvement (65).

These findings highlight the support caregivers require from health care professionals and family/friends to not only manage the emotional and physical burden of caregiving (66), but also cognitive and behavioral symptoms that can greatly impact on their caregiving experience.

DISCUSSION

Assessment and management of cognitive and behavioral symptoms forms the larger goal of preservation of quality of life in both ALS patients and caregivers. Timely assessment of cognitive and behavioral symptoms has important prognostic and therapeutic implications. The presence of dysexecutive symptoms is not only likely to impact on patient and caregiver psychological well-being but also decision-making, adherence to life-sustaining interventions, and capacity to engage and benefit from non-pharmacological interventions. Additionally, cognitive and behavioral symptoms may exist before full blown motor symptoms (67) and, therefore, the ability to make informed decisions may be effected early in the disease course. While treatments for symptomatic management in ALS is often most beneficial if initiated early [e.g., (68)] and clinicians value proactive decisions (69), failure to identify cognitive and behavioral symptoms may mean that patients are not fully supported by their health care team and caregivers to undertake informed decision-making that is in accordance with their current personal philosophy and values (70).

The provision of practical support by ALS specialists is known to facilitate adherence in ALS. Increased educational training and adaptation facilitates adherence to non-invasive ventilation (71); telemonitoring decreases emergency room visits and hospital admissions, and follow-up care between clinical visits increase adherence to clinical recommendations (36, 72). Support from other ALS patients through online platforms can also increase treatment adherence such as with medication adherence (73).

It is also essential to recognize the importance of caregivers in the management of ALS from an early stage, informing them about the possibility of burden, offering them health care support, and monitoring their well-being over time (74). Weisser et al. (75) showed that the needs of ALS caregivers were multiple, including practical, social, and psychological needs. A model of coping was subsequently proposed integrating resilience, burden, needs, and rewards (75). An intervention to reduce maladaptive coping strategies has also been found to improve well-being in caregivers of patients with ALS (76). Furthermore, the use of technological approaches (e.g., telemedicine) for ALS patients and their caregivers that live in remote and rural areas which have reduced access to health care services may be especially beneficial (77). Provision of training for health care professionals to help patients and caregivers during the advanced stages of the disease would also ensure that important factors such as fatigue, stress, and ethical challenges related to end-of-life care are adequaly addressed (78).

To the best of our knowledge, there are currently no evidence-based studies which examine interventions to manage the cognitive and behavioral symptoms of ALS patients, though there are a few that examine caregiver burden in response to behavioral symptoms (79). In the absence of such evidence, it is possible to extrapolate findings from intervention studies in non-ALS populations as possible non-pharmacological interventions for cognitive and behavioral symptoms in ALS. Behavioral variant FTD and cognitively impaired ALS show similar cognitive profiles, although cognitive deficits are more severe in patients with behavioral variant FTD in most domains (4). In both disorders, considerable impairment in social cognition, fluency and verbal memory is found, whereas impairment of visual memory and attention is less prominent (3, 4). Due to the similarity of symptoms, studies examining management of behavioral variant FTD may be relevant to ALS, though caution should be used in extrapolating their conclusions.

Environmental management has shown promise in addressing cognitive/behavioral symptoms of FTD patients (80). For example, reducing noise and stimulation, lessening clutter, or simplifying social situations can help patient's better focus on a nominated task or response (80, 81). Removing access to problematic stimuli or modifying public outings to reduce the opportunity for inappropriate interactions are also effective FTD-specific environmental manipulations (80, 81), which could also be implemented when working with ALS patients presenting symptoms of disinhibition or loss of social cognition.

Though the research on behavioral modification in FTD is also limited and consists mainly of case studies and reports, clinicians have typically focused on disinhibition, apathy and compulsive behaviors (80, 82). In a few specific cases, behavioral interventions successfully reduced behaviors that were most distressing for patients' and caregivers', improved the relationship between patients' and caregivers', and helped to prevent the patients from being institutionalized (82, 83). Two case reports used behavior theory techniques including reducing stimuli, introducing new non-verbal cues, and creating reward systems (82, 83). Similarly, Tailored Activities Programs have been shown to reduce agitation in behavioral variant FTD patients (83–85). Support groups for family caregivers have also proved helpful (in person and when using online live streams) and most effective when caregivers are experiencing similar behaviors and challenges with the patient (86, 87).

There are limitations to understanding the impact of cognitive and behavioral changes on patients with ALS and their caregivers. The majority of published studies have been completed in developed countries and thus results cannot be extrapolated to all countries. Also, many of these studies do not take into consideration the various socioeconomic variables attributable to the patient and caregivers daily experience with ALS, such as the individual's wealth or their country's health care system.

Despite the clinical necessity of an intervention to manage cognitive and behavioral symptoms, there has been a lack of research on the topic which further widens the gap between research and practice. Drawing from interventions in dementia, there is a large landscape of possible, untested interventions for cognitive and behavioral symptoms of ALS. Early and comprehensive management of cognitive and behavioral symptoms not only promotes holistic care of patients but would also further enhance caregiver's psychological well-being and likely to reduce the healthcare and societal burden of these symptoms due to poor intervention adherence and avoidable hospitalizations.

AUTHOR CONTRIBUTIONS

JC, SH, PL, and KD wrote the manuscript. EM edited it and had manuscript oversight.

FUNDING

JC holds a National Health and Medical Research Council of Australia Postgraduate Research Scholarship (APP1092891). SH holds a National Health and Medical Research Council of Australia-Dementia Research Development Fellowship. PL is funded by CONICYT/FONDAP 15150012, CONICYT/FONDECYT regular 1160940. KD is funded by MND Scotland. EM holds a grant from the Motor Neurone Disease Association UK.

REFERENCES

1. Kiernan MC, Vucic S, Cheah BC, Turner MR, Eisen A, Hardiman O, et al. Amyotrophic lateral sclerosis. *Lancet.* (2011) 377:942–55. doi: 10.1016/S0140-6736(10)61156-7
2. Turner MR, Hardiman O, Benatar M, Brooks BR, Chio A, de Carvalho M, et al. Controversies and priorities in amyotrophic lateral sclerosis. *Lancet Neurol.* (2013) 12:310–22. doi: 10.1016/S1474-4422(13)70036-X
3. Strong MJ, Abrahams S, Goldstein LH, Woolley S, McLaughlin P, Snowden J, et al. Amyotrophic lateral sclerosis - frontotemporal spectrum disorder (ALS-FTSD): revised diagnostic criteria. *Amyotr Lateral Scler Frontotemporal Degener.* (2017) 18:153–74. doi: 10.1080/21678421.2016.1267768
4. Beeldman E, Raaphorst J, Klein Twennaar M, Govaarts R, Pijnenburg YAL, de Haan RJ, et al. The cognitive profile of behavioural variant FTD and its similarities with ALS: a systematic review and meta-analysis. *J Neurol Neurosurg Psychiatry.* (2018) 89:995–1002. doi: 10.1136/jnnp-2017-317459
5. Goldstein LH, Abrahams S. Changes in cognition and behaviour in amyotrophic lateral sclerosis: nature of impairment and implications for assessment. *Lancet Neurol.* (2013) 12:368–80. doi: 10.1016/S1474-4422(13)70026-7
6. Phukan J, Pender NP, Hardiman O. Cognitive impairment in amyotrophic lateral sclerosis. *Lancet Neurol.* (2007) 6:994–1003. doi: 10.1016/S1474-4422(07)70265-X
7. Raaphorst J, Beeldman E, De Visser M, De Haan RJ, Schmand B. A systematic review of behavioural changes in motor neuron disease. *Amyotroph Lateral Scler.* (2012) 13:493–501. doi: 10.3109/17482968.2012.656652
8. Raaphorst J, de Visser M, Linssen WH, de Haan RJ, Schmand B. The cognitive profile of amyotrophic lateral sclerosis: a meta-analysis. *Amyotroph Lateral Scler.* (2010) 11:27–37. doi: 10.3109/17482960802645008
9. Miller RG, Jackson CE, Kasarskis EJ, England JD, Forshew D, Johnston W, et al. Practice parameter update: the care of the patient with amyotrophic lateral sclerosis: multidisciplinary care, symptom management, and cognitive/behavioral impairment (an evidence-based review): report of the Quality Standards Subcommittee of the American Academy of Neurology. *Neurology.* (2009) 73:1227–33. doi: 10.1212/WNL.0b013e3181bc01a4
10. Rabkin J, Goetz R, Murphy JM, Factor-Litvak P, Mitsumoto H, Group ACS. Cognitive impairment, behavioral impairment, depression, and wish to die in an ALS cohort. *Neurology.* (2016) 87:1320–8. doi: 10.1212/WNL.0000000000003035
11. Wei Q, Zheng Z, Guo X, Ou R, Chen X, Huang R, et al. Association between depression and survival in Chinese amyotrophic lateral sclerosis patients. *Neurol Sci.* (2016) 37:557–63. doi: 10.1007/s10072-015-2472-y
12. Carelli L, Solca F, Faini A, Madotto F, Lafronza A, Monti A, et al. The complex interplay between depression/anxiety and executive functioning: insights from the ECAS in a large ALS population. *Front Psychol.* (2018) 9:450. doi: 10.3389/fpsyg.2018.00450
13. Chen D, Guo X, Zheng Z, Wei Q, Song W, Cao B, et al. Depression and anxiety in amyotrophic lateral sclerosis: correlations between the distress of patients and caregivers. *Muscle Nerve.* (2015) 51:353–7. doi: 10.1002/mus.24325
14. Cui F, Zhu W, Zhou Z, Ren Y, Li Y, Li M, et al. Frequency and risk factor analysis of cognitive and anxiety-depressive disorders in patients with amyotrophic lateral sclerosis/motor neuron disease. *Neuropsychiatr Dis Treat.* (2015) 11:2847–54. doi: 10.2147/NDT.S90520
15. Korner S, Kollewe K, Abdulla S, Zapf A, Dengler R, Petri S. Interaction of physical function, quality of life and depression in Amyotrophic lateral sclerosis: characterization of a large patient cohort. *BMC Neurol.* (2015) 15:84. doi: 10.1186/s12883-015-0340-2
16. Paganoni S, McDonnell E, Schoenfeld D, Yu H, Deng J, Atassi H, Atassi N. Functional Decline is Associated with Hopelessness in Amyotrophic Lateral Sclerosis (ALS). *J Neurol Neurophysiol.* (2017) 8:423. doi: 10.4172/2155-9562.1000423
17. Poletti B, Solca F, Carelli L, Madotto F, Lafronza A, Faini A, et al. The validation of the italian edinburgh cognitive and behavioural ALS Screen (ECAS). *Amyotr Lateral Scler Frontotemporal Degener.* (2016) 17:489–98. doi: 10.1080/21678421.2016.1183679
18. Prado LGR, Bicalho ICS, Vidigal-Lopes M, Prado VGR, Gomez RS, de Souza LC, et al. Depression and anxiety in a case series of amyotrophic lateral sclerosis: frequency and association with clinical features. *Einstein.* (2017) 15:58–60. doi: 10.1590/s1679-45082017ao3870
19. Stephens HE, Lehman E, Raheja D, Yang C, Walsh S, Simmons Z. The role of mental health and self-efficacy in the pain experience of patients with amyotrophic lateral sclerosis. *Amyotr Lateral Scler Frontotemporal Degener.* (2016) 17:206–12. doi: 10.3109/21678421.2015.1131832
20. Thakore NJ, Pioro EP. Depression in ALS in a large self-reporting cohort. *Neurology.* (2016) 86:1031–8. doi: 10.1212/WNL.0000000000002465
21. Van Groenestijn AC, Schroder CD, Kruitwagen-Van Reenen ET, Van Den Berg LH, Visser-Meily JMA. Participation restrictions in ambulatory amyotrophic lateral sclerosis patients: physical and psychological factors. *Muscle Nerve.* (2017) 56:912–8. doi: 10.1002/mus.25574
22. Longinetti E, Mariosa D, Larsson H, Ye W, Ingre C, Almqvist C, et al. Neurodegenerative and psychiatric diseases among families with amyotrophic lateral sclerosis. *Neurology.* (2017) 89:578–85. doi: 10.1212/WNL.0000000000004179
23. Roos E, Mariosa D, Ingre C, Lundholm C, Wirdefeldt K, Roos PM, et al. Depression in amyotrophic lateral sclerosis. *Neurology.* (2016) 86:2271–7. doi: 10.1212/WNL.0000000000002671
24. Turner MR, Goldacre R, Talbot K, Goldacre MJ. Psychiatric disorders prior to amyotrophic lateral sclerosis. *Ann Neurol.* (2016) 80:935–8. doi: 10.1002/ana.24801
25. Caga J, Ramsey E, Hogden A, Mioshi E, Kiernan MC. A longer diagnostic interval is a risk for depression in amyotrophic lateral sclerosis. *Palliat Support Care.* (2015) 13:1019–24. doi: 10.1017/S1478951514000881
26. Londral A, Pinto A, Pinto S, Azevedo L, De Carvalho M. Quality of life in amyotrophic lateral sclerosis patients and caregivers: impact of assistive communication from early stages. *Muscle Nerve.* (2015) 52:933–41. doi: 10.1002/mus.24659
27. Lule D, Nonnenmacher S, Sorg S, Heimrath J, Hautzinger M, Meyer T, et al. Live and let die: existential decision processes in a fatal disease. *J Neurol.* (2014) 261:518–25. doi: 10.1007/s00415-013-7229-z
28. Maessen M, Veldink JH, Onwuteaka-Philipsen BD, Hendricks HT, Schelhaas HJ, Grupstra HF, et al. Euthanasia and physician-assisted suicide in amyotrophic lateral sclerosis: a prospective study. *J Neurol.* (2014) 261:1894–901. doi: 10.1007/s00415-014-7424-6
29. Pagnini F. Psychological wellbeing and quality of life in amyotrophic lateral sclerosis: a review. *Int J Psychol.* (2013) 48:194–205. doi: 10.1080/00207594.2012.691977
30. Simmons Z. Patient-Perceived Outcomes and Quality of Life in ALS. *Neurotherapeutics.* (2015) 12:394–402. doi: 10.1007/s13311-014-0322-x
31. Lule D, Ehlich B, Lang D, Sorg S, Heimrath J, Kubler A, et al. Quality of life in fatal disease: the flawed judgement of the social environment. *J Neurol.* (2013) 260:2836–43. doi: 10.1007/s00415-013-7068-y
32. Albrecht GL, Devlieger PJ. The disability paradox: high quality of life against all odds. *Soc Sci Med.* (1999) 48:977–88. doi: 10.1016/S0277-9536(98)00411-0
33. Radakovic R, Stephenson L, Colville S, Swingler R, Chandran S, Abrahams S. Multidimensional apathy in ALS: validation of the Dimensional Apathy Scale. *J Neurol Neurosurg Psychiatry.* (2016) 87:663–9. doi: 10.1136/jnnp-2015-310772
34. Santangelo G, Siciliano M, Trojano L, Femiano C, Monsurro MR, Tedeschi G, et al. Apathy in amyotrophic lateral sclerosis: insights from Dimensional Apathy Scale. *Amyotroph Lateral Scler Frontotemporal Degener.* (2017) 18:434–42. doi: 10.1080/21678421.2017.1313865
35. Bourke SC, Bullock RE, Williams TL, Shaw PJ, Gibson GJ. Noninvasive ventilation in ALS: indications and effect on quality of life. *Neurology.* (2003) 61:171–7. doi: 10.1212/01.WNL.0000076182.13137.38
36. Fullam T, Stephens HE, Felgoise SH, Blessinger JK, Walsh S, Simmons Z. Compliance with recommendations made in a multidisciplinary ALS clinic. *Amyotroph Lateral Scler Frontotemporal Degener.* (2015) 17:30–7. doi: 10.3109/21678421.2015.1074703
37. Giordana MT, Ferrero P, Grifoni S, Pellerino A, Naldi A, Montuschi A. Dementia and cognitive impairment in amyotrophic lateral sclerosis: a review. *Neurol Sci.* (2011) 32:9–16. doi: 10.1007/s10072-010-0439-6
38. Irwin D, Lippa CF, Swearer JM. Cognition and amyotrophic lateral sclerosis (ALS). *Am J Alzheimer's Dis Dementias.* (2007) 22:300–12. doi: 10.1177/1533317507301613

39. Witgert M, Salamone AR, Strutt AM, Jawaid A, Massman PJ, Bradshaw M, et al. Frontal-lobe mediated behavioral dysfunction in amyotrophic lateral sclerosis. *Eur J Neurol.* (2010) 17:103–10. doi: 10.1111/j.1468-1331.2009.02801.x
40. Woolley SC, Jonathan SK. Cognitive and behavioral impairment in amyotrophic lateral sclerosis. *Phys Med Rehabil Clin North Am.* (2008) 19:607–17, xi. doi: 10.1016/j.pmr.2008.04.002
41. Olney RK, Murphy J, Forshew D, Garwood E, Miller BL, Langmore S, et al. The effects of executive and behavioral dysfunction on the course of ALS. *Neurology.* (2005) 65:1774–7. doi: 10.1212/01.wnl.0000188759.87240.8b
42. Clawson LL, Cudkowicz M, Krivickas L, Brooks BR, Sanjak M, Allred P, et al. Randomized controlled trial of resistance and endurance exercise in amyotrophic lateral sclerosis. *Amyotroph Lateral Scler Frontotemporal Degener.* (2018) 19:250–8. doi: 10.1080/21678421.2017.1404108
43. Nicholson TT, Smith SB, Siddique T, Sufit R, Ajroud-Driss S, Coleman JM 3rd, et al. Respiratory pattern and tidal volumes differ for pressure support and volume-assured pressure support in amyotrophic lateral sclerosis. *Ann Am Thoracic Soc.* (2017) 14:1139–46. doi: 10.1513/AnnalsATS.201605-346OC
44. Introna A, D'Errico E, Modugno B, Scarafino A, Fraddosio A, Distaso E, et al. Adherence to riluzole in patients with amyotrophic lateral sclerosis: an observational study. *Neuropsychiatr Dis Treat.* (2018) 14:193–203. doi: 10.2147/NDT.S150550
45. Jacobs TL, Brown DL, Baek J, Migda EM, Funckes T, Gruis KL. Trial of early noninvasive ventilation for ALS: a pilot placebo-controlled study. *Neurology.* (2016) 87:1878–83. doi: 10.1212/WNL.0000000000003158
46. van Groenestijn AC, van de Port IG, Schroder CD, Post MW, Grupstra HF, Kruitwagen ET, et al. Effects of aerobic exercise therapy and cognitive behavioural therapy on functioning and quality of life in amyotrophic lateral sclerosis: protocol of the FACTS-2-ALS trial. *BMC Neurol.* (2011) 11:70. doi: 10.1186/1471-2377-11-70
47. Bertella E, Banfi P, Paneroni M, Grilli S, Bianchi L, Volpato E, et al. Early initiation of night-time NIV in an outpatient setting: a randomized non-inferiority study in ALS patients. *Eur J Phys Rehabil Med.* (2017) 53:892–9. doi: 10.23736/S1973-9087.17.04511-7
48. Jackson CE, Lovitt S, Gowda N, Anderson F, Miller RG, Bradley WG, et al. Factors correlated with NPPV use in ALS. *Amyotr Later Scler.* (2006) 7:80–5. doi: 10.1080/14660820500504587
49. Kim SM, Park KS, Nam H, Ahn SW, Kim S, Sung JJ, et al. Capnography for assessing nocturnal hypoventilation and predicting compliance with subsequent noninvasive ventilation in patients with ALS. *PLoS ONE.* (2011) 6:e17893. doi: 10.1371/journal.pone.0017893
50. Pinto AC, de Carvalho M, Evangelista T, Lopes A, Sales-Luis L. Nocturnal pulse oximetry: a new approach to establish the appropriate time for non-invasive ventilation in ALS patients. *Amyotr Later Scler Motor Neuron Disorders.* (2003) 4:31–5. doi: 10.1080/14660820310006706
51. Atassi N, Yerramilli-Rao P, Szymonifka J, Yu H, Kearney M, Grasso D, et al. Analysis of start-up, retention, and adherence in ALS clinical trials. *Neurology.* (2013) 81:1350–5. doi: 10.1212/WNL.0b013e3182a823e0
52. Thomas PT, Warrier MG, Sadasivan A, Balasubramanium B, Preethish-Kumar V, Nashi S, et al. Caregiver burden and quality of life of patients with amyotrophic lateral sclerosis in India. *Amyotroph Lateral Scler Frontotemporal Degener.* 19:606–10. doi: 10.1080/21678421.2018.1482353
53. Oh J, An JW, Oh KW, Oh SI, Kim JA, Kim SH, et al. [Depression and caregiving burden in families of patients with amyotrophic lateral sclerosis]. *J Korean Acad Nurs.* (2015) 45:202–10. doi: 10.4040/jkan.2015.45.2.202
54. Burke T, Elamin M, Galvin M, Hardiman O, Pender N. Caregiver burden in amyotrophic lateral sclerosis: a cross-sectional investigation of predictors. *J Neurol.* (2015) 262:1526–32. doi: 10.1007/s00415-015-7746-z
55. Burke T, Galvin M, Pinto-Grau M, Lonergan K, Madden C, Mays I, et al. Caregivers of patients with amyotrophic lateral sclerosis: investigating quality of life, caregiver burden, service engagement, and patient survival. *J Neurol.* (2017) 264:898–904. doi: 10.1007/s00415-017-8448-5
56. Burke T, Hardiman O, Pinto-Grau M, Lonergan K, Heverin M, Tobin K, et al. Longitudinal predictors of caregiver burden in amyotrophic lateral sclerosis: a population-based cohort of patient-caregiver dyads. *J Neurol.* (2018) 265:793–808. doi: 10.1007/s00415-018-8770-6
57. Galvin M, Corr B, Madden C, Mays I, McQuillan R, Timonen V, et al. Caregiving in ALS - a mixed methods approach to the study of Burden. *BMC Palliat Care.* (2016) 15:81. doi: 10.1186/s12904-016-0153-0
58. Bruletti G, Comini L, Scalvini S, Morini R, Luisa A, Paneroni M, et al. A two-year longitudinal study on strain and needs in caregivers of advanced ALS patients. *Amyotroph Lateral Scler Frontotemporal Degener* .(2015) 16:187–95. doi: 10.3109/21678421.2014.974616
59. Tramonti F, Bongioanni P, Leotta R, Puppi I, Rossi B. Age, gender, kinship and caregiver burden in amyotrophic lateral sclerosis. *Psychol Health Med.* (2015) 20:41–6. doi: 10.1080/13548506.2014.892627
60. Cui B, Cui L, Gao J, Liu M, Li X, Liu C, et al. Cognitive impairment in chinese patients with sporadic amyotrophic lateral sclerosis. *PLoS ONE.* (2015) 10:e0137921. doi: 10.1371/journal.pone.0137921
61. Bock M, Duong YN, Kim A, Allen I, Murphy J, Lomen-Hoerth C. Cognitive-behavioral changes in amyotrophic lateral sclerosis: screening prevalence and impact on patients and caregivers. *Amyotroph Lateral Scler Frontotemporal Degener.* (2016) 17:366–73. doi: 10.3109/21678421.2016.1165257
62. Tremolizzo L, Pellegrini A, Susani E, Lunetta C, Woolley SC, Ferrarese C, et al. Behavioural but not cognitive impairment is a determinant of caregiver burden in amyotrophic lateral sclerosis. *Eur Neurol.* (2016) 75:191–4. doi: 10.1159/000445110
63. Hsieh S, Leyton CE, Caga J, Flanagan E, Kaizik C, O'Connor CM, et al. The evolution of caregiver burden in frontotemporal dementia with and without amyotrophic lateral sclerosis. *J Alzheimers Dis.* (2016) 49:875–85. doi: 10.3233/JAD-150475
64. Andrews SC, Pavlis A, Staios M, Fisher F. Which behaviours? Identifying the most common and burdensome behaviour changes in amyotrophic lateral sclerosis. *Psychol Health Med.* (2017) 22:483–92. doi: 10.1080/13548506.2016.1164871
65. Watermeyer TJ, Brown RG, Sidle KC, Oliver DJ, Allen C, Karlsson J, et al. Impact of disease, cognitive and behavioural factors on caregiver outcome in amyotrophic lateral sclerosis. *Amyotroph Lateral Scler Frontotemporal Degener.* (2015) 16:316–23. doi: 10.3109/21678421.2015.1051990
66. Galvin M, Carney S, Corr B, Mays I, Pender N, Hardiman O. Needs of informal caregivers across the caregiving course in amyotrophic lateral sclerosis: a qualitative analysis. *BMJ Open.* (2018) 8:e018721. doi: 10.1136/bmjopen-2017-018721
67. Mioshi E, Caga J, Lillo P, Hsieh S, Ramsey E, Devenney E, et al. Neuropsychiatric changes precede classic motor symptoms in ALS and do not affect survival. *Neurology.* (2014) 82:149–55. doi: 10.1212/WNL.0000000000000023
68. Terzano C, Romani S. Early use of non invasive ventilation in patients with amyotrophic lateral sclerosis: what benefits? *Eur Rev Med Pharmacol Sci.* (2015) 19:4304–13.
69. Hogden A, Greenfield D, Nugus P, Kiernan MC. Engaging in patient decision-making in multidisciplinary care for amyotrophic lateral sclerosis: the views of health professionals. *Patient Prefer Adherence.* (2012) 6:691–701. doi: 10.2147/PPA.S36759
70. Hogden A, Greenfield D, Nugus P, Kiernan MC. What are the roles of carers in decision-making for amyotrophic lateral sclerosis multidisciplinary care? *Patient Prefer Adherence.* (2013) 7:171–81. doi: 10.2147/PPA.S40783
71. Volanti P, Cibella F, Sarva M, De Cicco D, Spanevello A, Mora G, et al. Predictors of non-invasive ventilation tolerance in amyotrophic lateral sclerosis. *J Neurol Sci.* (2011) 303:114–8. doi: 10.1016/j.jns.2010.12.021
72. Pinto A, Almeida JP, Pinto S, Pereira J, Oliveira AG, de Carvalho M. Home telemonitoring of non-invasive ventilation decreases healthcare utilisation in a prospective controlled trial of patients with amyotrophic lateral sclerosis. *J Neurol Neurosurg Psychiatry.* (2010) 81:1238–42. doi: 10.1136/jnnp.2010.206680
73. Wicks P, Mack Thorley E. Scaling PatientsLikeMe via a "Generalized Platform" for Members with Chronic Illness: web-based survey study of benefits *Arising.* (2018) 20:e175. doi: 10.2196/jmir.9909

74. de Wit J, Schroder CD, El Mecky J, Beelen A, van den Berg LH, Visser-Meily JMA. Support needs of caregivers of patients with amyotrophic lateral sclerosis: a qualitative study. *Palliat Support Care.* (2018) 5:1–7. doi: 10.1017/S1478951517001213
75. Weisser FB, Bristowe K, Jackson D. Experiences of burden, needs, rewards and resilience in family caregivers of people living with motor neurone disease/amyotrophic lateral sclerosis: a secondary thematic analysis of qualitative interviews. *Palliat Med.* (2015) 29:737–45. doi: 10.1177/0269216315575851
76. Siciliano M, Santangelo G, Trojsi F, Di Somma C, Patrone M, Femiano C, et al. Coping strategies and psychological distress in caregivers of patients with Amyotrophic Lateral Sclerosis (ALS). *Amyotroph Lateral Scler Frontotemporal Degener.* (2017) 18:367–77. doi: 10.1080/21678421.2017.1285316
77. Geronimo A, Wright C, Morris A, Walsh S, Snyder B, Simmons Z. Incorporation of telehealth into a multidisciplinary ALS Clinic: feasibility and acceptability. *Amyotroph Lateral Scler Frontotemporal Degener.* (2017) 18:555–61. doi: 10.1080/21678421.2017.1338298
78. Connolly S, Galvin M, Hardiman O. End-of-life management in patients with amyotrophic lateral sclerosis. *Lancet Neurol.* (2015) 14:435–42. doi: 10.1016/S1474-4422(14)70221-2
79. de Wit J, Bakker LA, van Groenestijn AC, van den Berg LH, Schroder CD, Visser-Meily JM, et al. Caregiver burden in amyotrophic lateral sclerosis: a systematic review. *Palliat Med.* (2018) 32:231–45. doi: 10.1177/0269216317709965
80. Barton C, Ketelle R, Merrilees J, Miller B. Non-pharmacological management of behavioral symptoms in frontotemporal and other dementias. *Curr Neurol Neurosci Rep.* (2016) 16:14. doi: 10.1007/s11910-015-0618-1
81. Merrilees J. A model for management of behavioral symptoms in frontotemporal lobar degeneration. *Alzheimer Dis Assoc Disord.* (2007) 21:S64–9. doi: 10.1097/WAD.0b013e31815bf774
82. Narumoto J, Miya H, Shibata K, Nakamae T, Okamura A, Matsuoka T, et al. Challenging behavior of patients with frontal dysfunction managed successfully with behavioral intervention. *Psychogeriatrics.* (2009) 9:147–50. doi: 10.1111/j.1479-8301.2009.00279.x
83. O'Connor CM, Clemson L, Brodaty H, Jeon YH, Mioshi E, Gitlin LN. Use of the Tailored Activities Program to reduce neuropsychiatric behaviors in dementia: an Australian protocol for a randomized trial to evaluate its effectiveness. *Int Psychogeriatr.* (2014) 26:857–69. doi: 10.1017/S1041610214000040
84. Gitlin LN, Winter L, Dennis MP, Hodgson N, Hauck WW. Targeting and managing behavioral symptoms in individuals with dementia: a randomized trial of a nonpharmacological intervention. *J Am Geriatr Soc.* (2010) 58:1465–74. doi: 10.1111/j.1532-5415.2010.02971.x
85. O'Connor CM, Clemson L, Brodaty H, Gitlin LN, Piguet O, Mioshi E. Enhancing caregivers' understanding of dementia and tailoring activities in frontotemporal dementia: two case studies. *Disabil Rehabil.* (2016) 38:704–14. doi: 10.3109/09638288.2015.1055375
86. Dowling GA, Merrilees J, Mastick J, Chang VY, Hubbard E, Moskowitz JT. Life enhancing activities for family caregivers of people with frontotemporal dementia. *Alzheimer Dis Assoc Disord.* (2014) 28:175–81. doi: 10.1097/WAD.0b013e3182a6b905
87. O'Connell ME, Crossley M, Cammer A, Morgan D, Allingham W, Cheavins B, et al. Development and evaluation of a telehealth videoconferenced support group for rural spouses of individuals diagnosed with atypical early-onset dementias. *Dementia.* (2014) 13:382–95. doi: 10.1177/14713012124 74143

19

Amyotrophic Lateral Sclerosis and Primary Biliary Cirrhosis Overlap Syndrome

Haibo Zhang[1], Yaling Liu[1,2], Zhenfei Li[1], Na Liang[1], Xiaomeng Zhou[1], Xiangyu Nie[1], Ting Zhang[1] and Weijing Qi[2,3]*

[1] Department of Neurology, The Second Hospital of Hebei Medical University, Shijiazhuang, China, [2] Key Laboratory of Neurology of Hebei Province, Shijiazhuang, China, [3] Department of Neurology, Baoding First Central Hospital of Hebei Province, Baoding, China

***Correspondence:**
Yaling Liu
lyldoctor@163.com*

Amyotrophic lateral sclerosis (ALS) is a disease of which the underlying etiology and pathogenesis are unknown. Numerous data indicate an important role of the immune system and mitochondrial function in the disease. Primary biliary cirrhosis (PBC) is an autoimmune liver disease resulting from a combination of genetic and environmental risk factors. Patients with PBC develop innate and adaptive immune reactions against mitochondrial antigens. Therefore, common mechanisms could exist in both diseases. We present two cases of ALS with PBC to explore the relationship between the two diseases from the immunological and mitochondrial aspects. Further attention should be given to immune-modulating therapy in ALS patients.

Keywords: amyotrophic lateral sclerosis, primary biliary cirrhosis, immunological mechanism, mitochondrial mechanism, ursodeoxycholic acid

INTRODUCTION

Primary biliary cirrhosis (PBC) is an autoimmune cholestatic disease characterized by the non-suppurative destruction of intrahepatic small bile ducts which can eventually progress to liver cirrhosis (1). It mainly affects middle-aged females, and the female to male ratio is about 10:1 (1). A diagnostic serum marker for PBC is an anti-mitochondrial antibody (AMA) which is positive in more than 90% of the patients (2). Autoimmunity plays an important role in the pathogenesis of PBC (3, 4).

Amyotrophic lateral sclerosis (ALS) is a progressive neurodegenerative disorder involved with the upper (brain, brainstem, and spinal cord) and lower (cranial nerve nuclei, anterior horn cells of spinal cord) motor neurons (5). It is characterized clinically by progressive muscle atrophy, muscle weakness, and respiratory insufficiency with a fatal course (6, 7). The median survival duration is 3–5 years after the onset of the disease, while 10% of the patients can survive for over 10 years (8). The proposed hypotheses for the pathogenesis include glutamate excitotoxicity (9), mitochondrial dysfunction (10), gene defects (11), free radical-mediated oxidative stress (12) and immunological mechanism (13). To date, many patients with ALS and immune diseases (multiple sclerosis, myasthenia gravis, etc) have been reported (14), but ALS concomitant with PBC hasn't been reported.

Here we firstly report two cases of ALS with PBC and analyze the possible relationship between them, mainly from immunological, and mitochondrial aspects.

CASE REPORTS

Case 1

A 47-year-old female was admitted to the office with limbs weakness and dysarthria in February 2017. She firstly presented with left upper limb weakness in October 2016. Her symptoms deteriorated rapidly, and 2 months later, she suffered from mild dysarthria and sometimes choking while drinking water, difficulty in lifting and fastening buttons, and walking <100 meters. She reported no weight loss during the last 4 months. She had no remarkable past medical history.

During hospitalization, her vitals were stable. On neurological physical examination, the patient had no obvious muscular atrophy but had fasciculations noted in bilateral bicep and tricep muscles. Power was Medical Research Council (MRC) grade 3/5 in the bilateral upper extremities and 4/5 in the lower extremities. Tendon reflexes were 4+ in all extremities. She had hyperpharyngeal reflex and palmomental reflex. Bilateral Hoffman signs were positive. Neither sensory nor cerebellar dysfunction were identified. A complete blood count, serum biochemical studies, thyroid function, tumor marker showed normal results. Hepatitis panel was negative. Antinuclear antibody (ANA) was positive at a titer of 1:3,200 and AMA was over 1:40. The laboratory test showed that levels of immunoglobulins were within normal limits and alexins were almost within normal range. To rule out Sjogren's syndrome, we ordered Saliva Flow Rate (SFR), corneal fluorescein staining (CFS), breaking up time (BUT), Schirmer I test (SIT), anti-Sjogren syndrome A (SSA) antibody, and anti-Sjogren syndrome B (SSB) antibody. The results were all negative. The magnetic resonance imaging (MRI) of the brain and cervical spinal cord showed no abnormalities. Her chest computed tomography (CT) showed multiple subpleural inflammatory nodules. Considering the absence of cough and fever, we advised her to have a regular examination. The upper abdominal CT was suggestive of splenomegaly and liver cirrhosis. It showed that the morphology of the liver was abnormal, the velamen was not smooth, and the surface was rough. Multiple enlarged lymph nodes were observed near porta hepatis. No expansion or stenosis was observed in the intrahepatic and extrahepatic bile ducts. Electromyography (EMG) showed active and chronic denervation in all limbs, and in the sternocleidomastoid and paraspinal muscles. Nerve conduction studies (NCS) revealed decreased compound muscle action potential (CMAP) amplitudes of right median and ulnar nerve. Ursodeoxycholic acid (UDCA), a hydrophilic tertiary bile acid as the first line treatment of PBC, and riluzole were prescribed. In the late follow-up by telephone, she showed bed-bound at home, dysphagia, and weight loss of 40 kg a year after the symptom's onset.

Case 2

The second case was a 64-year-old woman diagnosed with PBC in June 2010, when she started UDCA 750 mg/d. Some months later, she was started on endoscopic sclerotherapy and injection of cyanoacrylate glue for gastric fundal varices. In December 2017, gastroesophageal varicose vein ligation and stripping were demonstrated for uncontrolled gastric bleeding. She had a 3-year history of type 2 diabetes mellitus, treated by keeping an appropriate diet for blood sugar. She developed dysphonia and weakness of the hands 3 months before admission. The symptoms gradually progressed. Two months later, she presented weakness in her lower limbs, therefore, she was admitted to our hospital in May 2018. She had lost 10 kg of weight over 3 months. She had no family history of neurodegenerative diseases.

Upon physical examination, muscle atrophy was observed bilaterally in the first dorsal interosseous muscles and the thenar, hypothenar muscles. Fasciculations and atrophy were evident in the tongue. Power was MRC grade 3/5 in the upper limbs and 4/5 in the lower limbs bilaterally. Deep tendon reflexes were brisk in all extremities. Positive bilateral Hoffman signs and hyperreflexia in the pharyngeal muscles were observed. No abnormality was observed in sensations and cerebellar function. AMA (>1:40) and ANA (1:320) were both positive. Hepatitis markers were negative, so were tumor markers. The levels of white blood cell count (1.80*109/L), red blood cell count (3.11*1012/L), hemoglobin (105 g/L), and platelet (30*109/L) all decreased. The biochemical results showed aspartate aminotransferase (AST) 41.3U/L and total bilirubin (TBIL) 26.0 umol/L. Baseline data of the patient was as follows (**Table 1**). There were some lacunar infarctions in bilateral frontal, temporal lobes, and left basilar ganglia on brain MRI. A thyroid ultrasound scan showed small nodules on the left and right lobes (**Figure 1**). Clear lungs were observed on her chest CT. Abdominal ultrasound visualized out of proportion hepatic lobes, mild heterogeneous decrease in echogenicity of the portal vein consistent with mural thrombus, splenomegaly (**Figure 2**) and dilated splenic vein, neither biliary obstruction nor space-occupied lesions. The CMAP amplitudes of right median and ulnar nerve decreased on NCS. EMG revealed florid active denervation changes in bulbar muscles and all limbs. Lumbar puncture was not executed because of her low platelet count. She was given UDCA, riluzole, and edaravone (Radicava), a new medication for ALS in 2017 approved by Food and Drug Administration (FDA) (15). At the follow-up, she had indwelled gastric tube and difficulty in ambulation in 8 months.

DISCUSSION

Our patients both presented dysarthria and limbs weakness. One was a limb onset, while the other was bulbar. The disease courses were short. On physical examination, pharyngeal reflex, and tendon reflexes were active or hyperactive. EMG showed denervation changes in all 4 body segments including bulbar, cervical, lumbar, and paraspinal. The clinically-definite diagnosis of ALS requires the presence of combined upper (UMN) and lower motor neurons (LMN) signa, and/or symptoms in at least 3 body segments (16). Therefore, our patients were consistent with clinically-definite ALS.

The diagnosis of PBC requires the exclusion of other liver diseases, no evidence of extrahepatic biliary tract obstruction on imaging, and two of the three criteria are met:(i) AMA titer higher than 1:40, (ii) alkaline phosphatase (ALP) over 1.5 times normal upper limit for 24 weeks at least, (iii) characteristic

TABLE 1 | Baseline data of the patient in case 2.

Laboratory values	
Blood routine	**Hepatitis screening**
White blood cell count, $1.80*10^9$/L (3.50–9.50)	HBsAg ELISA Negative
Red blood cell count, $3.11*10^{12}$/L(3.80–5.10)	Anti-HCV ELISA Negative
Hemoglobin, 105 g/L (115–150)	Anti-HBc Total Negative
Platelet, $30*10^9$/L(125–350)	HIV ELISA Negative
Coagulation routine	**Immune indices**
International normalized ratio, 1.02 (0.80–1.20)	Immunoglobulin G, 15.5 g/L (7–16)
Activated partial thromboplastin time, 28.9s (25.4–38.4)	Immunoglobulin A, 2.21 g/L (0.7–4.0)
Thrombin time, 13.1 s (10.3–16.6)	Immunoglobulin M, 1.22 g/L (0.4–2.3)
Biochemistry	Antinuclear antibody, Positive (1:320)
Aspartate aminotransferase, 41.3 U/L (13–35)	Anti-mitochondrial antibody, Positive (>1:40)
Alanine aminotransferase, 31.4 U/L (7–40)	Alexin C3, 0.74 g/L (0.80–1.60 g/L)
r-Glutamyltransferase, 101 U/L (7–45)	Alexin C4, 0.18 g/L (0.16–0.38 g/L)
Alkaline phosphatase, 112 U/L (50–135)	**Thyroid function**
Albumin, 39.7 g/L (40–55)	Free triiodothyronine, 4.15 pmol/L (2.76–6.45)
Total bilirubin, 26.0 umol/L (3.4–17.1)	Free thyroxine, 12.80 pmol/L (8.75–22.00)
Creatinine, 48.1 umol/L (41–81)	Thyroid-stimulating hormone, 2.92 mIU/L (0.35–4.31)
Tumor marker	**Other indicators**
Alpha fetoprotein, <0.61 ng/ml(0–10.9)	Blood ammonia, 35 umol/L(9–30)
Carcino-embryonic antigen, 2.05 ng/ml(0–10)	Glycated hemoglobin, 8.00% (4.00–6.00)
Glycogen antigen CA125, 34.78 U/ml(0–35)	Folic acid, 3.43 ng/ml (>3.38)
Glycogen antigen CA199, 35.3 U/ml (0–37)	VitaminB12, 640 pg/ml (211–911)

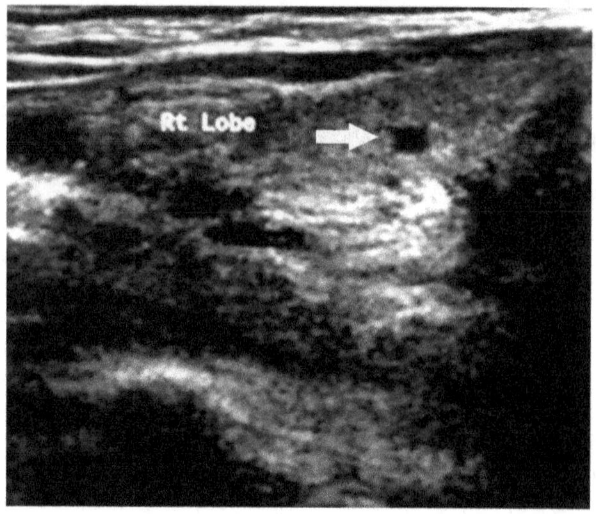

FIGURE 1 | Hypoechoic nodule of right lobe of thyroid (white arrow).

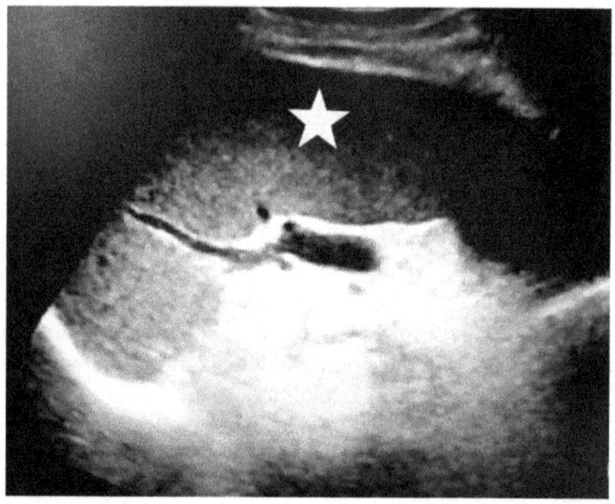

FIGURE 2 | Splenic enlargement (white asterisk).

liver histology, especially non-suppurative cholangitis and interlobular bile duct injury (17, 18). Our first patient was a middle-aged female diagnosed with PBC during hospitalization. Considering her negative results of hepatotropic virus, we ruled out cirrhosis caused by long-term hepatotropic virus infection. And no obstruction was found in extrahepatic bile duct on abdominal CT. AMA was positive in 95% of patients with PBC and ANA was 70%. In our case, AMA was positive (> 1:40) and ANA tire reached up to 1:3,200. The results of SFR, CFS, BUT, SIT, rheumatism factor, and lupus anticoagulant were all negative which excluded Sjogren's syndrome, systemic lupus erythematosus, and rheumatoid arthritis. The patient refused a liver biopsy. It had been found that up to 0.5% of the population in screening studies were AMA positive, typically, 50% of those having normal liver biochemistry (19). Our patient was initially diagnosed as PBC though her liver enzymes were normal. The second case had a history of PBC, and started a long-term use of UDCA. She presented end-stage liver performance, like liver cirrhosis, portal hypertension, hypersplenism, bleeding disorder, esophageal-gastric varices, and abnormal blood ammonia risk of hepatic encephalopathy (20).

It had been reported that 70% of PBC patients had extrahepatic diseases, but none with ALS. One study showed that PBC patients with overlapping characteristics of autoimmune hepatitis (AIH) would progress rapidly to cirrhosis and liver failure (21). Whereas, another study suggested that patients with superimposed features were more prone to develop esophageal varices, ascites and liver failure compared with typical PBC patients (22). Therefore, we analyzed the disease characteristics of ALS overlapped with PBC: (i) both patients were female, possibly due to the significant female susceptibility to PBC (1), and some scholars suggested that the gender difference might be related to the presence of genes to control immune tolerance on X chromosome (23) and sex hormone levels (24), (ii) both had a short course of disease, 4 and 3 months, respectively, (iii) clinical signs were involved with upper and LMN, and EMG showed wide denervation, (iv) in view of the follow-up, they both progressed quickly. The second patient might progress more rapidly than the first one as a consequence of end-stage liver disease.

The incidence of ALS ranges between 1.5 and 2.5 for 100,000 per year in the general population of the world (25) and the incidence of PBC is 4–40 per 100,000 people (26). Thus, the probability of co-occurrence of the two diseases in a single patient is statistically speaking very low, which may indicate common unknown mechanisms between the two diseases. The robust evidence points to a crucial role of urinary tract infection (UTI) caused by *Escherichia coli* (*E. coli*) in increasing the risk of PBC. *E. coli* infection is a key factor in the breaking of mitochondrial autoantigen immune tolerance, leading to the generation of specific AMA (27). Human PDC-E2 shares a significant homology with *E. coli* PDC-E2 which may reason for it. Besides, hepatocytes and bile epithelial cells in the liver of PBC patients express large amounts of human leucocyte antigen classes I and II molecules. Therefore, both CD4+ and CD8+ autoreactive T cells also play a crucial role in PBC (28). Thus, the pathogenesis of PBC is associated with the interaction between mitochondrial autoantigens and anti-mitochondrial antibodies and T cell-mediated toxicity (29). Changes in the immune system have also been observed in the spinal cord and cortical motor areas of ALS patients (30). The activity of CD8+ T cells could be found in both PBC and ALS. In the early stage, T cell subsets and M2 microglias are activated to prevent the neurodegenerative process. In the late stage, the activity of M1 microglia and CD8+ increases leading to decreased numbers of regulatory T cells. To some extent, the neurotoxic effect exceeds the neuroprotective effect, which results in the loss of neurons (31, 32). Association between the two diseases may be driven by dysregulation of the immune system particularly in CD8+ T cells.

The cumulative data shows that structural and functional abnormalities of mitochondria play an important role in ALS (33–35). PBC ensues from loss of mitochondrial antigen immune tolerance, and the mitochondrial autoantigens are found in all nucleated cells. Although it's said that the attack is predominantly for PDC-E2 expressed by bile epithelial cells, it is still under debate (36). Therefore, we speculate that immune attack of PBC may also impair other parts of the body, like motor neurons. Thus, (i) the normal process of electron transport chains is disturbed, causing less production of ATP (37), (ii) the destruction of Ca^{2+} homeostasis, resulting in synaptic dysfunction and neuronal damage (38), (iii) the apoptotic signaling is perturbed (39), leading to ALS. The hypothesis remains to be demonstrated.

With regards to treatment, UDCA is the approved medical treatment to reduce progression of disease in PBC and riluzole in ALS. However, there is no literature on specific medical doses in patients with ALS-PBC overlap syndrome. We recommended our patients to take the medications in regular doses and reexamine one time every 3 months, because most liver enzyme levels are elevated within the first 3 months of riluzole treatment (40). The patients responded satisfactorily except for intermittent nausea in the first patient. Her nausea was relieved by taking the drug in combination with food probably due to less abrupt rises in plasma concentrations. Our case report fills a gap in the researches on ALS-PBC overlap syndrome but the treatment about it has yet to be further studied. PBC is associated with immune-mediated destruction of intrahepatic bile ducts. In ALS, the immune system also plays a pivotal role. UDCA, as an immunomodulatory agent, protects cholangiocytes from bile acid toxicity in PBC patients and takes therapeutic effect on ALS (41). Recently, it has been showed that tauroursodeoxycholic acid (TUDCA) can slow progression in ALS patients (42). Compared with the first patient, our second one developed ALS after a long time with PBC, which may be related to her use of UDCA. Thus, we speculate that immune-modulating therapy for prior ALS, like UDCA, may have some protective or suppressive effect to delay the onset of motor neuron damage. However, it should be noted that this is still speculation based on a clinical phenomenon, and further studies are needed to verify the hypothesis.

CONCLUSION

The coexistence of ALS and PBC indicates a relationship between the two diseases from immunological and mitochondrial aspects. The pathomechanisms of them and the effects of immune-modulating therapy at an early stage before onset of ALS symptoms remain to be elucidated combined with more clinical data.

AUTHOR CONTRIBUTIONS

HZ: plan of the case reports, data acquisition and analysis, follow-up with patients, and writing of the initial manuscript. YL: work-up of the patients, investigation and organization of the work, manuscript review, and revision. ZL, NL, XZ, XN, TZ, and WQ: clinical investigations of patients, supplement to the argument, review, and revision.

FUNDING

This work was supported by the National Natural Sciences Foundation of China (NSFC) (81871001).

REFERENCES

1. Carey EJ, Ali AH, Lindor KD. Primary biliary cirrhosis. *Lancet.* (2015) 386:1565–75. doi: 10.1016/S0140-6736(15)00154-3
2. Invernizzi P, Lleo A, Podda M. Interpreting serological tests in diagnosing autoimmune liver diseases. *Semin Liver Dis.* (2007) 27:161–72. doi: 10.1055/s-2007-979469
3. Ma WT, Chang C, Gershwin ME, Lian ZX. Development of autoantibodies precedes clinical manifestations of autoimmune diseases: a comprehensive review. *J Autoimmun.* (2017) 83:95–112. doi: 10.1016/j.jaut.2017.07.003
4. Terziroli Beretta-Piccoli B, Stirnimann G, Cerny A, Semela D, Hessler R, Helbling B, et al. Geoepidemiology of primary biliary cholangitis: lessons from Switzerland. *Clin Rev Allergy Immunol.* (2018) 54:295–306. doi: 10.1007/s12016-017-8656-x
5. Rowland LP, Shneider NA. Amyotrophic lateral sclerosis. *N Engl J Med.* (2001) 344:1688–700. doi: 10.1056/NEJM200105313442207
6. Leigh PN, Abrahams S, Al-Chalabi A, Ampong MA, Goldstein LH, Johnson J, et al. The management of motor neurone disease. *J Neurol Neurosurg Psychiatr.* (2003) 74(Suppl 4):iv32–47. doi: 10.1136%2Fjnnp.74.suppl_4.iv32
7. Lyall RA, Donaldson N, Polkey MI, Leigh PN, Moxham J. Respiratory muscle strength and ventilatory failure in amyotrophic lateral sclerosis. *Brain.* (2001) 124:2000–13. doi: 10.1093/brain/124.10.2000
8. Pupillo E, Messina P, Logroscino G, Beghi E. Long-term survival in amyotrophic lateral sclerosis: a population-based study. *Ann Neurol.* (2014) 75, 287–97. doi: 10.1002/ana.24096
9. Zhao W, Xie W, Le W, Beers DR, He Y, Henkel JS, et al. Activated microglia initiate motor neuron injury by a nitric oxide and glutamate-mediated mechanism. *J Neuropathol Exp Neurol.* (2004) 63:964–77. doi: 10.1093/jnen/63.9.964
10. Cozzolino M, Ferri A, Valle C, Carri MT. Mitochondria and ALS: implications from novel genes and pathways. *Mol Cell Neurosci.* (2013) 55:44–9. doi: 10.1016/j.mcn.2012.06.001
11. Beleza-Meireles A, Al-Chalabi A. Genetic studies of amyotrophic lateral sclerosis: controversies and perspectives. *Amyotroph Lateral Scler.* (2009) 10:1–14. doi: 10.1080/17482960802585469
12. Carrì MT, Valle C, Bozzo F, Cozzolino M. Oxidative stress and mitochondrial damage: importance in non-SOD1 ALS. *Front Cell Neurosci.* (2015) 9:41. doi: 10.3389/fncel.2015.00041
13. Philips T, Robberecht W. Neuroinflammation in amyotrophic lateral sclerosis: role of glial activation in motor neuron disease. *Lancet Neurol.* (2011) 10:253–63. doi: 10.1016/S1474-4422(11)70015-1
14. Turner MR, Goldacre R, Ramagopalan S, Talbot K, Goldacre MJ. Autoimmune disease preceding amyotrophic lateral sclerosis: an epidemiologic study. *Neurology.* (2013) 81:1222–5. doi: 10.1212/WNL.0b013e3182a6cc13
15. Sawada H. Clinical efficacy of edaravone for the treatment of amyotrophic lateral sclerosis. *Exp Opin Pharmacother.* (2017) 18:735–38. doi: 10.1080/14656566.2017.1319937
16. de Carvalho M, Dengler R, Eisen A, England JD, Kaji R, Kimura J, et al. Electrodiagnostic criteria for diagnosis of ALS. *Clin Neurophysiol.* (2008) 119:497–503. doi: 10.1016/j.clinph.2007.09.143
17. Hirschfield GM, Dyson JK, Alexander GJM, Chapman MH, Collier J, Hübscher S, et al. The British Society of Gastroenterology/UKPBC primary biliary cholangitis treatment and management guidelines. *Gut.* (2018) 67:1–27. doi: 10.1136/gutjnl-2017-315259
18. Bowlus CL, Gershwin ME. The diagnosis of primary biliary cirrhosis. *Autoimmun Rev.* (2014) 13:441–4. doi: 10.1016/j.autrev.2014.01.041
19. Turchany JM, Uibo R, Kivik T, Van de Water J, Prindiville T, Coppel RL, et al. A study of antimitochondrial antibodies in a random population in Estonia. *Am J Gastroenterol.* (1997) 92:124–6. doi: 10.1007/s002619900154
20. Momah N, Silveira MG, Jorgensen R, Sinakos E, Lindor KD. Optimizing biochemical markers as endpoints for clinical trials in primary biliary cirrhosis. *Liver Int.* (2012) 32:790–5. doi: 10.1111/j.1478-3231.2011.02678.x
21. Chazouillères O, Wendum D, Serfaty L, Montembault S, Rosmorduc O, Poupon R. Primary biliary cirrhosis-autoimmune hepatitis overlap syndrome: clinical features and response to therapy. *Hepatology.* (1998) 28:296–301. doi: 10.1002/hep.510280203
22. Bairy I, Berwal A, Seshadri S. Autoimmune hepatitis - primary biliary cirrhosis overlap syndrome. *J Clin Diagn Res.* (2017) 11:OD07–9. doi: 10.7860/JCDR/2017/25193.10242
23. Kaplan MM, Bianchi DW. Primary biliary cirrhosis: for want of an X chromosome? *Lancet.* (2004) 363:505–6. doi: 10.1016/S0140-6736(04)15576-1
24. Schwinge D, Schramm C. Sex-related factors in autoimmune liver diseases. *Semin Immunopathol.* (2019) 41:165–75. doi: 10.1007/s00281-018-0715-8
25. Soriani MH, Desnuelle C. Epidemiology of amyotrophic lateral sclerosis. *Rev Neurol.* (2009) 165:627–40. doi: 10.1016/j.neurol.2009.04.004
26. Kim KA, Jeong SH. The diagnosis and treatment of primary biliary cirrhosis. *Kor J Hepatol.* (2011) 17:173–9. doi: 10.3350/kjhep.2011.17.3.173
27. Floreani A, Leung PS, Gershwin ME. Environmental basis of autoimmunity. *Clin Rev Allergy Immunol.* (2016) 50:287–300. doi: 10.1007/s12016-015-8493-8
28. Kita H, Matsumura S, He XS, Ansari AA, Lian ZX, Van de Water J, et al. Quantitative and functional analysis of PDC-E2-specific autoreactive cytotoxic T lymphocytes in primary biliary cirrhosis. *J Clin Invest.* (2002) 109:1231–40. doi: 10.1172/JCI14698
29. Gershwin ME, Ansari AA, Mackay IR, et al. Primary biliary cirrhosis: an orchestrated immune response against epithelial cells. *Immunol Rev.* (2000) 174:210–25. doi: 10.1034/j.1600-0528.2002.017402.x
30. Mantovani S, Garbelli S, Pasini A, Alimonti D, Perotti C, Melazzini M, et al. Immune system alterations in sporadic amyotrophic lateral sclerosis patients suggest an ongoing neuroinflammatory process. *J Neuroimmunol.* (2009) 210:73–9. doi: 10.1016/j.jneuroim.2009.02.012
31. Phani S, Re DB, Przedborski S. The role of the innate immune system in ALS. *Front Pharmacol.* (2012) 3:150. doi: 10.3389/fphar.2012.00150
32. Hovden H, Frederiksen JL, Pedersen SW. Immune system alterations in amyotrophic lateral sclerosis. *Acta Neurol. Scand.* (2013) 128:287–96. doi: 10.1111/ane.12125
33. Magrané J, Manfredi G. Mitochondrial function, morphology, and axonal transport in amyotrophic lateral sclerosis. *Antioxid Redox Signal.* (2009) 11:1615–26. doi: 10.1089/ars.2009.2604
34. Manfredi G, Xu Z. Mitochondrial dysfunction and its role in motor neuron degeneration in ALS. *Mitochondrion.* (2005) 5:77–87. doi: 10.1016/j.mito.2005.01.002
35. Sasaki S, Iwata M. Mitochondrial alterations in the spinal cord of patients with sporadic amyotrophic lateral sclerosis. *J Neuropathol Exp Neurol.* (2007) 66:10–6. doi: 10.1097/nen.0b013e31802c396b
36. Lleo A, Selmi C, Invernizzi P, Podda M, Coppel RL, Mackay IR, et al. Apotopes and the biliary specificity of primary biliary cirrhosis. *Hepatology.* (2009) 49:871–9. doi: 10.1002/hep.22736
37. Pasinelli P, Brown RH. Molecular biology of amyotrophic lateral sclerosis: insights from genetics. *Nat Rev Neurosci.* (2006) 7:710–23. doi: 10.1038/nrn1971
38. Jaiswal MK. Calcium, mitochondria, and the pathogenesis of ALS: the good, the bad, and the ugly. *Front Cell Neurosci.* (2013) 7:199. doi: 10.3389/fncel.2013.00199
39. Mattson MP. Apoptosis in neurodegenerative disorders. *Nat Rev Mol Cell Biol.* (2000) 1:120–9. doi: 10.1038/35040009
40. Lacomblez L, Bensimon G, Leigh PN, Guillet P, Meininger V. Dose-ranging study of riluzole in amyotrophic lateral sclerosis. Amyotrophic

Lateral Sclerosis/Riluzole Study Group II. *Lancet.* (1996) 347:1425–31. doi: 10.1016/S0140-6736(96)91680-3

41. Min JH, Hong YH, Sung JJ, Kim SM, Lee JB, Lee KW. Oral solubilized ursodeoxycholic acid therapy in amyotrophic lateral sclerosis: a randomized cross-over trial. *J Korean Med. Sci.* (2012) 27:200–6. doi: 10.3346/jkms.2012.27.2.200
42. Elia AE, Lalli S, Monsurro MR, Sagnelli A, Taiello AC, Reggiori B, et al. Tauroursodeoxycholic acid in the treatment of patients with amyotrophic lateral sclerosis. *Eur J Neurol.* (2016) 23:45–52. doi: 10.1111/ene.12664

20

The Clinical and Radiological Spectrum of Hippocampal Pathology in Amyotrophic Lateral Sclerosis

Foteini Christidi[1]*, Efstratios Karavasilis[2], Georgios Velonakis[2], Panagiotis Ferentinos[3], Michail Rentzos[1], Nikolaos Kelekis[2], Ioannis Evdokimidis[1] and Peter Bede[4]

[1] First Department of Neurology, Aeginition Hospital, National and Kapodistrian University of Athens, Athens, Greece, [2] Second Department of Radiology, General University Hospital "Attikon," National and Kapodistrian University of Athens, Athens, Greece, [3] Second Department of Psychiatry, General University Hospital "Attikon," National and Kapodistrian University of Athens, Athens, Greece, [4] Computational Neuroimaging Group, Academic Unit of Neurology, Trinity College Dublin, Dublin, Ireland

***Correspondence:**
Foteini Christidi
christidi.f.a@gmail.com

Hippocampal pathology in Amyotrophic Lateral Sclerosis (ALS) remains surprisingly under recognized despite compelling evidence from neuropsychology, neuroimaging and neuropathology studies. Hippocampal dysfunction contributes significantly to the clinical heterogeneity of ALS and requires structure-specific cognitive and neuroimaging tools for accurate *in vivo* evaluation. Recent imaging studies have generated unprecedented insights into the presymptomatic and longitudinal processes affecting this structure and have contributed to the characterisation of both focal and network-level changes. Emerging neuropsychology data suggest that memory deficits in ALS may be independent from executive dysfunction. In the era of precision medicine, where the development of individualized care strategies and patient stratification for clinical trials are key priorities, the comprehensive review of hippocampal dysfunction in ALS is particularly timely.

Keywords: hippocampus, amyotrophic lateral sclerosis, neuropathology, neuroimaging, cognition

INTRODUCTION

Amyotrophic lateral sclerosis (ALS) is relentlessly progressive neurodegenerative condition with considerable clinical heterogeneity (1). One of the key clinical dimensions of disease heterogeneity in ALS is the varying severity and profile of cognitive impairment. The quality of life implications of cognitive impairment in ALS and its impact on caregiver burden (2), compliance with assistive devices (3) and survival (4) are now universally recognized. The discovery of hexanucleotide expansions in *C9orf72* in 2011 (5) has given fresh momentum to neuropsychology research in ALS by confirming shared etiological factors between frontotemporal dementia (FTD) and ALS. The momentous conceptual advances in the neuropsychology of ALS have taken place in a remarkably short period of time, from sporadic observations, through the development of diagnostic criteria (6), to robust family aggregation (7) and genetic studies, to the development of disease-specific screening instruments (8, 9). The current consensus criteria (6) distinguish ALS with cognitive impairment; ALS with behavioral impairment; ALS with cognitive and behavioral impairment; ALS-FTD; ALS-dementia (non-FTD, i.e., Alzheimer dementia (AD), vascular dementia, mixed dementia). One of the most exciting aspects of ALS neuropsychology studies is their localization potential to specific anatomical circuits and that their observations are widely corroborated by neuropathology (10–12) and neuroimaging studies (13). Memory deficits in ALS have traditionally been regarded as atypical and considered suggestive of coexisting AD-type pathology. The recognition that memory deficits are part of the spectrum of ALS-associated cognitive impairment is relatively recent.

MEMORY IMPAIRMENT IN ALS

Early neuropsychology studies of ALS have predominantly examined frontal lobe-mediated neuropsychological domains, and highlighted executive dysfunction, impaired phonemic fluency, poor set shifting, reduced cognitive flexibility, impaired response inhibition, planning deficits, problem-solving difficulties, selective attention, and impaired social cognition (14). More recently, the spectrum of memory impairment has been specifically evaluated, including encoding and retrieval functions (primary memory system) (15, 16) and storage/consolidation domains (secondary memory system) (17). Furthermore, population-based studies identified cognitive phenotypes without executive impairment (18, 19). The description of episodic memory deficits without coexisting executive dysfunction in ALS drew attention to temporal lobe network dysfunction which has been elegantly corroborated by a series of neuropathology and neuroimaging studies (20).

ANATOMICAL OVERVIEW

The hippocampus (**Figure 1A**) is a bilaminar structure and consists of the cornu ammonis (CA) and the dentate gyrus (DG). Based on its cytoarchitecture and projections, the CA is further divided into four histological subfields, named CA1-CA4 by Lorente de No in his seminal paper (21). The dentate gyrus is a narrow, dorsally concave structure which envelops CA4. The cornu ammonis, the dentate gyrus, and the subiculum together form the "hippocampal formation" (**Figure 1B**). The subiculum is divided into the following segments: the prosubiculum, the subiculum proper, the presubiculum, and the parasubiculum.

Each segment of the hippocampal formation receives afferentation from its neighboring regions but these connections are not all bidirectional (22). For example, the "trisynaptic circuit" (23) is a unidirectional network, which arises from layer II of the entorhinal cortex, its axons perforate the subiculum, and form the "perforant pathway" (PP). Duvernoy (24) coined the term "polysynaptic pathway" for the intrinsic hippocampal circuitry, which refers to a circuit of at least four synapses that connect the entorhinal cortex, the dentate gyrus, the CA subfields, and the subiculum. A direct intrahippocampal pathway has also been identified, which originates from layer III of the entorhinal cortex and projects directly to the CA1 but not through the PP (25). The perforant pathway (**Figure 1C**) arises from layer II-III neurons of the lateral and medial entorhinal cortex (26), which is also the origin of the polysynaptic pathway (27). The PP perforates the subiculum to reach the dentate gyrus and the hippocampus proper, but minor projections also originate from the presubiculum and parasubiculum (28). The majority of the PP fibers reach the stratum moleculare of the dentate gyrus through the vestigial hippocampal sulcus (24). The PP contributes to the "Papez circuit" (26, 29, 30) which is relayed through the following structures; entorhinal cortex → dentate gyrus → hippocampus → hypothalamus → thalamus → cingulate cortex→ presubiculum → entorhinal cortex. In addition to the intrinsic hippocampal circuitry, there are numerous extrinsic hippocampal projections to subcortical and cortical regions (31). The main input to the hippocampus enters via the entorhinal area (31).

INSIGHTS FROM NEUROPATHOLOGY

Neuropathological changes have been consistently reported in the hippocampus in ALS (**Table 1**). Early reports highlighted ubiquitin-positive intraneuronal inclusions (32–35) in medial temporal structures, neuronal loss in the medial cortex of the temporal tip (36, 69) and focal depletion of pyramidal neurons in the pes hippocampi in both patients with and without dementia (33, 36, 69). A specific focus of interest in histopathological studies is the PP zone, which has been comprehensively studied in most neurodegenerative conditions, especially in AD. While AD is characterized by the extraneuronal deposits of the amyloid β-protein (Aβ) and the intraneuronal tauopathy (70), ALS is primarily associated with TAR DNA-binding protein 43 (TDP-43) deposits (71). ALS patients with and without dementia (37, 38) show neuropathological changes in the dentate gyrus and the outer lamina of the molecular layer where the PP terminals are distributed (26, 30, 72). In ALS, the molecular layer of the dentate gyrus is primarily affected, a pattern which is distinctly different from AD. The inner molecular layer, which is innervated by the CA4 (73), is the least affected layer in ALS (38). The intermediate layer, which receives projections from layer II of the medial entorhinal cortex, is affected (38), but the outer layer, is the most affected region in ALS (38). Despite considerable mesial temporal lobe involvement in both ALS and AD, the distribution of disease-specific inclusions is strikingly different. Neurofibrillary tangles in AD are mostly found in the entorhinal cortex and are positive for tau, whereas the main proteinopathy of ALS is TDP-43 and mostly affects the transentorhinal cortex (38).

It is now widely recognized that phosphorylated TDP-43 (pTDP-43) aggregates are the hallmark pathology of sporadic

Abbreviations: ALS, amyotrophic lateral sclerosis; ALSFRS-r, revised ALS functional rating scale revised; ALSnci, ALS with no cognitive impairment; aMCI, amnestic mild cognitive impairment; C9orf72 HRT, chromosome 9 open reading frame 72 hexanucleotide repeats; CA, cornu ammonis; DG, dentate gyrus; DTI, diffusion tensor imaging; DWI, diffusion weighted imaging; ECAS, Edinburgh cognitive and behavioral ALS screen; FTD, frontotemporal dementia; GM, gray matter; HARDI, high angular resolution diffusion imaging; HC, healthy control; MND, motor neuron disease; NeuroC, neurological controls; NODDI, neurite orientation dispersion and density imaging; PP, perforant pathway; PtwoCI, patients without cognitive impairment; PtwCI, patients with cognitive impairment; PtwoD, patients without dementia; PtwD, patients with dementia; TBSS, tract-based spatial statistics; VBM, voxel-based morphometry; WM, white matter; MRS, magnetic resonance spectroscopy.

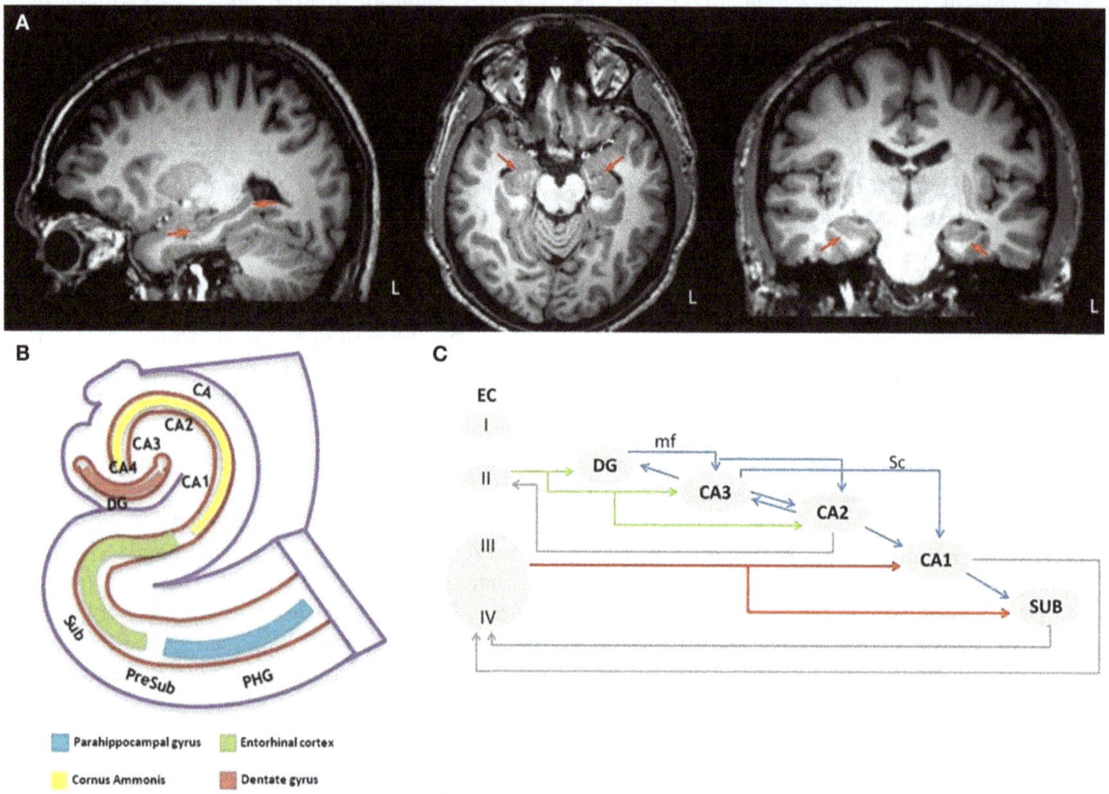

FIGURE 1 | Anatomical depiction of hippocampus on sagittal, axial and coronal plane of high resolution T1 image from a healthy control subject **(A)** and schematic representation of **(B)** the anatomy of the hippocampus-entorhinal cortex-parahippocampal gyrus system and **(C)** the intrahippocampal connections. L, left hemisphere; PHG, parahippocampal gyrus; PreSub, Presubiculum; Sub, Subiculum; CA, Cornu Ammonis; CA1-CA4, Cornu Ammonis subfields; DG, Dentate gyrus; EC, Entorhinal cortex; I-IV, Layer I-IV; mf, mossy fibers; Sc, Schaffer collaterals.

ALS (39, 74, 75). Based on post mortem observations, a sequential staging system of pTDP-43 pathology has been proposed, using stage-defining involvement of specific cortical and subcortical regions (12). According to this four-stage model of disease propagation, the PP is predominantly affected in stage IV. A three-stage model has also been suggested for PP degeneration (38) where stage I is the "inclusion stage" defined by TDP-43-positive cytoplasmatic inclusions appearing in the granular cells of the dentate gyrus, stage II is the "early perforant stage" where gliosis and neuronal loss of the transentorhinal cortex are observed, and stage III is the "advanced perforant stage" defined by the degeneration of the molecular layer of the dentate gyrus and neuronal loss in the transentorhinal cortex (38). The chronological stages of hippocampal pathology are closely linked to its structural anatomy, confirming that disease propagation occurs along connectivity patterns (76). The TDP-43 stages of ALS are in line with the notion that gray matter (GM) regions become sequentially involved via the WM pathways that connect them (77–79).

THE CONTRIBUTION OF NEUROIMAGING

Neuroimaging studies have already contributed meaningful structural, metabolic and functional insights in ALS (80, 81) and recent technological advances in imaging techniques offer unprecedented opportunities to characterize hippocampal changes *in vivo*. Following sporadic reports of hippocampal degeneration (82–85) in whole-brain exploratory studies, recent studies have specifically focused on the evaluation of this structure (43) (**Table 1**). Emerging imaging methods not only highlight hippocampal volume reductions, but have the potential to characterize specific sub-regions (78), shape changes (42), density alterations (20), progressive longitudinal changes (43), altered connectivity profiles, and functional changes (40, 46, 47).

Structural Neuroimaging

Computational neuroimaging techniques have consistently captured hippocampal GM changes which was initially thought to be more significant in ALS patients carrying the *C9orf72* hexanucleotide repeats (40), but later studies showed similarly extensive hippocampal degeneration in *C9orf72* negative ALS-FTD patients (78). Interestingly, unilateral hippocampal changes were not only captured in patients with cognitive impairment (42), but also in cognitively intact cohorts (41). Shape and density analyses of the hippocampus in ALS highlighted phenotype-specific patterns of hippocampal degeneration (42). A longitudinal study of hippocampus, which included a small (~6%) number of *C9orf72* positive patients, identified baseline

TABLE 1 | Research studies with hippocampal-related neuropathological, neuroimaging, or neuropsychological findings in ALS included in the present review.

References	Authors (Date)	Sample size	Diagnostic criteria	Genetic Status	Dementia	Cognitive status
NEUROPATHOLOGICAL STUDIES						
(32)	Wightman et al., 1992	33 ALS	N/A	N/A	Included	19 PtwoCI; 14 PtwCI-D*
(33)	Okamoto et al., 1991	27 ALS/50 HC	N/A	N/A	1 PtwD	N/A (1PtwD)*
(34)	Okamoto et al., 1992	10 MND	N/A	N/A	10 PtwD	Dementia*
(35)	Okamoto et al., 1996	2 ALS	N/A	N/A	N/A	Mental changes*
(36)	Nakano et al., 1993	54 ALS/35 non ALS	N/A	N/A	10 PtwD	44 PtwoD; 10 PtwD
(37)	Takeda et al., 2007	12 ALS	N/A	N/A	12 PtwD	Demented
(38)	Takeda et al., 2009	14 ALS	N/A	N/A	9 PtwD	9 PtwD* (6 PtwMI)
(39)	Brettschneider et al., 2012	102 ALS	El Escorial-R	N/A	12 PtwD	88 PtwoD; 12 PtwD; 2 unknown
(12)	Brettschneider et al., 2013	76 ALS	El Escorial-R	11 C9orf72(+)	5 PtwD	71 PtwoD*; 5 PtwD*
NEUROIMAGING STUDIES: STRUCTURAL GM						
(40)	Bede et al., 2013	39 ALS/44 HC	El Escorial	9 C9orf72(+)	N/A	Cognitive exam; Unspecified cognitive groups
(41)	Abdulla et al., 2014	58 ALS/29 HC	El Escorial-R	3 C9orf72(+)	N/A	Cognitive exam; Unspecified cognitive groups
(42)	Machts et al., 2015	67 ALS/ 39 HC	El Escorial-R	C9orf72(-)	7 PtwD	Cognitive exam; 42 PtwoCI; 18 PtwCI; 7 PtwFTD
(43)	Westeneng et al., 2015	112 ALS/60 HC	El Escorial-R	7 C9orf72(+)	N/A	N/A
(44)	Sage et al., 2007	28 ALS/26 HC	El Escorial	N/A	PtwoD	No behavioral or cognitive changes; Unspecified cognitive exam
(45)	Sage et al., 2009	28 ALS/26 HC	El Escorial	N/A	PtwoD	No behavioral or cognitive changes; Unspecified cognitive exam
NEUROIMAGING STUDIES: STRUCTURAL WM						
(46)	Barbagallo et al., 2014	24 ALS/22 HC	El Escorial-R	N/A	N/A	13 Pt cognitively examined; Unspecified cognitive groups
(47)	Thivard et al., 2007	15 ALS/25 HC	El Escorial-R	N/A	PtwoD	N/A
(48)	Prell et al., 2013	17 ALS/17 HC	El Escorial-R	N/A	PtwoD	No significant frontal or cognitive dysfunction; Unspecified cognitive exam
(49)	Keil et al., 2012	24 ALS/24 HC	El Escorial-R	N/A	PtwoD	No cognitive exam
(50)	Kassubek et al., 2014	111 ALS/74 HC	El Escorial-R	N/A	N/A	N/A
(51)	Christidi et al., 2017	42 ALS/25 HC	El Escorial-R	N/A	PtwoD	Cognitive exam; Memory impairment based on normative data; Unspecified cognitive groups
(52)	Steinbach et al., 2015	16 ALS/16HC	El Escorial-R	N/A	16 PtwD	Cognitive exam; Cognitive categories based on Phukan criteria#
NEUROIMAGING STUDIES: TASK fMRI						
(53)	Stoppel et al., 2014	14 ALS/14 HC	El Escorial-R	N/A	PtwoD	Cognitive exam; Memory impairment based on normative data; Cognitive categories based on Phukan criteria#
NEUROIMAGING STUDIES: RESTING-STATE fMRI						
(54)	Agosta et al., 2011	26 ALS/15 HC	El Escorial-R	N/A	PtwoD	N/A
(55)	Zhu et al., 2015	22 ALS/22 HC	El Escorial-R	N/A	PtwoD	Cognitive exam; Unspecified cognitive groups
(56)	Heimrath et al., 2014	9 ALS/11 HC	El Escorial-R	N/A	PtwoD	Cognitive exam; Unspecified cognitive groups
(57)	Loewe et al., 2017	64 ALS/38 HC	El Escorial-R	N/A	PtwoD	Cognitive exam; Specified cognitive groups#

(Continued)

TABLE 1 | Continued

References	Authors (Date)	Sample size	Diagnostic criteria	Genetic Status	Dementia	Cognitive status
NEUROPSYCHOLOGICAL STUDIES						
(58)	Abrahams et al., 1997	12 ALS/25 HC	N/A	N/A	N/A	Cognitive exam; Unspecified cognitive groups
(59)	Chari et al., 1996	50 MND/27 HC/23 NeuroC	El Escorial	N/A	PtwoD	Cognitive exam; Unspecified cognitive groups
(60)	Frank et al., 1997	74 ALS/56 HC	N/A	N/A	N/A	Cognitive exam; Unspecified cognitive groups
(61)	Hanagasi et al., 2002	20 ALS/13 HC	El Escorial	N/A	PtwoD	Cognitive exam; Unspecified cognitive groups
(62)	Iwasaki et al., 1990	18 ALS/15 HC	N/A	N/A	PtwoD	Cognitive exam; Unspecified cognitive groups
(63)	Ludolph et al., 1992	17 ALS/12 HC	N/A	N/A	PtwoD	Cognitive exam; Unspecified cognitive groups
(64)	Massman et al., 1996	146 ALS	El Escorial	N/A	N/A	Cognitive exam; Cognitive impairment based on normative data; Unspecified cognitive groups
(65)	Mantovan et al., 2003	20 ALS/20 HC	El Escorial	N/A	PtwoD	Cognitive exam; Unspecified cognitive groups
(66)	Christidi et al., 2012	22 ALS/22 HC	El Escorial-R	N/A	PtwoD	Cognitive exam; Unspecified cognitive groups
(67)	Machts et al., 2014	40 ALS/39 aMCI/40 HC	El Escorial-R	N/A	3 PtwD	Cognitive exam; Unspecified cognitive groups
(68)	Burke et al., 2017	203 ALS/117 HC	El Escorial-R	C9orf72(−)	30 PtwD	Cognitive exam; 117 PtwoCI; 56 PtwCI; 30 PtwD

*ALS, amyotrophic lateral sclerosis; HC, healthy control; MND, motor neuron disease; N/A, non-available; PtwoCI, patients without cognitive impairment; PtwCI-D, patients with cognitive impairment-dementia; PtwD, patients with dementia; PtwoD, patients without dementia; PtwMI, patients with memory impairment; PtwCI, patients with cognitive impairment; PtwFTD, patients with frontotemporal dementia; *unspecified cognitive status; #no comparison between cognitive groups; El Escorial-R, El Escorial revised criteria; C9orf72(+), C9orf72 positive status; GM, gray matter; WM, white matter.*

changes in the left presubiculum, and progressive CA2/3, CA4 and the left presubiculum involvement at follow-up (43).

While diffusion-weighted imaging (DWI) is primarily used to study white matter (WM) structures, there is increasing evidence that it may provide useful information on aspects of GM integrity (86). Evaluation of diffusion tensor imaging (DTI) metrics have consistently shown low fractional anisotropy (44, 49) and increased mean diffusivity in both hippocampal (44–47) and parahippocampal regions (48).

DTI has been initially used to characterize medial temporal lobe WM regions and later to assess limbic circuit integrity (i.e., fornix; uncinate fasciculus) (87–89). One of the most unique applications of hippocampal DTI in ALS however is the ability to reconstruct and evaluate of the PP. (50, 51). Based on *in vivo* assessments, these studies have not only confirmed previous neuropathological observations but also revealed structure-specific clinical correlations (51). The use of DWI-based PP imaging (90) has contributed to our understanding of impaired memory processing in a range of conditions from mild cognitive impairment, through AD, to traumatic brain injury (91–94). PP imaging is therefore a relatively well-established approach which has only recently been applied to ALS. A longitudinal tractography study of ALS (52) found increased connectivity between the visual cortex and medial temporal lobe regions which increased further at 3-month follow-up. Increased connectivity over time in ALS is not an isolated finding (95) and is often interpreted as a compensatory mechanism.

Functional Neuroimaging

There are relatively few paradigm-based functional magnetic resonance imaging (fMRI) studies specifically evaluating hippocampal function, but a longitudinal fMRI study identified increased novelty-evoked hippocampal activity over time (53). Resting-state studies have consistently captured increased connectivity between the left sensorimotor cortex and contralateral cortical regions including the parahippocampal gyrus (54). Additionally, increased low-frequency amplitudes have been observed in the right parahippocampal cortex (55). Increased functional connectivity was also identified between parahippocampal components of the default-mode network (56). In a relatively large sample of ALS patients with only minor cognitive changes, (57) decreased functional connectivity was identified between temporal lobe structures, including hippocampal and parahippocampal regions. This was thought to represent early metabolic disturbances before cell-loss occurs but highlight the fact that increased and decreased connectivity is both reported in fMRI studies of ALS.

INSIGHTS FROM NEUROPSYCHOLOGY

Contrary to the consensus around executive dysfunction in ALS (96–99), there are strikingly inconsistent reports about the incidence of memory impairment in ALS (**Table 1**). Intact memory function, mild dysfunction, executive function mediated memory impairment, and moderate memory deficits have all been reported (58–65, 97). The primary substrate of amnestic deficits is still under investigation. Most studies agree that the primary deficit is in encoding-retrieval (65) which is often linked to frontal dysfunction, attention, and other executive-based processes (65–68). However, recognition deficits and memory consolidation difficulties are likely to be just as important (66). Compelling evidence also exist for pure episodic memory dysfunction based on impaired picture recall, word list-learning, pair associations, and story-recall. These observations would suggest that memory impairment in non-demented ALS patients cannot be exclusively attributed to executive dysfunction (100–102).

In a combined neuroimaging-neuropsychology study, abnormal immediate and delayed recall scores were identified in 23% of non-demented ALS patients (102). While the ALS cohort of this study did not exhibit reduced hippocampal volumes in comparison to healthy controls, their memory performance correlated with hippocampal volumes. These findings are echoed by other studies which rely on volumetric analyses and verbal list-learning test and report significant correlations between the hippocampal volumes and verbal memory indices such as total learning, delayed recall, and recognition (41).

While direct clinico-radiological correlations are often regarded as contentious (103), a positive association has been reported between verbal memory indices and hippocampal volumes in several ALS subgroups, including ALSci and ALS-FTD (42). DTI studies have consistently revealed correlations between memory performance and memory-associated WM tracts such as the fornix (88), the uncinate fasciculus (87, 88), and the hippocampal PP (51). Emerging reports of similar episodic memory performance in ALS and amnestic mild cognitive impairment patients (67) corroborates neuropathological findings of comparable PP changes (37, 38).

Testing Recommendations

Traditionally, the assessment of episodic memory includes tests for immediate and delayed recall, and performance evaluated from a learning, retention and recognition perspective. More recently, distinct memory processes are specifically assessed, such as encoding, consolidation, and retrieval. (104–106) List-learning tests (e.g., California Verbal Learning Test; Rey Auditory Verbal Learning Test; Hopkins Verbal Learning Test etc.) are particularly useful to assess hippocampus-mediated verbal memory dysfunction in ALS. These tests enable the clinician to evaluate immediate recall, delayed recall, and recognition and can be readily interpreted in terms of encoding, consolidation, and retrieval performance (66). Story-recall tests, such as the Wechsler-Memory Scale, are also sensitive to detect episodic memory impairment and ideally, both list-learning and story-recall should be performed to comprehensively evaluate episodic memory in ALS. The accurate assessment of visual episodic memory is often confounded by motor disability in in ALS or by coexisting executive dysfunction which may affect the organization and encoding of complex figures (e.g., Rey-Osterreith Complex Figure Test). The limitations of short, non-ALS, cognitive screening tools such as MMSE; ACE; MoCA are widely recognized in the ALS research community, as these tests have been developed for other neurodegenerative conditions. The administration of ALS specific screening tools (ECAS, ALS-CBS) should be followed by specialist neuropsychological evaluation if memory impairment is identified or reported by the patient or caregiver.

DISCUSSION

The synthesis of insights from neuropathology, neuroimaging and neuropsychology enables the systematic discussion of structural and functional aspects of hippocampal degeneration in ALS and helps to integrate focal pathology into a network perspective.

While hippocampal pathology used to be primarily evaluated in ALS patients with comorbid dementia (34, 37, 38), recent studies have increasingly focused on non-demented patient cohorts (12, 32, 69, 71). With the increased recognition of neuropsychological deficits beyond executive dysfunction, imaging studies of ALS have gradually started to evaluate mesial temporal lobe structures and memory domains have now been incorporated in ALS-specific cognitive screening tools (8). The targeted evaluation of memory function and reliance on more sophisticated indices of episodic memory (65–68) not only help to characterize the heterogeneity of cognitive profiles but also confirm that pure episodic memory dysfunction is not uncommon in ALS and can be detected in the absence of FTD.

Despite the momentous advances in characterizing hippocampal degeneration in ALS, considerable shortcomings and inconsistencies can be identified. The commonest problem is sample size limitations followed by the inclusion of poorly characterized patients. The comprehensive neuropsychological assessment of patients is paramount and administering screening tests alone is not sufficient. Reliance on non-ALS specific batteries, such as Addenbrooke's Cognitive Examination, Mini-Mental State Examination, Montreal Cognitive Assessment, is not sufficient to characterize ALS-associated cognitive change. A common shortcoming of ALS neuropsychology papers is overlooking the confounding effect of medications which affect cognitive performance. Anticholinergics commonly used for sialorrhea, tricyclic antidepressants, opiates, benzodiazepines are all widely used in ALS and have a significant impact on attention, registration, and recall. Other disease-specific confounding factors such as hypoxia, hypercapnia, physical discomfort, fatigue, apathy, low mood, depression also need careful consideration. Despite established consensus criteria (6) different batteries are used in different centers to test memory. There is a paucity of reports where caregivers or family members are interviewed about the sort of memory impairment they may have observed. A few targeted questions if the patient gets lost in familiar places, misplaces items, forgets names, or dates etc. may be worth asking from the caregivers. Given the strikingly quick progression rates observed in ALS compared to other neurodegenerative conditions, resource allocation, care planning, assessment of capacity may be important at an early stage of the disease. ALS patients have to make a number of important financial, personal, and end-of-life decisions which may or may not be affected by memory impairment.

The practice of excluding patients with dementia in neuroimaging studies (44, 47, 49, 55) to evaluate clinically homogenous samples may also be counterintuitive. More recent imaging papers include comprehensive cognitive testing (55–57) which aids the interpretation of extra-motor changes (107). The lack of cognitive profiling of the healthy controls in many neuroimaging studies also precludes robust statistics as only the patient group is then used for correlative analyses. Often, reference normative neuropsychology data are used for the interpretation of patient's memory performance, data which is independent from the given study and originate from volunteers who have not been scanned as part of the given study. The patients' neuroimaging data on the other hand are contrasted to scans of controls who had no detailed neuropsychological evaluation. This unfortunately is a common study design, which essentially uses a different imaging and neuropsychology control group. Another common shortcoming of ALS neuroimaging studies is the lack of adjustment for education, which may impact on both structural and functional imaging data (80). A binary, comparative study design of patients versus controls and the contrasting of two clinically or genetically defined cohorts is not entirely satisfactory either. The inclusion of mimic cohorts, or a "disease-control" group with an alternative neurodegenerative condition such as MCI, AD, or Parkinson disease would also be desirable. The selection bias of relatively well patients who are able to lie flat in the scanner and able to make the journey to a radiology department is seldom acknowledged. It is conceivable that progressive hippocampal changes occur as the disease progresses, but these patients are no longer able to partake in imaging studies. Clinical trial designs are not only hampered by late recruitment of clinically heterogeneous cohorts, but they overwhelmingly rely on motor, respiratory, nutritional markers (108–110). Patient stratification based on cognitive performance prior to inclusion and monitoring performance during the trial seems essential, especially given the survival implications of cognitive impairment (3, 4, 111).

Despite initial enthusiasm that hexanucleotide repeats account for most of the ALS-FTD cohort (112, 113), it has quickly become apparent that *C9orf72* hexanucleotide repeats only explain a minority of ALS-FTD cases (114). Emerging studies confirm that a subgroup of *C9orf72* negative patients may show neuroanatomical alterations similar to the ones observed in patients carrying the hexanucleotide expansion. Furthermore, temporal lobe changes have been captured in asymptomatic hexanucleotide carriers, who also exhibited subcortical gray matter degeneration prior to symptom onset (115).

Existing multimodal studies which combine neuroimaging and neurocognitive measures either support a close association between anatomical changes and memory performance or highlight a relative dissociation between the two methods. This inconsistency is epitomized by reports of absent neuroimaging changes in patients with established memory deficits and the detection of significant hippocampal changes in patients with mild memory impairment (41, 42, 102). Based on the shortcomings of existing hippocampal studies in ALS, future studies should include large sample sizes, disease-controls, longitudinal designs, paradigm-based fMRI, comprehensive neuropsychological profiling, "disease-controls," anatomical corrections for education, and genetic screening for mutations implicated in ALS, FTD, and AD. Furthermore, reliance on high directional diffusion models such as neurite orientation dispersion and density imaging (NODDI), high angular resolution diffusion imaging (HARDI), or Q-ball imaging may be desirable to characterize early WM alterations in parahippocampal regions. Finally, combined imaging and post-mortem studies may provide a validation of the *in vivo* findings.

In conclusion, hippocampal pathology is a clinically and academically relevant field of ALS research which has gained unprecedented momentum in recent years and is likely to contribute important further insights in the coming years.

AUTHOR CONTRIBUTIONS

The paper was drafted by FC, EK, and PB and has been reviewed for intellectual content by GV, PF, MR, NK, and IE.

ACKNOWLEDGMENTS

We acknowledge the generosity and kindness of our patients for participating in ALS imaging studies worldwide. PB is supported by the Health Research Board (HRB—Ireland; HRB EIA-2017-019), the Irish Institute of Clinical Neuroscience IICN—Novartis Ireland Research Grant, the Iris O'Brien Foundation, the Perrigo Clinician-Scientist Research Fellowship, and the Research Motor Neuron (RMN-Ireland) Foundation.

REFERENCES

1. Brooks BR, Miller RG, Swash M, Munsat TL, World Federation of Neurology Research Group on Motor Neuron Diseases. El Escorial revisited: Revised criteria for the diagnosis of amyotrophic lateral sclerosis. *Amyotroph Lateral Scler Other Motor Neuron Disord.* (2000) 1:293–9. doi: 10.1080/146608200300079536
2. Burke T, Elamin M, Galvin M, Hardiman O, Pender N. Caregiver burden in amyotrophic lateral sclerosis: a cross-sectional investigation of predictors. *J Neurol.* (2015) 262:1526–32. doi: 10.1007/s00415-015-7746-z
3. Olney RK, Murphy J, Forshew D, Garwood E, Miller BL, Langmore S, et al. The effects of executive and behavioral dysfunction on the course of ALS. *Neurology* (2005) 65:1774–7. doi: 10.1212/01.wnl.0000188759.87240.8b
4. Elamin M, Phukan J, Bede P, Jordan N, Byrne S, Pender N, et al. Executive dysfunction is a negative prognostic indicator in patients with ALS without dementia. *Neurology* (2011) 76:1263–9. doi: 10.1212/WNL.0b013e318214359f
5. DeJesus-Hernandez M, Mackenzie Ian R, Boeve Bradley F, Boxer Adam L, Baker M, Rutherford Nicola J, et al. Expanded GGGGCC hexanucleotide

repeat in noncoding region of C9ORF72 causes chromosome 9p-linked FTD and ALS. *Neuron.* (2011) 72:245–56. doi: 10.1016/j.neuron.2011.09.011

6. Strong MJ, Abrahams S, Goldstein LH, Woolley S, McLaughlin P, Snowden J, et al. Amyotrophic lateral sclerosis - frontotemporal spectrum disorder (ALS-FTSD): Revised diagnostic criteria. *Amyotroph Lateral Scler Other Motor Neuron Disord.* (2017) 18:153–74. doi: 10.1080/21678421.2016.1267768
7. O'Brien M, Burke T, Heverin M, Vajda A, McLaughlin R, Gibbons J, et al. Clustering of neuropsychiatric disease in first-degree and second-degree relatives of patients with amyotrophic lateral sclerosis. *JAMA Neurol.* (2017) 74:1425–30. doi: 10.1001/jamaneurol.2017.2699
8. Abrahams S, Newton J, Niven E, Foley J, Bak TH. Screening for cognition and behaviour changes in ALS. *Amyotroph Lateral Scler Other Motor Neuron Disord.* (2014) 15:9–14. doi: 10.3109/21678421.2013.805784
9. Woolley SC, York MK, Moore DH, Strutt AM, Murphy J, Schulz PE, et al. Detecting frontotemporal dysfunction in ALS: utility of the ALS Cognitive Behavioral Screen (ALS-CBS). *Amyotroph Lateral Scler.* (2010) 11:303–11. doi: 10.3109/17482961003727954
10. Saberi S, Stauffer JE, Schulte DJ, Ravits J. Neuropathology of amyotrophic lateral sclerosis and its variants. *Neurol Clin.* (2015) 33:855–76. doi: 10.1016/j.ncl.2015.07.012
11. Fatima M, Tan R, Halliday GM, Kril JJ. Spread of pathology in amyotrophic lateral sclerosis: assessment of phosphorylated TDP-43 along axonal pathways. *Acta Neuropathol Commun.* (2015) 3:47. doi: 10.1186/s40478-015-0226-y
12. Brettschneider J, Del Tredici K, Toledo JB, Robinson JL, Irwin DJ, Grossman M, et al. Stages of pTDP-43 pathology in amyotrophic lateral sclerosis. *Annals Neurol.* (2013) 74:20–38. doi: 10.1002/ana.23937
13. Turner MR, Verstraete E. What does imaging reveal about the pathology of amyotrophic lateral sclerosis? *Curr Neurol Neurosci Rep.* (2015) 15:45. doi: 10.1007/s11910-015-0569-6
14. Murphy J, Henry R, Lomen-Hoerth C. Establishing subtypes of the continuum of frontal lobe impairment in amyotrophic lateral sclerosis. *Arch Neurol.* (2007) 64:330–4. doi: 10.1001/archneur.64.3.330
15. Beeldman E, Raaphorst J, Klein Twennaar M, de Visser M, Schmand BA, de Haan RJ. The cognitive profile of ALS: a systematic review and meta-analysis update. *J Neurol Neurosurg Psychiatry* (2016) 87:611–9. doi: 10.1136/jnnp-2015-310734
16. Raaphorst J, de Visser M, Linssen WH, de Haan RJ, Schmand B. The cognitive profile of amyotrophic lateral sclerosis: a meta-analysis. *Amyotroph Lateral Scler.* (2010) 11:27–37. doi: 10.3109/17482960802645008
17. Papanicolaou AC. *The Amnesias A Clinical Textbook of Memory Disorders.* New York, NY: Oxford University Press (2006).
18. Phukan J, Elamin M, Bede P, Jordan N, Gallagher L, Byrne S, et al. The syndrome of cognitive impairment in amyotrophic lateral sclerosis: a population-based study. *J Neurol Neurosurg Psychiatry* (2012) 83:102–8. doi: 10.1136/jnnp-2011-300188
19. Montuschi A, Iazzolino B, Calvo A, Moglia C, Lopiano L, Restagno G, et al. Cognitive correlates in amyotrophic lateral sclerosis: a population-based study in Italy. *J Neurol Neurosurg Psychiatry* (2015) 86:168–73. doi: 10.1136/jnnp-2013-307223
20. Bede P, Bokde A, Elamin M, Byrne S, McLaughlin RL, Jordan N, et al. Grey matter correlates of clinical variables in amyotrophic lateral sclerosis (ALS): a neuroimaging study of ALS motor phenotype heterogeneity and cortical focality. *J Neurol Neurosurg Psychiatry* (2013) 84:766–73. doi: 10.1136/jnnp-2012-302674
21. Lorente De Nó R. Studies on the structure of the cerebral cortex. II. Continuation of the study of the ammonic system. *J für Psychol Neurol.* (1934) 46:113–77.
22. Hjorth-Simonsen A. Some intrinsic connections of the hippocampus in the rat: an experimental analysis. *J Comp Neurol.* (1973) 147:145–61. doi: 10.1002/cne.901470202
23. Andersen P, Bliss TV, Lomo T, Olsen LI, Skrede KK. Lamellar organization of hippocampal excitatory pathways. *Acta physiologica Scandinavica.* (1969) 76:4a–5a.
24. Duvernoy HM, Cattin F, Risold P-Y. *The Human Hippocampus.* New York, NY: Springer (2013).
25. Du F, Whetsell WOJr, Abou-Khalil B, Blumenkopf B, Lothman EW, Schwarcz R. Preferential neuronal loss in layer III of the entorhinal cortex in patients with temporal lobe epilepsy. *Epilepsy Res.* (1993) 16:223–33. doi: 10.1016/0920-1211(93)90083-J
26. Hjorth-Simonsen A, Jeune B. Origin and termination of the hippocampal perforant path in the rat studied by silver impregnation. *J Comp Neurol.* (1972) 144:215–32. doi: 10.1002/cne.901440206
27. Amaral DG, Insausti R, Cowan WM. The entorhinal cortex of the monkey: I. Cytoarchitectonic organization. *J Comp Neurol.* (1987) 264:326–55. doi: 10.1002/cne.902640305
28. Kohler C. Intrinsic projections of the retrohippocampal region in the rat brain. I. The subicular complex. *J Comp Neurol.* (1985) 236:504–22. doi: 10.1002/cne.902360407
29. Papez JW. A proposed mechanism of emotion. *Arch Neurol Psychiatry* (1937) 38:725–43. doi: 10.1001/archneurpsyc.1937.02260220069003
30. Witter MP, Amaral DG. Entorhinal cortex of the monkey: V. Projections to the dentate gyrus, hippocampus, and subicular complex. *J Comp Neurol.* (1991) 307:437–59. doi: 10.1002/cne.903070308
31. Brodal P. *The Central Nervous System - Structure and Function.* New York, NY: Oxford University Press (2010).
32. Wightman G, Anderson VE, Martin J, Swash M, Anderton BH, Neary D, et al. Hippocampal and neocortical ubiquitin-immunoreactive inclusions in amyotrophic lateral sclerosis with dementia. *Neurosci Lett.* (1992) 139:269–74. doi: 10.1016/0304-3940(92)90569-S
33. Okamoto K, Hirai S, Yamazaki T, Sun XY, Nakazato Y. New ubiquitin-positive intraneuronal inclusions in the extra-motor cortices in patients with amyotrophic lateral sclerosis. *Neurosci Lett.* (1991) 129:233–6. doi: 10.1016/0304-3940(91)90469-A
34. Okamoto K, Murakami N, Kusaka H, Yoshida M, Hashizume Y, Nakazato Y, et al. Ubiquitin-positive intraneuronal inclusions in the extramotor cortices of presenile dementia patients with motor neuron disease. *J Neurol.* (1992) 239:426–30. doi: 10.1007/BF00856806
35. Okamoto K, Hirai S, Amari M, Sakurai A. Electron micrograph of ubiquitin-positive intraneuronal inclusions in the extra-motor cortices in patients with amyotrophic lateral sclerosis. *Neuropathology* (1996) 16:112–6. doi: 10.1111/j.1440-1789.1996.tb00165.x
36. Nakano I. Temporal lobe lesions in amyotrophic lateral sclerosis with or without dementia: a neuropathological study. *Neuropathology* (1993) 13:215–27. doi: 10.1111/j.1440-1789.1993.tb00200.x
37. Takeda T, Uchihara T, Mochizuki Y, Mizutani T, Iwata M. Memory deficits in amyotrophic lateral sclerosis patients with dementia and degeneration of the perforant pathway A clinicopathological study. *J Neurol Sci.* (2007) 260:225–30. doi: 10.1016/j.jns.2007.05.010
38. Takeda T, Uchihara T, Arai N, Mizutani T, Iwata M. Progression of hippocampal degeneration in amyotrophic lateral sclerosis with or without memory impairment: distinction from Alzheimer disease. *Acta Neuropathol.* (2009) 117:35–44. doi: 10.1007/s00401-008-0447-2
39. Brettschneider J, Libon DJ, Toledo JB, Xie SX, McCluskey L, Elman L, et al. Microglial activation and TDP-43 pathology correlate with executive dysfunction in amyotrophic lateral sclerosis. *Acta Neuropathol.* (2012) 123:395–407. doi: 10.1007/s00401-011-0932-x
40. Bede P, Elamin M, Byrne S, McLaughlin RL, Kenna K, Vajda A, et al. Basal ganglia involvement in amyotrophic lateral sclerosis. *Neurology* (2013) 81:2107–15. doi: 10.1212/01.wnl.0000437313.80913.2c
41. Abdulla S, Machts J, Kaufmann J, Patrick K, Kollewe K, Dengler R, et al. Hippocampal degeneration in patients with amyotrophic lateral sclerosis. *Neurobiol Aging* (2014) 35:2639–45. doi: 10.1016/j.neurobiolaging.2014.05.035
42. Machts J, Loewe K, Kaufmann J, Jakubiczka S, Abdulla S, Petri S, et al. Basal ganglia pathology in ALS is associated with neuropsychological deficits. *Neurology* (2015) 85:1301–9. doi: 10.1212/WNL.0000000000002017
43. Westeneng HJ, Verstraete E, Walhout R, Schmidt R, Hendrikse J, Veldink JH, et al. Subcortical structures in amyotrophic lateral sclerosis. *Neurobiol Aging* (2015) 36:1075–82. doi: 10.1016/j.neurobiolaging.2014.09.002

44. Sage CA, Peeters RR, Gorner A, Robberecht W, Sunaert S. Quantitative diffusion tensor imaging in amyotrophic lateral sclerosis. *NeuroImage* (2007) 34:486–99. doi: 10.1016/j.neuroimage.2006.09.025
45. Sage CA, Van Hecke W, Peeters R, Sijbers J, Robberecht W, Parizel P, et al. Quantitative diffusion tensor imaging in amyotrophic lateral sclerosis: revisited. *Hum Brain Mapp.* (2009) 30:3657–75. doi: 10.1002/hbm.20794
46. Barbagallo G, Nicoletti G, Cherubini A, Trotta M, Tallarico T, Chiriaco C, et al. Diffusion tensor MRI changes in gray structures of the frontal-subcortical circuits in amyotrophic lateral sclerosis. *Neurol Sci.* (2014) 35:911–8. doi: 10.1007/s10072-013-1626-z
47. Thivard L, Pradat P-F, Lehericy S, Lacomblez L, Dormont D, Chiras J, et al. Diffusion tensor imaging and voxel based morphometry study in amyotrophic lateral sclerosis: relationships with motor disability. *J Neurol Neurosurg Psychiatry* (2007) 78:889–92. doi: 10.1136/jnnp.2006.101758
48. Prell T, Peschel T, Hartung V, Kaufmann J, Klauschies R, Bodammer N, et al. Diffusion tensor imaging patterns differ in bulbar and limb onset amyotrophic lateral sclerosis. *Clin Neurol Neurosurg.* (2013) 115:1281–7. doi: 10.1016/j.clineuro.2012.11.031
49. Keil C, Prell T, Peschel T, Hartung V, Dengler R, Grosskreutz J. Longitudinal diffusion tensor imaging in amyotrophic lateral sclerosis. *BMC Neurosci.* (2012) 13:141. doi: 10.1186/1471-2202-13-141
50. Kassubek J, Muller HP, Del Tredici K, Brettschneider J, Pinkhardt EH, Lule D, et al. Diffusion tensor imaging analysis of sequential spreading of disease in amyotrophic lateral sclerosis confirms patterns of TDP-43 pathology. *Brain* (2014) 137(Pt 6):1733–40. doi: 10.1093/brain/awu090
51. Christidi F, Karavasilis E, Zalonis I, Ferentinos P, Giavri Z, Wilde EA, et al. Memory-related white matter tract integrity in amyotrophic lateral sclerosis: an advanced neuroimaging and neuropsychological study. *Neurobiol Aging* (2017) 49:69–78. doi: 10.1016/j.neurobiolaging.2016.09.014
52. Steinbach R, Loewe K, Kaufmann J, Machts J, Kollewe K, Petri S, et al. Structural hallmarks of amyotrophic lateral sclerosis progression revealed by probabilistic fiber tractography. *J Neurol.* (2015) 262:2257–70. doi: 10.1007/s00415-015-7841-1
53. Stoppel CM, Vielhaber S, Eckart C, Machts J, Kaufmann J, Heinze HJ, et al. Structural and functional hallmarks of amyotrophic lateral sclerosis progression in motor- and memory-related brain regions. *Neuroimage Clin.* (2014) 5:277–90. doi: 10.1016/j.nicl.2014.07.007
54. Agosta F, Valsasina P, Absinta M, Riva N, Sala S, Prelle A, et al. Sensorimotor functional connectivity changes in amyotrophic lateral sclerosis. *Cereb Cortex* (2011) 21:2291–8. doi: 10.1093/cercor/bhr002
55. Zhu W, Fu X, Cui F, Yang F, Ren Y, Zhang X, et al. ALFF value in right parahippocampal gyrus acts as a potential marker monitoring amyotrophic lateral sclerosis progression: a neuropsychological, voxel-based morphometry, and resting-state functional MRI study. *J Mol Neurosci.* (2015) 57:106–13. doi: 10.1007/s12031-015-0583-9
56. Heimrath J, Gorges M, Kassubek J, Muller HP, Birbaumer N, Ludolph AC, et al. Additional resources and the default mode network: evidence of increased connectivity and decreased white matter integrity in amyotrophic lateral sclerosis. *Amyotroph Lateral Scler Other Motor Neuron Disord.* (2014) 15:537–45. doi: 10.3109/21678421.2014.911914
57. Loewe K, Machts J, Kaufmann J, Petri S, Heinze HJ, Borgelt C, et al. Widespread temporo-occipital lobe dysfunction in amyotrophic lateral sclerosis. *Sci Rep.* (2017) 7:40252. doi: 10.1038/srep40252
58. Abrahams S, Goldstein LH, Al-Chalabi A, Pickering A, Morris RG, Passingham RE, et al. Relation between cognitive dysfunction and pseudobulbar palsy in amyotrophic lateral sclerosis. *J Neurol Neurosurg Psychiatry* (1997) 62:464–72. doi: 10.1136/jnnp.62.5.464
59. Chari G, Shaw PJ, Sahgal A. Nonverbal visual attention, but not recognition memory of learning, processes are impaired in motor neurone disease. *Neuropsychologia* (1996) 34:377–85. doi: 10.1016/0028-3932(95)00122-0
60. Frank B, Haas J, Heinze HJ, Stark E, Munte TF. Relation of neuropsychological and magnetic resonance findings in amyotrophic lateral sclerosis: evidence for subgroups. *Clin Neurol Neurosurg.* (1997) 99:79–86. doi: 10.1016/S0303-8467(97)80001-7
61. Hanagasi HA, Gurvit IH, Ermutlu N, Kaptanoglu G, Karamursel S, Idrisoglu HA, et al. Cognitive impairment in amyotrophic lateral sclerosis: evidence from neuropsychological investigation and event-related potentials. *Brain Res Cogn Brain Res.* (2002) 14:234–44. doi: 10.1016/S0926-6410(02)00110-6
62. Iwasaki Y, Kinoshita M, Ikeda K, Takamiya K, Shiojima T. Cognitive impairment in amyotrophic lateral sclerosis and its relation to motor disabilities. *Acta Neurol Scand.* (1990) 81:141–3. doi: 10.1111/j.1600-0404.1990.tb00950.x
63. Ludolph AC, Langen KJ, Regard M, Herzog H, Kemper B, Kuwert T, et al. Frontal lobe function in amyotrophic lateral sclerosis: a neuropsychologic and positron emission tomography study. *Acta Neurol Scand.* (1992) 85:81–9. doi: 10.1111/j.1600-0404.1992.tb04003.x
64. Massman PJ, Sims J, Cooke N, Haverkamp LJ, Appel V, Appel SH. Prevalence and correlates of neuropsychological deficits in amyotrophic lateral sclerosis. *J Neurol Neurosurg Psychiatry* (1996) 61:450–5. doi: 10.1136/jnnp.61.5.450
65. Mantovan MC, Baggio L, Dalla Barba G, Smith P, Pegoraro E, Soraru G, et al. Memory deficits and retrieval processes in ALS. *Eur J Neurol.* (2003) 10:221–7. doi: 10.1046/j.1468-1331.2003.00607.x
66. Christidi F, Zalonis I, Smyrnis N, Evdokimidis I. Selective attention and the three-process memory model for the interpretation of verbal free recall in amyotrophic lateral sclerosis. *J Int Neuropsychol Soc.* (2012) 18:809–18. doi: 10.1017/S1355617712000562
67. Machts J, Bittner V, Kasper E, Schuster C, Prudlo J, Abdulla S, et al. Memory deficits in amyotrophic lateral sclerosis are not exclusively caused by executive dysfunction: a comparative neuropsychological study of amnestic mild cognitive impairment. *BMC Neurosci.* (2014) 15:83. doi: 10.1186/1471-2202-15-83
68. Burke T, Lonergan K, Pinto-Grau M, Elamin M, Bede P, Madden C, et al. Visual encoding, consolidation, and retrieval in amyotrophic lateral sclerosis: executive function as a mediator, and predictor of performance. *Amyotroph Lateral Scler Other Motor Neuron Disord.* (2017) 18:193–201. doi: 10.1080/21678421.2016.1272615
69. Nakano I, Iwatsubo T, Hashizume Y, Mizutani T, Mannen T. Amyotrophic lateral sclerosis: lesions in the apical cortex and some deeper structures of the temporal lobes. *Neuropathology* (1992) 12:69–77.
70. Goedert M, Spillantini MG. A century of Alzheimer's disease. *Science* (2006) 314:777–81. doi: 10.1126/science.1132814
71. Janssens J, Van Broeckhoven C. Pathological mechanisms underlying TDP-43 driven neurodegeneration in FTLD-ALS spectrum disorders. *Hum Mol Genet.* (2013) 22:R77–87. doi: 10.1093/hmg/ddt349
72. Steward O. Topographic organization of the projections from the entorhinal area to the hippocampal formation of the rat. *J Comp Neurol.* (1976) 167:285–314. doi: 10.1002/cne.901670303
73. Ishizuka N, Weber J, Amaral DG. Organization of intrahippocampal projections originating from CA3 pyramidal cells in the rat. *J Comp Neurol.* (1990) 295:580–623. doi: 10.1002/cne.902950407
74. Geser F, Brandmeir NJ, Kwong LK, Martinez-Lage M, Elman L, McCluskey L, et al. Evidence of multisystem disorder in whole-brain map of pathological TDP-43 in amyotrophic lateral sclerosis. *Arch neurology.* (2008) 65:636–41. doi: 10.1001/archneur.65.5.636
75. Geser F, Prvulovic D, O'Dwyer L, Hardiman O, Bede P, Bokde AL, et al. On the development of markers for pathological TDP-43 in amyotrophic lateral sclerosis with and without dementia. *Prog Neurobiol.* (2011) 95:649–62. doi: 10.1016/j.pneurobio.2011.08.011
76. Schmidt R, de Reus MA, Scholtens LH, van den Berg LH, van den Heuvel MP. Simulating disease propagation across white matter connectome reveals anatomical substrate for neuropathology staging in amyotrophic lateral sclerosis. *NeuroImage* (2016) 124(Pt A):762–9. doi: 10.1016/j.neuroimage.2015.04.005
77. Braak H, Brettschneider J, Ludolph AC, Lee VM, Trojanowski JQ, Del Tredici K. Amyotrophic lateral sclerosis–a model of corticofugal axonal spread. *Nat Rev Neurol.* (2013) 9:708–14. doi: 10.1038/nrneurol.2013.221
78. Bede P, Omer T, Finegan E, Chipika RH, Iyer PM, Doherty MA, et al. Connectivity-based characterisation of subcortical grey matter pathology in frontotemporal dementia and ALS: a multimodal neuroimaging study. *Brain Imag Behav.* (2018) doi: 10.1007/s11682-018-9837-9. [Epub ahead of print].

79. Bak TH, Chandran S. What wires together dies together: verbs, actions and neurodegeneration in motor neuron disease. *Cortex* (2012) 48:936–44. doi: 10.1016/j.cortex.2011.07.008
80. Bede P, Hardiman O. Lessons of ALS imaging: Pitfalls and future directions - a critical review. *Neuroimage Clin.* (2014) 4:436–43. doi: 10.1016/j.nicl.2014.02.011
81. Turner MR, Agosta F, Bede P, Govind V, Lulé D, Verstraete E. Neuroimaging in amyotrophic lateral sclerosis. *Biomarkers Med.* (2012) 6:319–37. doi: 10.2217/bmm.12.26
82. Anderson VE, Cairns NJ, Leigh PN. Involvement of the amygdala, dentate and hippocampus in motor neuron disease. *J Neurol Sci.* (1995) 129(Suppl):75–8. doi: 10.1016/0022-510X(95)00069-E
83. Grosskreutz J, Kaufmann J, Fradrich J, Dengler R, Heinze HJ, Peschel T. Widespread sensorimotor and frontal cortical atrophy in Amyotrophic Lateral Sclerosis. *BMC Neurol.* (2006) 6:17. doi: 10.1186/1471-2377-6-17
84. Kato Y, Matsumura K, Kinosada Y, Narita Y, Kuzuhara S, Nakagawa T. Detection of pyramidal tract lesions in amyotrophic lateral sclerosis with magnetization-transfer measurements. *Am J Neuroradiol.* (1997) 18: 1541–7.
85. Neumann M, Sampathu DM, Kwong LK, Truax AC, Micsenyi MC, Chou TT, et al. Ubiquitinated TDP-43 in frontotemporal lobar degeneration and amyotrophic lateral sclerosis. *Science* (2006) 314:130–3. doi: 10.1126/science.1134108
86. den Heijer T, der Lijn F, Vernooij MW, de Groot M, Koudstaal PJ, van der Lugt A, et al. Structural and diffusion MRI measures of the hippocampus and memory performance. *NeuroImage* (2012) 63:1782–9. doi: 10.1016/j.neuroimage.2012.08.067
87. Christidi F, Zalonis I, Kyriazi S, Rentzos M, Karavasilis E, Wilde EA, et al. Uncinate fasciculus microstructure and verbal episodic memory in amyotrophic lateral sclerosis: a diffusion tensor imaging and neuropsychological study. *Brain Imag Behav.* (2014) 8:497–505. doi: 10.1007/s11682-013-9271-y
88. Sarro L, Agosta F, Canu E, Riva N, Prelle A, Copetti M, et al. Cognitive functions and white matter tract damage in amyotrophic lateral sclerosis: a diffusion tensor tractography study. *Am J Neuroradiol.* (2011) 32:1866–72. doi: 10.3174/ajnr.A2658
89. Sato K, Aoki S, Iwata NK, Masutani Y, Watadani T, Nakata Y, et al. Diffusion tensor tract-specific analysis of the uncinate fasciculus in patients with amyotrophic lateral sclerosis. *Neuroradiology* (2010) 52:729–33. doi: 10.1007/s00234-010-0653-1
90. Augustinack JC, Helmer K, Huber KE, Kakunoori S, Zollei L, Fischl B. Direct visualization of the perforant pathway in the human brain with *ex vivo* diffusion tensor imaging. *Front Hum Neurosci.* (2010) 4:42. doi: 10.3389/fnhum.2010.00042
91. Christidi F, Bigler ED, McCauley SR, Schnelle KP, Merkley TL, Mors MB, et al. Diffusion tensor imaging of the perforant pathway zone and its relation to memory function in patients with severe traumatic brain injury. *J Neurotrauma* (2011) 28:711–25. doi: 10.1089/neu.2010.1644
92. Kalus P, Slotboom J, Gallinat J, Mahlberg R, Cattapan-Ludewig K, Wiest R, et al. Examining the gateway to the limbic system with diffusion tensor imaging: the perforant pathway in dementia. *Neuroimage* (2006) 30:713–20. doi: 10.1016/j.neuroimage.2005.10.035
93. Rogalski EJ, Murphy CM, deToledo-Morrell L, Shah RC, Moseley ME, Bammer R, et al. Changes in parahippocampal white matter integrity in amnestic mild cognitive impairment: a diffusion tensor imaging study. *Behav Neurol.* (2009) 21:51–61. doi: 10.1155/2009/408037
94. Yassa MA, Muftuler LT, Stark CE. Ultrahigh-resolution microstructural diffusion tensor imaging reveals perforant path degradation in aged humans *in vivo*. *Proc Natl Acad Sci USA.* (2010) 107:12687–91. doi: 10.1073/pnas.1002113107
95. Menke RA, Proudfoot M, Wuu J, Andersen PM, Talbot K, Benatar M, et al. Increased functional connectivity common to symptomatic amyotrophic lateral sclerosis and those at genetic risk. *J Neurol Neurosurg Psychiatry* (2016) 87:580–8. doi: 10.1136/jnnp-2015-311945
96. Ringholz GM, Appel SH, Bradshaw M, Cooke NA, Mosnik DM, Schulz PE. Prevalence and patterns of cognitive impairment in sporadic ALS. *Neurology* (2005) 65:586–90. doi: 10.1212/01.wnl.0000172911.39167.b6
97. Abe K, Fujimura H, Toyooka K, Sakoda S, Yorifuji S, Yanagihara T. Cognitive function in amyotrophic lateral sclerosis. *J Neurol Sci.* (1997) 148:95–100. doi: 10.1016/S0022-510X(96)05338-5
98. Abrahams S, Leigh PN, Harvey A, Vythelingum GN, Grise D, Goldstein LH. Verbal fluency and executive dysfunction in amyotrophic lateral sclerosis (ALS). *Neuropsychologia* (2000) 38:734–47. doi: 10.1016/S0028-3932(99)00146-3
99. Kew JJ, Goldstein LH, Leigh PN, Abrahams S, Cosgrave N, Passingham RE, et al. The relationship between abnormalities of cognitive function and cerebral activation in amyotrophic lateral sclerosis. A neuropsychological and positron emission tomography study. *Brain* (1993) 116 (Pt 6):1399–423. doi: 10.1093/brain/116.6.1399
100. Gallassi R, Montagna P, Ciardulli C, Lorusso S, Mussuto V, Stracciari A. Cognitive impairment in motor neuron disease. *Acta Neurol Scand.* (1985) 71:480–4. doi: 10.1111/j.1600-0404.1985.tb03231.x
101. Strong MJ, Grace GM, Orange JB, Leeper HA, Menon RS, Aere C. A prospective study of cognitive impairment in ALS. *Neurology* (1999) 53:1665–70. doi: 10.1212/WNL.53.8.1665
102. Raaphorst J, van Tol MJ, de Visser M, van der Kooi AJ, Majoie CB, van den Berg LH, et al. Prose memory impairment in amyotrophic lateral sclerosis patients is related to hippocampus volume. *Eur J Neurol.* (2015) 22:547–54. doi: 10.1111/ene.12615
103. Verstraete E, Turner MR, Grosskreutz J, Filippi M, Benatar M. Mind the gap: the mismatch between clinical and imaging metrics in ALS. *Amyotroph Lateral Scler Other Motor Neuron Disord.* (2015) 16:524–9. doi: 10.3109/21678421.2015.1051989
104. Cattie JE, Woods SP, Arce M, Weber E, Delis DC, Grant I. Construct validity of the item-specific deficit approach to the California verbal learning test (2nd Ed) in HIV infection. *Clin Neuropsychol.* (2012) 26:288–304. doi: 10.1080/13854046.2011.653404
105. Wright MJ, Woo E, Schmitter-Edgecombe M, Hinkin CH, Miller EN, Gooding AL. The item-specific deficit approach to evaluating verbal memory dysfunction: rationale, psychometrics, and application. *J Clin Exp Neuropsychol.* (2009) 31:790–802. doi: 10.1080/13803390802508918
106. Wright MJ, Schmitter-Edgecombe M, Woo E. Verbal memory impairment in severe closed head injury: the role of encoding and consolidation. *J Clin Exp Neuropsychol.* (2010) 32:728–36. doi: 10.1080/13803390903512652
107. Bede P, Querin G, Pradat PF. The changing landscape of motor neuron disease imaging: the transition from descriptive studies to precision clinical tools. *Curr Opin Neurol.* (2018). doi: 10.1097/WCO.0000000000000569. [Epub ahead of print].
108. Kaufmann P, Levy G, Montes J, Buchsbaum R, Barsdorf AI, Battista V, et al. Excellent inter-rater, intra-rater, and telephone-administered reliability of the ALSFRS-R in a multicenter clinical trial. *Amyotroph Lateral Scler.* (2007) 8:42–6. doi: 10.1080/17482960600888156
109. Gooch CL, Pullman SL, Shungu DC, Ulug AM, Chane S, Gordon PH, et al. Motor unit number estimation (MUNE) in diseases of the motor neuron: utility and comparative analysis in a multimodal biomarker study. *Suppl Clin Neurophysiol.* (2009) 60:153–62. doi: 10.1016/S1567-424X(08)00015-9
110. Blasco H, Patin F, Descat A, Garcon G, Corcia P, Gele P, et al. A pharmaco-metabolomics approach in a clinical trial of ALS: identification of predictive markers of progression. *PLoS ONE* (2018) 13:e0198116. doi: 10.1371/journal.pone.0198116
111. Elamin M, Bede P, Byrne S, Jordan N, Gallagher L, Wynne B, et al. Cognitive changes predict functional decline in ALS A population-based longitudinal study. *Neurology* (2013) 80:1590–7. doi: 10.1212/WNL.0b013e31828f18ac
112. Byrne S, Elamin M, Bede P, Shatunov A, Walsh C, Corr B, et al. Cognitive and clinical characteristics of patients with amyotrophic lateral sclerosis carrying a C9orf72 repeat expansion: a population-based cohort study. *Lancet Neurol.* (2012) 11:232–40. doi: 10.1016/S1474-4422(12)70014-5

113. Bede P, Bokde ALW, Byrne S, Elamin M, McLaughlin RL, Kenna K, et al. Multiparametric MRI study of ALS stratified for the C9orf72 genotype. *Neurology* (2013) 81:361–9. doi: 10.1212/WNL.0b013e31829c5eee
114. Omer T, Finegan E, Hutchinson S, Doherty M, Vajda A, McLaughlin RL, et al. Neuroimaging patterns along the ALS-FTD spectrum: a multiparametric imaging study. *Amyotroph Lateral Scler Other Motor Neuron Disord.* (2017) 18:611–23. doi: 10.1080/21678421.2017.1332077
115. Walhout R, Schmidt R, Westeneng HJ, Verstraete E, Seelen M, van Rheenen W, et al. Brain morphologic changes in asymptomatic C9orf72 repeat expansion carriers. *Neurology* (2015) 85:1780–8. doi: 10.1212/WNL.0000000000002135

21

Metabolic Disturbances in the Striatum and Substantia Nigra in the Onset and Progression of MPTP-Induced Parkinsonism Model

Yi Lu[1,2†], Xiaoxia Zhang[1,2†], Liangcai Zhao[2], Changwei Yang[2], Linlin Pan[2], Chen Li[2], Kun Liu[1], Guanghui Bai[1], Hongchang Gao[2] and Zhihan Yan[1]**

[1] *Department of Radiology, The Second Affiliated Hospital and Yuying Children's Hospital of Wenzhou Medical University, Wenzhou, China,*
[2] *Institute of Metabonomics & Medical NMR, School of Pharmaceutical Sciences, Wenzhou Medical University, Wenzhou, China*

Correspondence:
Hongchang Gao
gaohc27@wmu.edu.cn
Zhihan Yan
zhihanyan@hotmail.com
†Co-first authors.

Metabolic confusion has been linked to the pathogenesis of Parkinson's disease (PD), while the dynamic changes associated with the onset and progression of PD remain unclear. Herein, dynamic changes in metabolites were detected from the initiation to the development of 1-Methyl-4-phenyl-1,2,3,6-tetrahydropyridine (MPTP) -induced Parkinsonism model to elucidate its potential metabolic mechanism. *Ex vivo* ^{1}H nuclear magnetic resonance (NMR) spectroscopy was used to measure metabolite changes in the striatum and substantia nigra (SN) of mice at 1, 7, and 21 days after injection of MPTP. Metabolomic analysis revealed a clear separation of the overall metabolites between PD and control mice at different time points. Glutamate (Glu) in the striatum was significantly elevated at induction PD day 1 mice, which persisted to day 21. N-acetylaspartate (NAA) increased in the striatum of induction PD mice on days 1 and 7, but no significant difference was found in striatum on day 21. Myo-Inositol (mI) and taurine (Tau) were also disturbed in the striatum in induction PD day 1 mice. Additionally, key enzymes in the glutamate-glutamine cycle were significantly increased in PD mice. These findings suggest that neuron loss and motor function impairment in induction PD mice may be linked to overactive glutamate-glutamine cycle and altered membrane metabolism.

Keywords: Parkinson's disease, ^{1}H NMR, striatum, metabolism, neurotransmitter

INTRODUCTION

Parkinson's disease (PD) is one of the most common neurodegenerative diseases found in the aging population. As the worldwide population ages and life expectancy increases, the number of people with PD is expected to rise by more than 50% by 2030 (Kalia and Lang, 2015). The attendant motor disorders, such as resting tremor, rigidity, bradykinesia or slowness, gait disturbance, and postural instability, significantly decrease the quality of life (Fasano et al., 2012). As individuals have an increased life span, increased PD and its treatment can lead to a severe burden to patients, caregivers, and social health institutions (Nagy et al., 2012).

A metabolic abnormality was previously implicated in the pathogenesis of PD. Dopamine (DA) and its metabolites, 3, 4-dihydroxyphenylacetic (DOPAC), and homovanillic acid (HVA), are critical in the physiopathology of PD with motor dyskinesia and were used to validate the pharmacology of L-Dopa and other therapies (Smith et al., 2014). Tryptophan, serotonin, and the serotonin metabolite 5-HIA were also thought to be related to the psychiatric symptoms of PD (Hatano et al., 2016). However, dopamine modulators can cause serious side effects and often lose effectiveness. The discovery of other metabolites that are altered in the pathogenesis of the neurodegeneration may be involved in the underlying molecular pathways of PD, such as oxidative stress, inflammation, and glial reactions (Dawson and Dawson, 2003; Niranjan, 2014).

Wen et al. (2015) found in a PD rat model with 6-hydroxydopamine (6-OHDA) lesions showed significantly decreased acetylcholine (ACh) and moderately decreased noradrenaline (NA) concentrations in the ventrolateral thalamic nucleus. Ma et al. (2015) revealed that regional glucose metabolism changed in parkinsonism non-human primates by FDG PET. Alterations in the bilirubin-to-biliverdin ratio and ergothioneine in the serum indicate altered oxidative stress intensity, suggesting elevated oxidative stress and/or insufficient ability for scavenging free radicals, as was shown in the work of Hatano et al. (2016). Therefore, studying metabolic changes in cerebral metabolites at the molecular level could uncover novel pathophysiologic mechanisms involved in PD.

Proton nuclear magnetic resonance (^{1}H NMR)-based metabolomics, a powerful approach to study the brain energy metabolism and neurotransmission, has been widely used in psychosis (Chitty et al., 2015), brain tumor (Zhang et al., 2014), and other cerebral diseases. Compared to other metabolomics analytical techniques, NMR has some unique advantages, such as minimal sample processing, robust reproducibility, and high throughput (Lei and Powers, 2013). Using this approach, our previous work showed disturbances of glutamate (Glu), glutamine (Gln), and γ-Aminobutyric acid (GABA) in the Gln-Glu-GABA cycle (GGC) in the striatum of PD rats (Zheng et al., 2015). Although the metabolic abnormality had been previously found to be involved in the pathogenesis of PD, dynamic changes associated with the onset and progression of PD remain to be investigated.

To comprehensively profile changes in metabolites associated with the onset and progression of PD, we used 1-Methyl-4-phenyl-1,2,3,6-tetrahydropyridine (MPTP)-induced PD mice, the most widely accepted dopaminergic neurotoxin used in rodents for studying the progression and mechanisms involved in PD (Jackson-Lewis and Przedborski, 2007). With the goals of exploring the cerebral metabolic bases of the occurrence and development of PD, NMR-based metabolomics was performed to study the kinetic changes in metabolites in the striatum and substantia nigra (SN) of MPTP-induced PD mice.

RESULTS

TH Neuronal Contents and Behavioral Performance

Tyrosine hydroxylase (TH) can be used to label dopaminergic afferents and is commonly used to verify the success of a PD model (Jackson-Lewis and Przedborski, 2007). Microscopic examinations identified representative TH-positive neurons in the SN and striatum from control and induction PD day 1 mice (**Figure 1A**). MPTP administration led to a significant reduction in the number of TH-positive cells in the SN compared with the control group (1,142 ± 122 vs. 3,213 ± 348, $p < 0.001$), demonstrating the successful establishment of the PD model (**Figure 1B**).

Mice were subjected to an open field test 1 day before modeling, and then 1 and 7 days after the injection of MPTP or normal saline (**Figure 2A**). Significant reductions in the movement path, activity time, and total distance were observed in the PD group at different time points (**Figures 2B–D**). In addition, the immobility time in the PD group was significantly increased compared to control mice (**Figure 2E**). These behavioral findings are consistent with the formation of lesions and motor symptoms in MPTP-induced Parkinsonism mice model.

NMR-Based Metabolic Profiling of the Striatum of Mice

To further characterize dynamic changes of metabolites that occur during PD progression, we performed an unbiased metabolic analysis of striatum and SN tissues from control and induction PD mice at different time points. Representative ^{1}H NMR spectra of striatum extracts obtained from control and induction PD mice are shown in **Figure 3**. Assignments presented in **Figure 3D** were based on our previously published work (Gao et al., 2007) using the 600 MHz library of Chenomx NMR suite 7.0 (Chenomx Inc., Edmonton, Canada). The ^{1}H NMR spectra of brain tissue extracts allows for the simultaneous measurement of the numbers of endogenous metabolites, including Glu, GABA, Gln, lactate (Lac), alanine (Ala), N-acetyl aspartate (NAA), succinate (Suc), aspartate (Asp), creatine (Cre), choline (Cho), taurine (Tau), glycine (Gly), and myo-inostitol (mI).

NMR spectra were normalized to the internal standard TSP concentration to evaluate the relative content of metabolites and binned to reduce data dimensions for further metabolomic analyses. We conducted a Partial Least Squares-Discriminant Analysis (PLS-DA), a method that incorporates elements from principal component analysis, regression, and linear discriminant analysis, which revealed a clear separation of the overall metabolite levels in the right striatum between induction PD mice and control mice on days 1, 7, and 21 (**Figure 4**). Further evaluation of the metabolome using a corresponding loading plot, shown with color-coded correlation coefficients ($|r|$) of metabolites, revealed changed levels of Glu, Gln, NAA, Asp, mI, Cre, and Ala, indicating that neurotransmitter regulation and other metabolites disturbances could be involved in the progression of PD.

Metabolite Changes in Various Brain Regions

For univariate statistical analysis, relative concentrations of specific metabolites were calculated for each subject by subtracting the integrals of the signals. Levels of all identified metabolites in the right striatum and SN are shown in **Figure 5**.

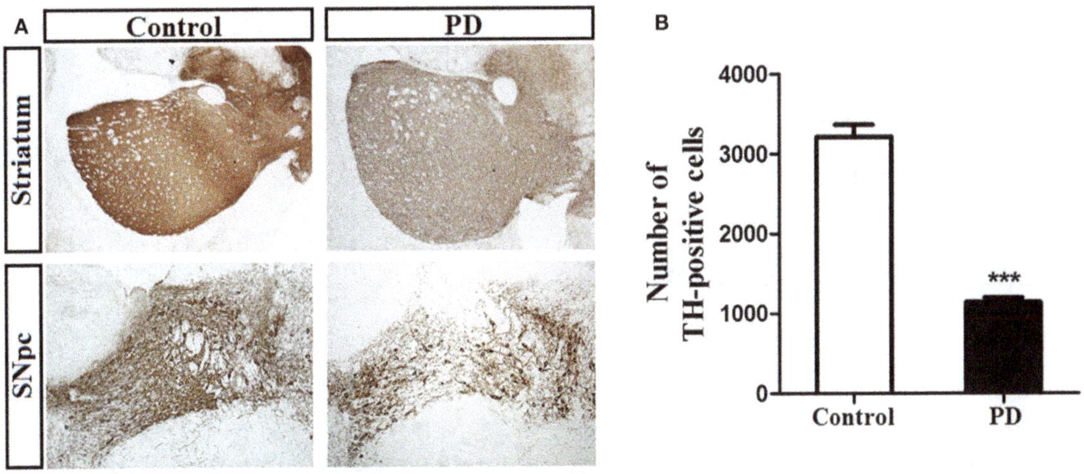

FIGURE 1 | Immunohistochemical staining of tyrosine hydroxylase (TH) in the substantia nigra pars compacta (SNpc) and striatum. **(A)** Illustration of toxicity of MPTP on TH in both SNpc and striatum at the first day after the last treatment. **(B)** MPTP administration induced a significant decrease (64%) number of TH-positive neurons in SNpc of PD group compared with control group (3,213 ± 348 vs. 1,142 ± 122). Bar represented means ± *SD* of three mice per group (***$p < 0.001$).

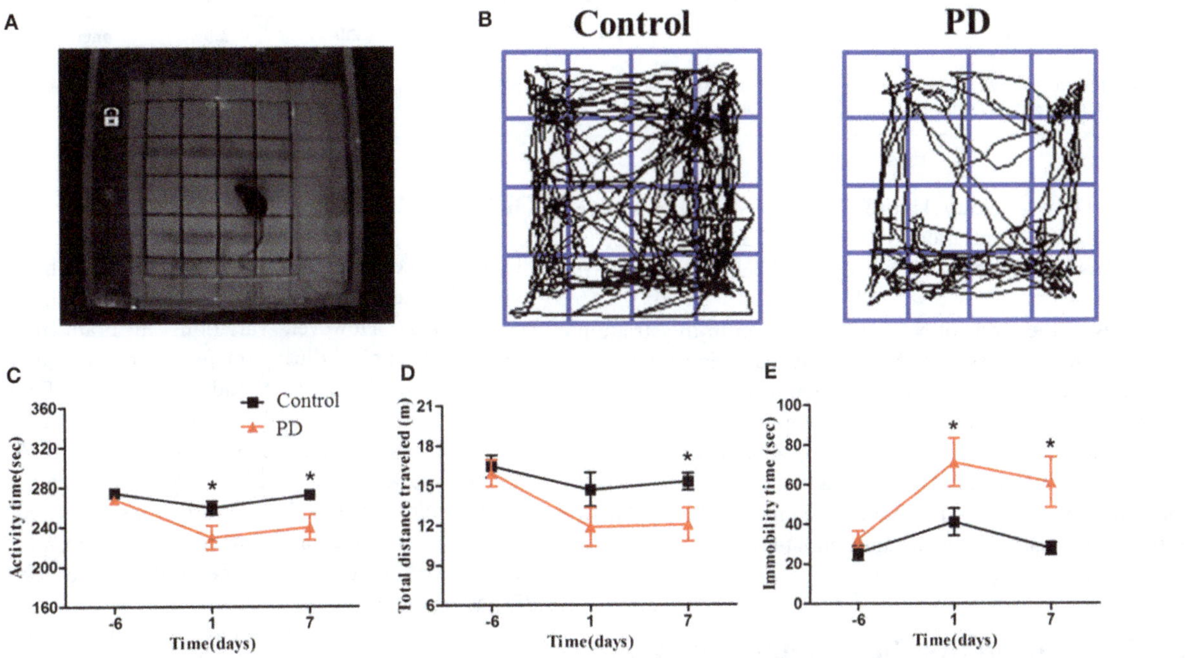

FIGURE 2 | MPTP deteriorated Behavioral alteration of mice in the open field test. **(A)** The open field test was conducted in the chamber measuring 25 × 25 × 45 cm with an automated video tracking system. **(B)** Representative examples of movement path was selected at 1 day after last treatment. The activity time, total distance traveled and immobility time **(C–E)** were recorded and analyzed at 3 time points (6 days before the last treatment, 1 and 7 days after the last treatment). All data were shown as means ± SEM, *$p < 0.05$.

In the right striatum of induction PD mice at day 1 (**Figure 5A**), compared with the control group we found higher levels of neurotransmitters, including Glu (32.72 ± 2.90 vs. 29.55 ± 1.59, $p = 0.041$) and Gln (20.46 ± 1.97 vs. 17.78 ± 0.53, $p = 0.009$), the neuronal marker NAA (28.73 ± 2.93 vs. 25.30 ± 2.07, $p = 0.041$) and the antioxidant Tau (39.99 ± 0.91 vs. 37.39 ± 2.30, $p = 0.027$). By contrast, levels of the energy-related metabolite Ala decreased (5.16 ± 0.32 vs. 6.03 ± 0.51, $p = 0.006$). In the induction PD day 7 group (**Figure 5B**), metabolic profiles revealed higher levels of NAA (32.23 ± 1.64 vs. 29.34 ± 1.91, $p = 0.014$), Glu (36.00 ± 1.15 vs. 33.38 ± 2.34, $p = 0.024$), and Asp (6.32 ± 0.40 vs. 5.86 ± 0.23, $p = 0.033$). In addition, higher levels of Glu (35.25 ± 2.54 vs. 31.98 ± 1.84, $p = 0.029$) and Tau (40.42 ± 1.08 vs. 37.53 ± 1.86, $p = 0.008$) were detected in the

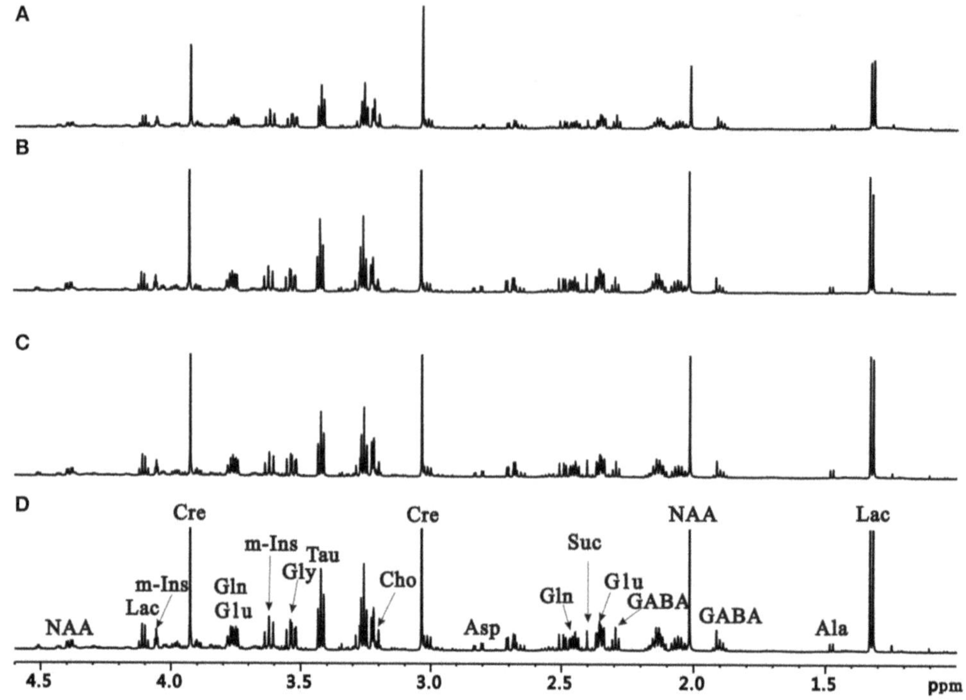

FIGURE 3 | Representative 1H NMR spectra of the right striatum extracts obtained from the control group at the first day after administration **(A)** and induction PD group, respectively at 1 day **(B)**, 7 days **(C)**, and 21 days **(D)**.

induction PD day 21 group (**Figure 5C**). In the SN, PD mice were marked by high concentrations of NAA (38.55 ± 0.93 vs. 37.55 ± 0.47, $p = 0.048$) and Gln (21.55 ± 1.53 vs. 19.72 ± 0.80, $p = 0.031$; **Figure 5D**).

Changes in the levels of NAA, Glu, and Gln in the striatum throughout the progression of MPTP-induced Parkinsonism are shown in **Figure 6**. NAA levels were significantly higher in the induction PD day 1 and 7 groups compared to the control group, while no difference was observed at induction PD day 21. Meanwhile, Glu levels were elevated at day 1, then reached a maximum at day 7, and remained elevated until day 21. In addition, Gln levels were significantly elevated at day 1, but not at days 7 or 21.

Key Enzymes in the Glutamate-Glutamine Cycle

The metabolic changes in Glu and Gln in PD mice suggested that the GGC was involved in the progression of MPTP-induced Parkinsonism. To further explore the reasons whereby GGC influenced PD in mice, levels of selected key enzymes involved in this cycle, including GS and GLS, were measured. GS, an ubiquitous enzyme present in the astroglial cytoplasm and involved in the formation of Gln from Glu (Hertz et al., 1999), was shown to be elevated in the subcortex of PD mice (**Figure 7**). In addition, a similar result was shown in the GLS, which was consistent with the increased conversion of Gln into Glu. Collectively, these findings suggest that an overactive GGC could be observed during the progression of MPTP-induced PD in mice.

DISCUSSION

PD, a multi-centric neurodegenerative disorder, has been shown to be associated with disturbed systemic metabolism (Bogdanov et al., 2008). However, variations in brain metabolites at different time points during the progression remain to be firmly established. In this present study, we used MPTP-induced PD mice to investigate dynamic changes in metabolite levels using high resolution *ex vivo* ^{1}H NMR spectroscopy. Metabolomics analysis showed that multiple time- and region-dependent neurochemical metabolite perturbations occurred, including NAA, Glu, Gln, mI, and Tau in the striatum and SN. These changes could be involved in the initiation and development of PD pathogenesis.

NAA has been widely used as a marker of neuronal density as its concentration is reduced in cases of neuronal loss (Delli Pizzi et al., 2013). However, in this present study, we found that MPTP administration significantly elevated NAA in the striatum in induction PD day 1 and 7 mice, as well as in the SN in induction PD day 1 mice. Previously, we showed (Gao et al., 2013) that 6-OHDA rats showed a trend for increased NAA in the striatum. This present study went a step further and showed that NAA returned to normal levels in the striatum in induction PD day 21 mice by assessing metabolite changes at different time points during PD progression. The recovery of NAA was consistent with early studies in both people with PD and PD model animals (Lewis et al., 2012; Groger et al., 2013; Zhou et al., 2014). It is possible that temporary increase in NAA levels may be a consequence of the stress response to the drug or, more

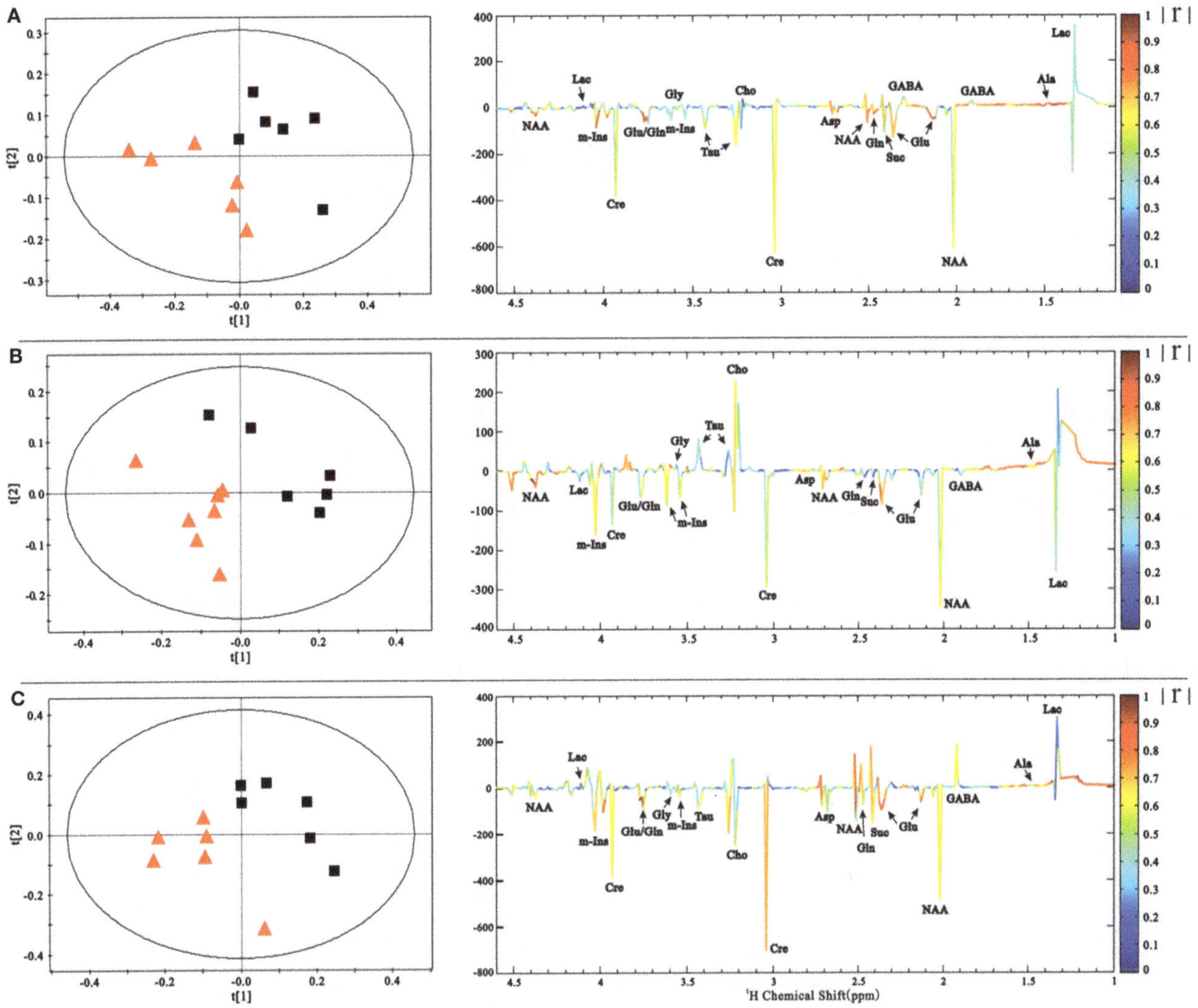

FIGURE 4 | PLS-DA scores plot based on the ^{1}H NMR spectra of the right striatum samples showed that PD group (▲) is clearly separated from control group (■) at 1, 7, and 21 days **(A–C)**. The coefficient-coded loading plots corresponding to PLS-DA revealed the metabolites with large intensities responsible for the discrimination of the corresponding score plots.

specifically, might compensate for the loss of dopaminergic neurons.

Glu is the major excitatory neurotransmitter in the mammalian central nervous system (CNS), which can be functionally invoked in virtually all activities of the nervous system (Lewerenz and Maher, 2015). In our present study, Glu levels in the striatum of induction PD day 1, 7, and 21 mice and the SN of induction PD day 1 mice were significantly increased compared with control rats. Similarly, our previous study also reported increased synthesis of Glu in the striatum of 6-OHDA rats (Gao et al., 2013). Both higher or lower levels of Glu can be noxious, as excessive Glu can stimulate activation of the N-methyl-D-aspartic acid (NMDA) receptor and induce excitatory toxicity (Grohm et al., 2012). In neurons, acute exposure to glutamate causes Parkin translocation to mitochondria in a calcium- and N-methyl-D-aspartate (NMDA) receptor-dependent manner, which disrupts some dynamic properties of mitochondria (Van Laar et al., 2015). Many studies in people with PD and animal models of PD have shown that mitochondrial dysfunction might be a defect that occurs early in the pathogenesis of PD (Subramaniam and Chesselet, 2013). Thus, we assume that the excitatory toxicity of Glu accumulation impairs mitochondrial function, and represents one of the potential metabolic mechanisms of PD.

GGC is one of the most important pathways involved in the metabolic coupling of astrocytes and neurons (Gallo and Ghiani, 2000). Changes in astrocyte-mediated GGC have been reported to be involved in the etiology of several neurodegenerative diseases, including epilepsy (Barker-Haliski and White, 2015), amyotrophic lateral sclerosis (ALS) (Sako et al., 2016), Alzheimer's disease (AD) (Chen et al., 2016), and Huntington's disease (HD) (Buren et al., 2016). Our present

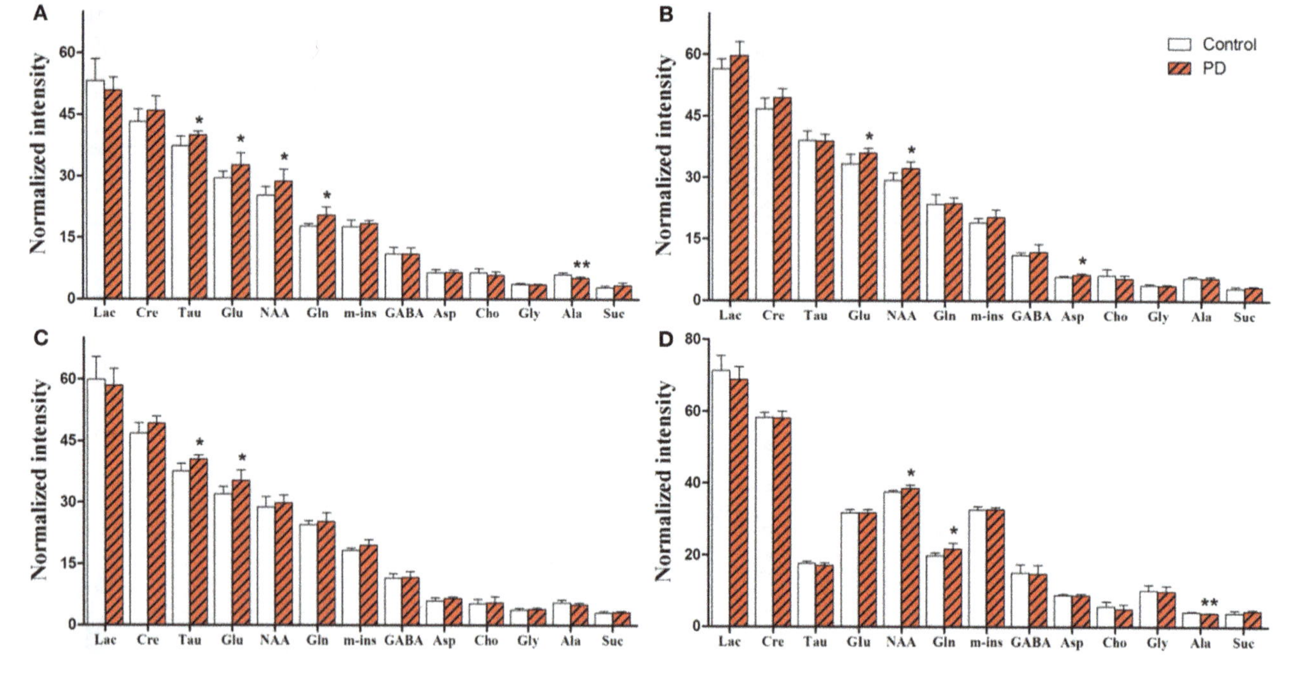

FIGURE 5 | Metabolic alterations obtained from the striatum of induction PD day 1, 7, 21 group **(A–C)** and the substantia nigra of induction PD day 1 group **(D)**, respectively. The results are expressed as mean ± *SD*, $^{*}p < 0.05$, $^{**}p < 0.01$.

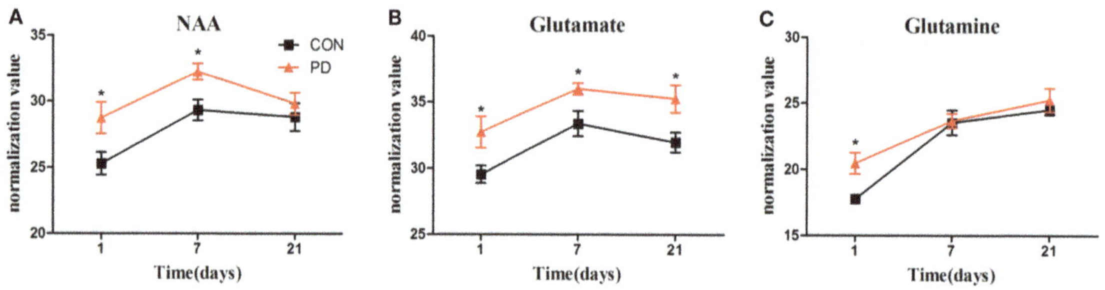

FIGURE 6 | Changes in the levels of NAA **(A)**, Glu **(B)**, and Gln **(C)** obtained from ^{1}H NMR spectra of right striatum samples collected from PD and control group of 1, 7, and 21 days after last administration. The results were expressed as means ± SD, $^{*}p < 0.05$.

findings showed that levels of Gln significantly increased in induction PD day 1 mice, while no significant change in Gln levels were observed in induction PD day 7 and 21 mice in the striatum or SN. Meanwhile, the cycle-related enzymes (i.e., both GLS and GS) in the subcortex were significantly increased. We, therefore, hypothesize that this phenomenon could serve as a temporary strategy to protect neurons from Glu excitotoxic injury after the injection of MPTP when the balance of the GGC was rapidly compromised, as Glu levels only increased in the striatum. Considering previous studies and our current measurements of metabolites and enzymes, we speculate that the GGC is involved in metabolism mechanisms related to PD, and could be a potential target in the treatment or prevention of neuron loss and/or motor function impairment in PD.

Myoinositol (MI), one of most abundant metabolites in the human brain, acts to maintain glial cell volumes as an osmolyte. Additionally, activated glia with enlarged cell volumes tends to have an elevated mI (Chang et al., 2013). Although there was no significant change in mI between the PD and control group mice, we found the normalized mI value was always slightly higher in the striatum of MPTP-induced PD mice, especially in induction PD day 21 mice ($p = 0.067$). This finding suggested that glia may be activated at later stages in the MPTP-induced Parkinsonism model, which is in accord with the opinion of Niranjan (2014) that a glial reaction participates in the cascade of events leading to neuronal degeneration in PD.

Tau is considered the major organic osmolyte, in addition to mI, that can regulate brain osmotic adaption (Lien et al., 1991). Our study showed that Tau is significantly elevated in the striatum and SN by MPTP in induction PD day 1 and 21 mice. Additionally, the changes in Tau

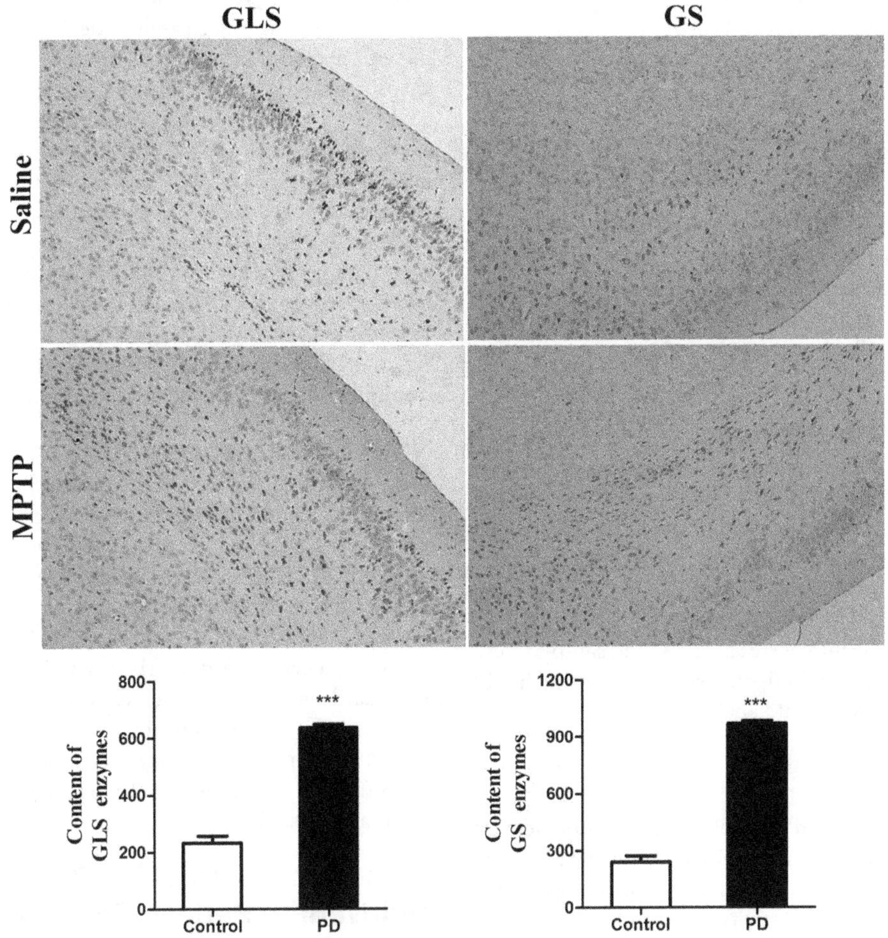

FIGURE 7 | Key enzymes were disturbed by MPTP in the disordered cycle of Glu-Gln-GABA. The deep dyed brown cytoplasm was represented as GLS and GS enzymes, by immunohistochemical staining. Content of GLS and GS enzymes were expressed as means ± SD, ***$p < 0.001$.

and mI indicated that osmolarity disorder occurs in the brain of PD mice. Furthermore, Tau was thought to have antioxidant properties and be able to reduce oxidative stress (Di Leo et al., 2004). These changes may represent a defense mechanism whereby increased Tau protects against the toxicity of MPTP, which can destroy the function of mitochondria and result in oxidative damage in the pathogenesis of PD.

Our study had several potential limitations for obtaining insights into the dynamic pathological mechanism leading to the development of PD. Indeed, people with PD at different severity levels would be the ideal subjects. However, the differentiation of these patients is not usually clinically feasible. In this present study, the MPTP mice model was used as an alternative to investigate changes in the metabolites underlying PD in a longitudinal study, from the initial to the final stages, which made it easy to control for the uniform state of disease. In addition, this present study adopted *in vitro* ^{1}H NMR for metabolomics analyses of mice brain, as it allowed for straightforward comparisons with the *in vivo* MRS results. Further work will be required to confirm whether these dynamic alterations of metabolism occur in the brains of people with PD, from the proximal to the distal stages, using *in vivo* MRS.

In conclusion, our results demonstrate that the neuron loss and motor function impairment related with PD might be linked to an overactive GGC and altered membrane metabolism. The increased Glu, accompanied by an overactive GGC, can induce excitatory toxicity and impaired mitochondrial function in the brain, which may be strongly associated with the pathogenesis of PD. The change in NAA was more likely to have occurred to compensate for the loss of dopaminergic neurons. In addition, altered osmolality and activated glia may also be involved in the mechanism driving the onset of PD, as reflected by the changes in mI and Tau. Notably, more evidence is needed to identify the exact mechanisms involved that lead to the observed changes in Glu, Gln, and GABA concentrations, and to test those metabolites as novel therapeutic targets to arrest or ameliorate PD progression.

MATERIALS AND METHODS

Animals

Male C57BL/6 mice (the SLAC Laboratory Animal Co. Ltd. Shanghai, China), weighing between 20 and 26 g, were housed 5 per cage under the standard laboratory conditions (controlled temperature/humidity condition, a normal 12/12-h light/dark schedule with the lights on at 08:00 a.m.). They were given free access to standard chow and water during whole experimental process. All animal handling and surgery were performed in accordance with standard animal protection guidelines and were approved by the Institutional Animal Care and Use Committee of Wenzhou Medical College (wydw2016-0128).

Preparation and Treatment

After adapting to the environment for a week, 60 mice were randomly divided into control and PD groups. Mice in PD groups were injected intraperitoneally (i.p.) 30 mg/kg MPTP-HCl (M0896, Sigma-Aldrich) daily for 5 consecutive days (Jackson-Lewis and Przedborski, 2007), while the mice in control group received equal volume of normal saline. At 1, 7, and 21 days after the last injection, the mice were sacrificed and samples were harvested immediately. All brain tissues were frozen using liquid nitrogen and stored at −80°C until analysis.

Behavioral Test

Open-field test was performed to evaluate locomotor activity when mice were exposed to the novel environment. Standard protocol was conducted in a dark sound-attenuating apparatus to avoid outside interference. Activity was limited in the test chamber (25 × 25 × 45 cm) with white smooth floor divided by black lines into 16 equal squares 4 × 4. Behavior test was carried out between 19:00 and 21:00. Mice from control 21 day and induction PD day 21 groups were gently placed in the center of the chamber and allowed to move freely for 5 min. The total distance traveled, number of activity, activity time and immobility time were analyzed using an automated video tracking system DigBehv Animal Behavior Video-tracking System (Shanghai Jiliang Software Technology Co. Ltd. China) (Jing et al., 2011).

Immunohistochemical Staining

Three mice of subgroup were processed for immunohistochemical studies. The brains were carefully removed and serial coronal sections (5 μm) of striatum and substantia nigra (SN) were mounted on slides. The stained was handled in accordance with the instruction of immunohistochemical Kit (KIT-9710, Fuzhou Maixin Biotech. Co. Ltd. Fujian, China). Primary antibodies were: Tyrosine Hydroxylase (TH, as marker of DA terminals, 1:750, ab112, abcam), Glutaminase (GS, 1:50, ab156876, abcam), and Glutamine synthetase (GLS, 1:50, SCB). Images were obtained and analyzed using a fluorescence microscope (Nikon, Tokyo, Japan). Control sections in which primary antibodies or secondary antibodies were omitted showed no labeled cells.

Sample Preparation

Mice were sacrificed by decapitation, specimens of mesencephalon and bilateral striatum were dissected rapidly, snap-frozen in liquid nitrogen, and stored at −80°C until analysis. The metabolite extraction was referred to our previous method (ref). The frozen tissues were weighed into an Eppendorf tube. Following the homogenization by electric homogenizer with ice-cold methanol (4.0 mL/g) and ultrapure water (0.85 mL/g; (Beckonert et al., 2007)), the mixture was homogenized again with 2 mL/g of chloroform and 0.85 mL/g of ultrapure water using a vortex mixer, placed on ice for 15 min, and centrifuged at 10,000 g for 15 min at 4°C. Finally, the supernatant was carefully transferred into a new Eppendorf tube, lyophilized for 24 h, and stored at −80°C until NMR analysis.

NMR Spectroscopy

The lyophilized extract was redissolved in 0.5 mL of D_2O containing 0.2 mM of TSP for NMR spectroscopy. D_2O provided a field-frequency lock, and TSP was used as the chemical shift reference. ^1H NMR spectra was acquired on a Bruker AVANCE III 600 MHz NMR spectrometer with a 5-mm TXI probe (Bruker BioSpin, Rheinstetten, Germany) at 298 K. The one-dimensional 1H NMR spectra of right striatum and SN were acquired using a standard single-pulse sequence with water signal presaturation (ZGPR). The acquisition time was 2.65 s per scan, and an additional 6 s relaxation delay was used to ensure full relaxation 128 transients were collected into 64 K data points with a spectral width of 12,000 Hz.

Data Processing of NMR Spectra and Multivariate Pattern Recognition

In all NMR spectra, the phase and baseline were corrected manually and referenced to the chemical shift of the methyl peak of lactate (CH_3, 1.33 ppm) using Topspin (v2.1 pl4, Bruker Biospin, Germany). The spectra (5.90–4.50 ppm) containing the residual peak from the suppressed water resonance was set to the zero integral in the analysis. The remaining spectral segments were normalized to the total sum of the spectral intensity to partially compensate for differences in concentration of the many metabolites in the samples. Then spectra (0.5–10.0 ppm) were data-reduced to 1,100 integrated regions of 0.01 ppm width for multivariate pattern recognition analysis by SIMCA-P+ 12.0 software (Umetrics, Umea, Sweden).The supervised projection to latent structure discriminant analysis, Partial least squares-discriminant analysis (PLS-DA), was carried out for classifying the samples according to their common spectral characteristics as described previously (Liu et al., 2013). And another data-reduced to 7,334 integrated regions of 0.0015 ppm width corresponding to the region of δ 10 to 0.5 for quantitative analysis.

Statistical Analysis

Metabolite intensities relative to the sum of the total spectral integral among groups were calculated. Repeated measures ANOVA were used to compare the data from control and PD mice at different time points. For statistical comparison between two groups, Independent sample *t*-test was used. Statistical analyses were performed using SPSS (version 22, IBM, USA). The normality was assessed by the Kolmogorov–Smirnov test. Data are expressed as mean ± SE, and a significance level of 0.05 was used.

AUTHOR CONTRIBUTIONS

YL and XZ data collection, statistical analyses and the initial draft of the manuscript. LP, KL and GB performed the experiments and reviewed the manuscript. LZ, CY, and CL contributed to the data discussion, and edited the manuscript. HG and ZY are the guarantors of this work and, as such, had full access to all the data in the study and takes responsibility for the integrity of the data and the accuracy of the data analysis.

ACKNOWLEDGMENTS

This work was supported by the National Natural Science Foundation of China (Nos. 81771386, 21575105, 81400863, 81171306), and the Natural Science Foundation of Zhejiang Provincial (Nos. LY14H090014, LY15H180010, and LY16H180009).

REFERENCES

1. Barker-Haliski, M., and White, H. S. (2015). Glutamatergic mechanisms associated with seizures and epilepsy. *Cold Spring Harb. Perspect. Med.* 5:a022863. doi: 10.1101/cshperspect.a022863
2. Beckonert, O., Keun, H. C., Ebbels, T. M. D., Bundy, J. G., Holmes, E., Lindon, J. C., et al. (2007). Metabolic profiling, metabolomic and metabonomic procedures for NMR spectroscopy of urine, plasma, serum and tissue extracts. *Nat. Protoc.* 2, 2692–2703. doi: 10.1038/nprot.2007.376
3. Bogdanov, M., Matson, W. R., Wang, L., Matson, T., Saunders-Pullman, R., Bressman, S. S., et al. (2008). Metabolomic profiling to develop blood biomarkers for Parkinson's disease. *Brain* 131(Pt 2), 389–396. doi: 10.1093/brain/awm304
4. Buren, C., Parsons, M. P., Smith-Dijak, A., and Raymond, L. A. (2016). Impaired development of cortico-striatal synaptic connectivity in a cell culture model of Huntington's disease. *Neurobiol. Dis.* 87, 80–90. doi: 10.1016/j.nbd.2015.12.009
5. Chang, L. D., Munsaka, S. M., Kraft-Terry, S., and Ernst, T. (2013). Magnetic resonance spectroscopy to assess neuroinflammation and neuropathic pain. *J. Neuroimmune Pharmacol.* 8, 576–593. doi: 10.1007/s11481-013-9460-x
6. Chen, S. Q., Cai, Q., Shen, Y. Y., Xu, C. X., Zhou, H., and Zhao, Z. (2016). Hydrogen proton magnetic resonance spectroscopy in multidomain amnestic mild cognitive impairment and vascular cognitive impairment without dementia. *Am. J. Alzheimers Dis. Other Demen.* 31, 422–429. doi: 10.1177/1533317515628052
7. Chitty, K. M., Lagopoulos, J., Hickie, I. B., and Hermens, D. F. (2015). Hippocampal glutamatergic/NMDA receptor functioning in bipolar disorder: a study combining mismatch negativity and proton magnetic resonance spectroscopy. *Psychiatry Res.* 233, 88–94. doi: 10.1016/j.pscychresns.2015.05.002
8. Dawson, T. M., and Dawson, V. L. (2003). Molecular pathways of neurodegeneration in Parkinson's disease. *Science* 302, 819–822. doi: 10.1126/science.1087753
9. Delli Pizzi, S., Rossi, C., Di Matteo, V., Esposito, E., Guarnieri, S., Mariggio, M. A., et al. (2013). Morphological and metabolic changes in the nigro-striatal pathway of synthetic proteasome inhibitor (PSI)-treated rats: a MRI and MRS study. *PLoS ONE* 8:e56501. doi: 10.1371/journal.pone.0056501
10. Di Leo, M. A., Santini, S. A., Silveri, N. G., Giardina, B., Franconi, F., and Ghirlanda, G. (2004). Long-term taurine supplementation reduces mortality rate in streptozotocin-induced diabetic rats. *Amino Acids* 27, 187–191. doi: 10.1007/s00726-004-0108-2
11. Fasano, A., Daniele, A., and Albanese, A. (2012). Treatment of motor and non- motor features of Parkinson's disease with deep brain stimulation. *Lancet Neurol.* 11, 429–442. doi: 10.1016/S1474-4422(12)70049-2
12. Gallo, V., and Ghiani, C. A. (2000). Glutamate receptors in glia: new cells, new inputs and new functions. *Trends Pharmacol. Sci.* 21, 252–258. doi: 10.1016/S0165-6147(00)01494-2
13. Gao, H., Xiang, Y., Sun, N., Zhu, H., Wang, Y., Liu, M., et al. (2007). Metabolic changes in rat prefrontal cortex and hippocampus induced by chronic morphine treatment studied *ex vivo* by high resolution 1H NMR spectroscopy. *Neurochem. Int.* 50, 386–394. doi: 10.1016/j.neuint.2006.09.012
14. Gao, H. C., Zhu, H., Song, C. Y., Lin, L., Xiang, Y., Yan, Z. H., et al. (2013). Metabolic changes detected by *ex vivo* high resolution 1H NMR spectroscopy in the striatum of 6-OHDA-induced Parkinson's rat. *Mol. Neurobiol.* 47, 123–130. doi: 10.1007/s12035-012-8336-z
15. Groger, A., Bender, B., Wurster, I., Chadzynski, G. L., Klose, U., and Berg, D. (2013). Differentiation between idiopathic and atypical parkinsonian syndromes using three-dimensional magnetic resonance spectroscopic imaging. *J. Neurol. Neurosurg. Psychiatry* 84, 644–649. doi: 10.1136/jnnp-2012-302699
16. Grohm, J., Kim, S. W., Mamrak, U., Tobaben, S., Cassidy-Stone, A., Nunnari, J., et al. (2012). Inhibition of Drp1 provides neuroprotection *in vitro* and *in vivo*. *Cell Death Differ.* 19, 1446–1458. doi: 10.1038/cdd.2012.18
17. Hatano, T., Saiki, S., Okuzumi, A., Mohney, R. P., and Hattori, N. (2016). Identification of novel biomarkers for Parkinson's disease by metabolomic technologies. *J. Neurol. Neurosurg. Psychiatry* 87, 295–301. doi: 10.1136/jnnp-2014-309676
18. Hertz, L., Dringen, R., Schousboe, A., and Robinson, S. R. (1999). Astrocytes: glutamate producers for neurons. *J. Neurosci. Res.* 57, 417–428. doi: 10.1002/(SICI)1097-4547(19990815)57:4<417::AID-JNR1>3.0.CO;2-N Jackson-Lewis, V., and Przedborski, S. (2007). Protocol for the MPTP mouse model of Parkinson's disease. *Nat. Protoc.* 2, 141–151. doi: 10.1038/nprot.2006.342
19. Jing, L., Luo, J., Zhang, M., Qin, W. J., Li, Y. L., Liu, Q., et al. (2011). Effect of the histone deacetylase inhibitors on behavioural sensitization to a single morphine exposure in mice. *Neurosci. Lett.* 494, 169–173. doi: 10.1016/j.neulet.2011.03.005
20. Kalia, L. V., and Lang, A. E. (2015). Parkinson's disease. *Lancet* 386, 896–912. doi: 10.1016/S0140-6736(14)61393-3
21. Lei, S., and Powers, R. (2013). NMR metabolomics analysis of Parkinson's Disease. *Curr. Metab.* 1, 191–209. doi: 10.2174/2213235X113019990004
22. Lewerenz, J., and Maher, P. (2015). Chronic glutamate toxicity in neurodegenerative diseases-what is the evidence? *Front. Neurosci.* 9:469. doi: 10.3389/fnins.2015.00469
23. Lewis, S. J., Shine, J. M., Duffy, S., Halliday, G., and Naismith, S. L. (2012). Anterior cingulate integrity: executive and neuropsychiatric features in Parkinson's disease. *Mov. Disord.* 27, 1262–1267. doi: 10.1002/mds.25104
24. Lien, Y. H., Shapiro, J. I., and Chan, L. (1991). Study of brain electrolytes and organic osmolytes during correction of chronic hyponatremia. Implications for the pathogenesis of central pontine myelinolysis. *J. Clin. Invest.* 88, 303–309. doi: 10.1172/JCI115292
25. Liu, K., Ye, X. J., Hu, W. Y., Zhang, G. Y., Bai, G. H., Zhao, L. C., et al. (2013). Neurochemical changes in the rat occipital cortex and hippocampus after repetitive and profound hypoglycemia during the neonatal period: an *ex vivo* H-1 magnetic resonance spectroscopy study. *Mol. Neurobiol.* 48, 729–736. doi: 10.1007/s12035-013-8446-2
26. Ma, Y., Johnston, T. H., Peng, S., Zuo, C., Koprich, J. B., Fox, S. H., et al. (2015). Reproducibility of a Parkinsonism-related metabolic brain network in non-human primates: a descriptive pilot study with FDG PET. *Mov. Disord.* 30, 1283–1288. doi: 10.1002/mds.26302
27. Nagy, C. L., Bernard, M. A., and Hodes, R. J. (2012). National institute on aging at middle ageuits past, present, and future. *J. Am. Geriatr. Soc.* 60, 1165–1169. doi: 10.1111/j.1532-5415.2012.03994.x
28. Niranjan, R. (2014). The role of inflammatory and oxidative stress mechanisms in the pathogenesis of Parkinson's Disease: focus on astrocytes. *Mol. Neurobiol.* 49, 28–38. doi: 10.1007/s12035-013-8483-x
29. Sako, W., Abe, T., Izumi, Y., Harada, M., and Kaji, R. (2016). The ratio of N-acetyl aspartate to glutamate correlates with disease duration of amyotrophic lateral sclerosis. *J. Clin. Neurosci.* 27, 110–113. doi: 10.1016/j.jocn.2015.08.044
30. Smith, M. L., King, J., Dent, L., Mackey, V., Muthian, G., Griffin, B., et al. (2014). Effects of acute and sub-chronic L-dopa therapy on striatal L-dopa methylation and dopamine oxidation in an MPTP mouse model of Parkinsons disease. *Life Sci.* 110, 1–7. doi: 10.1016/j.lfs.2014.05.014

31. Subramaniam, S. R., and Chesselet, M. F. (2013). Mitochondrial dysfunction and oxidative stress in Parkinson's disease. *Prog. Neurobiol.* 106, 17–32. doi: 10.1016/j.pneurobio.2013.04.004
32. Van Laar, V. S., Roy, N., Liu, A., Rajprohat, S., Arnold, B., Dukes, A. A., et al. (2015). Glutamate excitotoxicity in neurons triggers mitochondrial and endoplasmic reticulum accumulation of Parkin, and, in the presence of N-acetyl cysteine, mitophagy. *Neurobiol. Dis.* 74, 180–193. doi: 10.1016/j.nbd.2014.11.015
33. Wen, P., Li, M., Xiao, H., Ding, R., Chen, H., Chang, J., et al. (2015). Low-frequency stimulation of the pedunculopontine nucleus affects gait and the neurotransmitter level in the ventrolateral thalamic nucleus in 6-OHDA Parkinsonian rats. *Neurosci. Lett.* 600, 62–68. doi: 10.1016/j.neulet.2015. 06.006
34. Zhang, Z., Zeng, Q., Liu, Y., Li, C., Feng, D., and Wang, J. (2014). Assessment of the intrinsic radiosensitivity of glioma cells and monitoring of metabolite ratio changes after irradiation by 14. 7-T high-resolution (1)H MRS. *NMR Biomed.* 27, 547–552. doi: 10.1002/nbm.3091
35. Zheng, H., Zhao, L., Xia, H., Xu, C., Wang, D., Liu, K., et al. (2015). NMR-based metabolomics reveal a recovery from metabolic changes in the striatum of 6-OHDA-induced rats treated with basic fibroblast growth factor. *Mol. Neurobiol.* 53, 6690–6697. doi: 10.1007/s12035-015-9579-2
36. Zhou, B., Yuan, F. Z., He, Z., and Tan, C. L. (2014). Application of proton magnetic resonance spectroscopy on substantia nigra metabolites in Parkinson's disease. *Brain Imaging Behav.* 8, 97–101. doi: 10.1007/s11682-013-9251-2

22

Structural Connectivity Alterations in Amyotrophic Lateral Sclerosis: A Graph Theory Based Imaging Study

Etienne Fortanier[1,2,3], Aude-Marie Grapperon[1,2,3], Arnaud Le Troter[1,3], Annie Verschueren[1,2,3], Ben Ridley[1,3], Maxime Guye[1,3], Shahram Attarian[2,4], Jean-Philippe Ranjeva[1,3] and Wafaa Zaaraoui[1,3]*

[1] Aix Marseille Univ, CNRS, CRMBM, Marseille, France, [2] APHM, Hôpital de la Timone, Referral Centre for Neuromuscular Diseases and ALS, Marseille, France, [3] APHM, Hôpital de la Timone, CEMEREM, Marseille, France, [4] Aix Marseille Univ, INSERM, GMGF, Marseille, France

***Correspondence:**
Aude-Marie Grapperon
aude-marie.grapperon@ap-hm.fr

Background: Amyotrophic lateral sclerosis (ALS) is a relentlessly progressive neurodegenerative disorder. Diffusion magnetic resonance imagining (MRI) studies have consistently showed widespread alterations in both motor and non-motor brain regions. However, connectomics and graph theory based approaches have shown inconsistent results. Hub-centered lesion patterns and their impact on local and large-scale brain networks remain to be established. The objective of this work is to characterize topological properties of structural brain connectivity in ALS using an array of local, global and hub-based network metrics.

Materials and Methods: Magnetic resonance imagining data were acquired from 25 patients with ALS and 26 age-matched healthy controls. Structural network graphs were constructed from diffusion tensor MRI. Network-based statistics (NBS) and graph theory metrics were used to compare structural networks without *a priori* regions of interest.

Results: Patients with ALS exhibited global network alterations with decreased global efficiency (Eglob) ($p = 0.03$) and a trend of reduced whole brain mean degree ($p = 0.05$) compared to controls. Six nodes showed significantly decreased mean degree in ALS: left postcentral gyrus, left interparietal and transverse parietal sulcus, left calcarine sulcus, left occipital temporal medial and lingual sulcus, right precentral gyrus and right frontal inferior sulcus ($p < 0.01$). Hub distribution was comparable between the two groups. There was no selective hub vulnerability or topological reorganization centered on these regions as the hub disruption index (κ) was not significant for the relevant metrics (degree, local efficiency and betweenness centrality). Using NBS, we identified an impaired motor subnetwork of 11 nodes and 10 edges centered on the precentral and the paracentral nodes ($p < 0.01$). Significant clinical correlations were identified between degree in the frontal area and the disease progression rate of ALS patients ($p < 0.01$).

Conclusion: Our study provides evidence that alterations of structural connectivity in ALS are primarily driven by node degree and white matter tract degeneration within an extended network around the precentral and the paracentral areas without hub-centered reorganization.

Keywords: ALS, MRI, connectivity, DTI, hub, graph theory

INTRODUCTION

Amyotrophic lateral sclerosis (ALS) is a neurodegenerative motor neuron disorder characterized by progressive upper and lower motor neuron degeneration, leading to severe motor disability and death due to respiratory failure within few years (Kiernan et al., 2011). While the etiology of ALS remains elusive, ALS is now widely regarded as a multisystem disorder with considerable extra-motor involvement (Al-Chalabi et al., 2016; Christidi et al., 2018). Neuroimaging studies in ALS have consistently captured clinico-radiological correlations in the central nervous system (Cirillo et al., 2012; Bede and Hardiman, 2014).

Structural changes are relatively difficult to ascertain in ALS with conventional, clinical magnetic resonance imagining (MRI) sequences, therefore research studies rely on quantitative techniques, such as diffusion tensor imaging (DTI; Grolez et al., 2016), cortical thickness mapping (Schuster et al., 2017; Consonni et al., 2019) or MRI spectroscopy (Kalra, 2019). DTI studies have highlighted fractional anisotropy (FA) reductions in both motor and extra-motor regions (Foerster et al., 2013) and FA proved to be a sensitive DTI metric for both diagnostic (Tang et al., 2015; Bede et al., 2017) and progression modeling (Menke et al., 2012; Müller et al., 2016). Tractography studies in ALS readily detect white matter tract degeneration principally in the corticospinal tracts (Agosta et al., 2010). These studies have described anatomical patterns of white matter degeneration, but the impact of focal white matter changes on brain network integrity has not been fully characterized to date (Bede, 2017).

Structural connectivity studies based on graph theory offer a valuable tool to analyze the topological organization of cerebral networks and elucidate how different brain regions relate to each other (Bullmore and Sporns, 2009). In connectomics, cortical and subcortical brain regions can be parcellated in nodes with white matter tracts between them representing the edges of a mathematical graph. The human connectome has been extensively studied with graph theory in physiological and pathological contexts and it exhibits non-random features such as the presence of highly connected regions, named hubs (Achard, 2006). Connectivity hubs of the human brain support integrative processing and adaptive behaviors with high metabolic demands and represent vulnerable foci of neurodegeneration (Buckner et al., 2009; van den Heuvel et al., 2013; Proudfoot et al., 2019).

In ALS, few structural connectivity studies have reported both motor (Verstraete et al., 2011) and extra-motor node impairment (Verstraete et al., 2014; Buchanan et al., 2015; Dimond et al., 2017) and corticobasal connectivity is seldom evaluated specifically (Bede et al., 2018). However, due to methodological differences, the findings of these studies are inconsistent; some authors have described decreased (Dimond et al., 2017), while others reported preserved global efficiency (Buchanan et al., 2015). While many brain disorders, such as Alzheimer disease (Buckner et al., 2009; Verstraete et al., 2011) or schizophrenia (Rubinov and Bullmore, 2013) exhibit a hub-centered pattern, this finding is not evident in ALS connectivity studies (Crossley et al., 2014). It is still not clear if the clinical manifestations of ALS are primarily driven by white matter degeneration or by hub topology alterations.

Accordingly, the main objective of this prospective MRI study, is the characterization of structural connectivity in ALS using graph theory methods at different scales: global, local (nodal) and network analysis using statistical methods such as the Network-based Statistics (NBS; Zalesky et al., 2010) allowing us to analyze both cortical and white matter integrity.

MATERIALS AND METHODS

Ethics

This prospective imaging study was approved by the regional Ethics Committee (Sud Mediterranee I). All subjects provided informed consent in accordance with the principles of the Declaration of Helsinki.

Participants

Twenty-five consecutive patients with ALS, diagnosed according to the revised El Escorial criteria (Brooks et al., 2000), were recruited from the ALS Center of Marseille University Hospital, France. Comorbid neurological conditions or coexisting frontotemporal dementia (FTD; Rascovsky et al., 2011) were considered as exclusion criteria. Twenty-six healthy volunteers were also recruited as radiological controls. Healthy controls had no history of prior head injuries, neurological or psychiatric diagnoses and had a normal clinical examination.

Clinical Evaluation

All ALS patients underwent a standardized clinical examination on the day of the MRI. The recorded demographic and clinical parameters included: disease duration, site of onset, revised ALS functional rating scale (ALSFRS-R) scores (Cedarbaum et al., 1999) and disease progression rate defined as (48-ALSFRS-R)/disease duration (months).

Abbreviations: ALS: amyotrophic lateral sclerosis; ALSFRS-R: revised ALS functional rating scale; BC: betweenness centrality; CSF: cerebrospinal fluid; DTI: diffusion tensor imaging; Eglob: global efficiency; Eloc: local efficiency; FA: fractional anisotropy; FTD: frontotemporal dementia; NBS: network-based statistics; ROI: region of interest.

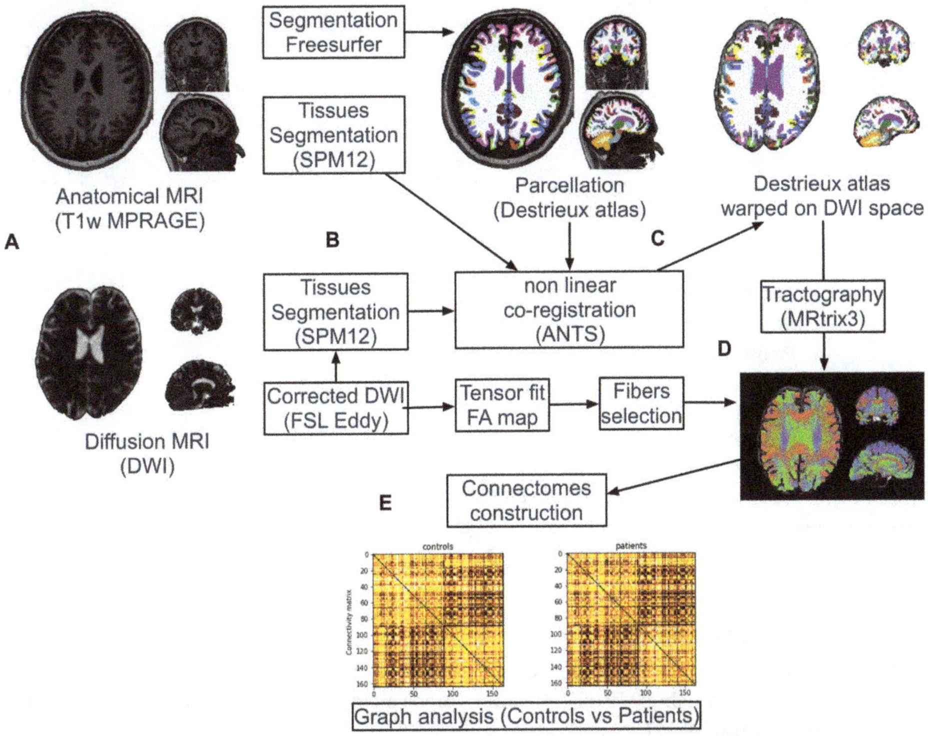

FIGURE 1 | Pipeline of image processing and graph analysis. T1w and diffusion MRI sequences were acquired from all patients and controls **(A)**. Following automatic parcellation of the structural images into cortical and subcortical regions **(B)**, the two set of images were non-linearly co-registered **(C)**. White matter tracts were reconstructed based on diffusion data using the probabilistic algorithm of MRtrix **(D)**. Individual brain network maps were generated using nodes and white matter connections resulting in a FA-weighted connectivity matrix for each subject. Graph analyses were performed on the FA-based connectivity matrix **(E)**.

MRI Acquisition

Magnetic resonance imagining data were acquired on a 3T MAGNETOM Verio system (Siemens, Erlangen, Germany) using a 32-channel phased-array ^{1}H head coil. The protocol included a high-resolution ^{1}H T1-weighted (T1w) 3D-Magnetization-Prepared Rapid Acquisition Gradient-Echo (MPRAGE) sequence (TE/TR/TI = 3/2300/0.9 ms, 160 slices, resolution of $1 \times 1 \times 1$ mm^3, acquisition time = 6 min), and a single shot echo-planar imaging DTI sequence (64 encoding directions, $b = 1000$ s/mm^2 and b0, TE = 95 ms, TR = 10700 ms, slice thickness 2 mm, 60 contiguous slices, resolution of 2×2 mm^2, acquisition time = 12 min). A T2-weighted 3D-Fluid-Attenuated Inversion Recovery (FLAIR) sequence (TE/TR/TI = 395/5000/1800 ms, 160 slices, $1 \times 1 \times 1$ mm^3 spatial resolution, acquisition time = 6 min) was also performed in both patients and controls and systematically reviewed to ensure the absence of vasculopathic white matter abnormalities which may affect focal diffusivity parameters.

Image Processing (Figure 1)

Anatomical Cortical and Subcortical Parcellation

Cortical and subcortical brain regions of each subject were parcellated using the Freesurfer software[1] (v5.0) with the Destrieux atlas, based on the T1w MPRAGE images to obtain 164 regions of interest (Destrieux et al., 2010). Subcortical regions included the thalamus, caudate nucleus, putamen, pallidum, hippocampus, amygdala, nucleus accumbens and ventral diencephalon.

Co-registration Between T1w Images and Diffusion Images

Tissues-type segmentation was performed based on T1w and b0 diffusion images using the Statistical Parameters Mapping software[2] (SPM12) to extract cerebrospinal fluid (CSF) maps (**Figure 1B**). T1w and b0 CSF maps were used as source and target images, respectively, to estimate geometric distortions with a non-linear registration procedure (Syn Model of ANTs library (Avants et al., 2008; **Figure 1C**). The resulting deformation map obtained from this co-registration was applied on the parcellation mask (Destrieux labels). Nearest neighbor interpolation was applied on the mask to keep the integer values of the original labels.

Diffusion Image Preprocessing

Each diffusion dataset was aligned to its b0 image using affine registration to correct for head movement and Eddy-currents using FSL[3] (version 5.0.8, FMRIB Software Library, Destrieux et al., 2010).

[1]http://surfer.nmr.mgh.harvard.edu

[2]https://www.fil.ion.ucl.ac.uk/spm/software/spm12/

[3]https://fsl.fmrib.ox.ac.uk

TABLE 1 | Demographic and clinical parameters of ALS patients and controls.

Demographic and clinical variables		ALS patients	Healthy controls	P-value
n (male/female)		25 (16/9)	26 (15/11)	0.64
Age mean ± SD (years)		55 ± 10	51 ± 10	0.17
Handedness (right/left)		23/2	21/5	0.24
Disease duration mean ± SD; [range] (months)		18 ± 15; [5–61]	N/A	N/A
Disease onset site	Spinal	*n* = 19 (left LL: *n* = 6, right LL: *n* = 7, left UL: *n* = 1, right UL: *n* = 5)	N/A	N/A
	Bulbar	*n* = 6	N/A	N/A
Revised El-Escorial criteria	Definite	*n* = 5	N/A	N/A
	Probable	*n* = 10	N/A	N/A
	Probable Laboratory Supported	*n* = 5	N/A	N/A
	Possible	*n* = 5	N/A	N/A
ALSFRS-R mean ± SD; [range]		39 ± 6; [23–47]	N/A	N/A
Disease progression rate mean ± SD; [range]		0.9 ± 0.9; [0.1–3.6]	N/A	N/A

ALSFRS-R, revised ALS functional rating scale; LL, lower limb; N/A, not applicable; UL, upper limb.

Tractography and Connectomes Construction

White matter tracts were reconstructed adopting a whole-brain probabilistic fibertracking approach using MRtrix[4] (Brain Research Institute, Melbourne, Australia). The method has been previously presented in detailed (Besson et al., 2014). A combined bi-hemispheric white matter mask was 1 mm dilated and defined as the region of interest (ROI) for the tracking algorithm (**Figure 1D**). One million fibers were then generated from all voxels included in this ROI with a probabilistic tracking algorithm [tckgen command, FOD model (Behrens et al., 2003)]. The algorithm generated one million fibers with a minimum length of 20 mm. Default tracking parameters included a minimum radius of curvature of 1 mm, a FOD cutoff of 0.1 and a step size of 0.2 mm. Finally, FA values were interpolated at each point of the fibers and the FA-based connectivity matrix (size 164 × 164) were generated from all streamlines and the parcellation mask (164 labels) previously warped in the diffusion dataset space (tck2connectome command, MRtrix) (**Figure 1E**).

Network Construction and Graph Theory Based Analysis

We modeled the structural undirected brain network of each participant using the reconstructed white matter tracts and the parcellated brain regions obtained in the previous steps (Bullmore and Sporns, 2009). Each region was used to define a node of a network graph. Edges were determined by tractography streamlines connecting any pair of nodes. An edge was considered present between two nodes if a streamline was generated with start and end points in each region. Network metrics were computed using the Brain Connectivity Toolbox (Rubinov and Bullmore, 2013). We investigated measures of global network architecture of each subject with global efficiency and mean degree. Local structural alterations were evaluated based on local efficiency, degree and betweenness centrality of each region.

[4]http://www.brain.org.au/software/

TABLE 2 | Global network analysis.

Graph metrics	ALS patients	Healthy controls	P-value
Eglob	0.3395	0.3507	0.0348
Degree mean ± SD	106.15 ± 29.77	111.46 ± 29.10	0.0523
Eloc mean ± SD	0.3775 ± 0.0249	0.3854 ± 0.0244	0.12
BC mean ± SD	169.80 ± 245.61	170.06 ± 209.02	0.98

Statistical significance was set at $p < 0.05$. Eglob, global efficiency; Eloc, local efficiency; BC, betweenness centrality.

As defined by Rubinov and Sporns (2010), global efficiency (Eglob) is the average inverse shortest path length in a network and is inversely related to the characteristic path length. It is a metric of functional integration that reflects on the brain's ability for specialized processing across distributed brain areas. Node degree is defined as the number of edges connected to the node and is a fundamental basic network measure to assess the central role of a brain region among a network.

Mean degree of the whole network was also computed and defined for one subject as the mean of each node degree of this subject. Betweenness centrality (BC) is the fraction of all shortest paths in the network that pass-through a given node. The local efficiency (Eloc) is the global efficiency computed on the neighborhood of the nodes.

Hub Analysis

In connectomics, hubs are described as highly connected nodes with topological centrality and a critical role in integrative processes and adaptive behaviors. Hubs are typically defined as nodes with the highest degree, i.e., a degree one standard deviation higher than the average degree of all nodes in the studied population (van den Heuvel and Sporns, 2011; Llufriu et al., 2017).

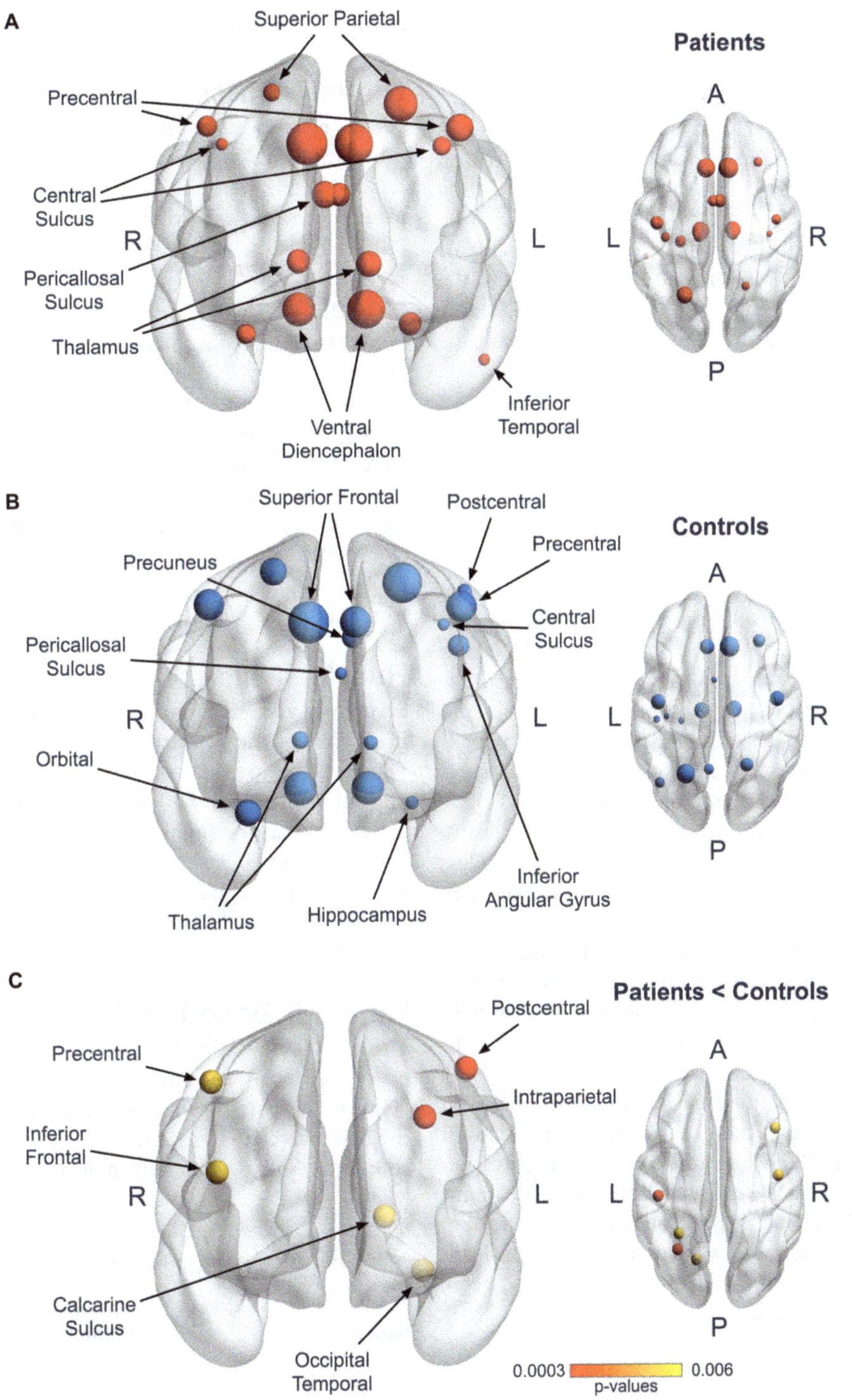

FIGURE 2 | Hubs in ALS patients and controls. Panels **(A,B)** represent coronal and axial views illustrating the hubs in patients (**A**, red) and controls (**B**, blue). The size of the nodes is proportional to their degree values. Panel **(C)** shows the 6 nodes with significantly reduced mean degree in patients at the Bonferroni corrected threshold (red, $p < 0.0003$) and at the 1/n exploratory threshold (yellow, $p < 0.006$).

To assess if the topologic reorganization was more prevalent in hubs, we also calculated the hub disruption index, κ, as defined by Achard (Achard, 2006). κ index is the gradient of a straight line, plotting the mean value at each node in the healthy controls group (x-axis) versus the difference between patient and control groups at each node, for any given metric (y-axis). For example, a negative κ index, crossing the zero line on the y-axis, reveals a trend for high-value regions in controls to decrease in the studied subject, and low-value nodes to increase.

Network Based Statistics

Considering a 164-node network, 26732 network connections can theoretically be generated. As a result, standard statistical tests for nodal analyses may be underpowered after correcting for multiple comparisons. Accordingly, we used the NBS approach to identify impaired subnetworks in patients compared to controls. The NBS methodology improves the statistical power by controlling for type I error (Zalesky et al., 2010). The NBS network was computed using the parameters detailed in a previous ALS study (Verstraete et al., 2011) permitting the identification of an altered network derived from the FA-based connectome. The mean FA of each tract of this isolated subnetwork was calculated for each subject and the total FA sum (NBS FA sum) was compared between the two groups.

Statistical Analyses

Statistical analyses were performed using JMP 9.0.1, SAS Institute Inc (JMP®, Version 9. SAS Institute Inc., Cary, NC, 1989–2019). Group characteristics were compared using the non-parametric Kruskal-Wallis test for age and Chi-squared test for gender and handedness. Differences in global connectivity between patient and control groups were assessed using pairwise non-parametric Wilcoxon signed-rank tests for multiple comparisons with uncorrected $p < 0.05$ being considered statistically significant. For each node, group differences in the mean degree, Eloc, and Eglob were also explored with non-parametric Wilcoxon tests ($p < 0.05$).

At the nodal scale, we used two thresholds to study differences between patients and controls: a first $p = 0.05/164 = 0.0003$ threshold corresponding to Bonferroni corrections applied with 164 brain regions, and a p exploratory threshold 1/n ($p < 0.006$) (Ridley et al., 2015).

The connectivity metrics with significant differences between patients and controls were then correlated with clinical parameters including ALSFRS-R score and disease progression rate, using a Spearman Rank test with multiple corrections. A $p < 0.0125$ for global metrics (Eglob and mean degree) and a $p < 0.004$ for local metrics (6 nodes with significant connectivity differences between patients and controls) were considered statistically significant.

RESULTS

Demographic and Clinical Parameters

The demographic and clinical profile of the participants is presented in **Table 1**. Twenty-five patients with ALS (mean age 55; SD 10 years; 16 males and 9 females, 2 left-handed) and 26 healthy controls (mean age 51; SD 10 years; 15 males and 11 females, 5 left-handed) were included. There was no statistical difference in age ($p = 0.17$), gender ($p = 0.64$) and handedness ($p = 0.24$) between the study groups. The mean ALSFRS-R score in the ALS cohort was 39 ± 6.

Global Metrics

Global network analyses are presented in **Table 2**. Compared to controls, ALS patients showed a significant decrease in Eglob (0.3395 vs. 0.3507, $p = 0.0348$). A trend of reduced mean degree of the whole brain was found in ALS patients (106.15 vs. 111.46, $p = 0.0523$).

Nodal Analysis

Using the Bonferroni corrected threshold, we found a significant decrease in ALS patients for the left postcentral gyrus ($p < 0.0001$) and for the left interparietal and transverse parietal sulcus ($p < 0.0001$) mean degree. No significant differences were identified in Eloc or BC in any nodes at this threshold. Furthermore, using the exploratory threshold, we found a significant decrease in the mean degree of the left calcarine sulcus ($p = 0.0021$), the left occipital temporal medial and lingual sulcus ($p = 0.0009$), the right precentral gyrus ($p = 0.0021$) and the right frontal inferior sulcus ($p = 0.0009$) (**Figure 2C** and **Table 3**).

Hub Analysis

Seventeen regions among 164 were defined as hubs both in patients and controls. The results are illustrated in **Figure 2**. Three hubs in controls were not identified as hubs in ALS patients: the left precuneus, the left parietal inferior angular gyrus and the left postcentral gyrus (**Figure 3**), but regarding the hub disruption index, no significant differences were found in κ-Eloc ($p = 0.1270$), κ-BC ($p = 0.6511$) or κ-degree ($p = 0.6647$) (**Figure 4**).

Network-Based Statistics

Network-based statistics highlighted a subnetwork (11 nodes, 10 edges) of impaired connectivity in the ALS group ($p = 0.015$) (**Figure 5**). This network included the left precentral gyrus, the left paracentral gyrus, the left caudate nucleus, the left suborbital sulcus, the left inferior temporal sulcus, the left

TABLE 3 | Significant mean degree nodes differences between ALS patients and controls.

Nodes	ALS patients	Healthy controls	*P*-value [a,b]
Left postcentral gyrus	133.64 ± 9.30	142.35 ± 8.16	0.0001[a]
Left interparietal and transverse parietal sulcus	126.68 ± 12.93	138.81 ± 7.93	0.0001[a]
Right precentral gyrus	139.52 ± 9.88	147.31 ± 6.83	0.0021[b]
Right frontal inferior sulcus	98.04 ± 15.00	110.69 ± 11.94	0.0009[b]
Left calcarine sulcus	76.52 ± 19.76	96.69 ± 21.03	0.0021[b]
Left occipital temporal medial and lingual sulcus	97.36 ± 12.13	109.11 ± 13.15	0.0009[b]

Values are reported as mean ± SD. [a]Statistical significance was set using Bonferroni corrections based on 164 brain regions ($p < 0.0003$). [b]Statistical significance was set using an exploratory threshold 1/n ($p < 0.006$).

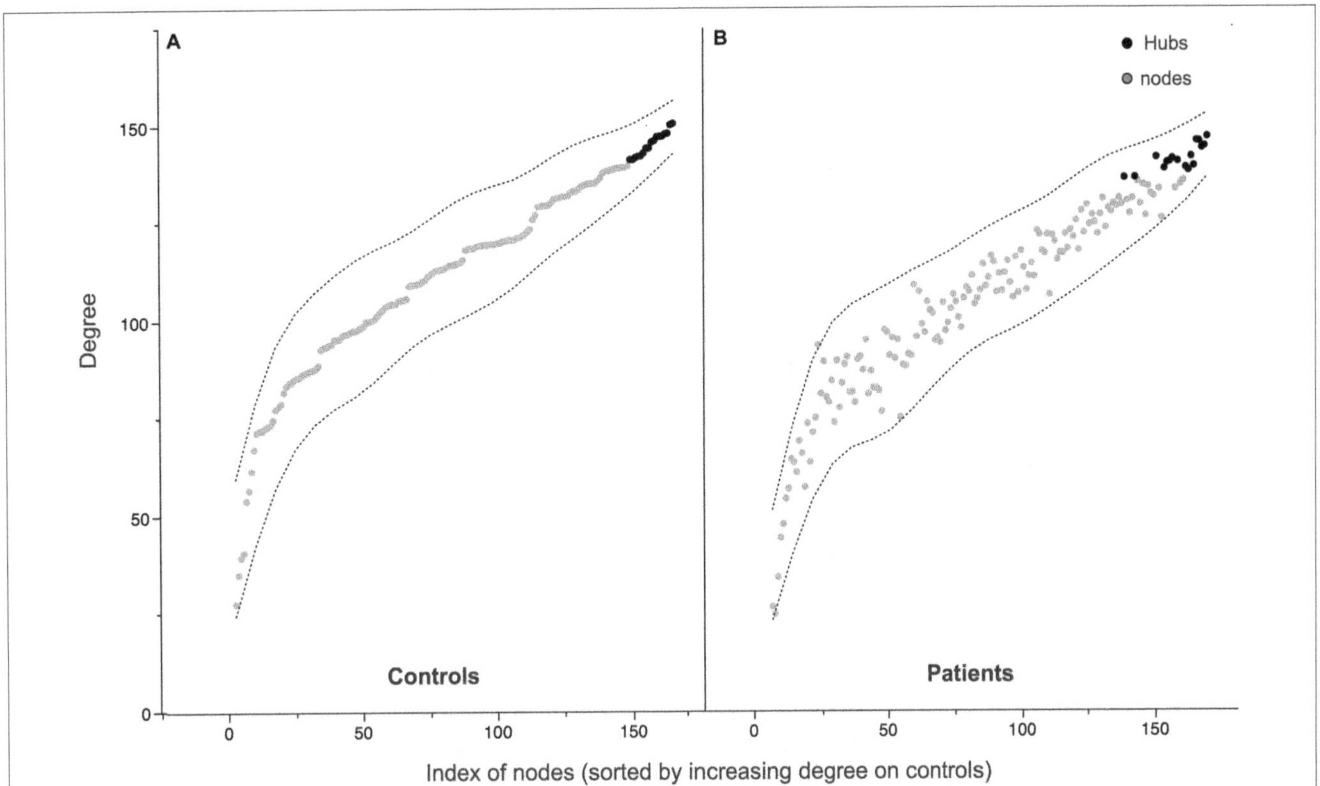

FIGURE 3 | Hub distribution patterns among controls **(A)** and patients **(B)**. Hubs were defined as nodes with a degree one standard deviation higher than the average node degree. 17 hubs were identified in patients and 17 hubs in controls. Nodes **(A,B)** are sorted out by increasing values of degree in controls showing similar distribution.

cingulate marginal gyrus, the right middle frontal gyrus, the right pallidum, the right accumbens area, the right anterior cingulate gyrus and sulcus and the right inferior superior parietal gyrus. The total FA sum of the edges in this subnetwork (NBS FA sum) was significantly reduced in ALS compared to controls ($p < 0.0001$).

Correlation Between Connectivity Metrics and Clinical Parameters

Among the six nodes identified in the Nodal Analysis results section, degree in the right frontal inferior sulcus was correlated with the disease progression rate ($p = 0.0089$, rho = −0.5396) and a trend of association was also identified with ALSFRS-R scores ($p = 0.0456$, rho = 0.4033).

No significant correlations were found between the other nodes and ALSFRS-R score or disease progression rate. There were no significant associations between Eglob and ALSFRS-R score or disease progression rate.

DISCUSSION

This study provides evidence of disease-specific structural connectivity changes in ALS. We report global efficiency reductions in structural networks in ALS characterized by a significant decrease in Eglob and a trend of mean degree reduction. The use of the graph theory enables a topological study of the entire cerebral network, without targeting *a priori* regions of interest. Our results are in line with the reports of decreased of Eglob in previous studies (Zhang et al., 2019). Our findings also support the notion of widespread, multisystem, multi-network degeneration in ALS which has been conceived based on other structural (Keil et al., 2012; Menke et al., 2012; Bede et al., 2016; Müller et al., 2016) and functional methods (Agosta et al., 2011; Douaud et al., 2011; Geevasinga et al., 2017; Dukic et al., 2019; Nasseroleslami et al., 2019). Reduced global connectivity underpins the impaired integration of multiple cerebral circuits in ALS, which may be driven by long-range connectivity changes (He et al., 2009). Previous structural connectivity studies did not capture significant reductions in global parameters (Verstraete et al., 2011; Buchanan et al., 2015) which may be explained by differences in post processing pipelines which were used to generate structural connectomes (deterministic fiber tracking algorithm, number of tracts or different parcellation atlas).

At a local scale, we evaluated parcellated brain regions with multiple metrics (Eloc, degree and betweenness centrality) to determine if the global disturbances were due to the alteration of specific nodes. Nodal analysis demonstrated a significant reduction of degree in 6 out of 164 regions in ALS patients. These six nodes are located in pathognomonic brain regions closely associated with ALS. Precentral and frontal structural degeneration is a hallmark feature of ALS confirmed by a

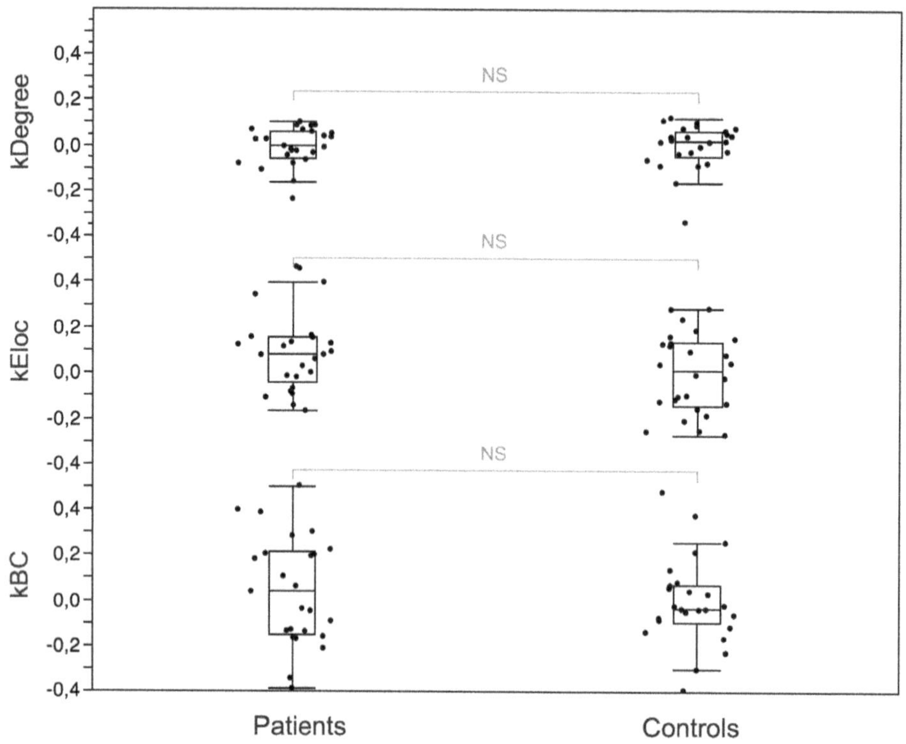

FIGURE 4 | Hub disruption index. The box plots show the κ index of each subject for 3 metrics: κ-degree, κ-Eloc, κ-BC. No significant differences were identified between ALS patients and controls. Differences were considered significant at $p < 0.05$ for each metric.

multitude of cortical gray and subcortical white matter studies (Kasper et al., 2014; Schuster et al., 2016; Mazón et al., 2018). The intraparietal sulcus is part of the supplementary motor areas which is also affected in ALS based on both functional and structural studies (Abidi et al., 2019). The involvement of the temporal lingual sulcus may be the substrate of the spectrum of cognitive changes observed in ALS (Abrahams et al., 2004; Phukan et al., 2007). Intrahemispheric connectivity alterations and the degeneration of the sensorimotor network have also been previously reported in ALS by studies demonstrating widespread pre- and postcentral FA reductions (Rose et al., 2012).

To explore internodal interactions, we used NBS (Zalesky et al., 2010). This tool permits the integrated analysis of a subgroup of nodes that belongs to a single altered network. In our study, we identified an impaired subnetwork centered on motor nodes: precentral, paracentral and frontal gyri. This subnetwork is comparable to the ones described in previous studies (Verstraete et al., 2011; Buchanan et al., 2015). Our finding of parietal and temporal lobe involvement is in line with recently proposed pathological staging systems (Brettschneider et al., 2013), and longitudinal connectivity studies (Verstraete et al., 2014).

Interestingly, no major topological reorganization of hubs was evidenced in ALS in the present study. The human connectome is known to follow characteristic topological patterns based on hubs, defined by a subnetwork of highly connected nodes with a high number of tracts playing a central role in the brain's structural architecture. Due to their anatomical position and their high metabolic demands, these regions are considered particularly vulnerable in many neurological and psychiatric disorders (Buckner et al., 2009; Sharma et al., 2011; Rubinov and Bullmore, 2013; Gollo et al., 2018). Previous studies have shown that the selective hub degeneration occurs in a disease-specific pattern in several neurological and psychiatric conditions such as Alzheimer's disease or schizophrenia (Crossley et al., 2014). Hub pathology in ALS, however, has not been specifically investigated to date and no graph theory based structural studies have been performed to evaluate the distribution of hubs and the extent to which they are reorganized in ALS patients relative to controls. We showed here that both the number and the distribution of hubs are similar between patients and controls. To our knowledge, this first use of the hub disruption index in ALS demonstrating the absence of hub reorganization, suggests that disease propagation in ALS does not follow hub-based patterns. Despite motor network changes evidenced by the NBS analysis, the precentral nodes kept their hub properties. Impairment of the global efficiency seems to be related to local structural abnormalities rather than a complex compensatory hub reorganization as reported in other disorders such as multiple sclerosis and epilepsy (Ridley et al., 2015; Faivre et al., 2016; Tur et al., 2018).

Noteworthy, we found associations between structural connectivity metrics and clinical parameters, such as disease

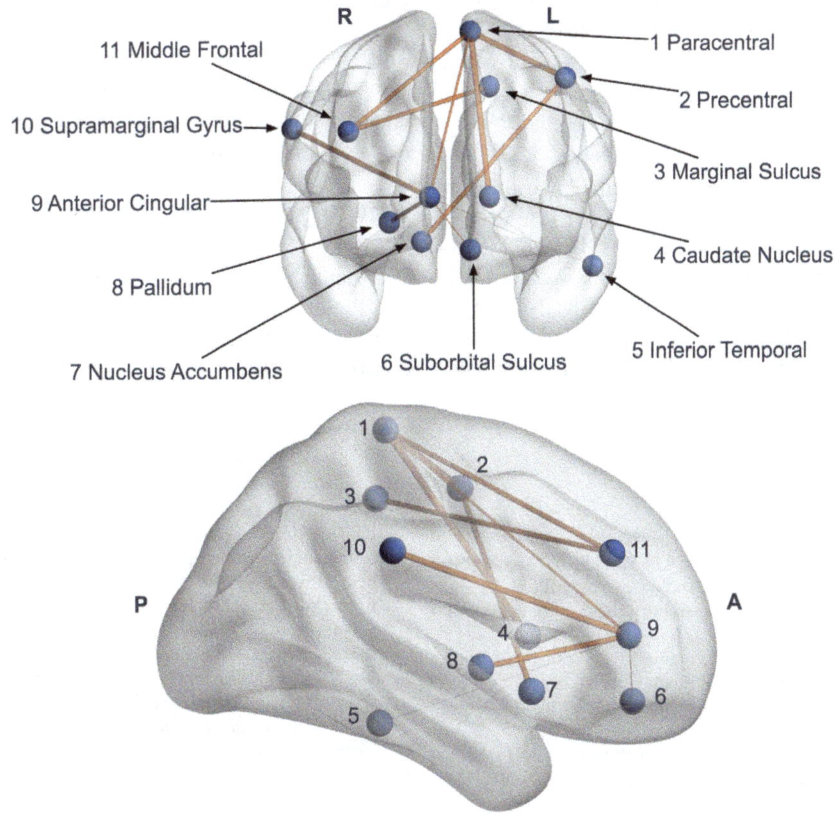

FIGURE 5 | Network based statistics (NBS) impaired subnetwork. Coronal and sagittal views of impaired subnetwork nodes and interconnections identified by NBS (11 nodes and 10 edges). Edge diameter is based on the FA reduction (the larger connections are the more affected, with significant FA reduction).

progression rate and ALSFRS-R score. Correlations between brain imaging metrics and clinical parameters are often difficult to establish in ALS (Chipika et al., 2019) because motor disability is not merely due to upper but also lower motor neuron degeneration and the considerable clinical heterogeneity of the disease precludes direct clinico-radiological associations (Verstraete et al., 2015). It is therefore not surprising that no direct correlations were identified between clinical parameters and global connectivity measures. Node degree and their white matter integrity indexes seem to better explain the clinical deficits observed in ALS.

This study is not without limitations. The sample size of our ALS cohort is relatively limited which did not allow the phenotypic stratification of ALS patients into subgroups. Nonetheless, our study presents compelling evidence that graph-analyses and connectomics provide meaningful non-invasive insights into the degenerative changes of ALS. Furthermore, genetic information was not available for all patients which is a limitation as certain ALS genotypes may be associated with specific white matter alterations and more extensive network impairment (Menke et al., 2016; Floeter and Gendron, 2018). The lack of standardized cognitive evaluation is another limitation given the evidence of phenotype-specific morphometric changes along the ALS-FTD continuum (Omer et al., 2017). Future studies should therefore include ALS-FTD patients and ALS patients with behavioral and executive dysfunction to characterize the connectivity signature of these cognitive phenotypes. An additional limitation is the significantly higher proportion of male ALS patients in the present study. Given the evidence of gender-associated developmental and radiological features in ALS and healthy populations (Menzler et al., 2011; Vivekananda et al., 2011; Bede et al., 2014), future connectivity studies should seek to recruit gender-balanced cohorts.

CONCLUSION

In conclusion, our structural connectivity study highlights a diffuse, non-focal network impairment in ALS without selective hubs vulnerability or topological network reorganization. These results suggest that clinical manifestations in ALS could be more driven by tract degeneration than by hub topology alterations. Based on these observations, a prospective longitudinal study is required to characterize dynamic progressive connectivity changes. Recent imaging studies have shown evidence of considerable presymptomatic structural changes in ALS-associated mutation carriers (Schuster et al., 2015; Querin et al., 2019). A connectomic analysis of such cohorts could identify early network alterations in the most vulnerable circuits and provide invaluable insights on disease propagation.

AUTHOR CONTRIBUTIONS

All authors contributed scientifically to this manuscript. Clinical evaluations were performed by A-MG, AV, and SA. The methodological design was optimized by A-MG, MG, J-PR, and WZ. Image processing was undertaken by EF, AL, and BR. Data analyses were conducted by EF, A-MG, BR, J-PR, and WZ. The manuscript was drafted by EF, A-MG, and WZ. All co-authors have reviewed the manuscript for intellectual content.

FUNDING

This research was funded by APHM (AORC Junior 2014 program) and by ANR (grant ANR-15-CE19-0019-01). CRMBM is a laboratory member of the France Life Imaging network (grant ANR-11-INBS-0006).

ACKNOWLEDGMENTS

We thank L. Pini, C. Costes, P. Viout, and S. Confort-Gouny for their contribution to MRI data acquisition. We also thank H. Kribich, N. Mispeleare, and V. Gimenez for their logistical support.

REFERENCES

1. Abidi, M., Marco, G., Couillandre, A., Feron, M., Mseddi, E., Termoz, N., et al. (2019). Adaptive functional reorganization in amyotrophic lateral sclerosis: coexisting degenerative and compensatory changes. *Eur. J. Neurol.* doi: 10.1111/ ene.14042 [Epub ahead of print].
2. Abrahams, S., Goldstein, L. H., Simmons, A., Brammer, M., Williams, S. C. R., Giampietro, V., et al. (2004). Word retrieval in amyotrophic lateral sclerosis: a functional magnetic resonance imaging study. *Brain* 127, 1507–1517. doi: 10.1093/brain/awh170
3. Achard, S. (2006). A resilient, low-frequency, small-world human brain functional network with highly connected association cortical hubs. *J. Neurosci.* 26, 63–72. doi: 10.1523/JNEUROSCI.3874-05.2006
4. Agosta, F., Pa gani, E., Petrolini, M., Caputo, D., Perini, M., Prelle, A., et al. (2010). Assessment of white matter tract damage in patients with amyotrophic lateral sclerosis: a diffusion tensor MR imaging tractography study: fig 1. *AJNR Am. J. Neuroradiol.* 31, 1457–1461. doi: 10.3174/ajnr.A2105
5. Agosta, F., Valsasina, P., Absinta, M., Riva, N., Sala, S., Prelle, A., et al. (2011). Sensorimotor functional connectivity changes in amyotrophic lateral sclerosis. *Cereb. Cortex* 21, 2291–2298. doi: 10.1093/cercor/bhr002
6. Al-Chalabi, A., Hardiman, O., Kiernan, M. C., Chiò, A., Rix-Brooks, B., and van den Berg, L. H. (2016). Amyotrophic lateral sclerosis: moving towards a new classification system. *Lancet Neurol.* 15, 1182–1194. doi: 10.1016/S1474-4422(16)30199-5
7. Avants, B., Epstein, C., Grossman, M., and Gee, J. (2008). Symmetric diffeomorphic image registration with cross-correlation: evaluating automated labeling of elderly and neurodegenerative brain. *Med. Image Anal.* 12, 26–41. doi: 10.1016/ j.media.2007.06.004
8. Bede, P. (2017). Deciphering neurodegeneration: a paradigm shift from focality to connectivity. *Neurology* 89, 1758–1759. doi: 10.1212/ WNL.0000000000004582 Bede, P., Elamin, M., Byrne, S., and Hardiman, O. (2014). Sexual dimorphism in ALS: exploring gender-specific neuroimaging signatures. *Amyotroph Lateral Scler Frontotemporal Degener* 15, 235–243. doi: 10.3109/21678421.2013.865749 Bede, P., and Hardiman, O. (2014). Lessons of ALS imaging: pitfalls and future directions — a critical review. *NeuroImage* 4, 436–443. doi: 10.1016/j.nicl.2014.02.011
9. Bede, P., Iyer, P. M., Finegan, E., Omer, T., and Hardiman, O. (2017). Virtual brain biopsies in amyotrophic lateral sclerosis: diagnostic classification based on in vivo pathological patterns. *NeuroImage* 15, 653–658. doi: 10.1016/j.nicl. 2017.06.010
10. Bede, P., Iyer, P. M., Schuster, C., Elamin, M., Mclaughlin, R. L., Kenna, K., et al. (2016). The selective anatomical vulnerability of ALS: 'disease-defining' and 'disease-defying' brain regions. *Amyotroph. Lateral Scler. Frontotemporal Degener.* 17, 561–570. doi: 10.3109/21678421.2016.1173702
11. Bede, P., Omer, T., Finegan, E., Chipika, R. H., Iyer, P. M., Doherty, M. A., et al. (2018). Connectivity-based characterisation of subcortical grey matter pathology in frontotemporal dementia and ALS: a multimodal neuroimaging study. *Brain Imag. Behav.* 12, 1696–1707. doi: 10.1007/s11682-018-9837-9
12. Behrens, T. E. J., Woolrich, M. W., Jenkinson, M., Johansen-Berg, H., Nunes, R. G., Clare, S., et al. (2003). Characterization and propagation of uncertainty in diffusion-weighted MR imaging. *Magn. Reson. Med.* 50, 1077–1088. doi: 10.1002/mrm.10609
13. Besson, P., Dinkelacker, V., Valabregue, R., Thivard, L., Leclerc, X., Baulac, M., et al. (2014). Structural connectivity differences in left and right temporal lobe epilepsy. *NeuroImage* 100, 135–144. doi: 10.1016/j. neuroimage.2014.04.071
14. Brettschneider, J., Del Tredici, K., Toledo, J. B., Robinson, J. L., Irwin, D. J., Grossman, M., et al. (2013). Stages of pTDP-43 pathology in amyotrophic lateral sclerosis: ALS Stages. *Ann. Neurol.* 74, 20–38. doi: 10.1002/ana.23937
15. Brooks, B. R., Miller, R. G., Swash, M., and Munsat, T. L. (2000). El Escorial revisited: revised criteria for the diagnosis of amyotrophic lateral sclerosis. *Amyotroph. Lateral Scler. Other Motor Neuron Disord.* 1, 293–299. doi: 10.1080/ 146608200300079536
16. Buchanan, C. R., Pettit, L. D., Storkey, A. J., Abrahams, S., and Bastin, M. E. (2015). Reduced structural connectivity within a prefrontal-motor-sub cortical network in amyotrophic lateral sclerosis: reduced Structural Connectivity in ALS. *J. Magn. Reson. Imag.* 41, 1342–1352. doi: 10.1002/jmri.24695
17. Buckner, R. L., Sepulcre, J., Talukdar, T., Krienen, F. M., Liu, H., Hedden, T., et al. (2009). Cortical hubs revealed by intrinsic functional connectivity: mapping, assessment of stability, and relation to alzheimer's disease. *J. Neurosci.* 29, 1860–1873. doi: 10.1523/JNEUROSCI.5062-08.2009
18. Bullmore, E., and Sporns, O. (2009). Complex brain networks: graph theoretic al analysis of structural and functional systems. *Nat. Rev. Neurosci.* 10, 186–198. doi: 10.1038/nrn2575
19. Cedarbaum, J. M., Stambler, N., Malta, E., Fuller, C., Hilt, D., Thurmond, B., et al. (1999). The ALSFRS-R: a revised ALS functional rating scale that incorporates assessments of respiratory function. *J. Neurol. Sci.* 169, 13–21. doi: 10.1016/ S0022-510X(99)00210-5
20. Chipika, R. H., Finegan, E., Li Hi Shing, S., Hardiman, O., and Bede, P. (2019). Tracking a fast-moving disease: longitudinal markers, monitoring, and clinical trial endpoints in ALS. *Front. Neurol.* 10:229. doi: 10.3389/fneur.2019.00229
21. Christidi, F., Karavasilis, E., Rentzos, M., Kelekis, N., Evdokimidis, I., and Bede, P. (2018). Clinical and radiological markers of extra-motor deficits in amyotrophic lateral sclerosis. *Front. Neurol.* 9:1005. doi: 10.3389/ fneur.2018.01005
22. Cirillo, M., Esposito, F., Tedeschi, G., Caiazzo, G., Sagnelli, A., Piccirillo, G., et al. (2012). Widespread microstructural white matter involvement in amyotrophic lateral sclerosis: a whole-brain DTI study. *AJNR Am. J. Neuroradiol.* 33, 1102– 1108. doi: 10.3174/ajnr.A2918
23. Consonni, M., Cappa, S. F., Dalla Bella, E., Contarino, V. E., and Lauria, G. (2019). Cortical correlates of behavioural change in amyotrophic lateral sclerosis.
24. *J. Neurol. Neurosurg. Psychiatry* 90, 380–386. doi: 10.1136/jnnp-2018-318619 Crossley, N. A., Mechelli, A., Scott, J., Carletti, F., Fox, P. T., McGuire, P., et al.
25. (2014). The hubs of the human connectome are generally implicated in the anatomy of brain disorders. *Brain* 137, 2382–2395. doi: 10.1093/brain/awu132
26. Destrieux, C., Fischl, B., Dale, A., and Halgren, E. (2010). Automatic parcellation of human cortical gyri and sulci using standard anatomical nomenclature. *NeuroImage* 53, 1–15. doi: 10.1016/j.neuroimage.2010.06.010
27. Dimond, D., Ishaque, A., Chenji, S., Mah, D., Chen, Z., Seres, P., et al. (2017). White matter structural network abnormalities underlie executive dysfunction in amyotrophic lateral sclerosis: structural disconnectivity and cognition in ALS. *Hum. Brain Mapp.* 38, 1249–1268. doi: 10.1002/hbm.23452

28. Douaud, G., Filippini, N., Knight, S., Talbot, K., and Turner, M. R. (2011). Integration of structural and functional magnetic resonance imaging in amyotrophic lateral sclerosis. *Brain* 134, 3470–3479. doi: 10.1093/brain/awr279
29. Dukic, S., McMackin, R., Buxo, T., Fasano, A., Chipika, R., Pinto-Grau, M., et al. (2019). Patterned functional network disruption in amyotrophic lateral sclerosis. *Hum. Brain Mapp.* doi: 10.1002/hbm.24740 [Epub ahead of print].
30. Faivre, A., Robinet, E., Guye, M., Rousseau, C., Maarouf, A., Le Troter, A., et al. (2016). Depletion of brain functional connectivity enhancement leads to disability progression in multiple sclerosis: a longitudinal resting-state fMRI study. *Mult. Scler* 22, 1695–1708. doi: 10.1177/1352458516628657
31. Floeter, M. K., and Gendron, T. F. (2018). Biomarkers for amyotrophic lateral sclerosis and frontotemporal dementia associated with hexanucleotide expansion mutations in C9orf72. *Front. Neurol.* 9:1063. doi: 10.3389/fneur.2018.01063
32. Foerster, B. R., Welsh, R. C., and Feldman, E. L. (2013). 25 years of neuroimaging in amyotrophic lateral sclerosis. *Nat. Rev. Neurol.* 9, 513–524. doi: 10.1038/nrneurol.2013.153
33. Geevasinga, N., Korgaonkar, M. S., Menon, P., Van den Bos, M., Gomes, L., Foster, S., et al. (2017). Brain functional connectome abnormalities in amyotrophic lateral sclerosis are associated with disability and cortical hyperexcitability. *Eur. J. Neurol.* 24, 1507–1517. doi: 10.1111/ene.13461
34. Gollo, L. L., Roberts, J. A., Cropley, V. L., Di Biase, M. A., Pantelis, C., Zalesky, A., et al. (2018). Fragility and volatility of structural hubs in the human connectome. *Nat. Neurosci.* 21, 1107–1116. doi: 10.1038/s41593-018-0188-z
35. Grolez, G., Moreau, C., Danel-Brunaud, V., Delmaire, C., Lopes, R., Pradat, P. F., et al. (2016). The value of magnetic resonance imaging as a biomarker for amyotrophic lateral sclerosis: a systematic review. *BMC Neurol.* 16:155. doi: 10.1186/s12883-016-0672-6
36. He, Y., Dagher, A., Chen, Z., Charil, A., Zijdenbos, A., Worsley, K., et al. (2009). Impaired small-world efficiency in structural cortical networks in multiple sclerosis associated with white matter lesion load. *Brain* 132, 3366–3379. doi: 10.1093/brain/awp089
37. Kalra, S. (2019). Magnetic resonance spectroscopy in ALS. *Front. Neurol.* 10:482. doi: 10.3389/fneur.2019.00482
38. Kasper, E., Schuster, C., Machts, J., Kaufmann, J., Bittner, D., Vielhaber, S., et al. (2014). Microstructural white matter changes underlying cognitive and behavioural impairment in ALS – an *in vivo* study using DTI. *PLoS One* 9:e114543. doi: 10.1371/journal.pone.0114543
39. Keil, C., Prell, T., Peschel, T., Hartung, V., Dengler, R., and Grosskreutz, J. (2012). Longitudinal diffusion tensor imaging in amyotrophic lateral sclerosis. *BMC Neurosci.* 13:141. doi: 10.1186/1471-2202-13-141
40. Kiernan, M. C., Vucic, S., Cheah, B. C., Turner, M. R., Eisen, A., Hardiman, O., et al. (2011). Amyotrophic lateral sclerosis. *Lancet* 377, 942–955. doi: 10.1016/S0140-6736(10)61156-7
41. Llufriu, S., Martinez-Heras, E., Solana, E., Sola-Valls, N., Sepulveda, M., Blanco, Y., et al. (2017). Structural networks involved in attention and executive functions in multiple sclerosis. *NeuroImage* 13, 288–296. doi: 10.1016/j.nicl.2016.11.026
42. Mazón, M., Vázquez Costa, J. F., Ten-Esteve, A., and Martí-Bonmatí, L. (2018). Imaging biomarkers for the diagnosis and prognosis of neurodegenerative diseases. example of amyotrophic lateral sclerosis. *Front. Neurosci.* 12:784. doi: 10.3389/fnins.2018.00784
43. Menke, R. A. L., Abraham, I., Thiel, C. S., Filippini, N., Knight, S., Talbot, K., et al. (2012). Fractional anisotropy in the posterior limb of the internal capsule and prognosis in amyotrophic lateral sclerosis. *Arch. Neurol.* 69:1493. doi: 10.1001/ archneurol.2012.1122
44. Menke, R. A. L., Proudfoot, M., Wuu, J., Andersen, P. M., Talbot, K., Benatar, M., et al. (2016). Increased functional connectivity common to symptomatic amyotrophic lateral sclerosis and those at genetic risk. *J. Neurol. Neurosurg. Psychiatry* 87, 580–588. doi: 10.1136/jnnp-2015-31 1945
45. Menzler, K., Belke, M., Wehrmann, E., Krakow, K., Lengler, U., Jansen, A., et al. (2011). Men and women are different: diffusion tensor imaging reveals sexual dimorphism in the microstructure of the thalamus, corpus callosum and cingulum. *Neuroimage* 54, 2557–2562. doi: 10.1016/j.neuroimage.2010.11.029
46. Müller, H.-P., Turner, M. R., Grosskreutz, J., Abrahams, S., Bede, P., Govind, V., et al. (2016). A large-scale multicentre cerebral diffusion tensor imaging study in amyotrophic lateral sclerosis. *J. Neurol. Neurosurg. Psychiatry* 87, 570–579. doi: 10.1136/jnnp-2015-311952
47. Nasseroleslami, B., Dukic, S., Broderick, M., Mohr, K., Schuster, C., Gavin, B., et al. (2019). Characteristic increases in EEG connectivity correlate with changes of structural MRI in amyotrophic lateral sclerosis. *Cereb. Cortex* 29, 27–41. doi: 10.1093/cercor/bhx301
48. Omer, T., Finegan, E., Hutchinson, S., Doherty, M., Vajda, A., McLaughlin, R. L., et al. (2017). Neuroimaging patterns along the ALS-FTD spectrum: a multiparametric imaging study. *Amyotrop. Lateral Scler. Frontotemporal Degener.* 18, 611–623. doi: 10.1080/21678421.2017.1332077
49. Phukan, J., Pender, N. P., and Hardiman, O. (2007). Cognitive impairment in amyotrophic lateral sclerosis. *Lancet Neurol.* 6, 994–1003. doi: 10.1016/S1474-4422(07)70265-X
50. Proudfoot, M., Bede, P., and Turner, M. R. (2019). Imaging cerebral activity in amyotrophic lateral sclerosis. *Front. Neurol.* 9:1148. doi: 10.3389/fneur.2018.01148
51. Querin, G., Bede, P., El Mendili, M. M., Li, M., Pélégrini-Issac, M., Rinaldi, D., et al. (2019). Presymptomatic spinal cord pathology in *c9orf72* mutation carriers: a longitudinal neuroimaging study. *Ann. Neurol.* 86, 158–167. doi: 10.1002/ana. 25520
52. Rascovsky, K., Hodges, J. R., Knopman, D., Mendez, M. F., Kramer, J. H., Neuhaus, J., et al. (2011). Sensitivity of revised diagnostic criteria for the behavioural variant of frontotemporal dementia. *Brain* 134, 2456–2477. doi: 10.1093/brain/ awr179
53. Ridley, B. G. Y., Rousseau, C., Wirsich, J., Le Troter, A., Soulier, E., Confort-Gouny, S., et al. (2015). Nodal approach reveals differential impact of lateralized focal epilepsies on hub reorganization. *NeuroImage* 118, 39–48. doi: 10.1016/j.neuroimage.2015.05.096
54. Rose, S., Pannek, K., Bell, C., Baumann, F., Hutchinson, N., Coulthard, A., et al. (2012). Direct evidence of intra- and interhemispheric corticomotor network degeneration in amyotrophic lateral sclerosis: an automated MRI structural connectivity study. *NeuroImage* 59, 2661–2669. doi: 10.1016/j.neuroimage.2011.08.054
55. Rubinov, M., and Bullmore, E. (2013). Schizophrenia and abnormal brain network hubs. *Dialog. Clin. Neurosci.* 15, 339–349.
56. Rubinov, M., and Sporns, O. (2010). Complex network measures of brain connectivity: uses and interpretations. *NeuroImage* 52, 1059–1069. doi: 10.1016/j.neuroimage.2009.10.003
57. Schuster, C., Elamin, M., Hardiman, O., and Bede, P. (2015). Presymptomatic and longitudinal neuroimaging in neurodegeneration—from snapshots to motion picture: a systematic review. *J. Neurol. Neurosurg. Psychiatry* 86, 1089–1096. doi: 10.1136/jnnp-2014-309888
58. Schuster, C., Elamin, M., Hardiman, O., and Bede, P. (2016). The segmental diffusivity profile of amyotrophic lateral sclerosis associated white matter degeneration. *Eur. J. Neurol.* 23, 1361–1371. doi: 10.1111/ene.13038
59. Schuster, C., Hardiman, O., and Bede, P. (2017). Survival prediction in amyotrophic lateral sclerosis based on MRI measures and clinical characteristics. *BMC Neurol.* 17:73. doi: 10.1186/s12883-017-0854-x
60. Sharma, K. R., Saigal, G., Maudsley, A. A., and Govind, V. (2011). 1H MRS of basal ganglia and thalamus in amyotrophic lateral sclerosis. *NMR Biomed.* 24, 1270–1276. doi: 10.1002/nbm.1687
61. Tang, M., Chen, X., Zhou, Q., Liu, B., Liu, Y., Liu, S., et al. (2015). Quantitative assessment of amyotrophic lateral sclerosis with diffusion tensor imaging in 3.0T magnetic resonance. *Int. J. Clin. Exp. Med.* 8, 8295–8303.
62. Tur, C., Eshaghi, A., Altmann, D. R., Jenkins, T. M., Prados, F., Grussu, F., et al. (2018). Structural cortical network reorganization associated with early conversion to multiple sclerosis. *Sci. Rep.* 8:10715. doi: 10.1038/s41598-018- 29017-1
63. van den Heuvel, M. P., and Sporns, O. (2011). Rich-club organization of the human connectome. *J. Neurosci.* 31, 15775–15786. doi: 10.1523/JNEUROSCI.3539-11. 2011
64. van den Heuvel, M. P., Sporns, O., Collin, G., Scheewe, T., Mandl, R. C. W., Cahn, W., et al. (2013). Abnormal rich club organization and functional brain dynamics in schizophrenia. *JAMA Psychiatry* 70:783. doi: 10.1001/jamapsychiatry.2013.1328
65. Verstraete, E., Turner, M. R., Grosskreutz, J., Filippi, M., and Benatar, M. (2015). Mind the gap: the mismatch between clinical and imaging metrics in ALS. *Amyotrop. Lateral Scler. Frontotemporal Degener.* 16, 524–529. doi: 10.3109/ 21678421.2015.1051989
66. Verstraete, E., Veldink, J. H., Mandl, R. C. W., van den Berg, L. H., and van den Heuvel, M. P. (2011). Impaired structural motor connectome in amyotrophic lateral sclerosis. *PLoS One* 6:e24239. doi: 10.1371/journal.pone.0024239
67. Verstraete, E., Veldink, J. H., van den Berg, L. H., and van den Heuvel, M. P. (2014). Structural brain network imaging shows expanding disconnection of the motor system in amyotrophic lateral sclerosis: expanding motor disconnection in ALS. *Hum. Brain Mapp.* 35, 1351–1361. doi: 10.1002/hbm.22258
68. Vivekananda, U., Manjalay, Z.-R., Ganesalingam, J., Simms, J., Shaw, C. E., Leigh, P. N., et al. (2011). Low index-to-ring finger length ratio in sporadic ALS supports prenatally defined motor neuronal vulnerability.

69. *J. Neurol. Neurosurg. Psychiatry* 82, 635–637. doi: 10.1136/jnnp.2010.237412
70. Zalesky, A., Fornito, A., and Bullmore, E. T. (2010). Network-based statistic: identifying differences in brain networks. *NeuroImage* 53, 1197–1207. doi: 10.1016/j.neuroimage.2010.06.041
71. Zhang, Y., Qiu, T., Yuan, X., Zhang, J., Wang, Y., Zhang, N., et al. (2019). Abnormal topological organization of structural covariance networks in amyotrophic lateral sclerosis. *NeuroImage* 21:101619. doi: 10.1016/j.nicl.2018.101619

23

Developing a Neuroimaging Biomarker for Amyotrophic Lateral Sclerosis: Multi-Center Data Sharing and the Road to a "Global Cohort"

Robert Steinbach†, Nayana Gaur†, Beatrice Stubendorff, Otto W. Witte and Julian Grosskreutz*

Hans Berger Department of Neurology, Jena University Hospital, Jena, Germany

***Correspondence:**
Robert Steinbach
robert.steinbach@med.uni-jena.de

†These authors have contributed equally to this work and share first authorship

Neuroimaging in Amyotrophic Lateral Sclerosis (ALS) has steadily evolved from an academic exercise to a powerful clinical tool for detecting and following pathological change. Nevertheless, significant challenges need to be addressed for the translation of neuroimaging as a robust outcome-metric and biomarker in quality-of-care assessments and pharmaceutical trials. Studies have been limited by small sample sizes, poor replication, incomplete patient characterization, and substantial differences in data collection and processing. This has been further exacerbated by the substantial heterogeneity associated with ALS. Multi-center transnational collaborations are needed to address these methodological limitations and achieve representation of rare phenotypes. This review will use the example of the Neuroimaging Society in ALS (NiSALS) to discuss the set-up of a multi-center data sharing ecosystem and the flow of information between various stakeholders. NiSALS' founding objective was to establish best practices for the acquisition and processing of MRI data and establish a structure that allows continuous data sharing and therefore augments the ability to fully describe patients. The practical challenges associated with such a system, including quality control, legal, ethical, and logistical constraints, will be discussed, as will be recommendations for future collaborative endeavors. We posit that "global cohorts" of well-characterized sub-populations within the disease spectrum are needed to fully understand the complex interplay between neuroimaging and other clinical metrics used to study ALS.

Keywords: amyotrophic lateral sclerosis, MRI, data-sharing, NiSALS, quality-control, harmonization, multi-center

INTRODUCTION

Acknowledging the Inherent Heterogeneity in ALS

It is widely accepted that amyotrophic lateral sclerosis (ALS) is a multifactorial disease, with an etiology that extends far beyond the selective vulnerability of motor neurons. Heterogeneity stemming from site-of- and age-at-onset, survival, genetic predictors, and the presence of frontotemporal dementia has severely constrained therapeutic translation (1). Precision biomarkers provide frameworks for early detection, tracking, and patient stratification, ensuring that treatment effects are not occluded by phenotypic variability. Today, neuroimaging in ALS isn't limited to merely structural-functional correlations and is on par with traditional "wet" biomarkers when it comes to group- and individual-level analyses (2, 3). Neuroimaging represents a crucial addition to the current repertoire of outcome metrics used in clinical trials; this includes respiratory measures, muscle strength, and the Revised Amyotrophic Functional Rating Scale (ALSFRS-R), the ambiguity of which has been previously reported (4).

NiSALS: Why Data-Sharing Is the Way Forward for ALS Research

Given the underlying complexity, low prevalence, and poor patient longevity, larger, multi-layered data sets are needed to capture the full spectrum of pathological signatures in ALS and develop population-specific markers. Such data sets can only be generated through well co-ordinated, multi-center efforts. In the wider neurodegenerative field, ventures like the Alzheimer's Disease Neuroimaging Initiative (ADNI) have demonstrated the analytical power of transnational collaborations. ADNI was launched in 2004 as a multi-site, longitudinal study to develop biomarkers for Alzheimer's Disease. To date, over 1,700 publications spanning several topics have resulted from ADNI data (5–7). ADNI has inspired similar initiatives in various neurodegenerative conditions, including ALS. "Sampling and Biomarker Optimization in ALS and other Motor Neuron Diseases" (SOPHIA) was the most comprehensive of these efforts and ran from 2012 to 2016, with ~2.4 million EUR in funding (http://www.neurodegenerationresearch.eu/fileadmin/Project_Fact_Sheets/PDFs/Biomarkers/SOPHIA_Fact_Sheet.pdf). It was conceived with the goal of harmonizing optimal methodologies for biomarker identification, thereby providing a pan-European framework within which existing and future endeavors could integrate. By consolidating expertise from over 15 leading European centers, SOPHIA helped establish the Progeny database: a web-based sampling infrastructure for the streamlined collection of clinical, neurophysiological, imaging, and bio sample-based data. Furthermore, the development of a centralized repository system for MRI data as part of SOPHIA led to the establishment of The Neuroimaging Society in Amyotrophic Lateral Sclerosis (NiSALS). The first NiSALS meeting (Oxford 2010) recognized the need for quality-controlled and harmonized MRI data and led to the publication of consensus guidelines on data acquisition (8). Annual meetings have since cemented NiSALS' role as an international consortium fostering neuroimaging as a key tool for understanding ALS. Today, a growing number of centers across Europe, North America, and Australia are NiSALS members, and are actively contributing data and hosting symposiums.

Each year has brought its own set of hurdles and achievements, showing that large-scale efforts like NiSALS rather than being monolithic, have the capacity to continuously adjust to the needs of the scientific community (9, 10). This review, while not exhaustive, will use NiSALS to illustrate the stakeholders and processes involved in multi-center data sharing. We hope to demonstrate that the associated challenges, while not insignificant, are surmountable, and that only global cohorts can generate the volume and variety of data needed to understand complex disorders like ALS.

THE NiSALS ECOSYSTEM: A GENERAL OVERVIEW

NiSALS' primary goal was always to function as a self-sustaining entity that provides the ALS community with the tools needed to advance neuroimaging-based research. The establishment of a secure central repository and the institution of a formally elected steering committee (http://nisals.net/?page_id=159) were significant first steps. The committee is responsible for the democratic governance of NiSALS activities, including making timely project and data-transfer decisions, event management, and liaising with third-party stakeholders. The general flow of data and stakeholder-interactions is depicted in **Figure 1**. Participating centers can continuously upload MRI data into a designated repository slot. Folders are available for the collection of additional clinical data that can be integrated into the server architecture for appropriate dissemination. However, individual centers are responsible for (a) obtaining approval for data sharing from the relevant ethics committee or review board and (b) appropriate data coding. Contributing centers are provided with guides, accessible through the NiSALS webpage, that include recommended packages of established freeware imaging resources to ensure thorough data de-identification prior to upload. The uploaded data then undergoes an additional round of pseudonymization (discussed in Section Data De-identification) for complete legal compliance. Crucially, each center has exclusive read/write access to their own data, in addition to having read-only access to common information areas. The repository creates individual data root trees to prevent users from accessing data domains that aren't theirs. The exact repository content for each contributor is kept confidential to add credence to the NiSALS curation mechanisms.

Figure 1 shows that the centralized communication hub (overseen by the NiSALS co-ordinator and repository curator) is essential for the streamlined running of the platform. Given the dynamic data sharing that NiSALS entails, the hub serves as a liaison point for all stakeholders, especially since data generators have expressed a desire for continuous feedback on data content and usage. The co-ordinator is also responsible for organizing annual NiSALS meetings and collection of associated materials.

The NiSALS webpage (https://nisals.net/) is an indispensable platform tool. It is used for administrative duties, including member and event management, compiling support documentation, and regularly updating legal compliance notices. The website also serves as an entry-point for interested

---

Abbreviations: ADNI, Alzheimer's Disease Neuroimaging Initiative; ALS, Amyotrophic Lateral Sclerosis; ALSFRS-R, Amyotrophic Lateral Sclerosis Functional Rating Scale Revised; DICOM, Digital Imaging and Communications in Medicine; DTI, Diffusion Tensor Imaging; MRI, Magnetic Resonance Imaging; NiSALS, Neuroimaging Society in Amyotrophic Lateral Sclerosis; QC, Quality Control; SOPHIA, Sampling and Biomarker Optimization in ALS and other Motor Neuron Diseases.

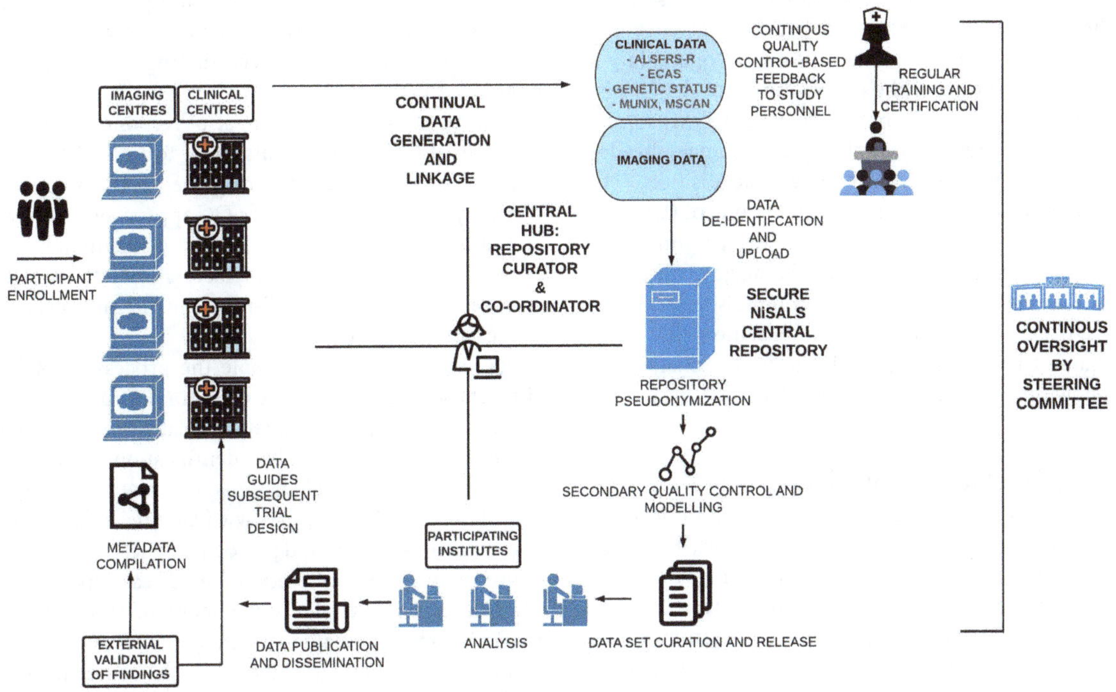

FIGURE 1 | Visual Schematic of the NiSALS ecosystem, including representations of future recommendations.

stakeholders, and is crucial for bolstering outreach. In the future, the webpage will contain teaching materials and enable center-specific repository content viewing.

LEGAL FRAMEWORKS AND DATA-SHARING

Central to any data-sharing effort is the cultivation of trust. All data-handling procedures are therefore in accordance with the NiSALS bylaws, which are designed to be collaborative and transparent. The bylaws recognize that all users need to be treated equally and should shoulder both the costs and benefits associated with embargo-free data sharing. Data sharing within NiSALS most closely resembles the "learned intermediary" model (11). Briefly, the model stipulates that an independent panel reviews applications and grants access to data primarily on the basis of applicant expertise and the quality of the proposed research. Within NiSALS, all applications are reviewed by the steering committee. Applicants must clearly detail (1) intended scientific analyses, (2) expected time-line to completion, and (3) specifications of required data in a project proposal. Successful applicants are bound by a stringent data-sharing agreement i.e., a legal mechanism to enforce NiSALS' core bylaws. Of note, are the following specifics:

1) Following publication, the released data set has to be destroyed
2) The released data set cannot be shared with third parties
3) Any additional analyses must first be vetted by the aforementioned application process.

Crucially, NiSALS recognizes that ownership of uploaded data permanently resides with the uploading center, regardless of which stage in the data-handling cycle the data is at. Thus, contributors also have the right to have their data removed from the repository upon written request.

As with any scientific undertaking, there arises the question of publications. NiSALS encourages collaborators to define and agree in writing to authorship roles prior to project commencement. Authorship credit should be in keeping with the guidelines developed by the International Committee of Medical Journal Editors. Responsible data generators should be offered contributory roles, regardless of the volume of data used. Finally, authors must reference NiSALS in resulting publications.

In summary, NiSALS operates with maximum practicability to ensure that (a) the immense benefits of sharing data outweigh the potential risks and (b) there is no disproportionate burden on data generators. Of note, when working with multiple stakeholders across geographical locations, it is unlikely that a "one size fits all" data-sharing agreement can be developed, as the judiciary requirements vastly vary between and within countries and institutions. Similar repositories should ensure that while their legal frameworks are exacting, they should be broad enough to facilitate the desired results.

DATA DE-IDENTIFICATION

As within other research domains, data sharing within neuroimaging is a constant balance between protecting confidentiality and sharing information to facilitate in-depth analyses. Multi-centre initiatives add further complexity, as individuals have to be universally identifiable, with seamless linkage of their participation across various projects.

Substantial efforts in bolstering technical inter-operability in diagnostic imaging resulted in the establishment of the "Digital Imaging and Communications in Medicine" (DICOM) format. NiSALS adopted it for repository uploads, as the image-headers specify the parameters used during image acquisition. This information is needed for subsequent quality-control (QC) and harmonization procedures as it is essential for determining which parameters are most likely to have disturbed image quality or be most relevant during multi-center data comparison. However, all original DICOM-files also contain information that needs to be safeguarded to maintain participant confidentiality. De-identification within NiSALS is conducted in two basic steps explained below.

Basic DICOM Pseudonymization

DICOM files are first pseudonymized by removing information linked to participant identity. As mentioned above, individual contributing centers are responsible for ensuring this prior to uploading data. Further, private DICOM-header fields that are modality- and vendor-dependent must be removed (12, 13). NiSALS' internal naming conventions require that all uploaded files use local center-specific pseudonyms; this allows contributors to (a) keep track of uploaded data, (b) continuously provide additional data sets, and (c) link insights from the analysis process back to the original data set.

Internal Repository Pseudonymization

Data within the repository are also subjected to secondary internal checks prior to being released for analyses. These checks include the removal of identifiable facial structures (defacing) and auxiliary whole-DICOM header de-identification (14). The latter is always in keeping with the current recommendations by the National Electrical Manufacturers Association that regularly lists relevant public header fields (15). Any center-specific information is implicitly removed, as researchers using the data should be blinded to its source of origin. All study participants are allocated a unique NiSALS-generated internal pseudonym. As centers subsequently submit associated data, it is essential to maintain linkage through these layers. Therefore, NiSALS' requires all additional data to be submitted to the repository following the same pipeline of pseudonym generation, thus allowing integration with the individual participant.

QUALITY CONTROL PROCEDURES

As a first layer of QC, robust mechanisms are needed to prevent inclusion of corrupted MRI data in subsequent analyses. While being susceptible to obvious errors (e.g., extinction-artifacts), images in a multi-center set-up can also be compromised by scanner-hardware/software and modality-specific factors that may result in bias further downstream (16–18). Manual analysis and exclusion/inclusion of data sets by a trained rater is time- and labor-intensive, and contingent on rater expertise. Conversely, while automated QC procedures may overcome inter- and intra-rater variability, their applicability to one distinct data-set may not necessarily be transferable to new data acquired from different sites, thereby still necessitating visual checks by human operators (19).

Contributing centers are also responsible for complying with initial QC requirements prior to upload to minimize the risk of corrupted data entering the repository. Subsequently, modality- and analysis-specific QC approaches are applied to the stored data. Here, the challenge lies in identifying artefacts and correcting for scanner-specific factors prior to the data entering a multi-center analysis, whilst minimizing time expenditure and potential manual bias.

QC mechanisms that enable the processing of large multi-site data sets have been developed for T1 data. First, covariance screening of image parameters related to inhomogeneity or noise is conducted for outlier identification. Hereafter, software-based preprocessing algorithms for raw T1 images (e.g., as available with SPM; https://www.fil.ion.ucl.ac.uk/spm/) facilitate correction of scanner- and protocol-induced systematic artefacts, whilst minimizing alteration of disease-specific signatures. Mathematical models like Mahalanobis distance analysis can help minimize and eliminate software-bias and overcorrection when identifying technical artefacts in multi-center data sets. These models provide a meta-analysis of image quality parameters, indicating which data sets are similar and amenable to pooling as illustrated in **Figure 2**. Ultimately, all algorithmic solutions involve compromise between correction and the biological signal and therefore need to be continuously improved with feedback from all users, which is naturally extremely resource-intensive.

Similar QC procedures have been adopted by the NiSALS DTI Study Group; these include the automated exclusion of particular gradient directions in single DTI data sets (20, 21) and correction for acquisition-derived eddy-current-induced geometric distortions (20). The NiSALS DTI Study Group used these QC procedures to correct 442 single DTI data sets (from 8 contributing ALS centers) for artefacts like susceptibility-induced geometric warping, participant motion and chemical shift, prior to further analysis (10).

CROSS-PLATFORM MRI INTERPRETATION AND HARMONIZATION

As discussed above, multi-center-studies suffer from poor data comparability, owing to scanner-hardware/software differences. For instance, a study using MRI scans of the same subjects taken at different sites showed that DTI-derived values (e.g., fractional anisotropy) showed moderate reproducibility between different scanners, while particular higher field strengths and enlarged acquisition resolutions decreased inter-center variability (22).

Even if different sites use identical scanners, variance can still arise from differences in derived structural and functional imaging information; however, harmonization can improve comparability (23, 24). Processing procedures used at different sites can also contribute to variability. Therefore, as with ADNI, standardized MRI-data sets that rely on harmonized acquisition

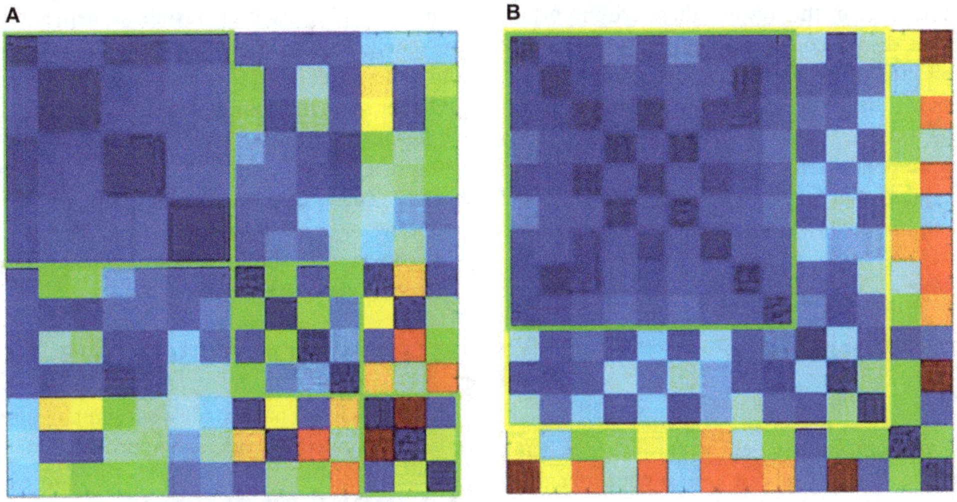

FIGURE 2 | Mahalanobis distance analysis of quality parameters for T1-weighted images of 14 ALS centers. **(A)** Shows the Mahalanobis distances of the raw T1 data, revealing 3 clusters of centers, which although internally homogenous (green squares) could not be pooled into one large data set. **(B)** Shows the effect of preprocessing. This allows pooling of T1 data from additional centers with good (green square) or acceptable homogeneity (yellow square). However, 2 centers although homogenous with each other, could not be pooled with the other data sets (shown in the last 2 rows or right-most columns, respectively).

schemes and have undergone QC are needed to support direct comparisons of different processing methods.

The majority of MRI-centric publications in ALS are offset by low sample sizes and high phenotypic heterogeneity within disease cohorts (3). One of NiSALS' core objectives was to define rules for MRI acquisition to help maximize accuracy and comparability and thereby enlarge study sample sizes. The published consensus guidelines therefore detail essential and desirable recommendations for T1, DTI, functional MRI and spectroscopy data acquisition (8).

ADNI uses a cross-platform calibration procedure that utilizes traveling phantoms for data harmonization (25). Certainly, implementing a comparable procedure for ALS centers on a global scale would require a substantially larger investment of financial and human resources, partly due to the lower prevalence of ALS (26). Therefore, NiSALS' current harmonization efforts focus on (a) ensuring that previously acquired neuroimaging data meets standards for multi-center analyses and (b) using feedback to maximize acquisition accuracy. Ultimately, MRI acquisition, and harmonization protocols need to be diligently updated to reflect the latest technical advances.

Although current uploads primarily include DTI and T1 data (~1,000 participants for the latter), NiSALS welcomes the integration of multi-modal imaging techniques and combined structural-functional approaches and hopes to collect and disseminate data that reflects the full breadth of neuroimaging methods currently available. However, appropriate set-ups for the acquisition and use of these modalities also need to be concurrently developed if they are to be used for multi-site projects (9).

CLINICAL DATA LINKAGE

Owing to its complexity, ALS cannot be studied as a homogenous disease. In-depth multi-modal data are required for the classification of clinical, neuropsychological and imaging-based phenotypes of sporadic disease and genetic variants. This is particularly relevant when developing neuroimaging biomarkers. Incomplete patient characterization has limited several neuroimaging-based studies; the lack of clinical data constrains both accurate distinction of ALS from disease mimics and understanding of pathophysiology and progression. To fully understand the degree to which MRI and other modalities can assess disease activity and quantitate functional progression, they have to be placed within the framework of core clinical data and other biomarkers. The latter is crucial as individual biomarkers display different patterns across the disease course and in different clinical phenotypes; this has been well described for Alzheimer's Disease (27).

Naturally, this is contingent on available resources and NiSALS therefore advises contributing centers on clinical data to submit alongside MRI data sets; these have been previously published (https://www.encals.eu/wp-content/uploads/2016/09/2015-01-14-ALS-Core-clinical-dataset.pdf). In particular, NiSALS recognizes the importance of genotyping individuals and studying mutation carriers in presymptomatic disease phases to understand how genetic factors may influence the behavior of different markers (9).

Further, although data from healthy and disease controls is being continuously uploaded to the repository and requested in project proposals, both NiSALS and future efforts need to rigorously tackle the lack of longitudinal data from these subjects.

Although a detailed consideration of disease progression models is beyond the scope of this review, these are important tools for describing the disease course, particularly when clinical data cannot be collected at regular time-points for patients. Models can also help identify center-dependent and independent biological components. For instance, the newly developed D50 model enables random sampling of patients, comparisons between different progressor types and the placement of biomarker profiles within the functional time course of patients (28, 29).

FUTURE DIRECTIONS AND CONCLUSIONS

ALS, although highly heterogeneous, has the advantage of being measurably progressive. It is crucial to tap into neuroimaging's potential and use quantitative tools like MRI to describe the disease and understand its spread. Efforts like NiSALS can help the community develop and execute high-level data sharing, facilitate the replication of results and avoid unnecessary duplication of efforts. The ecosystem described here provides a structure for continuous QC and feedback that can help identify markers that are readily transferable to both the clinic and industry. Indeed, NiSALS hopes to establish well-defined collaborations with industrial partners looking to develop neuroimaging as an outcome metric for clinical trials. NiSALS can also offer its experience in implementing best practices, efficiently executing research, and disseminating results for the benefit of the neurodegenerative community. Future efforts must build on this momentum and endeavor to make the exercise more patient-centric by boosting engagement with them and communicating scientific results to them and the lay population. Stakeholders should also consider collecting meta-data on the outcomes of data sharing and how the process can be modified to better serve the community's needs.

Resources must also be directed toward building comprehensive, well-characterized multimodal biomarker panels. These can help expand the role of imaging beyond reductive clinico-structural correlations to a precision tool that can capture subtle pathological changes in population and individual-level analyses.

AUTHOR CONTRIBUTIONS

All authors listed have made a substantial, direct and intellectual contribution to the work, and approved it for publication.

ACKNOWLEDGMENTS

The present study was supported by the German Bundesministerium für Bildung und Forschung (BMBF) grant SOPHIA and OnWEBDuals to JG under the aegis of the EU Joint Programme—Neurodegenerative Disease Research (JPND) and a BMBF grant PYRAMID to JG in the framework of the ERANET E-RARE program. Support was also received from the Motor Neurone Disease Association (MNDA) and Deutsche Gesellschaft für Muskelkranke (DGM). We extend our thanks to Robert Dahnke and Prof. Christian Gaser for their support. Finally, we are grateful to the community of ALS patients and their caregivers, without whom this work would not be possible. Icons in **Figure 1** were sourced from the FlatIcon webpage.

REFERENCES

1. Sabatelli M, Conte A, Zollino M. Clinical and genetic heterogeneity of amyotrophic lateral sclerosis. *Clin Genet.* (2013) 83:408–16. doi: 10.1111/cge.12117
2. Bede P, Hardiman O. Lessons of ALS imaging: pitfalls and future directions - a critical review. *Neuroimage Clin.* (2014) 4:436–43. doi: 10.1016/j.nicl.2014.02.011
3. Chio A, Pagani M, Agosta F, Calvo A, Cistaro A, Filippi M. Neuroimaging in amyotrophic lateral sclerosis: insights into structural and functional changes. *Lancet Neurol.* (2014) 13:1228–40. doi: 10.1016/S1474-4422(14)70167-X
4. Franchignoni F, Mora G, Giordano A, Volanti P, Chio A. Evidence of multidimensionality in the ALSFRS-R Scale: a critical appraisal on its measurement properties using Rasch analysis. *J Neurol Neurosurg Psychiatry* (2013) 84:1340–5. doi: 10.1136/jnnp-2012-304701
5. Carrillo MC, Bain LJ, Frisoni GB, Weiner MW. Worldwide Alzheimer's disease neuroimaging initiative. *Alzheimers Dement.* (2012) 8:337–42. doi: 10.1016/j.jalz.2012.04.007
6. Weiner MW, Veitch DP, Aisen PS, Beckett LA, Cairns NJ, Cedarbaum J, et al. Impact of the alzheimer's disease neuroimaging initiative, 2004 to 2014. *Alzheimers Dement.* (2015) 11:865–84. doi: 10.1016/j.jalz.2015.04.005
7. Weiner MW, Veitch DP, Aisen PS, Beckett LA, Cairns NJ, Green RC, et al. Recent publications from the alzheimer's disease neuroimaging initiative: reviewing progress toward improved AD clinical trials. *Alzheimers Dement.* (2017) 13:e1–e85. doi: 10.1016/j.jalz.2016.11.007
8. Turner MR, Grosskreutz J, Kassubek J, Abrahams S, Agosta F, Benatar M, et al. Towards a neuroimaging biomarker for amyotrophic lateral sclerosis. *Lancet Neurol.* (2011) 10:400–3. doi: 10.1016/S1474-4422(11)70049-7
9. Filippi M, Agosta F, Grosskreutz J, Benatar M, Kassubek J, Verstraete E, et al. Progress towards a neuroimaging biomarker for amyotrophic lateral sclerosis. *Lancet Neurol.* (2015) 14:786–8. doi: 10.1016/S1474-4422(15)00134-9
10. Muller HP, Turner MR, Grosskreutz J, Abrahams S, Bede P, Govind V, et al. A large-scale multicentre cerebral diffusion tensor imaging study in amyotrophic lateral sclerosis. *J Neurol Neurosurg Psychiatry* (2016) 87:570–9. doi: 10.1136/jnnp-2015-311952
11. Antman E. Data sharing in research: benefits and risks for clinicians. *BMJ* (2014) 348:g237. doi: 10.1136/bmj.g237
12. Aryanto KY, Oudkerk M, van Ooijen PM. Free DICOM de-identification tools in clinical research: functioning and safety of patient privacy. *Eur Radiol.* (2015) 25:3685–95. doi: 10.1007/s00330-015-3794-0
13. Moore SM, Maffitt DR, Smith KE, Kirby JS, Clark KW, Freymann JB, et al. De-identification of medical images with retention of scientific research value. *Radiographics* (2015) 35:727–35. doi: 10.1148/rg.2015140244
14. Leung KY, van der Lijn F, Vrooman HA, Sturkenboom MC, Niessen WJ. IT Infrastructure to support the secondary use of routinely acquired clinical imaging data for research. *Neuroinformatics* (2015) 13:65–81. doi: 10.1007/s12021-014-9240-7
15. Freymann JB, Kirby JS, Perry JH, Clunie DA, Jaffe CC. Image data sharing for biomedical research–meeting HIPAA requirements for De-identification. *J Digit Imaging* (2012) 25:14–24. doi: 10.1007/s10278-011-9422-x
16. Abdulkadir A, Mortamet B, Vemuri P, Jack CRJr, Krueger G, Kloppel S, et al. Effects of hardware heterogeneity on the performance of

SVM Alzheimer's disease classifier. *Neuroimage* (2011) 58:785–92. doi: 10.1016/j.neuroimage.2011.06.029

17. Reuter M, Tisdall MD, Qureshi A, Buckner RL, van der Kouwe AJW, Fischl B. Head motion during MRI acquisition reduces gray matter volume and thickness estimates. *Neuroimage* (2015) 107:107–15. doi: 10.1016/j.neuroimage.2014.12.006
18. Vogelbacher C, Mobius TWD, Sommer J, Schuster V, Dannlowski U, Kircher T, et al. The Marburg-Munster Affective Disorders Cohort Study (MACS): a quality assurance protocol for MR neuroimaging data. *Neuroimage* (2018) 172:450–60. doi: 10.1016/j.neuroimage.2018.01.079
19. Esteban O, Birman D, Schaer M, Koyejo OO, Poldrack RA, Gorgolewski KJ. MRIQC: Advancing the automatic prediction of image quality in MRI from unseen sites. *PLoS ONE* (2017) 12:e0184661. doi: 10.1371/journal.pone.0184661
20. Shen Y, Larkman DJ, Counsell S, Pu IM, Edwards D, Hajnal JV. Correction of high-order eddy current induced geometric distortion in diffusion-weighted echo-planar images. *Magn Reson Med.* (2004) 52:1184–9. doi: 10.1002/mrm.20267
21. Muller HP, Sussmuth SD, Landwehrmeyer GB, Ludolph A, Tabrizi SJ, Kloppel S, et al. Stability effects on results of diffusion tensor imaging analysis by reduction of the number of gradient directions due to motion artifacts: an application to presymptomatic Huntington's disease. *PLoS Curr.* (2011) 3:RRN1292. doi: 10.1371/currents.RRN1292
22. Grech-Sollars M, Hales PW, Miyazaki K, Raschke F, Rodriguez D, Wilson M, et al. Multi-centre reproducibility of diffusion MRI parameters for clinical sequences in the brain. *NMR Biomed.* (2015) 28:468–85. doi: 10.1002/nbm.3269
23. Veenith TV, Carter E, Grossac J, Newcombe VF, Outtrim JG, Lupson V, et al. Inter subject variability and reproducibility of diffusion tensor imaging within and between different imaging sessions. *PLoS ONE* (2013) 8:e65941. doi: 10.1371/journal.pone.0065941
24. Veenith TV, Mada M, Carter E, Grossac J, Newcombe V, Outtrim J, et al. Comparison of inter subject variability and reproducibility of whole brain proton spectroscopy. *PLoS ONE* (2014) 9:e115304. doi: 10.1371/journal.pone.0115304
25. Gunter JL, Bernstein MA, Borowski BJ, Ward CP, Britson PJ, Felmlee JP, et al. Measurement of MRI scanner performance with the ADNI phantom. *Med Phys.* (2009) 36:2193–205. doi: 10.1118/1.3116776
26. de Pedro-Cuesta J, Rabano A, Martinez-Martin P, Ruiz-Tovar M, Alcalde-Cabero E, Almazan-Isla J, et al. Comparative incidence of conformational, neurodegenerative disorders. *PLoS ONE* (2015) 10:e0137342. doi: 10.1371/journal.pone.0137342
27. Jack CR Jr, Knopman DS, Jagust WJ, Shaw LM, Aisen PS, Weiner MW, et al. Hypothetical model of dynamic biomarkers of the Alzheimer's pathological cascade. *Lancet Neurol.* (2010) 9:119–28. doi: 10.1016/S1474-4422(09)70299-6
28. Poesen K, De Schaepdryver M, Stubendorff B, Gille B, Muckova P, Wendler S, et al. Neurofilament markers for ALS correlate with extent of upper and lower motor neuron disease. *Neurology* (2017) 88:2302–9. doi: 10.1212/WNL.0000000000004029
29. Gaur N, Stubendorff B, Witte OW, Grosskreutz J. P46. Modelling individual amyotrophic lateral sclerosis (ALS) disease courses in the PRO-ACT data base using the D50 progression model. *Clin Neurophysiol.* (2018) 129:e86. doi: 10.1016/j.clinph.2018.04.684

Permissions

All chapters in this book were first published by Frontiers; hereby published with permission under the Creative Commons Attribution License or equivalent. Every chapter published in this book has been scrutinized by our experts. Their significance has been extensively debated. The topics covered herein carry significant findings which will fuel the growth of the discipline. They may even be implemented as practical applications or may be referred to as a beginning point for another development.

The contributors of this book come from diverse backgrounds, making this book a truly international effort. This book will bring forth new frontiers with its revolutionizing research information and detailed analysis of the nascent developments around the world.

We would like to thank all the contributing authors for lending their expertise to make the book truly unique. They have played a crucial role in the development of this book. Without their invaluable contributions this book wouldn't have been possible. They have made vital efforts to compile up to date information on the varied aspects of this subject to make this book a valuable addition to the collection of many professionals and students.

This book was conceptualized with the vision of imparting up-to-date information and advanced data in this field. To ensure the same, a matchless editorial board was set up. Every individual on the board went through rigorous rounds of assessment to prove their worth. After which they invested a large part of their time researching and compiling the most relevant data for our readers.

The editorial board has been involved in producing this book since its inception. They have spent rigorous hours researching and exploring the diverse topics which have resulted in the successful publishing of this book. They have passed on their knowledge of decades through this book. To expedite this challenging task, the publisher supported the team at every step. A small team of assistant editors was also appointed to further simplify the editing procedure and attain best results for the readers.

Apart from the editorial board, the designing team has also invested a significant amount of their time in understanding the subject and creating the most relevant covers. They scrutinized every image to scout for the most suitable representation of the subject and create an appropriate cover for the book.

The publishing team has been an ardent support to the editorial, designing and production team. Their endless efforts to recruit the best for this project, has resulted in the accomplishment of this book. They are a veteran in the field of academics and their pool of knowledge is as vast as their experience in printing. Their expertise and guidance has proved useful at every step. Their uncompromising quality standards have made this book an exceptional effort. Their encouragement from time to time has been an inspiration for everyone.

The publisher and the editorial board hope that this book will prove to be a valuable piece of knowledge for researchers, students, practitioners and scholars across the globe.

List of Contributors

Soichiro Shimizu, Daisuke Hirose, Hirokuni Hatanaka, Naoto Takenoshita, Yoshitsugu Kaneko, Yusuke Ogawa, Hirofumi Sakurai and Haruo Hanyu
Department of Geriatric Medicine, Tokyo Medical University, Tokyo, Japan

Veronique Marchand-Pauvert
Laboratoire d'Imagerie Biomédicale, CNRS, INSERM, Sorbonne Université, Paris, France

Giorgia Querin
Laboratoire d'Imagerie Biomédicale, CNRS, INSERM, Sorbonne Université, Paris, France
APHP, Département de Neurologie, Centre Référent SLA, Hôpital Pitié-Salpêtrière, Paris, France

Peter Bede
Laboratoire d'Imagerie Biomédicale, CNRS, INSERM, Sorbonne Université, Paris, France
APHP, Département de Neurologie, Centre Référent SLA, Hôpital Pitié-Salpêtrière, Paris, France
Computational Neuroimaging Group, Academic Unit of Neurology, Trinity College Dublin, Dublin, Ireland

Pierre-Francois Pradat
Laboratoire d'Imagerie Biomédicale, CNRS, INSERM, Sorbonne Université, Paris, France
APHP, Département de Neurologie, Centre Référent SLA, Hôpital Pitié-Salpêtrière, Paris, France
Northern Ireland Centre for Stratified Medicine, Biomedical Sciences Research Institute Ulster University, C-TRIC, Altnagelvin Hospital, Londonderry, United Kingdom

Thierry Burnouf
Graduate Institute of Biomedical Materials and Tissue Engineering, College of Biomedical Engineering, Taipei Medical University, Taipei, Taiwan
International PhD Program in Biomedical Engineering, College of Biomedical Engineering, Taipei Medical University, Taipei, Taiwan
International PhD Program in Cell Therapy and Regeneration Medicine, College of Medicine, Taipei Medical University, Taipei, Taiwan

David Devos
Department of Medical Pharmacology, Lille University, INSERM UMRS_1171, University Hospital Center, LICEND COEN Center, Lille, France
Department of Neurology, Lille University, INSERM UMRS_1171, University Hospital Center, LICEND COEN Center, Lille, France

Flore Gouel, Anne-Sophie Rolland and Jean-Christophe Devedjian
Department of Medical Pharmacology, Lille University, INSERM UMRS_1171, University Hospital Center, LICEND COEN Center, Lille, France

Siw Johannesen, Sebastian Peters, Anne-Louise Meyer, Tina Kammermaier, Eva Wirkert, Tim-Henrik Bruun, Wilhelm Schulte-Mattler and Ulrich Bogdahn
Department of Neurology, University Hospital Regensburg, Regensburg, Germany

Bettina Budeus and Armin Schneider
Lifedatascience Consulting, Schriesheim, Germany

Sabine Iberl, Wolfgang Herr and Jochen Grassinger
Department of Hematology, Internal Medicine III, University Hospital Regensburg, Regensburg, Germany

Verena C. Samara
Stanford Neuroscience Health Center, Palo Alto, CA, United State

Greig Joilin and Majid Hafezparast
School of Life Sciences, University of Sussex, Brighton, United Kingdom

P. Nigel Leigh and Sarah F. Newbury
Brighton and Sussex Medical School, University of Sussex, Brighton, United Kingdom

Philippe Corcia
Université de Tours, Inserm U1253, Tours, France
Centre Constitutif SLA, CHRU Bretonneau, Tours, France
Federation des centres SLA de Tours et Limoges, LITORALS, Tours, France

Pierre-François Pradat
Département des Maladies du Système Nerveux, Centre Référent Maladie Rare SLA, Hôpital de la Pitié-Salpétrière, Paris, France
Laboratoire d'Imagerie Biomédicale, Sorbonne Université, CNRS, INSERM, Paris, France
Northern Ireland Centre for Stratified Medicine, Biomedical Sciences Research Institute Ulster University, C-TRIC, Altnagelvin Hospital, Londonderry, United Kingdom

Hélène Blasco
Université de Tours, Inserm U1253, Tours, France
Service de Biochimie et Biologie Moléculaire, CHRU de Tours, Tours, France

Sophie Foggin, Raquel Mesquita-Ribeiro, Federico Dajas-Bailador and Rob Layfield
School of Life Sciences, University of Nottingham Medical School, Nottingham, United Kingdom

Maria-Letizia Campanari, Annis-Rayan Bourefis and Edor Kabashi
Sorbonne Université, Université Pierre et Marie Curie, Université de Paris 06, Unité Mixte 75, Institut National de la Santé et de la Recherche Médicale (INSERM) Unité 1127, Centre National de la Recherche Scientifique, Unité Mixte de Recherche 7225 Institut du Cerveau et de la Moelle Épinière, Paris, France
Imagine Institute, INSERM Unité 1163, Paris Descartes Université, Paris, France

Zhilin Huang, Youna Xie, Weineng Chen, Simei Long, Zhong Pei and Xiaoli Yao
Department of Neurology, National Key Clinical Department and Key Discipline of Neurology, Guangdong Key Clinical Laboratory for Diagnosis and Treatment of Major Neurological Diseases, The First Affiliated Hospital, Sun Yat-sen University, Guangzhou, China

Qiang Liu, Yu Peng and Huanxing Su
State Key Laboratory of Quality Research in Chinese Medicine, Institute of Chinese Medical Sciences, University of Macau, Macao, China

Jiaying Dai
Comprehensive Department, Sun Yat-sen Memorial Hospital affiliated to Sun Yat-sen University, Guangzhou, China

Susana Pinto
Instituto de Fisiologia-Instituto de Medicina Molecular, Faculdade de Medicina, Universidade de Lisboa, Lisbon, Portugal

Mamede de Carvalho
Instituto de Fisiologia-Instituto de Medicina Molecular, Faculdade de Medicina, Universidade de Lisboa, Lisbon, Portugal
Department of Neurosciences and Mental Health, Hospital de Santa Maria-CHLN, Lisbon, Portugal

Michael Swash
Instituto de Fisiologia-Instituto de Medicina Molecular, Faculdade de Medicina, Universidade de Lisboa, Lisbon, Portugal
Barts and the London School of Medicine, Queen Mary University of London, London, United Kingdom

Sheena Chew and Nazem Atassi
Department of Neurology, Harvard Medical School, Neurological Clinical Research Institute, Massachusetts General Hospital, Boston, MA, United States

Venkateswaran Rajagopalan
Department of Electrical and Electronics Engineering, Birla Institute of Technology and Science, Pilani, Hyderabad, India
Department of Biomedical Engineering, ND2, Lerner Research Institute, Cleveland Clinic, Cleveland, OH, United States

Erik P. Pioro
Department of Neurology, Neuromuscular Center, Neurological Institute, Cleveland Clinic, Cleveland, OH, United States
Department of Neurosciences, Lerner Research Institute, Cleveland Clinic, Cleveland, OH, United States

Rangariroyashe Hannah Chipika, Eoin Finegan, Stacey Li Hi Shing, Orla Hardiman and Peter Bede
Computational Neuroimaging Group, Biomedical Sciences Institute, Trinity College Dublin, Dublin, Ireland

Lulé and Albert C. Ludolph
Department of Neurology, University of Ulm, Ulm, Germany

Andrea Kübler
Interventional Psychology, Psychology III, University of Würzburg, Würzburg, Germany

Malcolm Proudfoot
Nuffield Department of Clinical Neurosciences, University of Oxford, Oxford, United Kingdom

Peter Bede
Computational Neuroimaging Group, Academic Unit of Neurology, Trinity College Dublin, Dublin, Ireland

Martin R. Turner
Nuffield Department of Clinical Neurosciences, University of Oxford, Oxford, United Kingdom
Wellcome Centre for Integrative Neuroimaging, University of Oxford, Oxford, United Kingdom

Udaya Geetha Vijayakumar, Vanessa Milla, Mei Yu Cynthia Stafford, Anthony J. Bjourson, William Duddy and Stephanie Marie-Rose Duguez
Northern Ireland Center for Stratified Medicine, Biomedical Sciences Research Institute, Londonderry, United Kingdom

Hsiao Shan Cho
Department of Neurology, Shuang Ho Hospital, Taipei Medical University, New Taipei City, Taiwan

Li Kai Huang
Department of Neurology, Shuang Ho Hospital, Taipei Medical University, New Taipei City, Taiwan
Graduate Institute of Humanities in Medicine, Taipei Medical University, Taipei, Taiwan

Yao Tung Lee
Department of Psychiatry, Shuang Ho Hospital, Taipei Medical University, New Taipei City, Taiwan
Department of Psychiatry, School of Medicine, College of Medicine, Taipei Medical University, Taipei, Taiwan

Lung Chan and Chien Tai Hong
Department of Neurology, Shuang Ho Hospital, Taipei Medical University, New Taipei City, Taiwan
Department of Neurology, School of Medicine, College of Medicine, Taipei Medical University, Taipei, Taiwan

Jashelle Caga
Sydney Medical School, University of Sydney, Camperdown, NSW, Australia
Brain & Mind Centre, University of Sydney, Camperdown, NSW, Australia

Sharpley Hsieh
Faculty of Health and Behavioural Sciences, School of Psychology, University of Queensland, QLD, Australia

Patricia Lillo
Departamento de Neurología Sur/Neurociencia, Facultad de Medicina, Universidad de Chile & Geroscience Center for Brain Health and Metabolism, Santiago, Chile

Kaitlin Dudley and Eneida Mioshi
School of Health Sciences, University of East Anglia, Norwich, United Kingdom

Haibo Zhang, Zhenfei Li, Na Liang, Xiaomeng Zhou, Xiangyu Nie and Ting Zhang
Department of Neurology, The Second Hospital of Hebei Medical University, Shijiazhuang, China

Yaling Liu
Department of Neurology, The Second Hospital of Hebei Medical University, Shijiazhuang, China
Key Laboratory of Neurology of Hebei Province, Shijiazhuang, China

Weijing Qi
Key Laboratory of Neurology of Hebei Province, Shijiazhuang, China
Department of Neurology, Baoding First Central Hospital of Hebei Province, Baoding, China

Foteini Christidi, Michail Rentzos and Ioannis Evdokimidis
First Department of Neurology, Aeginition Hospital, National and Kapodistrian University of Athens, Athens, Greece

Peter Bede
Computational Neuroimaging Group, Academic Unit of Neurology, Trinity College Dublin, Dublin, Ireland

Efstratios Karavasilis, Georgios Velonakis and Nikolaos Kelekis
Second Department of Radiology, General University Hospital "Attikon," National and Kapodistrian University of Athens, Athens, Greece

Panagiotis Ferentinos
Second Department of Psychiatry, General University Hospital "Attikon," National and Kapodistrian University of Athens, Athens, Greece

Kun Liu, Guanghui Bai and Zhihan Yan
Department of Radiology, The Second Affiliated Hospital and Yuying Children's Hospital of Wenzhou Medical University, Wenzhou, China

Yi Lu and Xiaoxia Zhang
Department of Radiology, The Second Affiliated Hospital and Yuying Children's Hospital of Wenzhou Medical University, Wenzhou, China
Institute of Metabonomics & Medical NMR, School of Pharmaceutical Sciences, Wenzhou Medical University, Wenzhou, China

Liangcai Zhao, Changwei Yang, Linlin Pan, Chen Li and Hongchang Gao
Institute of Metabonomics & Medical NMR, School of Pharmaceutical Sciences, Wenzhou Medical University, Wenzhou, China

Shahram Attarian
APHM, Hôpital de la Timone, Referral Centre for Neuromuscular Diseases and ALS, Marseille, France
Aix Marseille Univ, INSERM, GMGF, Marseille, France

Arnaud Le Troter, Ben Ridley, Maxime Guye, Jean-Philippe Ranjeva and Wafaa Zaaraoui
Aix Marseille Univ, CNRS, CRMBM, Marseille, France
APHM, Hôpital de la Timone, CEMEREM, Marseille, France

Etienne Fortanier, Aude-Marie Grapperon and Annie Verschueren
Aix Marseille Univ, CNRS, CRMBM, Marseille, France
APHM, Hôpital de la Timone, Referral Centre for Neuromuscular Diseases and ALS, Marseille, France
APHM, Hôpital de la Timone, CEMEREM, Marseille, France

Robert Steinbach, Nayana Gaur, Beatrice Stubendorff, Otto W. Witte and Julian Grosskreutz
Hans Berger Department of Neurology, Jena University Hospital, Jena, Germany

Index

A

Adult Myopathy Assessment Tool, 9-10

Alzheimer Disease, 2, 6, 193, 208

Amyloid, 1-6, 82, 93, 96, 102, 187

Amyotrophic Lateral Sclerosis, 10, 14-16, 23-28, 39-42, 49-51, 55-59, 64-66, 68, 70-72, 74, 80, 82-84, 89-92, 98, 101-104, 110-113, 122-130, 135-138, 145-152, 158-167, 173-174, 177-180, 184-187, 190, 192-195, 201, 207-208, 216-220, 224-225

Androgen Receptor, 7, 70, 72

Autophagy, 65-66, 71-72, 154, 158, 160-162

Axonopathy, 66, 71, 105

B

Betweenness Centrality, 207-208, 210, 213

Biomarker, 1-5, 7-9, 11-12, 14-15, 27-29, 39, 41, 43, 47-50, 52-53, 55-60, 63, 65, 92, 99-103, 112, 114, 118-129, 138, 142, 144, 147, 149-151, 153-154, 156-158, 163-166, 195, 217, 219-220, 224

C

Cardiovascular Diseases, 54, 157

Central Nervous System, 16, 39, 47, 49, 59, 69, 75, 92-93, 100, 104, 128, 158, 171, 193, 201, 208

Cerebrospinal Fluid, 1, 5-6, 34, 41-42, 47, 49-50, 52, 56, 64, 68, 72, 113, 126-128, 151, 154, 159, 163-165, 208-209

Cholinesterase Inhibitors, 168

Circadian Rhythm Dysfunction, 74, 77-80, 82

Cognitive Abilities Screening Instrument, 168, 170

Cognitive Dysfunction, 144, 169, 189, 194

Computed Tomography, 1-3, 113

Corticospinal Tract, 104, 109-111, 120, 138, 144

Cyanobacteria, 74-75, 77-82

Cytokines, 19, 27, 29, 32-33, 37-39, 41, 68, 118, 171-172

D

Dopamine, 1-3, 6, 99, 103, 197-198, 206

E

El Escorial Criteria, 28, 67, 71, 153, 208

Electromyography, 100, 105, 113, 120, 181

Electrophysiology, 9, 113, 145, 150

Encephalography, 138-139, 142

Epilepsy, 53, 193, 201, 205, 214, 216

F

Forced Vital Capacity, 10, 52, 86-87, 90, 113, 120, 125

Fractional Anisotropy, 93, 97, 105-106, 123, 190, 208, 217, 222

Frontal Hypometabolism, 2-3, 11, 99

Frontotemporal Dementia, 3, 5, 47, 59, 65-66, 70-71, 82, 92-93, 98, 102, 104-105, 127-128, 138, 141, 147, 160-162, 173-174, 178-179, 186-187, 190, 194, 208, 216-217, 219

G

Genetic Testing, 69, 72

Glial Cells, 25, 67, 78-79, 103, 154

Global Efficiency, 207-208, 210, 213-214

Glutamate Excitotoxicity, 37, 51, 67, 153, 180, 206

Granulocyte-colony Stimulating Factor, 17, 24, 26-28, 39-40

Graph Theory, 141-142, 145, 207-208, 210, 213-214

Gray Matter, 11, 14, 95, 97, 106, 109, 113, 120, 122, 146, 166, 187-188, 190

Gut Microflora, 81

H

Hematopoietic Stem Cells, 22, 27-30, 32-34, 36-37

Hippocampus, 2, 95-96, 186-188, 191, 193, 195, 205, 209

Homeostasis, 11, 28, 40, 53, 81, 131, 164, 183

Homocysteine, 53, 56, 151, 154, 158, 164-165, 171-172

Hypercapnia, 84-86, 191

Hypoxemia, 84-86

K

Kennedy's Disease, 7, 13-15, 68, 120, 141

L

Leukocytosis, 30, 34

Local Efficiency, 207-208, 210

M

Magnetic Resonance Imaging, 1-2, 14, 68, 72, 93, 100, 102, 104, 110, 112-113, 125, 146-148, 150, 181, 216-217, 220

Magnetoencephalography, 142, 148-150

Maximal Expiratory Pressure, 87-88

Maximal Inspiratory Pressure, 86-87, 113, 125

Mesenchymal Stromal Cells, 19, 22, 26

Metabolomics, 51-57, 121, 127, 165, 195, 198, 200, 203, 205-206

Metalloproteinases, 68, 72

Methylation, 160, 163, 171, 206

Mood Disorders, 74

Motor Neurons, 7, 9, 15-16, 24-25, 42, 56, 59, 66-68, 71-72, 74, 82, 85, 89, 92-93, 103, 110, 152-154, 157, 159, 162, 166, 180-181, 219

Myasthenia Gravis, 8, 10, 70, 72, 164, 180

N

Nerve Conduction Study, 68

Network-based Statistics, 207, 212

Neural Progenitor Cells, 19, 24

Neural Stem Cells, 19-20, 22-26, 28, 37, 39
Neurodegenerative Diseases, 1-5, 16, 23, 50, 75, 82, 145, 154, 157, 161, 163, 181, 197, 201, 205
Neuroimaging, 1-7, 28, 34, 38, 68, 72, 92-93, 98, 100-102, 104-106, 110, 112-114, 120-123, 127, 129, 138, 142, 146-147, 186-196, 208, 216-217, 219-221, 223-225
Neuromuscular Junctions, 66, 154
Neuropathology, 122, 162, 186-187, 191, 193-194
Neurotransmitter, 93, 197-198, 201, 206
Nuclear Magnetic Resonance, 113, 197-198

O
Osmolyte, 202
Oxidative Stress, 23, 37, 40, 51-53, 56, 68, 72, 92-93, 98-100, 103, 153, 159-160, 164-165, 180, 184, 198, 203, 205-206

P
Parkinson's Disease, 6, 23, 26, 47, 56, 63, 65, 74-75, 82-83, 99-100, 103, 120, 164, 197, 205-206
Parkinsonism, 3, 6, 83, 98-99, 103, 124, 197-198, 200, 202, 205
Peak Cough Flow, 85, 91
Pharmacodynamic Biomarker, 92, 99-102, 126
Positron Emission Tomography, 1-2, 92-93, 100, 102-103, 113, 138, 146, 194-195
Primary Biliary Cirrhosis, 180, 184
Primary Lateral Sclerosis, 68, 102, 108, 110, 113, 123, 139, 141, 143, 146
Proteostasis, 59, 63, 154, 161
Pseudonymization, 220, 222

R
Respiratory Insufficiency, 84, 86, 89, 121, 125, 131, 133, 180

S
Schizophrenia, 79, 208, 214, 217
Spinal Muscular Atrophy, 13-14, 63, 65, 68-69, 72, 113, 128, 162
Substantia Nigra, 99, 197-199, 202, 204, 206

T
Tractography, 106-107, 111, 123, 190, 194-195, 208, 210, 216
Transcranial Magnetic Stimulation, 92, 105, 113, 124, 138
Transdiaphragmatic Pressure, 85, 87
Tyrosine Hydroxylase, 198-199

U
Upper Motor Neuron, 86, 92-93, 98, 104, 110, 112-113, 126, 143, 148
Ursodeoxycholic Acid, 180-181, 185

V
Videofluoroscopy, 9-10

W
White Matter, 4, 11, 14, 40, 68, 93, 97, 100, 103, 105, 107-108, 110-111, 122-123, 127, 145, 171, 190, 194-195, 208-210, 214-217

www.ingramcontent.com/pod-product-compliance
Lightning Source LLC
LaVergne TN
LVHW082201200926
848484LV00008B/2194